CLINICAL HANDBOOK FOR

BRUNNER & SUDDARTH'S
Textbook of Medical-Surgical Nursing

Edition
13

Wolters Kluwer | Lippincott Williams & Wilkins
Health
Philadelphia · Baltimore · New York · London
Buenos Aires · Hong Kong · Sydney · Tokyo

Publisher: Lisa McAllister
Executive Editor: Sherry Dickinson
Product Development Editor: Roxanne Halpine Ward
Editorial Assistant: Dan Reilly
Design Coordinator: Joan Wendt
Production Project Manager: Cynthia Rudy
Manufacturing Coordinator: Karin Duffield
Prepress Vendor: Aptara, Inc.

13th edition

Library of Congress Cataloging-in-Publication Data

Clinical handbook for Brunner & Suddarth's textbook of medical-surgical nursing. – Edition 13.
   p. ; cm.
  Preceded by: Handbook for Brunner & Suddarth's textbook of medical-surgical nursing. 12th ed. c2010.
  Includes bibliographical references and index.
  ISBN 978-1-4511-4667-7
  I. Hinkle, Janice L. Brunner & Suddarth's textbook of medical-surgical nursing. Complemented by (work): II. Handbook for Brunner & Suddarth's textbook of medical-surgical nursing. Preceded by (work):
  [DNLM: 1. Nursing Care–Handbooks. 2. Perioperative Nursing–Handbooks. WY 49]
  RT41
  617′.0231–dc23

2013033687

LWW.com

Mary R. Perrecone, MSN, CRRN, CNN
Nurse Manager, Chronic Pediatric and Acute Adult Dialysis Unit
Albany Medical Center
Albany, New York

Cathleen E. Shannon, CPNP-PC, MSN, BSN, RN
Pediatric Nurse Practitioner
Potomac, Maryland

Kathy Batton, PhD
Instructor
Associate Degree Nursing
Hinds Community College
Jackson, Mississippi

Diane Booker, MSN, RN
Assistant Professor
Department of Nursing
Brookdale Community College
Lincroft, New Jersey

Angela Brindowski, MSN
Clinical Assistant Professor
Department of Nursing
Carroll University
Waukesha, Wisconsin

Lynette Debellis, MA, RN
Assistant Professor Nursing-
    Curriculum Chairperson
Department of Nursing
Westchester Community
    College
Valhalla, New York

Jalibun Earp, PhD, ARNP,
    FNP-BC, CNE
Professor
School of Nursing
Florida A&M University
Tallahassee, Florida

Darlene Gattens, BSN,
    MN, CNE
Instructor
School of Nursing
The Western Pennsylvania
    Hospital
Pittsburgh, Pennsylvania

Hilary Gersbach, MS
Instructor
Nursing and Allied Health
Norfolk State University
Norfolk, Virginia

Stephen Gilliam, PhD
Assistant Professor
BioBehavioral Nursing
Georgia Regents University
Athens, Georgia

Jacqueline Guhde, MSN,
    RN, CNS
Senior Instructor
College of Health Professions
The University of Akron
Akron, Ohio

Melissa Humfleet, EdS,
    MSN, RN
Instructor
Department of Nursing
Lincoln Memorial University
Harrogate, Tennessee

Debra Kantor, PhD
Assistant Professor
Department of Nursing
Molloy College
Rockville Centre, New York

Susan Kelly, MSN, MS, RN
Clinical Instructor
Acute & Tertiary Care
  Department
University of Pittsburgh
  School of Nursing
Pittsburgh, Pennsylvania

Vicki Kerwin, MSN
Assistant Professor
Department of Nursing
Fairmont State University
Fairmont, West Virginia

Gabrielle King, MSN, RN
Clinical Nursing Instructor
Department of Nursing
Wayne Community College
Goldsboro, North Carolina

Rhonda Koenig, MSN
Associate Professor
Department of Nursing
Sinclair Community College
Dayton, Ohio

Phyllis Magaletto, MSN,
  RN, BC
Instructor First Year
Department of Nursing
Cochran School of Nursing
Yonkers, New York

Elisa Mangosing-Lemmon,
  MSN
Nursing Faculty
School of Professional Nursing
Riverside School of
  Professional Nursing
Newport News, Virginia

Patricia Martin, MSN
Associate Professor
Department of Nursing
West Kentucky Community
  and Technical College
Paducah, Kentucky

Janis McMillan, MSN, RN
Nursing Faculty
Department of Nursing
Coconino Community College
Flagstaff, Arizona

Anna Moore, MSN
Associate Professor
School of Nursing and Allied
  Health
J. Sargeant Reynolds
  Community College
Richmond, Virginia

Vicky O'Neil, DNP
Associate Professor
Department of Nursing
Dixie State College of Utah
George, Utah

Diana Paladino, MSN
Director, BSN Program
Department of Nursing
Carlow University
Pittsburgh, Pennsylvania

Erayna Paquet, MSN
Assistant Professor
Department of Nursing
North Central Michigan
    College
Petoskey, Michigan

Carswella Phillips, DNP
Nursing Instructor/ARNP
Department of Nursing
Florida A&M University
Tallahassee, Florida

Beth Pippin, MSN, RN,
    FNP-BC
Professor of Nursing
Program Leader, ADN
Department of Nursing
Lord Fairfax Community
    College
Middletown, Virginia

Donna Polverini, MSN, CNE
Associate Professor
Department of Nursing
American International
    College
Springfield, Massachusetts

Janet Reagor, PhD
Assistant Professor
Department of Nursing
Avila University
Kansas City, Missouri

Amanda Reichert, RN, MS, MSN
Faculty
Department of Nursing
Georgia Perimeter College
Clarkston, Georgia

Ellis Siegel, MN
Professor
Nursing and Allied Health
Norfolk State University
Norfolk, Virginia

Annette Stacy, MSN
Associate Professor
Department of Nursing
Arkansas State University
State University, Arkansas

Nancy Steffen, MSN, ADN
Instructor
Department of Nursing
Century College
White Bear Lake, Montana

Sandy Strouse, MSN, RN
Faculty
Department of Nursing
Riverside School of Health
    Careers
Newport News, Virginia

Billy Tart, MSN
Instructor
Department of Nursing
Wayne Community College
Goldsboro, North Carolina

Kim Tinsley, MSN, CNE
RN Director
Department of Nursing
North Arkansas College
Harrison, Arkansas

Christina Tomkins, MSN
Assistant Professor
Department of Nursing
Misericordia University
Dallas, Pennsylvania

This *Clinical Handbook for Brunner & Suddarth's Textbook of Medical-Surgical Nursing*, 13th edition, is a concise clinical reference designed for use by nursing students and professionals. Perfect for use across multiple health care settings, the *Clinical Handbook* presents need-to-know information on nearly 200 commonly encountered diseases and disorders, organized alphabetically with tabbed pages for speedy reference.

Organization

The consistent and easy-to-use outline format enables readers to gain quick access to vital information on

- Pathophysiology
- Clinical Manifestations
- Assessment and Diagnostic Findings
- Medical, Surgical, and Pharmacologic Management
- Nursing Management according to the Nursing Process

For readers requiring more in-depth information, the *Clinical Handbook* is completely cross-referenced to chapters in *Brunner & Suddarth's Textbook of Medical-Surgical Nursing*, 13th edition.

Special Features

The *Clinical Handbook* places special emphasis on home- and community-based nursing practice, patient education, and expected outcomes of care. Additional features include the following:

Gerontologic Considerations—Thumbnail descriptions and interventions related to the care of the older adult population, whose health care needs continue to expand at a rapid rate.

Quality and Safety Nursing Alerts—Tips for best clinical practice and red-flag safety warnings about priority care issues and hazardous or potentially life-threatening situations.

Tables and **Boxes**—At-a-glance presentations of additional information such as diagnostic findings and measurements.

Appendices—Ideal for use in clinicals or in practice, on the unit, at home, or in the community. These include the following:

- Important lab values
- Current nursing diagnoses

Mobile Format Available

The *Clinical Handbook* is available in print or as an enhanced ebook, offering full access to the handbook's quick-reference content, along with instant search capability to quickly locate information needed on the go! For more information, please visit **thePoint**.

We hope you will find this *Clinical Handbook* to be helpful, and we wish you every success in your studies and future profession.

The Publisher

Contents

A

Acquired Immunodeficiency Syndrome (HIV Infection) 1
Acute Coronary Syndrome and Myocardial Infarction 16
Acute Respiratory Distress Syndrome 22
Addison's Disease (Adrenocortical Insufficiency) 25
Alzheimer's Disease 29
Amyotrophic Lateral Sclerosis 34
Anaphylaxis 36
Anemia 39
Anemia, Aplastic 43
Anemia, Iron-Deficiency 44
Anemia, Megaloblastic 46
Anemia, Sickle Cell 49
Aneurysm, Aortic 55
Aneurysm, Intracranial 58
Angina Pectoris 63
Aortic Insufficiency (Regurgitation) 68
Aortic Stenosis 70
Appendicitis 71
Arterial Embolism and Arterial Thrombosis 74
Arteriosclerosis and Atherosclerosis 77
Arthritis, Rheumatoid 78
Asthma 83
Asthma: Status Asthmaticus 89

B

Back Pain, Low 92
Bell's Palsy 95
Benign Prostatic Hyperplasia and Prostatectomy 97
Bone Tumors 100
Bowel Obstruction, Large 104
Bowel Obstruction, Small 105
Brain Abscess 107
Brain Tumors 109
Bronchiectasis 113
Burn Injury 114

C

Cancer 130
Cancer of the Bladder 147
Cancer of the Breast 149
Cancer of the Cervix 157
Cancer of the Colon and Rectum (Colorectal Cancer) 161
Cancer of the Endometrium 169
Cancer of the Esophagus 170
Cancer of the Kidneys (Renal Tumors) 173
Cancer of the Larynx 175
Cancer of the Liver 183
Cancer of the Lung (Bronchogenic Carcinoma) 186
Cancer of the Oral Cavity and Pharynx 190
Cancer of the Ovary 192
Cancer of the Pancreas 193
Cancer of the Prostate 196
Cancer of the Skin (Malignant Melanoma) 204
Cancer of the Stomach (Gastric Cancer) 208
Cancer of the Testis 214
Cancer of the Thyroid 216
Cancer of the Vagina 218
Cancer of the Vulva 219
Cardiac Arrest 221
Cardiomyopathies 223
Cataract 230
Cholelithiasis (and Cholecystitis) 233
Chronic Obstructive Pulmonary Disease 239
Cirrhosis, Hepatic 244
Constipation 248
Coronary Atherosclerosis 251
Crohn's Disease (Regional Enteritis) 252
Cushing Syndrome 254
Cystitis (Lower Urinary Tract Infection) 259

D

Dermatitis, Contact 264
Dermatitis, Exfoliative 265
Diabetes 267
Diabetes Insipidus 278
Diabetic Ketoacidosis 289
Diarrhea 285
Disseminated Intravascular Coagulation 288
Diverticular Disease 291

E

Empyema 296
Endocarditis, Infective 297
Endocarditis, Rheumatic 301
Endometriosis 302
Epididymitis 304
Epilepsies 306
Epistaxis (Nosebleed) 312
Esophageal Varices, Bleeding 314

F

Fractures 317

G

Gastritis 331
Glaucoma 335
Glomerulonephritis, Acute 338
Glomerulonephritis, Chronic 340
Gout 342
Guillain-Barré Syndrome (Polyradiculoneuritis) 344

H

Head Injury (Brain Injury) 350
Headache 361
Heart Failure 366
Hemophilia 373
Hepatic Encephalopathy and Hepatic Coma 377
Hepatic Failure, Fulminant 379
Hepatitis, Viral: Types A, B, C, D, E, and G 380
Hiatal Hernia 386
Hodgkin Lymphoma 389
Huntington Disease 392
Hyperglycemic Hyperosmolar Syndrome 394
Hypertension (and Hypertensive Crisis) 396
Hyperthyroidism (Graves' Disease) 403
Hypoglycemia (Insulin Reaction) 410
Hypoparathyroidism 413
Hypopituitarism 414
Hypothyroidism and Myxedema 415

I

Immune Thrombocytopenic Purpura 419
Impetigo 421

Increased Intracranial Pressure 423
Influenza 429

K
Kaposi's Sarcoma 431

L
Leukemia 433
Leukemia, Lymphocytic, Acute 440
Leukemia, Lymphocytic, Chronic 441
Leukemia, Myeloid, Acute 443
Leukemia, Myeloid, Chronic 446
Lung Abscess 447
Lymphedema and Elephantiasis 450
Lymphomas, Non-Hodgkin 452

M
Mastoiditis and Mastoid Surgery 455
Ménière's Disease 458
Meningitis 461
Mitral Regurgitation (Insufficiency) 465
Mitral Stenosis 466
Mitral Valve Prolapse 468
Multiple Myeloma 469
Multiple Sclerosis 473
Muscular Dystrophies 479
Musculoskeletal Trauma (Contusions, Strains, Sprains, and
    Joint Dislocations) 481
Myasthenia Gravis 483
Myocarditis 487

N
Nephritic Syndrome, Acute 489
Nephrotic Syndrome 491

O
Obesity and Bariatric Surgery 493
Obesity, Morbid 498
Osteoarthritis (Degenerative Joint Disease) 500
Osteomalacia 502
Osteomyelitis 504

Osteoporosis 507
Otitis Media, Acute 511
Otitis Media, Chronic 512

P

Pancreatitis, Acute 514
Pancreatitis, Chronic 519
Parkinson's Disease 521
Pelvic Infection (Pelvic Inflammatory Disease) 527
Pemphigus 530
Peptic Ulcer 534
Pericarditis (Cardiac Tamponade) 540
Perioperative Nursing Management 544
Peripheral Arterial Occlusive Disease 570
Peritonitis 572
Pharyngitis, Acute 575
Pharyngitis, Chronic 577
Pheochromocytoma 578
Pituitary Tumors 580
Pleural Effusion 582
Pleurisy 584
Pneumonia 585
Pneumothorax and Hemothorax 591
Polycythemia 594
Prostatitis 596
Pruritus 598
Psoriasis 601
Pulmonary Arterial Hypertension 605
Pulmonary Edema, Acute 608
Pulmonary Embolism 610
Pyelonephritis, Acute 616
Pyelonephritis, Chronic 618

R

Raynaud's Phenomenon and Other Acrosyndromes 620
Renal Failure, Acute 621
Renal Failure, Chronic (End-Stage Kidney Disease) 626

S

Seborrheic Dermatoses 631
Seizures 632
Sexually Transmitted Infections 635
Shock, Anaphylactic 643

Shock, Cardiogenic 645
Shock, Hypovolemic 647
Shock, Neurogenic 649
Shock, Septic 650
Spinal Cord Injury 653
Stroke, Hemorrhagic 662
Stroke, Ischemic 669
Syndrome of Inappropriate Antidiuretic Hormone
    Secretion 679
Systemic Lupus Erythematosus 680

T

Thrombocytopenia 684
Thyroid Storm (Thyrotoxic Crisis) 685
Thyroiditis, Acute 687
Thyroiditis, Chronic (Hashimoto's Thyroiditis) 688
Toxic Epidermal Necrolysis and Stevens-Johnson
    Syndrome 689
Transient Ischemic Attack 694
Trigeminal Neuralgia (*Tic Douloureux*) 696
Tuberculosis, Pulmonary 698

U

Ulcerative Colitis 702
Unconscious Patient 710
Urolithiasis (Nephrolithiasis) 717

V

Vein Disorders: Venous Thrombosis, Thrombophlebitis,
    Phlebothrombosis, and Deep Vein Thrombosis 723

Appendix A: Selected Lab Values 729
Appendix B: NANDA International Nursing Diagnoses
    2012–2014 732
Index 737

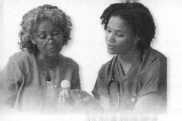

Acquired Immunodeficiency Syndrome
(HIV Infection)

Acquired immunodeficiency syndrome (AIDS) is defined as the most severe form of a continuum of illnesses associated with human immunodeficiency virus (HIV) infection. HIV belongs to a group of viruses known as *retroviruses*. These viruses carry their genetic material in the form of ribonucleic acid (RNA) rather than deoxyribonucleic acid. Infection with HIV occurs when it enters the host CD4 (T) cell and causes this cell to replicate viral RNA and viral proteins, which in turn invade other CD4 cells.

The stage of HIV disease is based on clinical history, physical examination, laboratory evidence of immune dysfunction, signs and symptoms, and infections and malignancies. The Centers for Disease Control and Prevention (CDC) standard case definition of AIDS categorizes HIV infection and AIDS in adults and adolescents on the basis of clinical conditions associated with HIV infection and CD4+ T-cell counts. Three stages of infected states have been denoted:

- Stage 1 or primary infection: acute/recent HIV infection, acute HIV syndrome: dramatic drops in CD4+ T lymphocyte counts >500
- Stage 2: HIV symptomatic: 200 to 499 CD4+ T lymphocytes/mm^3
- Stage 3: AIDS: fewer than 200 CD4+ T lymphocytes/mm^3

HIV Transmission

HIV is transmitted through bodily fluids by high-risk behaviors such as intercourse with an HIV-infected partner and IV or injection drug use. People who received transfusions of blood or blood products contaminated with HIV, children born to mothers with HIV infection, breast-fed infants of HIV-infected mothers, and health care workers exposed to needle-stick injury associated with an infected patient are also at risk.

Clinical Manifestations

Symptoms are widespread and may affect any organ system. Manifestations range from mild abnormalities in immune response without overt signs and symptoms to profound immunosuppression, life-threatening infection, malignancy, and the direct effect of HIV on body tissues.

Respiratory

- Shortness of breath, dyspnea, cough, chest pain, and fever are associated with opportunistic infections, such as those caused by *Pneumocystis jiroveci* (*Pneumocystis* pneumonia [PCP], the most common infection), *Mycobacterium avium-intracellulare*, cytomegalovirus (CMV), and *Legionella* species.
- HIV-associated tuberculosis occurs early in the course of HIV infection, often preceding a diagnosis of AIDS.

Gastrointestinal

- Loss of appetite
- Nausea and vomiting
- Oral and esophageal candidiasis (white patches, painful swallowing, retrosternal pain, and possibly oral lesions)
- Chronic diarrhea, possibly with devastating effects (e.g., profound weight loss, fluid and electrolyte imbalances, perianal skin excoriation, weakness, and inability to perform activities of daily living)

Wasting Syndrome (Cachexia)

- Multifactorial protein-energy malnutrition
- Profound involuntary weight loss exceeding 10% of baseline body weight
- Either chronic diarrhea (for more than 30 days) or chronic weakness and documented intermittent or constant fever with no concurrent illness
- Anorexia, diarrhea, gastrointestinal (GI) malabsorption, lack of nutrition and, for some patients, a hypermetabolic state

Oncologic

Certain types of cancer occur often in people with AIDS and are considered AIDS-defining conditions.

- Kaposi's sarcoma (KS) is the most common HIV-related malignancy and involves the endothelial layer of blood and lymphatic vessels (exhibiting a variable and aggressive course, ranging from localized cutaneous lesions to disseminated disease involving multiple organ systems).

- B-cell lymphomas are the second most common malignancy; they tend to develop outside the lymph nodes, most commonly in the brain, bone marrow, and GI tract. These types of lymphomas are characteristically of a higher grade, indicating aggressive growth and resistance to treatment.
- Invasive cervical cancer can occur.

Neurologic

HIV-associated neurocognitive disorders consist of cognitive impairment that is often accompanied by motor dysfunction and behavioral change.

- HIV-related peripheral neuropathy is common across the trajectory of HIV infection and may occur in a variety of patterns, with distal sensory polyneuropathy (DSPN) or distal symmetrical polyneuropathy the most frequently occurring type. DSPN can lead to significant pain and decreased function.
- HIV encephalopathy (formerly referred to as *AIDS dementia complex*) is a clinical syndrome that is characterized by a progressive decline in cognitive, behavioral, and motor functions. Symptoms include memory deficits, headache, difficulty in concentrating, progressive confusion, psychomotor slowing, apathy, and ataxia and, in later stages, global cognitive impairments, delayed verbal responses, a vacant stare, spastic paraparesis, hyperreflexia, psychosis, hallucinations, tremor, incontinence, seizures, mutism, and death.
- *Cryptococcus neoformans* is a fungal infection (fever, headache, malaise, stiff neck, nausea, vomiting, mental status changes, and seizures).
- Progressive multifocal leukoencephalopathy is a central nervous system demyelinating disorder (mental confusion, blindness, aphasia, muscle weakness, paresis, and death).
- Other common infections involving the nervous system include *Toxoplasma gondii*, CMV, and *Mycobacterium tuberculosis* infections.
- Central and peripheral neuropathies include vascular myelopathy, spastic paraparesis, ataxia, and incontinence.

Depressive

- Causes of depression are multifactorial and may include a history of pre-existing mental illness, neuropsychiatric disturbances, psychosocial factors, or response to the physical symptoms.

- People with HIV/AIDS who are depressed may experience irrational guilt and shame, loss of self-esteem, feelings of helplessness and worthlessness, and suicidal ideation.

Integumentary
- KS, herpes simplex, and herpes zoster viruses and various forms of dermatitis associated with painful vesicles
- Folliculitis, associated with dry flaking skin or atopic dermatitis (eczema or psoriasis)

Gynecologic
- Persistent recurrent vaginal candidiasis may be the first sign of HIV infection.
- Ulcerative sexually transmitted diseases, such as chancroid, syphilis, and herpes, are more severe in women with HIV.
- Human papillomavirus causes venereal warts and is a risk factor for cervical intraepithelial neoplasia, a cellular change that is frequently a precursor to cervical cancer.
- Women with HIV are 10 times more likely to develop cervical intraepithelial neoplasia.
- Women with HIV have a higher incidence of pelvic inflammatory disease and menstrual abnormalities (amenorrhea or bleeding between periods).

Assessment and Diagnostic Findings
Confirmation of HIV antibodies is conducted using enzyme immunoassay (formerly enzyme-linked immunosorbent assay), Western blot assay, and viral load tests such as target amplification methods. In addition to this HIV-1 antibody assay, two additional techniques are now available: the OraSure saliva test and the OraQuick Rapid HIV-1 antibody test.

Medical Management

Treatment of Opportunistic Infections
Guidelines for the treatment of opportunistic infections should be consulted for the most current recommendations. Immune function should improve with initiation of highly active antiretroviral therapy, resulting in faster resolution of the opportunistic infection.

Pneumocystis *Pneumonia*
- Trimethoprim-sulfamethoxazole (TMP-SMZ; Bactrim, Cotrim, Septra) is the treatment of choice for PCP; adjunctive corticosteroids should be started as early as possible (and certainly within 72 hours).

- Alternative therapeutic regimens (mild to moderate) include (1) dapsone and TMP; (2) primaquine plus clindamycin; and (3) atovaquone suspension.
- Alternative therapeutic regimens (moderate to severe) include (1) primaquine plus clindamycin or (2) IV pentamidine.
- Adverse effects include hypotension, impaired glucose metabolism leading to the development of diabetes from damage to the pancreas, renal damage, hepatic dysfunction, and neutropenia.

Mycobacterium Avium Complex

- HIV-infected adults and adolescents should receive chemoprophylaxis against disseminated *Mycobacterium avium* complex disease if they have a CD4+ count of fewer than 50 cells/mcL.
- Azithromycin (Zithromax) and clarithromycin (Biaxin) are the preferred prophylactic agents.
- Rifabutin (Mycobutin) is an alternative prophylactic agent, although drug interactions may make use of this agent difficult.

Cryptococcal Meningitis

- Current primary therapy for cryptococcal meningitis is IV amphotericin B with or without oral flucytosine (5-FC, Ancobon) or fluconazole (Diflucan).
- Serious potential adverse effects of amphotericin B include anaphylaxis, renal and hepatic impairment, electrolyte imbalances, anemia, fever, and severe chills.

Cytomegalovirus Retinitis

- Oral valganciclovir, IV ganciclovir, IV ganciclovir followed by oral valganciclovir, IV foscarnet, IV cidofovir, and the ganciclovir intraocular implant coupled with valganciclovir are all effective treatments for CMV retinitis.
- A common adverse reaction to ganciclovir is severe neutropenia, which limits the concomitant use of zidovudine (azidothymidine, Compound S, Retrovir).
- Common adverse reactions to foscarnet are nephrotoxicity, including acute renal failure, and electrolyte imbalances, including hypocalcemia, hyperphosphatemia, and hypomagnesemia, which can be life-threatening.
- Other common adverse effects include seizures, GI tract disturbances, anemia, phlebitis at the infusion site, and low back pain.
- Possible bone marrow suppression (producing a decrease in white blood cell [WBC] and platelet counts), oral

candidiasis, and liver and renal impairments require close monitoring.

Other Infections
Oral acyclovir (Zovirax), famciclovir (Famvir), or valacyclovir (Valtrex) may be used to treat infections caused by herpes simplex or herpes zoster. Esophageal or oral candidiasis is treated topically with clotrimazole (Mycelex) oral troches or nystatin suspension. Chronic refractory infection with candidiasis (thrush) or esophageal involvement is treated with ketoconazole (Nizoral) or fluconazole (Diflucan).

Prevention of Opportunistic Infections
- People with HIV infection who have a T-cell count of fewer than 200 cells/mm^3 should receive chemoprophylaxis with TMP-SMZ to prevent PCP.
- PCP prophylaxis can be safely discontinued in patients who are responding to highly active antiretroviral therapy (HAART) with a sustained increase in T lymphocytes.

Antidiarrheal Therapy
Therapy with octreotide acetate (Sandostatin), a synthetic analog of somatostatin, has been shown to be effective in managing chronic severe diarrhea.

Chemotherapy

Kaposi's Sarcoma
- Treatment goals are to reduce symptoms by decreasing the size of the skin lesions, to reduce discomfort associated with edema and ulcerations, and to control symptoms associated with mucosal or visceral involvement.
- Radiation therapy is effective as a palliative measure; alpha-interferon can lead to tumor regression and improved immune system function.
- IFN alfa-2b (Intron) is approved for use in AIDS-related KS.

Lymphoma
Successful treatment of AIDS-related lymphomas has been limited because of the rapid progression of these malignancies. Combination chemotherapy and radiation therapy regimens may produce an initial response, but it is usually short-lived.

Antidepressant Therapy
- Treatment of depression involves psychotherapy integrated with pharmacotherapy (antidepressants [e.g., imipramine,

desipramine, and fluoxetine] and possibly a psychostimulant [e.g., methylphenidate]).

- Electroconvulsive therapy may be an option for patients who have severe depression and do not respond to pharmacologic interventions.

Nutrition Therapy

A healthy diet tailored to meet the nutritional needs of the patient is important.

- Calorie counts should be obtained to evaluate nutritional status and initiate appropriate therapy for patients experiencing unexplained weight loss.
- Appetite stimulants can be used in patients with AIDS-related anorexia.
- Oral supplements may be used to supplement diets that are deficient in calories and protein.
- Patients with diarrhea should consume a diet low in fat, insoluble fiber, and caffeine, lactose-free, and high in soluble fiber.

Complementary and Alternative Modalities (CAM)

- Some patients may be interested in using complementary and alternative therapies such as humor, herbs, acupuncture, massage, or yoga. These therapies may be considered very important to the patient and should be viewed as such.
- The patient should report any forms of alternative therapies already in use to the primary health care provider to ensure that they do not interfere with other forms of treatment being considered.
- It is important that the patient become familiar with potential side effects of alternative therapies so that drug–drug interactions can be identified.

Supportive Care

- Nutritional support may be as simple as providing assistance in obtaining or preparing meals.
- Parenteral feedings may be required for advanced nutritional impairment resulting from decreased intake, wasting syndrome, or gastrointestinal malabsorption.
- IV fluid and electrolyte replacement can be used for imbalances from nausea, vomiting, and profuse diarrhea.
- Skin management of perianal skin excoriation or immobility entails thorough and meticulous skin care that involves regular turning, cleansing, and applications of medicated ointments and dressings.

- Pulmonary management can include oxygen therapy, relaxation training, and energy conservation techniques.

NURSING PROCESS

The Patient With HIV/AIDS

Assessment

Identify potential risk factors, including sexual practices and IV/injection drug use history. Assess physical and psychological status. Thoroughly explore factors affecting immune system functioning.

NUTRITIONAL STATUS
- Obtain dietary history.
- Identify factors that may interfere with oral intake, such as anorexia, nausea, vomiting, oral pain, or difficulty in swallowing.
- Assess the patient's ability to purchase and prepare food.
- Measure nutritional status by weight, anthropometric measurements (triceps skinfold measurement), and blood urea nitrogen (BUN), serum protein, albumin, and transferrin levels.

SKIN INTEGRITY
- Inspect skin and mucous membranes daily for breakdown, ulceration, and infection.
- Monitor oral cavity for redness, ulcerations, and creamy-white patches (candidiasis).
- Assess perianal area for excoriation and infection.
- Obtain wound cultures to identify infectious organisms.

RESPIRATORY STATUS
- Monitor for cough, sputum production, shortness of breath, orthopnea, tachypnea, and chest pain; assess breath sounds.
- Assess other parameters of pulmonary function (chest x-rays, arterial blood gases [ABGs], pulse oximetry, pulmonary function tests).

NEUROLOGIC STATUS
- Assess mental status as early as possible to provide a baseline. Note the level of consciousness and orientation to person, place, and time and the occurrence of memory lapses.

- Observe for sensory deficits, such as visual changes, headache, and numbness and tingling in the extremities.
- Observe for motor impairments, such as altered gait, paresis, or paralysis.
- Observe for seizure activity.

FLUID AND ELECTROLYTE BALANCE
- Examine skin and mucous membranes for turgor and dryness.
- Assess for dehydration by observing for increased thirst, decreased urine output, low blood pressure, weak rapid pulse, or urine's specific gravity.
- Monitor electrolyte imbalances. (Laboratory studies show low serum sodium, potassium, calcium, magnesium, and chloride levels.)
- Assess for signs and symptoms of electrolyte deficits, including altered mental status, muscle twitching, muscle cramps, irregular pulse, nausea and vomiting, and shallow respirations.

KNOWLEDGE LEVEL
- Evaluate patient's knowledge of disease and transmission.
- Assess level of knowledge of family and friends.
- Explore patient's reaction to the diagnosis of HIV infection or AIDS.
- Explore ways in which the patient has dealt with illness and major life stressors in the past.
- Identify patient's resources for support.

Diagnosis

NURSING DIAGNOSES
- Impaired skin integrity related to cutaneous manifestations of HIV infection, excoriation, and diarrhea
- Diarrhea related to enteric pathogens or HIV infection
- Risk for infection related to immunodeficiency
- Activity intolerance related to weakness, fatigue, malnutrition, impaired fluid and electrolyte balance, and hypoxia associated with pulmonary infections
- Altered thought processes related to shortened attention span, impaired memory, confusion, and disorientation associated with HIV encephalopathy
- Ineffective airway clearance related to infection, increased bronchial secretions, and decreased ability to cough related to weakness and fatigue

- Acute and chronic pain related to impaired perianal skin integrity secondary to diarrhea, KS, and peripheral neuropathy
- Imbalanced nutrition, less than body requirements, related to decreased oral intake
- Social isolation related to stigma of the disease, withdrawal of support systems, isolation procedures, and fear of infecting others
- Grieving related to changes in lifestyle and roles and unfavorable prognosis
- Deficient knowledge related to HIV infection, means of preventing HIV transmission, and self-care

COLLABORATIVE PROBLEMS/POTENTIAL COMPLICATIONS
- Opportunistic infections
- Impaired breathing or respiratory failure
- Wasting syndrome and fluid and electrolyte imbalance
- Adverse reaction to medications

Planning and Goals

Goals for the patient may include achievement and maintenance of skin integrity, resumption of usual bowel patterns, absence of infection, improved activity tolerance, improved thought processes, improved airway clearance, increased comfort, improved nutritional status, increased socialization, expression of grief, increased knowledge regarding disease prevention and self-care, and absence of complications.

Nursing Interventions

PROMOTING SKIN INTEGRITY
- Assess patient's skin and oral mucosa for changes in appearance, location and size of lesions, and evidence of infection and breakdown; encourage regular oral care.
- Encourage patient to balance rest and mobility whenever possible; assist immobile patients to change position every 2 hours.
- Use devices such as alternating-pressure mattresses and low-air-loss beds.
- Encourage patient to avoid scratching, to use nonabrasive and nondrying soaps, and to use nonperfumed skin moisturizers on dry skin; administer antipruritic agents, antibiotic medication, analgesic agents, medicated lotions, ointments, and dressings as prescribed; avoid excessive use of tape.

- Keep bed linen free of wrinkles, and avoid tight or restrictive clothing to reduce friction to skin.
- Advise patient with foot lesions to wear white cotton socks and shoes that do not cause feet to perspire.
- Assess patient's perianal region for impaired skin integrity and infection. Instruct patient to keep the area as clean as possible, to cleanse after each bowel movement, to use sitz bath or irrigation, and to dry the area thoroughly after cleaning.
- Assist debilitated patient in maintaining hygiene practices.
- Promote healing with prescribed topical ointments and lotions.

PROMOTING USUAL BOWEL PATTERNS
- Assess bowel patterns for diarrhea (frequency and consistency of stool, pain or cramping with bowel movements).
- Assess factors that increase frequency of diarrhea.
- Measure and document volume of liquid stool as fluid volume loss; obtain stool cultures.
- Educate patient about ways to decrease diarrhea (rest bowel, avoid foods that act as bowel irritants, including raw fruits and vegetables); encourage small, frequent meals.
- Administer prescribed medications, such as anticholinergic antispasmodic medications or opiates, antibiotic medications, and antifungal agents.
- Assess self-care strategies that the patient uses to control diarrhea.

PREVENTING INFECTION
- Instruct patient and caregivers to monitor for signs and symptoms of infection. Recommend strategies to avoid infection (upper respiratory tract infections).
- Monitor laboratory values that indicate the presence of infection, such as WBC count and differential; assist in obtaining culture specimens as ordered.
- Strongly urge patients and sexual partners to avoid exposure to body fluids and to use condoms for any sexual activities.
- Strongly discourage IV and injection drug use because of risk of other infections and transmission of HIV infection to the patient.
- Maintain strict aseptic technique for invasive procedures

> ### Quality and Safety Nursing Alert
>
> Observe universal precautions in all patient care. Educate colleagues and other health care workers to apply precautions to blood and all body fluids, secretions, and excretions except sweat (e.g., cerebrospinal fluid; synovial, pleural, peritoneal, pericardial, amniotic, and vaginal fluids; semen). Consider all body fluids to be potentially hazardous in emergency circumstances when differentiating between fluid types is difficult.

IMPROVING ACTIVITY TOLERANCE
- Monitor patient's ability to ambulate and perform daily activities.
- Assist in planning daily routines to maintain balance between activity and rest.
- Educate patient in energy conservation techniques (e.g., sitting while washing or preparing a meal).
- Decrease anxiety that contributes to weakness and fatigue by using measures such as relaxation and guided imagery.
- Collaborate with other health care team members to uncover and address factors associated with fatigue (e.g., epoetin alfa [Epogen] for fatigue related to anemia).

MAINTAINING COHERENT THOUGHT PROCESSES
- Assess the patient for alterations in mental status.
- Reorient the patient to person, place, and time as necessary; maintain and post a regular daily schedule.
- Provide instructions, and educate family to speak to the patient in a slow, simple, and clear manner.
- Provide night lights for bedroom and bathroom. Plan safe leisure activities that the patient previously enjoyed.

> ### Quality and Safety Nursing Alert
>
> Provide around-the-clock supervision as necessary for patients with HIV encephalopathy.

IMPROVING AIRWAY CLEARANCE
- At least daily, assess patient's respiratory status, mental status, and skin color.
- Assess and document presence of cough and quantity and characteristics of sputum; send specimen for analysis as ordered.

- Provide pulmonary therapy, such as coughing, deep breathing, postural drainage, percussion, and vibration, every 2 hours to prevent stasis of secretions and promote airway clearance.
- Assist patient into a position (high- or semi-Fowler's) that facilitates breathing and airway clearance.
- Encourage adequate rest to minimize energy expenditure and prevent fatigue.
- Evaluate patient's fluid volume status; encourage intake of 3 L daily.
- Provide humidified oxygen, suctioning, intubation, and mechanical ventilation as necessary.

RELIEVING PAIN AND DISCOMFORT
- Assess patient for quality and severity of pain associated with impaired perianal skin integrity, KS lesions, and peripheral neuropathy.
- Explore effects of pain on elimination, nutrition, sleep, affect, and communication, along with exacerbating and relieving factors.
- Encourage patient to use soft cushions or foam pads while sitting and topical anesthetics or ointments as prescribed.
- Educate patient to avoid irritating foods and to use antispasmodic agents and antidiarrheal preparations if necessary.
- Administer nonsteroidal anti-inflammatory agents and opiates, and use nonpharmacologic approaches, such as relaxation techniques.
- Administer opioids and tricyclic antidepressants, and recommend graduated compression stockings as prescribed to help alleviate neuropathic pain.

IMPROVING NUTRITIONAL STATUS
- Assess patient's weight; dietary intake; anthropometric measurements; and serum albumin, BUN, protein, and transferrin levels.
- Based on assessment of factors interfering with oral intake, implement specific measures to facilitate oral intake; consult a dietitian to determine nutritional requirements.
- Administer antiemetic medications to control nausea and vomiting; encourage patient to eat easy-to-swallow foods and avoid spicy or sticky food items and foods that are excessively hot or cold; encourage oral hygiene before and after meals.

- Encourage rest before meals; do not schedule meals after painful or unpleasant procedures.
- Educate patient about ways to supplement nutritional value of meals (e.g., add eggs, butter, milk).
- Provide enteral or parenteral feedings to maintain nutritional status, as indicated.

DECREASING SENSE OF SOCIAL ISOLATION

- Provide an atmosphere of acceptance and understanding of AIDS patients, their families, and partners.
- Assess patient's usual level of social interaction early to provide a baseline for monitoring changes in behavior.
- Encourage patient to express feelings of isolation and aloneness; assure patient that these feelings are not unique or abnormal.
- Educate patients, family, and friends that AIDS is not spread through casual contact.

COPING WITH GRIEF

- Help patient to explore and identify resources for support and mechanisms for coping.
- Encourage patient to maintain contact with family, friends, and coworkers and to continue usual activities whenever possible.
- Encourage patient to use local or national AIDS support groups and hotlines and to identify losses and deal with them when possible.

IMPROVING KNOWLEDGE OF HIV

- Educate patient and family about HIV infection, means of preventing HIV transmission, and appropriate self-care measures.
- Educate patient regarding the purpose of the medications, their correct administration, side effects, and strategies to manage or prevent side effects.
- Ensure that patient avoids others with active infections such as upper respiratory infections.

MONITORING AND MANAGING POTENTIAL COMPLICATIONS

- Opportunistic infections: Monitor for fever, malaise, difficulty in breathing, nausea or vomiting, diarrhea, difficulty in swallowing, and any occurrences of swelling or discharge. These symptoms should be reported to the health care provider immediately.

- Respiratory failure and impaired breathing: Monitor ABG values, oxygen saturation, respiratory rate and pattern, and breath sounds; provide suctioning and oxygen therapy; assist the patient on mechanical ventilation to cope with associated stress.
- Cachexia and wasting and fluid and electrolyte disturbances: Monitor weight gain or loss, skin turgor and dryness, ferritin levels, hemoglobin and hematocrit, and electrolytes. Assist in selecting foods that replenish electrolytes. Initiate measures to control diarrhea. Provide IV fluids and electrolytes as prescribed.
- Side effects of medications: Provide information about purpose, administration, side effects (those reportable to physician), and strategies to manage or prevent side effects of medications. Monitor laboratory test values.

PROMOTING HOME- AND COMMUNITY-BASED CARE
Educating Patients About Self-Care

- Thoroughly discuss the disease and all fears and misconceptions; instruct patient, family, and friends about the transmission of AIDS.
- Discuss precautions to prevent transmission of HIV: use of condoms during vaginal or anal intercourse; using dental dam or avoiding oral contact with the penis, vagina, or rectum; avoiding sexual practices that might cut or tear the lining of the rectum, vagina, or penis; and avoiding sexual contact with multiple partners, those known to be HIV-positive, those who use illicit injectable drugs, and those who are sexual partners of people who inject drugs.
- Educate patient and family about how to prevent disease transmission, including hand hygiene and methods of safely handling items soiled with bodily fluids.
- Instruct patient not to donate blood.
- Emphasize importance of taking medication as prescribed. Assist patient and caregivers in fitting the medication regimen into their lives.
- Educate patient in medication administration, including IV preparations.
- Educate patient in guidelines about infection, follow-up care, diet, rest, and activities.
- Instruct patient and family how to administer enteral or parenteral feedings, if applicable.
- Offer support and guidance in coping with this disease.

Continuing Care
- Refer patient and family for home care nursing or hospice for physical and emotional support.
- Assist family and caregivers in providing supportive care.
- Assist patient in administration of parenteral antibiotics, chemotherapy, nutrition, complicated wound care, and respiratory care.
- Provide emotional support to patient and family.
- Refer patient to community programs, housekeeping assistance, meals, transportation, shopping, individual and group therapy, support for caregivers, telephone networks for the homebound, and legal and financial assistance.
- Encourage patient and family to discuss end-of-life decisions.

Evaluation

EXPECTED PATIENT OUTCOMES
- Maintains skin integrity
- Resumes usual bowel habits
- Experiences no infections
- Maintains adequate level of activity tolerance
- Maintains usual thought processes
- Maintains effective airway clearance
- Experiences increased sense of comfort and less pain
- Maintains adequate nutritional status
- Experiences decreased sense of social isolation
- Progresses through grieving process
- Reports increased understanding of AIDS and participates in self-care activities as possible
- Remains free of complications

For more information, see Chapter 37 in Hinkle, J. L., & Cheever, K. H. (2014). *Brunner and Suddarth's textbook of medical-surgical nursing* (13th ed.). Philadelphia: Lippincott Williams & Wilkins.

Acute Coronary Syndrome and Myocardial Infarction

Acute coronary syndrome (ACS) is an emergent situation characterized by an acute onset of myocardial ischemia that results in myocardial death (i.e., myocardial infarction [MI]) if definitive interventions do not occur promptly. (Although the terms *coronary occlusion, heart attack,* and *myocardial infarction* are used synonymously, the preferred term is *myocardial infarction.*) The spectrum of ACS includes unstable angina, non–ST-segment elevation MI (NSTEMI), and ST-segment elevation MI (STEMI).

Pathophysiology

In unstable angina, blood flow in a coronary artery is reduced, often due to rupture of an atherosclerotic plaque. A clot begins to form, but the artery is not completely occluded. This is an acute situation that can result in chest pain and other symptoms and is sometimes referred to as *preinfarction angina* because the patient will likely have an MI if prompt interventions do not occur.

In an MI, plaque rupture and subsequent thrombus formation result in complete occlusion of the artery, leading to ischemia and necrosis of the myocardium supplied by that artery. Vasospasm (sudden constriction or narrowing) of a coronary artery, decreased oxygen supply (e.g., from acute blood loss, anemia, or low blood pressure), and increased demand for oxygen (e.g., from a rapid heart rate, thyrotoxicosis, or ingestion of cocaine) are other causes of MI. In each case, a profound imbalance exists between myocardial oxygen supply and demand. The area of infarction develops over minutes to hours; the expression "time is muscle" reflects the urgency of appropriate treatment to improve patient outcomes. An MI may be defined by the type, the location of the injury to the ventricular wall (anterior, inferior, posterior, or lateral wall), or by the point in time in the process of infarction (acute, evolving, old).

Clinical Manifestations

In many cases, the signs and symptoms of MI cannot be distinguished from those of unstable angina—hence, the evolution of the term *acute coronary syndrome.*

- Chest pain that occurs suddenly and continues despite rest and medication is the primary presenting symptom.
- Some patients have prodromal symptoms or a previous diagnosis of coronary artery disease (CAD), but about half report no previous symptoms.
- Patient may present with a combination of symptoms, including chest pain, shortness of breath, indigestion, nausea, and anxiety.

- Patient may have cool, pale, and moist skin; heart rate and respiratory rate may be faster than normal. These signs and symptoms, which are caused by stimulation of the sympathetic nervous system, may be present for only a short time or may persist.

Assessment and Diagnostic Findings

- Patient history (description of presenting symptom; history of previous illnesses and family health history, particularly of heart disease): History should also include information about patient's risk factors for heart disease.
- 12-lead electrocardiogram (ECG) within 10 minutes of pain onset or arrival at the emergency department: ECG findings are used to categorize the type of ACS (e.g., unstable angina, STEMI, or NSTEMI).
- Echocardiography to evaluate ventricular function, including wall motion and ejection fraction.
- Cardiac enzymes and biomarkers (creatine kinase iso-enzymes, myoglobin, and troponin).

Medical Management

The goals of medical management are to minimize myocardial damage, preserve myocardial function, and prevent complications such as lethal dysrhythmias and cardiogenic shock.

- Initial management includes supplemental oxygen, aspirin, nitroglycerin, and morphine.
- Reperfuse via emergency use of thrombolytic medications or percutaneous coronary intervention (PCI).
- Reduce myocardial oxygen demand and increase oxygen supply with medications, oxygen administration, and bed rest.
- Perform coronary artery bypass or minimally invasive direct coronary artery bypass (MIDCAB).
- After the patient with an MI is free of symptoms, initiate a multiphase cardiac rehabilitation program.

Pharmacologic Therapy

- Nitrates (nitroglycerin) to increase oxygen supply via vasodilation
- Anticoagulants (aspirin, unfractionated or low-molecular-weight heparin) to prevent clot formation
- Analgesic agents (morphine sulfate) to reduce pain and anxiety and to decrease workload of the heart
- Angiotensin-converting enzyme (ACE) inhibitors to decrease blood pressure and reduce oxygen demand of the

myocardium or, if ACE inhibitors not appropriate, an angiotensin receptor blocker (ARB)
- Beta-blocker if needed initially for dysrhythmias, or introduced within 24 hours of admission if not needed initially
- Thrombolytic medications (alteplase [t-PA, Activase] and reteplase [r-PA, TNKase]): must be administered as early as possible after the onset of symptoms, generally within 30 minutes of arrival; may be initiated when timely access to PCI therapy is not available

Emergent Percutaneous Coronary Intervention
- Patient with STEMI may be taken to the cardiac catheterization laboratory for an emergent PCI, usually within 60 minutes after arrival to the facility.
- PCI treats the underlying atherosclerotic lesion via balloon angioplasty, placement of stents, atherectomy, or brachytherapy to open the occluded vessel.

NURSING PROCESS

The Patient With ACS

Assessment
Obtain baseline data on current status of patient for comparison with ongoing status. Include history of chest pain or discomfort, difficulty breathing (dyspnea), palpitations, unusual fatigue, faintness (syncope), or other possible indicators of myocardial ischemia. Perform a focused physical assessment, which is crucial for detecting complications and any change in status. The examination should include the following:
- Assess level of consciousness.
- Evaluate chest pain (most important clinical finding).
- Assess heart rate and rhythm; dysrhythmias may indicate not enough oxygen to the myocardium.
- Assess heart sounds; S_3 can be an early sign of impending left ventricular failure.
- Measure blood pressure to determine response to pain and treatment; note pulse pressure, which may be narrowed after an MI, suggesting ineffective ventricular contraction.
- Assess peripheral pulses: rate, rhythm, and volume.
- Evaluate skin color and temperature.

- Auscultate lung fields at frequent intervals for signs of ventricular failure (crackles in lung bases).
- Assess bowel motility; mesenteric artery thrombosis is a potentially fatal complication.
- Observe urinary output and check for edema; an early sign of cardiogenic shock is hypotension with oliguria.
- Two IV lines are typically placed; examine IV lines and sites.

Diagnosis

NURSING DIAGNOSES

- Risk for decreased cardiac tissue perfusion related to reduced coronary blood flow
- Risk for imbalanced fluid volume
- Risk for ineffective peripheral tissue perfusion related to decreased cardiac output from left ventricular dysfunction
- Anxiety related to cardiac event and possible death
- Deficient knowledge about post-ACS self-care

COLLABORATIVE PROBLEMS/POTENTIAL COMPLICATIONS

- Acute pulmonary edema
- Heart failure
- Cardiogenic shock
- Dysrhythmias and cardiac arrest
- Pericardial effusion and cardiac tamponade

Planning and Goals

The major goals for the patient include relief of pain or ischemic signs (e.g., ST-segment changes) and symptoms, prevention of myocardial damage, maintenance of effective respiratory function, maintenance or attainment of adequate tissue perfusion, reduced anxiety, adherence to the self-care program, and early recognition of complications.

Nursing Interventions

RELIEVING PAIN AND OTHER SIGNS AND SYMPTOMS OF ISCHEMIA

- Administer oxygen in tandem with medication therapy to assist with relief of symptoms. (Inhalation of oxygen reduces pain associated with low levels of circulating oxygen.)
- Assess vital signs frequently as long as patient is experiencing pain.

- Assist patient to rest with the head of the bed elevated or in cardiac chair to decrease chest discomfort and dyspnea.

IMPROVING RESPIRATORY FUNCTION
- Assess respiratory function to detect early signs of complications.
- Monitor fluid volume status to prevent fluid overload.
- Encourage patient to breathe deeply and change position often to maintain effective ventilation throughout the lungs.

PROMOTING ADEQUATE TISSUE PERFUSION
- Keep patient on bed or chair rest to reduce myocardial oxygen consumption.
- Check skin temperature and peripheral pulses frequently to determine adequate tissue perfusion.

REDUCING ANXIETY
- Develop a trusting and caring relationship with patient; provide information to the patient and family in an honest and supportive manner.
- Ensure a quiet environment, prevent interruptions that disturb sleep, and provide spiritual support consistent with the patient's beliefs. Alternative therapies such as pet therapy have been shown to relax patients and reduce anxiety.
- Provide frequent and private opportunities to share concerns and fears.
- Provide an atmosphere of acceptance to help patient know that his or her feelings are realistic and normal.

MONITORING AND MANAGING COMPLICATIONS
Monitor closely for cardinal signs and symptoms that signal onset of complications including changes in cardiac rate and rhythm, heart sounds, blood pressure, chest pain, respiratory status, urinary output, skin color and temperature, mental status, ECG changes, and laboratory values.

PROMOTING HOME- AND COMMUNITY-BASED CARE
Educating Patients About Self-Care
- Identify the patient's priorities, provide adequate education about heart-healthy living, and facilitate the patient's involvement in a cardiac rehabilitation program.
- Work with the patient to develop a plan to meet specific needs to enhance compliance.
- Include caregivers and responsible family members in planning follow-up care.

Continuing Care
- Provide home care referral if warranted.
- Assist the patient with scheduling and keeping follow-up appointments and with adhering to the prescribed cardiac rehabilitation regimen.
- Provide reminders about follow-up monitoring, including periodic laboratory testing and ECGs, as well as general health screening.
- Monitor the patient's adherence to dietary restrictions and to prescribed medications.
- If the patient is receiving home oxygen, ensure that the patient is using the oxygen as prescribed and that appropriate home safety measures are maintained.
- If the patient has evidence of heart failure secondary to an MI, appropriate home care guidelines for the patient with heart failure are followed.

Evaluation

EXPECTED PATIENT OUTCOMES
- Experiences relief of angina
- Has stable cardiac and respiratory status
- Maintains adequate tissue perfusion
- Exhibits decreased anxiety
- Complies with self-care program
- Experiences absence of complications

For more information, see Chapter 27 in Hinkle, J. L., & Cheever, K. H. (2014). *Brunner and Suddarth's textbook of medical-surgical nursing* (13th ed.). Philadelphia: Lippincott Williams & Wilkins.

Acute Respiratory Distress Syndrome

Acute respiratory distress syndrome (ARDS) can be thought of as a spectrum of disease from its milder form of acute lung injury (ALI) to its most severe form of fulminant, life-threatening ARDS. ARDS is characterized by sudden and progressive pulmonary edema, increasing bilateral infiltrates, hypoxemia unresponsive to oxygen supplementation, and the absence of an elevated left atrial pressure. ARDS occurs when inflammatory triggers initiate the release of cellular and chemical mediators, causing injury to the alveolar capillary membrane in addition to other structural damage to the lungs. Factors associated with the development of ARDS include direct injury to the lungs (e.g., smoke inhalation) or indirect insult to the lungs (e.g., shock). ARDS has been associated with a mortality rate ranging from 25% to 58%, with the major cause of death in ARDS being nonpulmonary multiple organ dysfunction syndrome (MODS), often with sepsis.

Clinical Manifestations
- Rapid onset of severe dyspnea, less than 72 hours after an initiating event
- Possible intercostal retractions and crackles
- Arterial hypoxemia not responsive to oxygen supplementation
- Lung injury, which then progresses to fibrosing alveolitis with persistent, severe hypoxemia
- Increased alveolar dead space and decreased pulmonary compliance

Assessment and Diagnostic Findings
- Plasma brain natriuretic peptide (BNP) levels, to help differentiate ARDS from cardiogenic pulmonary edema
- Echocardiography

Medical Management
- Identify and treat the underlying condition; provide aggressive, supportive care (endotracheal intubation and mechanical ventilation; circulatory support, adequate fluid volume, and nutritional support).
- Use supplemental oxygen as the patient begins the initial spiral of hypoxemia.
- Monitor arterial blood gas (ABG) values, pulse oximetry, and pulmonary function testing.
- As disease progresses, use positive end-expiratory pressure (PEEP).
- Treat hypovolemia carefully; avoid overload. (Inotropic or vasopressor agents may be required.)

Pharmacologic Therapy
- There is no specific pharmacologic treatment for ARDS except supportive care. Numerous pharmacologic treatments are under investigation to stop the cascade of events leading to ARDS (e.g., surfactant replacement therapy, pulmonary antihypertensive agents, and antisepsis agents).

- Additional treatment for ARDS may include prone positioning, high-frequency oscillatory ventilation, and low-dose steroids administered within the first 14 days of the onset of symptoms.
- Neuromuscular blocking agents, sedative agents, and analgesic medications may be used to improve patient-ventilator synchronization; inhaled nitrous oxide may help to reduce ventilation–perfusion mismatch and improve oxygenation.

Nutritional Therapy
Provide nutritional support (35 to 45 kcal/kg daily).

Nursing Management

- Closely monitor the patient in an ICU; frequently assess effectiveness of treatment (e.g., oxygen administration, nebulizer therapy, chest physiotherapy, endotracheal intubation or tracheostomy, mechanical ventilation, suctioning, bronchoscopy).
- Consider other needs of the patient (e.g., positioning, anxiety, rest).
- Identify any problems with ventilation that may cause an anxiety reaction: tube blockage, other acute respiratory problems (e.g., pneumothorax, pain), a sudden decrease in the oxygen level, the level of dyspnea, or ventilator malfunction.
- Sedation may be required to decrease the patient's oxygen consumption, allow the ventilator to provide full support of ventilation, and decrease the patient's anxiety.
- If sedative agents do not work, paralytic agents (used for the shortest time possible) may be administered (with adequate sedation and pain management). Reassure the patient that paralysis is a result of the medication and is temporary, and describe the purpose and effects of the paralytic agents to the patient's family.
- Use peripheral nerve stimulators to assess nerve impulse transmissions at the neuromuscular junction of select skeletal muscles when neuromuscular blocking agents are used, in order to evaluate whether stimuli are effectively blocked.
- Closely monitor patients on paralytic agents: Ensure that the patient is not disconnected from the ventilator and that all ventilator and patient alarms are on at all times, provide

eye care, minimize complications related to neuromuscular blockade, and anticipate the patient's needs regarding pain and comfort.

> **Quality and Safety Nursing Alert**
>
> Nursing assessment is essential to minimize the complications related to neuromuscular blockade. The patient may have discomfort or pain but cannot communicate these sensations. Analgesia is usually administered concurrently with neuromuscular blocking agents.

For more information, see Chapter 23 in Hinkle, J. L., & Cheever, K. H. (2014). *Brunner and Suddarth's textbook of medical-surgical nursing* (13th ed.). Philadelphia: Lippincott Williams & Wilkins.

Addison's Disease
(Adrenocortical Insufficiency)

Addison's disease, or adrenocortical insufficiency, occurs when the adrenal cortex function is inadequate to meet a patient's need for cortical hormones. Autoimmune or idiopathic atrophy of the adrenal glands is responsible for the vast majority of cases. Other causes include surgical removal of both adrenal glands or infection (tuberculosis or histoplasmosis) of the adrenal glands. Inadequate secretion of adrenocorticotropic hormone (ACTH) from the primary pituitary gland also results in adrenal insufficiency. Therapeutic use of corticosteroids is the most common cause of adrenocortical insufficiency. Symptoms may also result from sudden cessation of exogenous adrenocortical hormonal therapy, which interferes with normal feedback mechanisms.

Clinical Manifestations

Addison's disease is characterized by muscle weakness, anorexia, GI symptoms, fatigue, emaciation, dark pigmentation of the mucous membranes and skin, hypotension, low blood glucose, low serum sodium, and high serum potassium. The onset usually occurs with nonspecific symptoms. Mental changes (depression, emotional liability, apathy, and confusion) are present in 20% to 40% of patients. In severe cases, disturbance of sodium and potassium metabolism may be marked by depletion of sodium and water and severe, chronic dehydration.

Addisonian Crisis
With disease progression and acute hypotension, addisonian crisis develops and is characterized by the following:

- Cyanosis and classic signs of circulatory shock: pallor, apprehension, rapid and weak pulse, rapid respirations, and low blood pressure
- Headache, nausea, abdominal pain, diarrhea, confusion, and restlessness
- Slight overexertion, exposure to cold, acute infections, or a decrease in salt intake possibly leading to circulatory collapse, shock, and death
- Stress of surgery or dehydration from preparation for diagnostic tests or surgery possible triggers for addisonian or hypotensive crisis

Assessment and Diagnostic Findings
- Greatly increased plasma ACTH (more than 22.0 pmol/L)
- Serum cortisol level lower than normal (less than 165 nmol/L) or in the low-normal range
- Decreased blood glucose (hypoglycemia) and sodium (hyponatremia) levels, increased serum potassium concentration (hyperkalemia), and increased white blood cell (WBC) count (leukocytosis)

Medical Management
Immediate treatment is directed toward combating circulatory shock:

- Restore blood circulation, administer fluids and corticosteroids, monitor vital signs, and place patient in a recumbent position with legs elevated.
- Administer IV hydrocortisone followed by 5% dextrose in normal saline.
- Vasopressor amines may be required if hypotension persists.
- Antibiotics may be administered if infection has precipitated adrenal crisis.
- Oral intake may be initiated as soon as tolerated.
- If adrenal gland does not regain function, lifelong replacement of corticosteroids and mineralocorticoids is required.
- Dietary intake should be supplemented with salt during times of GI losses of fluids through vomiting and diarrhea.

Nursing Management

Assessing the Patient
- Focus the health history and exam on presence of symptoms of fluid imbalance and stress.
- Monitor blood pressure and pulse rate as the patient moves from a lying, sitting, and standing position to assess for inadequate fluid volume.
- Assess skin color and turgor.
- Assess history of weight changes, muscle weakness, and fatigue.
- Ask patient and family about onset of illness or increased stress that may have precipitated crisis.

Monitoring and Managing Addisonian Crisis
- Monitor for signs and symptoms indicative of addisonian crisis, which can include shock; hypotension; rapid, weak pulse; rapid respiratory rate; pallor; and extreme weakness.
- Advise patient to avoid physical and psychological stressors such as cold exposure, overexertion, infection, and emotional distress.
- Immediately treat patient in addisonian crisis with IV administration of fluid, glucose, and electrolytes, especially sodium; with replacement of missing steroid hormones; and with vasopressors.
- Anticipate and meet patient's needs to promote return to a precrisis state.

Restoring Fluid Balance
- Encourage the patient to consume foods and fluids that assist in restoring and maintaining fluid and electrolyte balance.
- Along with the dietitian, help the patient to select foods high in sodium during GI tract disturbances and in very hot weather.
- Educate the patient and family to administer hormone replacement as prescribed and to modify the dosage during illness and other stressful situations.
- Provide written and verbal instructions about the administration of mineralocorticoid (Florinef) or corticosteroid (prednisone) as prescribed.

Improving Activity Tolerance
- Avoid unnecessary activities and stress that might precipitate a hypotensive episode.
- Detect signs of infection or presence of stressors that may have triggered the crisis.

- Explain the rationale for minimizing stress during acute crisis and increased activity.

Promoting Home- and Community-Based Care

Educating Patients About Self-Care

- Provide patient and family explicit verbal and written instructions about the rationale for replacement therapy and proper dosage.
- Educate patient and family about how to modify drug dosage and increase salt intake in times of illness, very hot weather, and stressful situations.
- Modify diet and fluid intake to maintain fluid and electrolyte balance.
- Provide patient and family with preloaded, single-injection syringes of corticosteroid for use in emergencies and instruct them in when and how to use.
- Advise patient to inform health care providers (e.g., dentists) of steroid use.
- Urge patient to wear a medical alert bracelet and to carry information at all times about the need for corticosteroids.
- Educate patient and family about the signs of excessive or insufficient hormone replacement.

Continuing Care

- If patient cannot return to work and family responsibilities after hospital discharge, refer patient to home care to ensure a safe environment; assess patient's recovery; monitor hormone replacement; and evaluate stress in the home.
- Assess patient's and family's knowledge about medication regimen compliance; emphasize the side effects of medications and dietary modifications.
- Assess patient's plans for regular medical follow-up to clinic or health care provider's office.
- Encourage the patient to wear medical identification for Addison's disease.
- Remind patient and family about the importance of health promotion activities and health screening.

Evaluation

Expected Patient Outcomes

- Decrease risk of injury
- Decrease risk of infection
- Increases participation in self-care activities
- Attains/maintains skin integrity

- Achieves improved body image
- Exhibits improved mental functioning
- Exhibits absence of complications

For more information, see Chapter 52 in Hinkle, J. L., & Cheever, K. H. (2014). *Brunner and Suddarth's textbook of medical-surgical nursing* (13th ed.). Philadelphia: Lippincott Williams & Wilkins.

Alzheimer's Disease

Alzheimer's disease (AD) is the fifth leading cause of death for older adults. AD is one of the most common types of dementia and is a progressive, irreversible, degenerative neurologic disease that begins insidiously and is characterized by gradual losses of cognitive function and disturbances in behavior and affect. It is important to note that AD is not a normal part of aging.

Although the greatest risk factor for AD is increasing age, many environmental, dietary, and inflammatory factors also may determine whether a person suffers from this cognitive disease. AD is a complex brain disorder caused by a combination of various factors that may include genetics, neurotransmitter changes, vascular abnormalities, stress hormones, circadian changes, head trauma, and the presence of seizure disorders.

AD can be classified into two types: familial or early-onset AD (which is rare and accounts for less than 10% of cases) and sporadic or late-onset AD.

Pathophysiology

Specific neuropathologic and biochemical changes are found in patients with AD. These include neurofibrillary tangles and senile or neuritic plaques. The neuronal damage occurs primarily in the cerebral cortex and results in decreased brain size. Similar changes are found in the normal brain tissue of older adults but to a lesser extent. Cells that use the neurotransmitter acetylcholine are principally affected by AD. At the biochemical level, the enzyme active in producing acetylcholine, which is specifically involved in memory processing, is decreased.

Clinical Manifestations

Symptoms are highly variable; some include the following:

- In early stages, forgetfulness and subtle memory loss may occur, such as small difficulties with work or social activities, but patients retain adequate cognitive function to compensate for the loss and continue to function independently.

Forgetfulness is manifested in many daily actions with progression of the disease (e.g., the patient gets lost in a familiar environment or repeats the same stories).

- Conversation becomes difficult, and word-finding difficulties occur.
- Ability to formulate concepts and think abstractly disappears.
- Patient may exhibit inappropriate impulsive behavior.
- Personality changes are evident; patient may become depressed, suspicious, paranoid, hostile, and combative.
- Speaking skills deteriorate to nonsense syllables; agitation and physical activity increase.
- Eventually, patient requires assistance with most activities of daily living (ADLs), including eating and toileting, because dysphagia and incontinence develop.
- Terminal stage may last for months or years during which the patient is usually immobile and requires total care.
- Death typically occurs as a result of complications of pneumonia, malnutrition, or dehydration.

Assessment and Diagnostic Findings

The definitive diagnosis of AD can be made only at autopsy. An accurate clinical diagnosis can be made in about 90% of cases by ruling out other causes of dementia or reversible causes of confusion.

- Clinical symptoms found through health history (including medical history, family history, social and cultural history, and medication history) and physical examination (including functional and mental health status; e.g., Geriatric Depression Scale and Mini-Mental Status Examination)
- Electroencephalography (EEG)
- CT scan
- MRI
- Diagnostic tests (complete blood cell count, chemistry profile, and vitamin B_{12} and thyroid hormone levels) and examination of the cerebrospinal fluid (CSF)

Medical Management

The primary goal is to manage the cognitive and behavioral symptoms. There is no cure for AD, but several medications have been introduced to slow its progression. For mild to moderate symptoms, cholinesterase inhibitors (CEIs), such as donepezil hydrochloride (Aricept), rivastigmine tartrate (Exelon), galantamine hydrobromide (Razadyne [formerly known as

Reminyl]), and tacrine (Cognex) may improve cognitive ability within 6 to 12 months of therapy. These drugs enhance acetylcholine uptake in the brain to maintain memory skills for a period of time. Combination CEI with memantine (Namenda) may also be useful for mild to moderate cognitive symptoms.

NURSING PROCESS

The Patient With AD

Assessment

Obtain a health history with mental status examination and physical examination, noting symptoms indicating dementia (e.g., asking the same question repeatedly or getting lost). Report findings to physician. As indicated, assist with diagnostic evaluation, promoting a calm environment to maximize patient safety and cooperation.

Diagnosis

NURSING DIAGNOSES

- Impaired thought processes related to decline in cognitive function
- Risk for injury related to decline in cognitive function
- Anxiety related to confused thought processes
- Imbalanced nutrition: less than body requirements, related to cognitive decline
- Activity intolerance related to imbalance in activity–rest pattern
- Deficient self-care, bathing and hygiene, feeding, toileting related to cognitive decline
- Impaired social interaction related to cognitive decline
- Deficient knowledge of family or caregiver related to care for patient as cognitive function declines
- Ineffective family processes related to decline in patient's cognitive function

Planning and Goals

Goals include promoting patient functioning, physical safety, adequate nutrition, and independence (in ADLs and self-care activities) for as long as possible; reducing anxiety and agitation; improving communication; balancing activity and rest;

providing socialization and intimacy; and supporting and educating family caregivers.

Nursing Interventions

SUPPORTING COGNITIVE FUNCTION

- Provide a calm, predictable environment to minimize confusion and disorientation.
- Limit environmental stimuli and establish a regular routine.
- Help patient to feel a sense of security with a quiet voice, speaking in a pleasant manner, and providing clear and simple explanations.
- Encourage the use of memory aids and cues such as clocks, calendars, and color-coding the doorway.
- Encourage active participation including social interaction and physical activity.

PROMOTING PHYSICAL SAFETY

- Provide a safe environment (whether at home or in the hospital) to allow patient to move about as freely as possible and to help relieve the family of worry about safety.
- Prevent falls and other injuries by removing obvious hazards, providing adequate lighting, and installing handrails in the home.
- Prohibit driving.
- Allow smoking only with supervision.
- Reduce wandering behavior with gentle persuasion and distraction or by placing the patient close to the nursing station. Supervise all activities outside the home to protect patient. Secure doors leading from the house, and ensure that the patient wears an identification bracelet or neck chain.
- Avoid restraints because they may increase agitation.

PROMOTING ADEQUATE NUTRITION

- Keep mealtimes simple and calm; avoid confrontations.
- Cut food into small pieces to prevent patient's choking, and convert liquids to gelatin to ease swallowing. Offer one dish at a time.
- Prevent burns by serving typically hot food and beverages warm.
- Use adaptive equipment or allow patient to eat with a spoon or with fingers if the patient lacks self-feeding coordination along with an apron or smock.

PROMOTING INDEPENDENCE IN SELF-CARE ACTIVITIES

- Simplify daily activities into short achievable steps so that patient experiences a sense of accomplishment.

- Occupational therapists can suggest ways to simplify tasks or recommend adaptive equipment.
- Maintain patient's personal dignity and autonomy.
- Encourage patient to make choices when appropriate and to participate in self-care activities as much as possible.

REDUCING ANXIETY AND AGITATION
- Provide constant emotional support to reinforce a positive self-image.
- When skill losses occur, adjust goals to fit patient's declining ability, and structure activities to help prevent agitation.
- Keep the environment simple, familiar, and noise-free; limit changes.
- Remain calm and unhurried, particularly if the patient is experiencing a combative, agitated state known as *catastrophic reaction* (overreaction to excessive stimulation).

IMPROVING COMMUNICATION
- Reduce noises and distractions.
- Use clear, easy-to-understand sentences to convey messages.
- Lists and simple written instructions, pointing to an object or use of nonverbal language, and tactile stimuli may be used to communicate, depending on the stage of dementia.

PROMOTING BALANCED ACTIVITY AND REST
- Assess and address any unmet underlying physical or psychological needs that may prompt sleep disturbances, wandering or other inappropriate behavior.
- Ensure that the patient participates in adequate physical exercise during the day.
- Offer music, warm milk, or a back rub to help the patient relax and fall asleep.
- To enhance nighttime sleep, provide sufficient opportunities for daytime exercise. Discourage long periods of daytime sleeping.

PROVIDING FOR SOCIALIZATION AND INTIMACY NEEDS
- Encourage visits, letters, and phone calls from family and friends (visits should be brief and nonstressful, with one or two visitors at a time).
- Encourage patient to participate in simple activities or hobbies.

- Advise patient that the nonjudgmental friendliness of a pet or care of plants can provide stimulation, comfort, and contentment as a satisfying activity and an outlet for energy.
- Encourage patient's spouse to talk about any sexual concerns and suggest sexual counseling if necessary.

SUPPORTING HOME- AND COMMUNITY-BASED CARE
- Be sensitive to the highly emotional issues that the family is confronting.
- Notify the local adult protective services agency if neglect or abuse is suspected.
- Refer family to the Alzheimer's Association for assistance with family support groups, respite care, and adult day care services.

Evaluation

EXPECTED PATIENT OUTCOMES
- Patient maintains cognitive, functional, and social interaction abilities for as long as possible.
- Patient remains free of injury.
- Patient participates in self-care activities as much as possible.
- Patient demonstrates minimal anxiety and agitation.
- Patient is able to communicate (verbally or nonverbally).
- Patient's socialization and intimacy needs are met.
- Patient receives adequate nutrition, activity, and rest.
- Patient and family caregivers are knowledgeable about condition and treatment and care regimens.

For more information, see Chapter 11 in Hinkle, J. L., & Cheever, K. H. (2014). *Brunner and Suddarth's textbook of medical-surgical nursing* (13th ed.). Philadelphia: Lippincott Williams & Wilkins.

Amyotrophic Lateral Sclerosis

Amyotrophic lateral sclerosis (ALS) is a disease of unknown cause in which there is a loss of motor neurons (nerve cells controlling muscles) in the anterior horns of the spinal cord and the motor nuclei of the lower brain stem. It is often referred to as *Lou Gehrig's disease*. As these cells die, the muscle fibers that they supply undergo atrophic changes.

Neuronal degeneration may occur in both upper and lower motor neuron systems. Possible causes of ALS include autoimmune disease, free radical damage, oxidative stress, and transmission of an autosomal dominant trait for familial ALS (5% to 10%). Death usually occurs from infection, respiratory failure, or aspiration. The average time from onset to death is about 3 to 5 years.

Clinical Manifestations

Clinical features of ALS depend on the location of the affected motor neurons, because specific neurons activate specific muscle fibers. The chief symptoms are fatigue, progressive muscle weakness, cramps, fasciculations (twitching), and incoordination.

Loss of Motor Neurons in Anterior Horns of Spinal Cord

- Progressive weakness and atrophy of the arms, trunk, or leg muscles occur.
- Spasticity occurs; deep tendon stretch reflexes are brisk and overactive.
- Rectum and bladder sphincters usually remain intact.

Weakness in Muscles Supplied by Cranial Nerves (25% of Patients in Early Stage)

- Difficulty talking, swallowing, and ultimately breathing
- Soft palate and upper esophageal weakness, causing liquids to be regurgitated through nose
- Impaired ability to laugh, cough, or blow the nose

Bulbar Muscle Impairment

- Progressive difficulty in speaking and swallowing, and aspiration
- Nasal voice and unintelligible speech
- Emotional liability
- Eventually, compromised respiratory function

Assessment and Diagnostic Findings

Diagnosis is based on signs and symptoms because no clinical or laboratory tests are specific for this disease. Electromyographic and muscle biopsy studies, MRI, and neuropsychological testing can assist in assessment and diagnosis.

Medical Management

No specific treatment for ALS is available. Symptom treatment includes the following:

- Riluzole (Rilutek), a glutamate antagonist, as a neuroprotective effect in early ALS
- Baclofen, dantrolene sodium, or diazepam for spasticity
- Modafinil (Provigil) possibly used for fatigue
- Mechanical ventilation (using negative-pressure ventilators) for alveolar hypoventilation; optional noninvasive positive-pressure ventilation
- Enteral feedings (percutaneous endoscopic gastrostomy [PEG]) for patients with aspiration or swallowing difficulties
- Decision about life support measures, made by the patient and family and based on a thorough understanding of the disease, prognosis, and implications of initiating such therapy
- Encouraging patient to complete an advance directive or "living will" to preserve autonomy

Nursing Management

The nursing care of the patient with ALS is generally the same as the basic care plan for patients with degenerative neurologic disorders (e.g., see Myasthenia Gravis in Section M). Encourage patient and family to contact the ALS Association for information and support.

For more information, see Chapter 70 in Hinkle, J. L., & Cheever, K. H. (2014). *Brunner and Suddarth's textbook of medical-surgical nursing* (13th ed.). Philadelphia: Lippincott Williams & Wilkins.

Anaphylaxis

Anaphylaxis, the most severe hypersensitivity reaction, is a clinical response to an immediate (type I hypersensitivity) immunologic reaction between a specific antigen and an antibody. The reaction results from a rapid release of IgE-mediated chemicals, which can induce a severe, life-threatening allergic reaction resulting in hypotension, bronchospasm, and cardiovascular collapse. Histamine, prostaglandins, and inflammatory leukotrienes are potent vasoactive mediators that are implicated in the vascular permeability changes, flushing, urticaria, angioedema, hypotension, and bronchoconstriction that characterize anaphylaxis. Substances that most commonly cause anaphylaxis include foods, medications, insect stings, and latex. Antibiotics (e.g., penicillin) and radiocontrast agents cause the most serious anaphylactic reactions. Closely related to anaphylaxis is a nonallergenic anaphylaxis (anaphylactoid) reaction.

Clinical Manifestations

Anaphylactic reactions produce a clinical syndrome that affects multiple organ systems. Reactions may be categorized as mild, moderate, or severe. The severity depends on the degree of allergy and the dose of allergen; type I hypersensitivity reactions may include both local and systemic reactions.

Mild

Symptoms include peripheral tingling, a warm sensation, fullness in the mouth and throat, nasal congestion, periorbital swelling, pruritus, sneezing, and tearing eyes. Symptoms begin within 2 hours of exposure.

Moderate

Symptoms include flushing, warmth, anxiety, and itching in addition to any of the milder symptoms. More serious reactions include bronchospasm and edema of the airways or larynx with dyspnea, cough, and wheezing. The onset of symptoms is the same as for a mild reaction.

Severe

Severe systemic reactions have an abrupt onset with the same signs and symptoms described previously. Symptoms progress rapidly to bronchospasm, laryngeal edema, severe dyspnea, cyanosis, and hypotension. Dysphagia, abdominal cramping, vomiting, diarrhea, and seizures can also occur. Cardiac arrest and coma may follow.

Assessment and Diagnostic Findings

Diagnostic evaluation of the patient with allergic disorders commonly includes blood tests (complete blood cell count [CBC] with differential, high total serum IgE levels), smears of body secretions, skin tests, and the radioallergosorbent test (RAST).

Prevention

Prevention by avoidance of allergens is of utmost importance. If avoidance of exposure to allergens is impossible, an auto-injection system for epinephrine (e.g., Epi-Pen Autoinjector) will be prescribed. The patient should be instructed to carry and administer epinephrine to prevent an anaphylactic reaction in the event of exposure to the allergen. Health care providers should always obtain a careful, comprehensive history of any sensitivities before administering medications. Reactions to allergens should be assessed and documented.

Venom immunotherapy may be given to people who are allergic to insect venom. Insulin-allergic patients with diabetes or penicillin-sensitive patients may require desensitization.

Medical Management

Respiratory and cardiovascular functions are evaluated and cardiopulmonary resuscitation (CPR) is initiated in cases of cardiac arrest. Supplemental oxygen is administered in high concentrations during CPR or when the patient is cyanotic, dyspneic, or wheezing. Patients with mild reactions need to be educated about the risk for recurrences. Patients with severe reactions need to be observed for 12 to 14 hours; patients at risk for adverse events include older patients and those with hypertension, arteriopathies, or known ischemic heart disease.

Pharmacologic Therapy

- Epinephrine, antihistamines, and corticosteroids may be given to prevent recurrences of the reaction and to relieve urticaria and angioedema.
- IV fluids (e.g., normal saline solution), volume expanders, and vasopressor agents are administered to maintain blood pressure and normal hemodynamic status; glucagon may be administered.
- Aminophylline and corticosteroids may also be administered to improve airway patency and function.

Nursing Management

- Assess patent's airway, breathing pattern, and vital signs; document any other signs of an allergic reaction.
- Observe patient for signs of edema or respiratory distress; prompt notification of the rapid response team and/or the provider is required.
- Explain to the patient who has recovered from anaphylaxis what occurred and educate the patient and family about avoiding future exposure to antigens and how to administer emergency medications to treat anaphylaxis.
- Instruct patient about antigens that should be avoided and about other strategies to prevent recurrence of anaphylaxis.
- Instruct patient and family how to use preloaded (auto-injector) syringes of epinephrine, if needed, and have the patient and family demonstrate correct administration.

For more information, see Chapter 38 in Hinkle, J. L., & Cheever, K. H. (2014). *Brunner and Suddarth's textbook of medical-surgical nursing* (13th ed.). Philadelphia: Lippincott Williams & Wilkins.

Anemia

Anemia is a condition in which the hemoglobin concentration is lower than normal; it reflects the presence of fewer than the normal number of erythrocytes within the circulation. As a result, the amount of oxygen delivered to body tissues is also diminished. Anemia is not a specific disease state but a sign of an underlying disorder. It is by far the most common hematologic condition. A physiologic approach classifies anemia according to whether the deficiency in erythrocytes is caused by a defect in their production (hypoproliferative anemia), by their destruction (hemolytic anemia), or by their loss (bleeding).

Clinical Manifestations

Aside from the severity of the anemia itself, several factors influence the development of anemia-associated symptoms: the rapidity with which the anemia has developed, the duration of the anemia (i.e., its chronicity), the metabolic requirements of the patient, other concurrent disorders or disabilities (e.g., cardiac, pulmonary, or renal disease), and complications or concomitant features of the condition that produced the anemia. In general, the more rapidly an anemia develops, the more severe are its symptoms. Pronounced symptoms of anemia include the following:

- Dyspnea, chest pain, muscle pain or cramping, tachycardia
- Weakness, fatigue, general malaise
- Hemoglobin level less than 11g/dL
- Pallor of the skin and mucous membranes (conjunctivae, oral mucosa)
- Jaundice (megaloblastic or hemolytic anemia)
- Smooth, red tongue (iron-deficiency anemia)
- Beefy, red, sore tongue (megaloblastic anemia)
- Angular cheilosis (ulceration of the corner of the mouth)
- Brittle, ridged, concave nails and pica (unusual craving for substances not normally considered food, such as starch, dirt, ice, etc.) are most often associated with iron-deficiency anemia.

Assessment and Diagnostic Findings

- Complete hematologic studies (e.g., hemoglobin, hematocrit, reticulocyte count, and red blood cell [RBC] indices, particularly the mean corpuscular volume [MCV] and RBC distribution width [RDW])
- Iron studies (serum iron level, total iron-binding capacity [TIBC], percent saturation, and ferritin)

- Serum vitamin B_{12} and folate levels; haptoglobin and erythropoietin levels
- Bone marrow aspiration
- Other studies as indicated to determine underlying hematologic condition or chronic illness.

Complications

General complications of severe anemia include heart failure, paresthesias, and delirium. Patients with underlying heart disease are far more likely to have angina or symptoms of heart failure than those without heart disease.

Medical Management

Management of anemia is directed toward correcting or controlling the cause of the anemia; if the anemia is severe, the erythrocytes that are lost or destroyed may be replaced with a transfusion of packed RBCs (PRBCs).

🍂 Gerontologic Considerations

Anemia is the most common hematologic condition affecting older patients. The impact of anemia on function is significant and may include decreased mobility, increased depression, increased risk of falling, and delirium when hospitalized. Prevalence increases particularly for those admitted to hospitals and long-term care facilities with increased risk for mortality when anemic for those with pre-existing renal or cardiac disease or for those who have had recent surgery.

NURSING PROCESS

The Patient With Anemia

Assessment

- Obtain a health history with a medication and alcohol intake history, including OTC drugs and herbal supplements; perform a physical examination.
- Ask patient about extent and type of symptoms experienced and impact of symptoms on lifestyle; medication history; alcohol intake; and athletic endeavors (extreme exercise).
- Obtain a family history of inherited anemias.
- Perform nutritional assessment: Ask about dietary habits resulting in nutritional deficiencies, such as those of iron, vitamin B_{12}, and folic acid.

- Obtain and monitor relevant laboratory test results; note changes.
- Assess cardiac status (for symptoms of increased workload or heart failure): tachycardia, palpitations, dyspnea, dizziness, orthopnea, exertional dyspnea, cardiomegaly, hepatomegaly, and peripheral edema.
- Assess patient for gastrointestinal function: nausea, vomiting, diarrhea, melena or dark stools, occult blood, anorexia, glossitis; women should be questioned about their menstrual periods (e.g., excessive menstrual flow, other vaginal bleeding) and the use of iron supplements during pregnancy.
- Assess patient for neurologic deficits (important with pernicious anemia): presence and extent of peripheral numbness and paresthesias, ataxia, poor coordination, confusion.

Diagnosis

NURSING DIAGNOSES

- Fatigue related to decreased hemoglobin and diminished oxygen-carrying capacity of the blood
- Imbalanced nutrition, less than body requirements, related to inadequate intake of essential nutrients
- Ineffective tissue perfusion related to inadequate hemoglobin and hematocrit
- Noncompliance with prescribed therapy

COLLABORATIVE PROBLEMS/POTENTIAL COMPLICATIONS

- Heart failure
- Angina
- Paresthesias
- Injury related to falls
- Depressed mood
- Confusion

Planning and Goals

The major goals for the patient may include decreased fatigue, attainment or maintenance of adequate nutrition, maintenance of adequate tissue perfusion, compliance with prescribed therapy, and absence of complications.

Nursing Interventions

MANAGING FATIGUE

- Assist patient to prioritize activities and establish a balance between activity and rest.

- Encourage patient with chronic anemia to maintain physical activity and exercise to prevent deconditioning.
- Assess patient for other conditions that can exacerbate fatigue, such as pain, depression, and sleep disturbance.

Maintaining Adequate Nutrition
- Encourage a healthy diet with essential nutrients, such as iron, vitamin B_{12}, folic acid, and protein.
- Instruct patient to avoid or limit intake of alcohol.
- Plan dietary education sessions for patient and family; consider cultural aspects of nutrition.
- Discuss nutritional supplements (e.g., vitamins, iron, folate, protein) as prescribed.

Maintaining Adequate Perfusion
- Monitor patient's vital signs and pulse oximeter readings closely, and adjust or withhold medications (antihypertensives) as indicated.
- Administer supplemental oxygen, transfusions, and IV fluids as ordered.

Promoting Compliance with Prescribed Therapy
- Discuss with patient the purpose of their medication, ways to take the medication and over what time period, and how to manage any side effects; ensure that patient knows that abruptly stopping some medications can have serious consequences.
- Assist the patient to incorporate the therapeutic plan into everyday activities, rather than merely giving patient a list of instructions.
- Provide patient assistance to obtain needed insurance coverage for expensive medications (e.g., growth factors) or to explore alternative ways to obtain these medications.

Monitoring and Managing Complications
- Assess patient with anemia for heart failure.
- Perform a neurologic assessment for patients with known or suspected megaloblastic anemia.
- Evaluate patient's gait, balance, and any complaint of paresthesias.

Evaluation

EXPECTED PATIENT OUTCOMES
- Reports less fatigue
- Attains and maintains adequate nutrition
- Maintains adequate perfusion
- Displays absence of complications

For more information, see Chapter 33 in Hinkle, J. L., & Cheever, K. H. (2014). *Brunner and Suddarth's textbook of medical-surgical nursing* (13th ed.). Philadelphia: Lippincott Williams & Wilkins.

Anemia, Aplastic

Aplastic anemia is a rare disease caused by a decrease in or damage to marrow stem cells, damage to the microenvironment within the marrow, and replacement of the marrow with fat. The precise etiology of aplastic anemia is unknown, but the body's T cells are hypothesized to mediate an inappropriate attack against the bone marrow, resulting in bone marrow aplasia (i.e., markedly reduced hematopoiesis). Significant neutropenia and thrombocytopenia (i.e., a deficiency of platelets) also occur. Aplastic anemia can be congenital or acquired, but most cases are idiopathic. Infections and pregnancy can trigger it, or it may be caused by certain medications, chemicals, or radiation damage. Agents that may produce marrow aplasia include benzene and benzene derivatives (e.g., paint remover). Certain toxic materials, such as inorganic arsenic, glycol ethers, plutonium, and radon, have also been implicated as potential causes.

Clinical Manifestations
- Infection and the symptoms of anemia (e.g., fatigue, pallor, dyspnea)
- Retinal hemorrhages
- Purpura (bruising)
- Repeated throat infections with possible cervical lymphadenopathy
- Possible lymphadenopathies and splenomegaly

Assessment and Diagnostic Findings
- Assess for medication or chemical ingestion in toxic amounts.

- Obtain diagnosis by a bone marrow aspirate that shows an extremely hypoplastic or even aplastic (very few to no cells) marrow replaced with fat.

Medical Management

- Those who are younger than 60 years, are otherwise healthy, and have a compatible donor can be cured of the disease by a hematopoietic stem cell transplant (HSCT).
- In others, the disease can be managed with immunosuppressive therapy, commonly using a combination of antithymocyte globulin (ATG) and cyclosporine or androgens.
- Supportive therapy plays a major role in the management of aplastic anemia. Any offending agent is discontinued. The patient is supported with transfusions of packed red blood cells (PRBCs) and platelets as necessary.

Nursing Management

See "Nursing Process" under Anemia for additional information.

- Assess patient carefully for signs of infection and bleeding, as patients with aplastic anemia are vulnerable to problems related to erythrocyte, leukocyte, and platelet deficiencies.
- Monitor patient for side effects of therapy, particularly for hypersensitivity reaction while administering ATG.
- If patient requires long-term cyclosporine therapy, monitor for long-term effects, including renal or liver dysfunction, hypertension, pruritus, visual impairment, tremor, and skin cancer.
- Carefully assess each new prescription for drug–drug interactions, as the metabolism of ATG is altered by many other medications.
- Ensure that patient understands the importance of not abruptly stopping immunosuppressive therapy.

For more information, see Chapter 33 in Hinkle, J. L., & Cheever, K. H. (2014). *Brunner and Suddarth's textbook of medical-surgical nursing* (13th ed.). Philadelphia: Lippincott Williams & Wilkins.

Anemia, Iron-Deficiency

Iron-deficiency anemia typically results when the intake of dietary iron is inadequate for hemoglobin synthesis. Iron-deficiency anemia is the most common type of anemia in all age groups, and it is the most common anemia in the world. The most common cause of iron-deficiency anemia in men and postmenopausal women is bleeding from ulcers, gastritis, inflammatory bowel disease, or GI tumors. The most common causes of iron-deficiency anemia in premenopausal women are menorrhagia (i.e., excessive menstrual bleeding) and pregnancy with inadequate iron supplementation. Patients with chronic alcoholism often have chronic blood loss from the GI tract, which causes iron loss and eventual anemia. Other causes include iron malabsorption, as is seen after gastrectomy or with celiac disease.

Clinical Manifestations
- Symptoms of anemia
- Symptoms in more severe or prolonged cases: smooth, sore tongue; brittle and ridged nails; angular cheilosis (mouth ulceration)

Assessment and Diagnostic Findings
- Bone marrow aspiration shows a low level or absence of iron.
- Laboratory values, including serum ferritin levels (indicates iron stores), blood cell count (hemoglobin, hematocrit, red blood cell [RBC] count, mean corpuscular volume [MCV]), serum iron level, and total iron-binding capacity.

Medical Management
- Obtain the patient's health history, which may reveal multiple pregnancies, GI bleeding, or pica.
- Search for the cause, which may be a curable GI cancer or uterine fibroids. Rule out other disease states, such as infection or inflammatory conditions.
- Test stool specimens for occult blood.
- People age 50 or older should have periodic colonoscopy, endoscopy, or x-ray examination of the GI tract to detect ulcerations, gastritis, polyps, or cancer.
- Administer prescribed iron preparations (oral, intramuscularly [IM], or IV).
- Have patient continue iron preparations for 6 to 12 months.

Nursing Management
See "Nursing Process" under Anemia for additional information.

- Administer iron IM or IV in some cases when oral iron is not absorbed, is poorly tolerated, or is needed in large amounts.
- Administer a small test dose before IM injection to avoid risk of anaphylaxis (greater with IM than with IV injections).

- Advise patient to take iron supplements an hour before meals. If gastric distress occurs, suggest taking the supplement with meals and, after symptoms subside, resuming between-meal schedule for maximum absorption.
- Inform patient that stool will become dark.
- Advise patient to take liquid forms of iron through a straw, to rinse the mouth with water, and to practice good oral hygiene after taking this medication.
- Provide preventive education, because iron-deficiency anemia is common in menstruating and pregnant women.
- Educate patient regarding foods high in iron (e.g., organs and other meats, beans, leafy green vegetables, raisins, molasses).
- Instruct patient to avoid taking antacids or dairy products with iron (diminishes iron absorption).
- Instruct patient to increase vitamin C intake (e.g., citrus fruits and juices, strawberries, tomatoes, broccoli) to enhance iron absorption.
- Provide nutritional counseling for those whose normal diet is inadequate.
- Encourage patient to continue iron therapy for total therapy time (6 to 12 months), even when fatigue is no longer present.

For more information, see Chapter 33 in Hinkle, J. L., & Cheever, K. H. (2014). *Brunner and Suddarth's textbook of medical-surgical nursing* (13th ed.). Philadelphia: Lippincott Williams & Wilkins.

Anemia, Megaloblastic

In the anemias caused by deficiencies of vitamin B_{12} or folic acid, identical bone marrow and peripheral blood changes occur because both vitamins are essential for normal DNA synthesis.

Pathophysiology

Folic Acid Deficiency

Folic acid is stored as compounds referred to as *folates*. The folate stores in the body are much smaller than those of vitamin B_{12}, and can be quickly depleted when the dietary intake of folate is deficient (within 4 months). Folate deficiency occurs in people who rarely eat uncooked vegetables. Alcohol increases folic acid requirements; folic acid requirements are also increased in patients with chronic hemolytic anemias and in women who are pregnant. Some patients with malabsorptive diseases of the small bowel may not absorb folic acid normally.

Vitamin B_{12} Deficiency

A deficiency of vitamin B_{12} can occur in several ways. Inadequate dietary intake is rare but can develop in strict vegetarians who consume no meat or dairy products. Faulty absorption from the GI tract is more common, as with conditions such as Crohn's disease or after ileal resection or gastrectomy. Chronic proton pump inhibitors may reduce gastric acid production inhibiting B_{12} absorption, as can the use of the drug metformin in managing diabetes. Another cause is the absence of intrinsic factor. A deficiency may also occur if disease involving the ileum or pancreas impairs absorption, resulting in pernicious anemia. The body normally has large stores of vitamin B_{12}, so years may pass before the deficiency results in anemia.

Clinical Manifestations

Symptoms of folic acid and vitamin B_{12} deficiencies are similar, and the two anemias may coexist. Symptoms are progressive, although the course of illness may be marked by spontaneous partial remissions and exacerbations.

- Gradual development of signs of anemia (weakness, listlessness, and fatigue)
- Possible development of a smooth, sore, red tongue and mild diarrhea (pernicious anemia)
- Mild jaundice, vitiligo, and premature graying
- Possible confusion; more often, paresthesias in the extremities and difficulty in keeping balance; loss of position sense
- Lack of neurologic manifestations with folic acid deficiency alone

Assessment and Diagnostic Findings

- Schilling test (primary diagnostic tool)
- Complete blood cell count (Hgb value as low as 4 to 5 g/dL, white blood cell [WBC] count 2,000 to 3,000/mm^3, platelet count fewer than 50,000/mm^3; very high mean corpuscular volume [MCV], usually exceeding 110 mcm^3)
- Serum levels of folate and vitamin B_{12} (folic acid deficiency and deficient vitamin B_{12})
- Measurement of methylmalonic acid levels in vitamin B_{12} deficiency

Medical Management: Folic Acid Deficiency

- Increase intake of folic acid in patient's diet and administer 1 mg folic acid daily.
- Administer IM folic acid for malabsorption syndromes.
- Prescribe additional supplements as necessary, because the amount in multivitamins may be inadequate to fully replace deficient body stores.
- Prescribe folic acid for patients with alcoholism as long as they continue to consume alcohol.

Medical Management: Vitamin B$_{12}$ Deficiency

- Provide vitamin B$_{12}$ replacement: Vegetarians can prevent or treat deficiency with oral supplements with vitamins or fortified soy milk; when the deficiency is due to the more common defect in absorption or the absence of intrinsic factor, replacement is by monthly intramuscular (IM) injections of vitamin B$_{12}$.
- A small amount of an oral dose of vitamin B$_{12}$ can be absorbed by passive diffusion, even in the absence of intrinsic factor, but large doses (2 mg/day) are required if vitamin B$_{12}$ is to be replaced orally.
- To prevent recurrence of pernicious anemia, vitamin B$_{12}$ therapy must be continued for life.

Nursing Management

See "Nursing Process" under Anemia for additional information.

- Assess patient at risk for megaloblastic anemia for clinical manifestations (e.g., inspect the skin, sclera, and mucous membranes for jaundice; note vitiligo and premature graying).
- Perform careful neurologic assessment (e.g., note gait and stability; cognitive function, test of position and vibration sense).
- Instruct patient about the chronicity of the disorder.
- Assess patient's need for assistive devices (e.g., canes, walkers) and need for support and guidance in managing activities of daily living and home environment.
- Ensure patient safety when position sense, coordination, and gait are affected.
- Refer patient for physical or occupational therapy as needed.
- When patient's sensation is altered, instruct patient to avoid excessive heat and cold.
- Advise patient to prepare bland, soft foods and to eat small amounts frequently.

- Explain that other nutritional deficiencies, such as alcohol-induced anemia, can induce neurologic problems.
- Instruct patient in complete urine collections for the Schilling test. Also explain the importance of the test and of complying with the collection.
- Teach patient about chronicity of the disorder and need for monthly vitamin B_{12} injections even when patient has no symptoms. Instruct patient how to self-administer injections, when appropriate.
- Stress importance of ongoing medical follow-up and screening, because gastric atrophy associated with pernicious anemia increases the risk of gastric carcinoma.

For more information, see Chapter 33 in Hinkle, J. L., & Cheever, K. H. (2014). *Brunner and Suddarth's textbook of medical-surgical nursing* (13th ed.). Philadelphia: Lippincott Williams & Wilkins.

Anemia, Sickle Cell

Sickle cell anemia is a severe hemolytic anemia resulting from the inheritance of the sickle hemoglobin (HbS) gene, which causes a defective hemoglobin molecule.

Pathophysiology

HbS acquires a crystal-like formation when exposed to low oxygen tension. HbS loses its round, biconcave disk shape and becomes a dehydrated, long, rigid, and sickle-shaped erythrocyte that lodges in small vessels and can obstruct blood flow. If ischemia or infarction results, the patient may have pain, swelling, and fever. The sickling process takes time; if the erythrocyte is again exposed to adequate amounts of oxygen (e.g., when it travels through the pulmonary circulation) before the membrane becomes too rigid, it can revert to a normal shape. For this reason, the "sickling crises" are intermittent. The HbS gene is inherited, with some people having the sickle cell trait (a carrier, inheriting one abnormal gene) and some having sickle cell disease (inheriting two abnormal genes). The HbS gene is inherited in people of African descent and, to a lesser extent, in people from the Mediterranean area, the Middle East, or aboriginal tribes of India. Sickle cell anemia is the most severe form of sickle cell disease.

Clinical Manifestations

Symptoms of sickle cell anemia vary and are based only somewhat on the amount of HbS. Symptoms and complications result from chronic hemolysis or thrombosis.

- Anemia reveals hemoglobin values in the range of 7 to 10 g/dL.
- Jaundice is characteristic, usually obvious in the sclera.
- Bone marrow expands in childhood, sometimes causing enlargement of bones of the face and skull.
- Tachycardia, cardiac murmurs, and often cardiomegaly are associated with chronic anemia.
- Dysrhythmias and heart failure may occur in adults.
- Virtually any organ may be affected by thrombosis; primary sites involve those areas with slower circulation, such as the spleen, lungs, and central nervous system.
- Severe pain occurs in various parts of the body. All tissues and organs are vulnerable and susceptible to hypoxic damage or ischemic necrosis.
- Sickle cell crisis may take the form of acute vaso-occlusive crisis, aplastic crisis, or sequestration crisis.
- Acute chest syndrome involves fever, cough, tachycardia, and new infiltrates seen on the chest x-ray.
- Pulmonary hypertension is a common sequela of sickle cell disease and often the cause of death.

Assessment and Diagnostic Findings

- The patient with sickle cell trait usually has a normal hemoglobin level, a normal hematocrit, and a normal blood smear.
- The patient with sickle cell anemia has a low hematocrit level and sickled cells on the peripheral smear. The diagnosis is confirmed by hemoglobin electrophoresis.
- Doppler echocardiography may be useful in identifying patients with elevated pulmonary artery pressures.
- High levels of the amino-terminal form of brain natriuretic peptide (BNP) can serve as a useful biomarker.

Medical Management

Treatment of sickle cell anemia is the focus of continued research. However, aside from the equally important aggressive management of symptoms and complications, currently few primary treatment modalities exist for sickle cell diseases.

- Hematopoietic stem cell transplantation (HSCT) may cure sickle cell anemia; however, it is available only to a small subset of affected patients either because of the lack of a compatible donor or because severe organ damage that may be already present in the patient is a contraindication for HSCT.

- Pharmacologic therapy includes hydroxyurea, a chemotherapy agent effective in increasing fetal hemoglobin (i.e., hemoglobin F) levels in patients with sickle cell anemia. Arginine may be useful in managing pulmonary hypertension and acute chest syndrome.
- Transfusion therapy has been shown to be highly effective in several situations (e.g., in an acute exacerbation of anemia, in the prevention of severe complications from anesthesia and surgery, and in improving the response to infection and in severe cases of acute chest syndrome).
- Pulmonary function is monitored, and pulmonary hypertension is treated early if found. Infections and acute chest syndrome are treated promptly with antibiotics. Incentive spirometry is performed to prevent pulmonary complications; bronchoscopy is performed to identify the source of pulmonary disease.
- Fluid restriction may be beneficial. Corticosteroids may be useful.
- Folic acid is administered daily for increased marrow requirement.
- Supportive care involves pain management (aspirin or nonsteroidal anti-inflammatory drugs, morphine, and patient-controlled analgesia), oral or IV hydration, physical and occupational therapy, physiotherapy, cognitive and behavioral intervention, and support groups.

NURSING PROCESS

The Patient With Sickle Cell Crisis

See "Nursing Process" under Anemia for additional information.

Assessment

- Identify precipitating factors for a crisis and measures used to prevent a crisis.
- Assess all body systems, with particular emphasis on pain (0-to-10 scale, quality, and frequency), swelling, fever (all joint areas and abdomen).
- Assess patient's fatigue with impact on current life style and quality.

- Carefully assess respiratory system, including breath sounds and oxygen saturation levels.
- Assess for signs of cardiac failure (edema, increased point of maximal impulse, and cardiomegaly [as seen on chest x-ray]).
- Elicit symptoms of cerebral hypoxia by careful neurologic examination.
- Assess for signs of dehydration and history of fluid intake; examine mucous membranes, skin turgor, urine output, serum creatinine, and blood urea nitrogen values.
- Assess for signs of any infectious process (examine chest and long bones and femoral head, because pneumonia and osteomyelitis are common).
- Monitor hemoglobin, hematocrit, and reticulocyte count and compare with baseline levels.
- Assess current and past history of medical management, particularly chronic transfusion therapy, hydroxyurea use, and prior treatment for infection.

Diagnosis

NURSING DIAGNOSES
- Acute pain and fatigue related to tissue hypoxia due to agglutination of sickled cells within blood vessels
- Risk for infection
- Risk for powerlessness related to illness-induced helplessness
- Deficient knowledge regarding prevention of crisis

COLLABORATIVE PROBLEMS/POTENTIAL COMPLICATIONS
- Hypoxia, ischemia, infection, and poor wound healing leading to skin breakdown and ulcers
- Dehydration
- Cerebrovascular accident (cerebrovascular accident, stroke)
- Anemia
- Acute and chronic renal failure
- Heart failure, pulmonary hypertension, and acute chest syndrome
- Impotence
- Poor compliance
- Substance abuse related to poorly managed chronic pain

Planning and Goals

The major goals for the patient are relief of pain, decreased incidence of crises, enhanced sense of self-esteem and power, and absence of complications.

Nursing Interventions

MANAGING PAIN

- Use patient's subjective description of pain and pain rating on a pain scale to guide the use of analgesic agents.
- Support and elevate any joint that is acutely swollen until swelling diminishes.
- Instruct patient about relaxation techniques, breathing exercises, and distraction to ease pain.
- When an acute painful episode has diminished, implement aggressive measures to preserve function (e.g., physical therapy, whirlpool baths, and transcutaneous nerve stimulation).

MANAGING FATIGUE

- Fatigue experienced can be acute or chronic in nature.
- Assist patient to balance between exercise and rest.
- Help patient develop strategies to cope with daily life demands in the setting of chronic fatigue.
- Maximize nutrition, hydration, healthy sleep cycles, and diminishing tissue hypoxia to minimize fatigue.

PREVENTING AND MANAGING INFECTION

- Monitor patient for signs and symptoms of infection.
- Initiate prescribed antibiotics promptly.
- Assess patient for signs of dehydration.
- Instruct patient to take prescribed oral antibiotics at home, if indicated, emphasizing the importance to complete the entire course of antibiotic therapy.

PROMOTING COPING SKILLS

- Enhance pain management to promote a therapeutic relationship based on mutual trust.
- Focus on patient's strengths rather than deficits to enhance effective coping skills.
- Provide opportunities for patient to make decisions about daily care to increase feelings of control.

MINIMIZING DEFICIENT KNOWLEDGE

- Educate patient about situations that can precipitate a sickle cell crisis and steps to take to prevent or diminish such crises (e.g., keep warm, maintain adequate hydration, avoid stressful situations).
- If hydroxyurea is prescribed for a woman of childbearing age, inform her that the drug can cause congenital harm to unborn children and advise about pregnancy prevention.

MONITORING AND MANAGING POTENTIAL
COMPLICATIONS

Management measures for many of the potential complications
are delineated in the previous sections; additional measures
should be taken to address the following issues.

Leg Ulcers
- Protect the patient's leg from trauma and contamination.
- Use scrupulous aseptic technique to prevent nosocomial
  infections.
- Referral to a wound–ostomy–continence nurse may facilitate
  healing and assist with prevention.

Priapism Leading to Impotence
- Instruct patient to empty the bladder at the onset of the
  attack, exercise and take a warm bath.
- Inform patient to seek medical attention if an episode persists
  more than 3 hours.

Chronic Pain and Substance Abuse
- Emphasize the importance of complying with the prescribed
  treatment plan.
- Promote trust with patient through adequate management of
  acute pain during episodes of crisis.
- Suggest to patient that receiving care from a single provider over time is much more beneficial than receiving
  care from rotating physicians and staff in an emergency
  department.
- When a crisis arises, emergency department staff should contact patient's primary health care provider for optimal management.
- Promote continuity of care and establish written contracts
  with patient.

PROMOTING HOME- AND COMMUNITY-BASED CARE
- Involve the patient and his or her family in education about
  the disease, treatment, assessment, and monitoring needed to
  detect complications.
- Advise health care providers, patients, and families to communicate regularly.
- Provide guidelines regarding when to seek urgent care.
- Provide follow-up care for patients with vascular access
  devices, if necessary, and include education about chelation
  therapy.

Evaluation

EXPECTED PATIENT OUTCOMES

- Reports control of pain and fatigue
- Absence of infection
- Expresses improved sense of control
- Increases knowledge about disease process
- Absence of complications

For more information, see Chapter 33 in Hinkle, J. L., & Cheever, K. H. (2014). *Brunner and Suddarth's textbook of medical-surgical nursing* (13th ed.). Philadelphia: Lippincott Williams & Wilkins.

Aneurysm, Aortic

An aneurysm is a localized sac or dilation formed at a weak point in the wall of an artery. It may be classified by its shape or form. The most common forms of aneurysms are saccular and fusiform. A saccular aneurysm projects from only one side of the vessel. If an entire arterial segment becomes dilated, a fusiform aneurysm develops. Very small aneurysms due to localized infection are called *mycotic aneurysms*. Historically, the cause of abdominal aortic aneurysm, the most common type of degenerative aneurysm, has been attributed to atherosclerotic changes in the aorta. Occasionally, in an aorta diseased by arteriosclerosis, a tear develops in the intima or the media degenerates, resulting in a dissection. Aneurysms are serious because they can rupture, leading to hemorrhage and death.

Thoracic aortic aneurysms occur most frequently in men between the ages of 50 and 70. The thoracic area is the most common site for the development of a dissecting aneurysm. About one-third of patients die from rupture. Abdominal aortic aneurysms are more common among Caucasians, affect men two to six times more often than women, and are most prevalent in older adult patients. Most of these aneurysms occur below the renal arteries (infrarenal aneurysms).

🍃 Gerontologic Considerations

Most abdominal aortic aneurysms occur in patients between age 60 and 90. Rupture is likely with coexisting hypertension and with aneurysms more than 6 cm wide. In most cases at this point, the chances of rupture are greater than the chance of death during surgical repair. If the older patient is considered at moderate risk of complications related to surgery or anesthesia, the aneurysm is not repaired until it is at least 5.5 cm (2 in) wide.

Clinical Manifestations

Thoracic Aortic Aneurysm
- Symptoms variable and dependent on how rapidly the aneurysm dilates and affects the surrounding intrathoracic structures; some patients asymptomatic
- Constant, boring pain, which may occur only when the patient is in the supine position (prominent symptom)
- Dyspnea, cough (paroxysmal and brassy)
- Hoarseness, stridor, or weakness or complete loss of the voice (aphonia)
- Dysphagia
- Dilated superficial veins on chest, neck, or arms
- Edematous areas on chest wall
- Cyanosis
- Unequal pupils

Abdominal Aortic Aneurysm
- Only about 40% of patients with abdominal aortic aneurysms have symptoms.
- The patient complains of "heart beating" in abdomen when lying down or a feeling of an abdominal mass or abdominal throbbing.
- Cyanosis and mottling of the toes can occur if aneurysm is associated with small cholesterol, platelet, or fibrin emboli.

Dissecting Aneurysm
- Sudden onset with severe and persistent pain described as "tearing" or "ripping" in anterior chest or back, extending to shoulders, epigastric area, or abdomen (may be mistaken for acute myocardial infarction [MI])
- Pallor, sweating, and tachycardia
- Blood pressure elevated or markedly different from one arm to the other

Assessment and Diagnostic Findings
- Thoracic aortic aneurysm: chest x-ray, CT angiography (CTA), and transesophageal echocardiography (TEE)
- Abdominal aortic aneurysm: palpation of pulsatile mass in the middle and upper abdomen (a systolic bruit may be heard over the mass); duplex ultrasonography or CTA to determine the size, length, and location of the aneurysm

- Dissecting aneurysm: arteriography, multidetector computed tomography angiography, (MDCTA), TEE, duplex ultrasonography, and magnetic resonance angiogram (MRA)

Medical Management

Pharmacologic therapy or surgical treatment depends on the type and size of the aneurysm. For a ruptured aneurysm, prognosis is poor, and surgery is performed immediately. When surgery can be delayed, medical measures include the following:

- Monitoring and control of systolic blood pressure between 90 and 120 mmHg with antihypertensive agents including diuretics, beta-blockers, ACE inhibitors, angiotensin II receptor antagonists, and calcium channel blockers.
- For a small aneurysm, ultrasonography conducted at 6-month follow-up to monitor and assess the need for surgical procedure

Surgical Management

An expanding or enlarging abdominal aortic aneurysm is likely to rupture. Surgery is the treatment of choice for abdominal aortic aneurysms more than 5.5 cm (2 in) wide or those that are enlarging; the standard treatment has been open surgical repair of the aneurysm by resecting the vessel and sewing a bypass graft in place. An alternative for treating an infrarenal abdominal aortic aneurysm is endovascular grafting, which involves the transluminal placement and attachment of a sutureless aortic graft prosthesis across an aneurysm.

Nursing Management

Preoperative Assessment

- Assessment is guided by anticipating a rupture (signs include persistent or intermittent back or abdominal pain that may be localized in the middle or lower abdomen or lower back) and by recognizing that the patient may have cardiovascular, cerebral, pulmonary, and renal impairment from atherosclerosis.
- Assess functional capacity of all organ systems.
- Assess patient for signs of heart failure, loud bruit, and high blood pressure.
- Implement medical therapies to stabilize physiologic function of the patient.

> **Quality and Safety Nursing Alert**
>
> Constant intense back pain, falling blood pressure, and decreasing hematocrit level are signs of a rupturing abdominal aortic aneurysm. Hematomas into the scrotum, perineum, flank, or penis indicate retroperitoneal rupture. Rupture into the peritoneal cavity is rapidly fatal.

Postoperative Assessment

- Obtain vital sign and Doppler assessment of peripheral pulses while patient is on bed rest with head of bed at 45 degrees, continuing to log roll until patient can ambulate.
- Frequently monitor patient's pulmonary, cardiovascular, renal, and neurologic status.
- Monitor patient for complications: arterial occlusion, hemorrhage (persistent coughing, sneezing, vomiting, or systolic blood pressure greater than 180 mm Hg), infection, ischemic bowel, renal failure, and impotence.
- Assess patient for skin changes, bleeding, pulsation, swelling, pain, and hematoma formation.
- Assess patient for adequate fluid intake by continuing IV infusion until patient resumes oral fluids.

For more information, see Chapter 30 in Hinkle, J. L., & Cheever, K. H. (2014). *Brunner and Suddarth's textbook of medical-surgical nursing* (13th ed.). Philadelphia: Lippincott Williams & Wilkins.

Aneurysm, Intracranial

An intracranial (cerebral) aneurysm is a dilation of the walls of a cerebral artery that develops as a result of weakness in the arterial wall. Its cause is unknown, but it may be due to atherosclerosis, a congenital defect of the vessel walls, hypertensive vascular disease, head trauma, or advancing age. Most commonly affected are the internal carotid, anterior or posterior cerebral, anterior or posterior communicating, and middle cerebral arteries. Symptoms are produced when the aneurysm presses on nearby cranial nerves or brain tissue or ruptures, causing subarachnoid hemorrhage. Prognosis depends on the age and neurologic condition of the patient, associated diseases, and the extent and location of the aneurysm.

Clinical Manifestations

- Neurologic deficits are similar to those of ischemic stroke.
- Vomiting, early sudden change in level of consciousness, and possibly focal seizures are seen more frequently in acute intracerebral hemorrhage (compared with ischemic stroke) due to frequent brain stem involvement.
- Rupture of the aneurysm causes sudden, unusually severe headache; often, loss of consciousness for a variable period; pain and rigidity of the back of the neck and spine; and visual disturbances (visual loss, diplopia, ptosis). Tinnitus, dizziness, and hemiparesis may also occur.
- If the aneurysm leaks blood and forms a clot, the patient may show little neurologic deficit or may have severe bleeding, resulting in cerebral damage followed rapidly by coma and death.

Assessment and Diagnostic Findings

CT scan or MRI, cerebral angiography, and lumbar puncture (in absence of increased intracranial pressure) are diagnostic procedures used to confirm an aneurysm. Toxicology testing for illicit drugs may be considered for patients younger than 40 years.

Prevention

- Primary prevention includes managing hypertension and ameliorating other significant modifiable risk factors.
- Additional risk factors include age, male gender, and excessive alcohol use.
- Stroke risk screenings can identify high-risk individuals and educate patients and the community about prevention and recognition.

Medical Management

Treatment goals are to allow the brain to recover from the initial insult (bleeding), prevent or minimize risk of rebleeding, and prevent or treat other complications. Management may consist of bed rest with sedation to prevent agitation and stress, management of vasospasm, and surgical or medical treatment to prevent re-bleeding. If the bleeding is caused by anticoagulation with warfarin, the International Normalized Ration (INR) may be corrected with fresh-frozen plasma and vitamin K. Reversing the anticoagulation effect of the newer anticoagulants is more complicated. If they occur, seizures are treated with antiepileptic drugs such as phenytoin (Dilantin); hyperglycemia should be treated to achieve the goal of normoglycemia. Measures to prevent venous thromboembolism are implemented. Analgesic agents are provided for head and neck pain; fever is treated with acetaminophen, iced saline boluses, and cooling blankets. Adequate control of hypertension will decrease risk of additional intracerebral bleeding.

Surgical Management

Surgical treatment of the patient with an unruptured aneurysm is an option to prevent bleeding in an unruptured aneurysm or further bleeding in an already ruptured aneurysm. An aneurysm may be excluded from the cerebral circulation by means of a ligature or a clip across its neck or reinforced by wrapping to provide support.

Primary intracerebral hemorrhage is not treated surgically. However, if the patient is showing signs of worsening neurologic exam, increased intracranial pressure, or signs of brain stem compression, surgical evacuation via a craniotomy is recommended.

NURSING PROCESS

The Patient With an Intracranial Aneurysm

Assessment

- Perform a complete neurologic assessment: level of patient's consciousness, pupillary reaction (sluggishness), motor and sensory function, cranial nerve deficits (extraocular eye movements, facial droop, ptosis), speech difficulties, visual disturbance, headache, nuchal rigidity, or other neurologic deficits.
- Document and report neurologic assessment findings, and reassess and report any changes in patient's condition; report changes immediately.
- Detect subtle changes, especially altered levels of consciousness (earliest signs of deterioration include mild drowsiness and slight slurring of speech).

Diagnosis

NURSING DIAGNOSES

- Ineffective tissue perfusion (cerebral) related to bleeding or vasospasm
- Disturbed sensory perception due to the restrictions of aneurysm precautions

- Anxiety due to illness and/or medically imposed restrictions (aneurysm precautions)

COLLABORATIVE PROBLEMS/POTENTIAL COMPLICATIONS
- Vasospasm
- Seizures
- Hydrocephalus
- Rebleeding
- Hyponatremia

Planning and Goals

Patient goals include improved cerebral tissue perfusion, relief of anxiety, and absence of complications.

Nursing Interventions

IMPROVING CEREBRAL TISSUE PERFUSION
- Monitor closely for neurologic deterioration, and maintain a neurologic flow record.
- Check blood pressure, pulse, level of consciousness, pupillary responses, and motor function hourly; monitor respiratory status and report changes immediately.
- Implement aneurysm precautions (immediate and absolute bed rest in a quiet, nonstressful setting; restrict visitors except for family).
- Elevate the head of the bed 15 to 30 degrees or as ordered.
- Avoid any activity that suddenly increases blood pressure or obstructs venous return (e.g., Valsalva maneuver, straining), instruct patient to exhale during voiding or defecation to decrease strain, eliminate caffeine, administer all personal care, and minimize external stimuli.
- Apply antiembolism stockings or sequential compression devices. Observe patient's legs for signs and symptoms of deep vein thrombosis tenderness, redness, swelling, warmth, and edema.

RELIEVING SENSORY DEPRIVATION
- Keep sensory stimulation to a minimum; no television or reading.
- Dim lighting is helpful as photophobia is common.
- Explain restrictions to help reduce patient's sense of isolation.

RELIEVING ANXIETY
- Inform patient of plan of care.
- Provide support and appropriate reassurance to patient and family.

MONITORING AND MANAGING POTENTIAL COMPLICATIONS

- Assess for and immediately report signs of possible vasospasm, which may occur several days after surgery or on the initiation of treatment (intensified headaches, decreased level of responsiveness, or evidence of aphasia or partial paralysis). Also administer calcium channel blockers or fluid-volume expanders as prescribed.
- Maintain seizure precautions. Also maintain airway and prevent injury if a seizure occurs. Administer antiseizure medications as prescribed (phenytoin [Dilantin] is medication of choice).
- Monitor for onset of symptoms of hydrocephalus, which may be acute (first 24 hours after hemorrhage), subacute (days later), or delayed (several weeks later). Report symptoms immediately: Acute hydrocephalus is characterized by sudden stupor or coma; subacute or delayed is characterized by gradual onset of drowsiness, behavioral changes, and ataxic gait.
- Monitor for and report symptoms of aneurysm rebleeding (occurs most often in the first 2 weeks). Symptoms include sudden severe headache, nausea, vomiting, decreased level of consciousness, and neurologic deficit. Administer medications as ordered.
- Hyponatremia: Monitor laboratory data often because hyponatremia (serum sodium level less than 135 mEq/L) affects up to 50% of patients. Report low levels persisting for 24 hours, as syndrome of inappropriate antidiuretic hormone or cerebral salt-wasting syndrome (kidneys cannot conserve sodium) may develop.

EDUCATING PATIENTS ABOUT SELF-CARE

- Provide patient and family with information to promote cooperation with the care and required activity restrictions and prepare them for patient's return home.
- Identify the causes of intracranial hemorrhage, its possible consequences, and the medical or surgical treatments that are implemented.
- Discuss the importance of interventions taken to prevent and detect complications (e.g., aneurysm precautions, close monitoring of patient).
- Education should include the use of assistive devices or home environmental changes to assist the patient with a disability at home.
- As indicated, facilitate patient's transfer to a rehabilitation unit or center.

CONTINUING CARE
- Urge patient and family to follow recommendations to prevent further complications and to schedule and keep follow-up appointments.
- Refer patient for home care if warranted, and encourage health promotion and screening practices.

Evaluation

EXPECTED PATIENT OUTCOMES
- Demonstrates stable neurologic status, vital signs, and respiratory patterns
- Demonstrates functional sensory perceptions
- Exhibits reduced anxiety level
- Is free of complications

For more information, see Chapter 67 in Hinkle, J. L., & Cheever, K. H. (2014). *Brunner and Suddarth's textbook of medical-surgical nursing* (13th ed.). Philadelphia: Lippincott Williams & Wilkins.

Angina Pectoris

Angina pectoris is a clinical syndrome characterized by paroxysms of pain or a feeling of pressure in the anterior chest. The cause is insufficient coronary blood flow, resulting in an inadequate supply of oxygen to meet the myocardial demand.

Pathophysiology

Angina is usually a result of atherosclerotic heart disease and is associated with a significant obstruction of a major coronary artery. Normally, the myocardium extracts a large amount of oxygen from the coronary circulation. When there is blockage in a coronary artery, flow cannot be increased to meet an increased myocardial demand and the resulting ischemia causes anginal pain. Factors affecting anginal pain are physical exertion, exposure to cold, eating a heavy meal, or stress or any emotion-provoking situation that increases blood pressure, heart rate, and myocardial workload. Unstable angina is not closely associated with the above and may occur at rest.

Clinical Manifestations

- Pain varies from a feeling of mild indigestion to a choking or heavy sensation in the upper chest; severity can range from discomfort to agonizing pain. The patient with diabetes may not experience severe pain with angina.

- Pain may be accompanied by severe apprehension and a feeling of impending death and is often retrosternal, deep in the chest behind the upper or middle third of the sternum.
- Discomfort is poorly localized and may radiate to the neck, jaw, shoulders, and inner aspect of the upper arms (usually the left arm).
- A feeling of weakness or numbness in the arms, wrists, and hands, as well as shortness of breath, pallor, diaphoresis, dizziness or lightheadedness, and nausea and vomiting may accompany the pain. Anxiety may occur with angina.
- An important characteristic of anginal pain is that it subsides when the precipitating cause is removed or with nitroglycerin.
- Women may have different or milder symptoms than men including nausea, vomiting, jaw pain, unusual fatigue, and discomfort in the upper back or abdomen.

Gerontologic Considerations

The older adult with angina may not exhibit a typical pain profile because of the diminished pain transmission that can occur with aging. Often, the presenting symptom in older adults is dyspnea. Sometimes, there are no symptoms ("silent" coronary artery disease [CAD]), making recognition and diagnosis a clinical challenge. Older patients should be encouraged to recognize their chest pain–like symptom (e.g., weakness) as an indication that they should rest or take prescribed medications.

Assessment and Diagnostic Findings

- Evaluation of clinical manifestations of pain and patient history
- 12-lead electrocardiogram (ECG) changes, stress testing, blood tests (including cardiac biomarkers)
- Echocardiogram, nuclear scan, or invasive procedures such as cardiac catheterization and coronary angiography

Medical Management

The objectives of the medical management of angina are to decrease the oxygen demand of the myocardium and to increase the oxygen supply. Medically, these objectives are met through pharmacologic therapy and control of risk factors. Alternatively, reperfusion procedures may be used to restore the blood supply to the myocardium. These include percutaneous coronary intervention (PCI) procedures (e.g., percutaneous transluminal coronary angioplasty [PTCA], intracoronary stents, and atherectomy) and coronary artery bypass graft (CABG) surgery.

Pharmacologic Therapy

- Nitrates, the standard of therapy (nitroglycerin)
- Beta-adrenergic blockers (metoprolol and atenolol)
- Calcium channel blockers, calcium ion antagonists (amlodipine and diltiazem)
- Antiplatelet and anticoagulant medications (aspirin, clopidogrel, prasugrel, unfractionated or low-molecular-weight heparin, glycoprotein [GP] IIb/IIIa agents [abciximab, tirofiban, eptifibatide])
- Oxygen therapy

NURSING PROCESS

The Patient With Angina

Assessment

Gather information about the patient's symptoms and activities, especially those that precede and precipitate attacks of angina pectoris. In addition, assess the patient's risk factors for CAD, the patient's response to angina, the patient's and family's understanding of the diagnosis, and adherence to the current treatment plan.

Diagnosis

NURSING DIAGNOSES
- Risk for decreased cardiac tissue perfusion
- Anxiety related to cardiac symptoms and possible death
- Deficient knowledge about underlying disease and methods for avoiding complications
- Noncompliance, ineffective management of therapeutic regimen related to failure to accept necessary lifestyle changes

COLLABORATIVE PROBLEMS/POTENTIAL COMPLICATIONS
Potential complications of angina include acute coronary syndrome (ACS) and myocardial infarction (MI), dysrhythmias, cardiac arrest, heart failure, and cardiogenic shock.

Planning and Goals

Goals include immediate and appropriate treatment when angina occurs, prevention of angina, reduction of anxiety, awareness of the disease process and understanding of the prescribed care, adherence to the self-care program, and absence of complications.

Nursing Interventions

TREATING ANGINA

- Take immediate action if patient reports pain or prodromal symptoms suggestive of cardiac ischemia, including sensations of indigestion or nausea, choking, heaviness, weakness or numbness in the upper extremities, dyspnea, or dizziness.
- Direct the patient to stop all activities and sit or rest in bed in a semi-Fowler's position to reduce the oxygen requirements of the ischemic myocardium.
- Measure vital signs and observe for signs of respiratory distress.
- Obtain a 12-lead ECG and place the patient on continuous cardiac monitoring.
- Administer nitroglycerin sublingually and assess the patient's response (repeat up to three doses).
- Administer oxygen therapy if the patient's respiratory rate is increased or if the oxygen saturation level is decreased.
- If the pain is significant and continues after these interventions, evaluate the patient further for acute MI and possibly transfer to a higher-acuity nursing unit.

REDUCING ANXIETY

- Explore implications that the diagnosis has for the patient.
- Provide essential information about the illness and methods of preventing progression.
- Explain the importance of following the prescribed directives for the ambulatory patient at home.
- Explore various stress reduction methods with the patient (e.g., music therapy).

PREVENTING PAIN

- Review the assessment findings, identify the level of activity that causes the patient's pain or prodromal symptoms, and plan the patient's activities accordingly (see the Factors That Trigger Angina Episodes box).
- If the patient has pain frequently or with minimal activity, alternate the patient's activities with rest periods. Balancing activity and rest is an important aspect of the educational plan for the patient and family.

Educating Patients About Self-Care

- The educational program for the patient with angina is designed so that the patient and family understand the illness, identify the symptoms of myocardial ischemia, state the actions to take when symptoms develop, and discuss methods to prevent chest pain and the advancement of CAD.
- The goals of education are to reduce the frequency and severity of anginal attacks, to delay the progress of the underlying disease if possible, and to prevent complications.
- Collaborate on a self-care program with patient, family, or friends.
- Plan activities to minimize angina episodes.
- Instruct the patient that any pain unrelieved within 15 minutes by the usual methods, including nitroglycerin, should be treated at the closest emergency center. The patient should call 911 for assistance.

Evaluation

Expected Patient Outcomes

- Reports that pain is relieved promptly
- Reports decreased anxiety
- Understands ways to avoid complications and demonstrates freedom from complications
- Complies with self-care program

For more information, see Chapter 27 in Hinkle, J. L., & Cheever, K. H. (2014). *Brunner and Suddarth's textbook of medical-surgical nursing* (13th ed.). Philadelphia: Lippincott Williams & Wilkins.

Factors That Trigger Angina Episodes

- Sudden or excessive physical exertion
- Exposure to cold
- Tobacco use
- Heavy meals
- Excessive weight
- Some over-the-counter drugs, such as diet pills, nasal decongestants, or drugs that increase heart rate and blood pressure
- Stress or emotion-provoking situations

Aortic Insufficiency (Regurgitation)

Aortic regurgitation is the flow of blood back into the left ventricle from the aorta during diastole. It may be caused by inflammatory lesions that deform the aortic valve leaflets or dilation of the aorta, preventing complete closure of the aortic valve, or it may result from infective or rheumatic endocarditis, congenital abnormalities, diseases such as syphilis, a dissecting aneurysm that causes dilation or tearing of the ascending aorta, blunt chest trauma, or deterioration of a surgically placed aortic valve.

Pathophysiology

In addition to the blood normally delivered by the left atrium, blood from the aorta returns to the left ventricle during diastole. This causes the left ventricle to dilate and eventually hypertrophy, resulting in increases in systolic pressure. Arteries attempt to compensate for the higher pressures by reflex vasodilation; the peripheral arterioles relax, reducing peripheral resistance and diastolic blood pressure.

Clinical Manifestations

- Asymptomatic development in most patients
- Earliest manifestation: increased force of heartbeat—that is, visible or palpable pulsations over the temporal arteries (head) and at the neck (carotid)
- Exertional dyspnea and fatigue
- Signs and symptoms of progressive left ventricular failure (e.g., orthopnea, paroxysmal nocturnal dyspnea)

Assessment and Diagnostic Findings

- High-pitched, blowing diastolic murmur heard best at the third or fourth intercostal space
- Widened pulse pressure
- Water-hammer (Corrigan's) pulse (pulse strikes the palpating finger with quick, sharp strokes and then suddenly collapses)
- Diagnosis confirmation by Doppler echocardiography (preferably 2-D Doppler and transesophageal), radionuclide imaging, ECG, MRI, and cardiac catheterization

Prevention

Prevention and treatment of bacterial infections is key. (See Endocarditis, Rheumatic in Section E.)

Medical Management
- Advise patient to avoid physical exertion, competitive sports, and isometric exercise.
- Treat dysrhythmias and heart failure.

Pharmacologic Therapy
Medications that are usually prescribed first for patients with symptoms of aortic regurgitation are vasodilators such as calcium channel blockers (e.g., felodipine, [Plendil], nifedipine [Adalat, Procardia]), ACE inhibitors (e.g., captopril [Capoten], enalapril [Vasotec], lisinopril [Prinivil, Zestril], and ramipril [Altace]), or hydralazine (Apresoline).

 Quality and Safety Nursing Alert

The calcium channel blockers diltiazem [Cardizem] and verapamil [Calan, Isoptin] are contraindicated for patients with aortic regurgitation as they decrease ventricular contractility and may cause bradycardia.

Surgical Management
The treatment of choice is aortic valve replacement or valvuloplasty, preferably performed before left ventricular failure occurs. Surgery is recommended for any patient with left ventricular hypertrophy, regardless of the presence or absence of symptoms.

Nursing Management
See Perioperative Nursing Management in Section P for additional information.

- Teach patient about wound care, diet, activity, medication, and self-care.
- Instruct patient on importance of antibiotic prophylaxis to prevent endocarditis.
- Reinforce all new information and self-care instructions for 4 to 8 weeks after the procedure.

For more information, see Chapter 28 in Hinkle, J. L., & Cheever, K. H. (2014). *Brunner and Suddarth's textbook of medical-surgical nursing* (13th ed.). Philadelphia: Lippincott Williams & Wilkins.

Aortic Stenosis

Aortic valve stenosis is the narrowing of the orifice between the left ventricle and the aorta. In adults, stenosis often is a result of degenerative calcifications, or it may be a result of rheumatic endocarditis, congenital malformations, or cusp calcification of unknown cause. Progressive narrowing of the valve orifice occurs over a period of several years to several decades.

Risk Factors

Diabetes, hypercholesterolemia, hypertension, and low levels of high-density lipoprotein cholesterol may be risk factors for degenerative changes of the valve. Congenital leaflet malformations or an abnormal number of leaflets (i.e., one or two rather than three) may be involved. Rheumatic endocarditis may also cause structural changes.

Pathophysiology

Progressive narrowing of the valve orifice causes an obstruction to the left ventricle emptying. The ventricular wall thickens in response (i.e., hypertrophies) and, when these compensatory mechanisms of the heart begin to fail, clinical signs and symptoms develop.

Clinical Manifestations

- Exertional dyspnea
- Orthopnea, paroxysmal nocturnal dyspnea (PND), and pulmonary edema
- Dizziness and syncope (fainting)
- Angina pectoris
- Possibly low blood pressure, though usually normal
- Low pulse pressure (30 mm Hg or less)

Assessment and Diagnostic Findings

- Physical examination: loud, rough, systolic murmur heard over the aortic area; vibration over the base of the heart; possible S_4 murmur
- 12-lead electrocardiogram (ECG) and echocardiogram
- Cardiac magnetic resonance (CMR) and computed tomography (CT) scanning
- Left-sided heart catheterization

> ### Quality and Safety Nursing Alert
>
> Graded exercise studies (stress tests) to assess exercise capacity are performed with caution for patients with aortic stenosis because of the high risk of precipitating ventricular tachycardia or fibrillation.

Prevention
Control modifiable risk factors to minimize any proliferative inflammatory responses (e.g., treat diabetes, hypertension, and elevated cholesterol, and stress avoidance of tobacco products).

Medical Management
Medications are prescribed to treat dysrhythmia or left ventricular failure. Patients who are symptomatic and are not surgical candidates may benefit from one- or two-balloon percutaneous valvuloplasty procedures with or without transcatheter aortic valve implantation (TAVI).

Surgical Management
Definitive treatment for aortic stenosis is surgical replacement of the aortic valve. The following procedures are also used:

- Valvuloplasty
- Commissurotomy (open or closed)
- Balloon valvuloplasty
- Annuloplasty
- TAVI
- Valve replacement with mechanical valves, tissue valves, or bioprostheses (heterografts [porcine, bovine, or equine], homografts [human from cadavers], or autografts [patient's own pulmonic valve])

Nursing Management
See Perioperative Nursing Management in Section P for additional information.

For more information, see Chapter 28 in Hinkle, J. L., & Cheever, K. H. (2014). *Brunner and Suddarth's textbook of medical-surgical nursing* (13th ed.). Philadelphia: Lippincott Williams & Wilkins.

Appendicitis

The appendix is a small, finger-like appendage attached to the cecum just below the ileocecal valve. Because it empties into the colon inefficiently and its lumen is small, it is prone to becoming obstructed and is vulnerable to infection (appendicitis). Appendicitis is the most common cause of acute inflammation in the right lower quadrant of the abdominal cavity and the most common cause of emergency abdominal surgery. Although it can occur at any age, it more commonly occurs between the ages of 10 and 30 years.

Pathophysiology

The appendix becomes inflamed and edematous as a result of becoming kinked or occluded by a fecalith (i.e., hardened mass of stool), tumor, lymphoid hyperplasia, or foreign body. Once obstructed, the resulting inflammatory process increases intraluminal pressure, causing pain that is localized to the right lower quadrant within a few hours. The appendix becomes ischemic, bacterial overgrowth occurs, and eventually gangrene can occur.

Clinical Manifestations

- Lower right quadrant pain is usually accompanied by low-grade fever, nausea, and sometimes vomiting; loss of appetite is common; constipation can occur.
- At McBurney's point (located halfway between the umbilicus and the anterior spine of the ilium), local tenderness occurs with pressure and some rigidity of the lower portion of the right rectus muscle.
- Rebound tenderness may be present; location of appendix dictates amount of tenderness, muscle spasm, and occurrence of constipation or diarrhea.
- Rovsing's sign can be elicited by palpating left lower quadrant, which paradoxically causes pain in right lower quadrant.
- Additional positive signs include psoas sign (i.e., pain that occurs on slow extension of the right thigh when patient is lying on the left side) or the obturator sign (i.e., pain that occurs with passive internal rotation of the flexed right thigh with the patient supine).
- If appendix ruptures, pain becomes more diffuse; abdominal distention develops from paralytic ileus, and condition worsens.

Assessment and Diagnostic Findings

- Diagnosis is based on a complete patient history and physical examination and laboratory and imaging tests; patients are usually younger, therefore, age is a crucial differential finding.

- Elevated white blood cell (WBC) count with an elevation of the neutrophils; abdominal radiographs, ultrasound studies, and CT scans may reveal right lower quadrant density or localized distention of the bowel.
- Urinalysis is usually obtained to rule out urinary tract infections; a pregnancy test may be ordered for women of childbearing potential to rule out ectopic pregnancy.

Gerontologic Considerations

In the older adult population, acute appendicitis is uncommon; signs and symptoms of appendicitis may vary greatly. Signs may be very vague and suggestive of bowel obstruction or another process; some patients may experience no symptoms until the appendix ruptures. Older adult patients should have an electrocardiogram and chest x-ray to rule out cardiac ischemia or pneumonia, respectively. The incidence of perforated appendix is higher in the older adult population because many do not seek health care as quickly as do younger people.

Medical Management

- Surgery (laparoscopic is the preferred method) is indicated if appendicitis is diagnosed and should be performed as soon as possible to decrease risk of perforation.
- Conservative, nonsurgical management for uncomplicated appendicitis (i.e., absence of perforation of the appendix, empyema/abscess formation, or fecal peritonitis) has been instituted in some instances with a reduced risk of complications and similar hospital stay; males are at a higher risk of recurrence with this approach.
- Antibiotics and IV fluids are administered until surgery is performed and postoperatively as prescribed.
- Analgesic agents can be given after diagnosis is made.

Complications of Appendectomy

- The major complication is perforation of the appendix, which can lead to peritonitis, abscess formation (collection of purulent material), or portal pylephlebitis.
- Perforation generally occurs 24 hours after the onset of pain. Symptoms include a fever of 37.7°C (100°F) or greater, a toxic appearance, and continued abdominal pain or tenderness. Patients with peritonitis are often found supine and motionless.

Nursing Management

- Nursing goals include relieving pain, preventing fluid volume deficit, reducing anxiety, eliminating infection due to the potential or actual disruption of the GI tract, maintaining skin integrity, and attaining optimal nutrition.
- Preoperatively, prepare patient for surgery, start IV line, administer antibiotic, and insert nasogastric tube (if evidence of paralytic ileus). Do not administer an enema or laxative (which could cause perforation).
- Postoperatively, place the patient in high Fowler's position, give narcotic analgesic as ordered, administer oral fluids when tolerated, give food as desired on day of surgery (if tolerated and bowel sounds are present). If the patient is dehydrated before surgery, administer IV fluids.
- If a drain is left in place at the area of the incision, monitor carefully for signs of intestinal obstruction, secondary hemorrhage, or secondary abscesses (e.g., fever, tachycardia, and increased leukocyte count).

Promoting Home- and Community-Based Care

Educating Patients About Self-Care

- Educate patient and family to care for the wound and perform dressing changes and irrigations as prescribed.
- Reinforce the need for follow-up appointment with surgeon.
- Discuss incision care and activity guidelines (i.e., avoiding heavy lifting until follow-up visit).
- Refer patient for home care nursing as indicated to assist with care and continued monitoring of complications and wound healing.

For more information, see Chapter 48 in Hinkle, J. L., & Cheever, K. H. (2014). *Brunner and Suddarth's textbook of medical-surgical nursing* (13th ed.). Philadelphia: Lippincott Williams & Wilkins.

Arterial Embolism and Arterial Thrombosis

Acute vascular occlusion may be caused by an embolus or acute thrombosis. Arterial emboli arise most commonly from thrombi that develop in the chambers of the heart as a result of atrial fibrillation, myocardial infarction (MI), infective endocarditis, or chronic heart failure. Acute arterial occlusions may result from iatrogenic injury, which can occur during insertion of invasive catheters such as those used for arteriography, percutaneous transluminal coronary angioplasty or stent placement, or an intra-aortic balloon pump. Other causes include IV drug abuse, trauma from a fracture, crush injury, and penetrating wounds that disrupt the arterial intima.

Arterial thrombosis is a slowly developing clot in a degenerated vessel that can itself occlude an artery. Thrombi also become detached and are carried from the left side of the heart into the arterial system, where they cause obstruction. The immediate effect is cessation of distal blood flow. Secondary vasospasm can contribute to ischemia. Emboli tend to lodge at arterial bifurcations and areas of atherosclerotic narrowing (cerebral, mesenteric, renal, and coronary arteries). Acute thrombosis frequently occurs in patients with pre-existing ischemic symptoms.

Clinical Manifestations
Acute arterial emboli symptoms depend primarily on the size of the embolus, the organ involved, and the state of the collateral vessels.

- Symptoms can generally be described as the six "P"s: pain, pallor, pulselessness, paresthesia, poikilothermia (coldness), and paralysis.
- The part of the limb below the occlusion is markedly colder and paler than the part above as a result of ischemia.

Acute thrombotic arterial occlusion symptoms are similar to those described for embolic occlusion. Treatment is more difficult with a thrombus because the arterial occlusion has occurred in a degenerated vessel and requires more extensive reconstructive surgery to restore flow than is required with an embolic event.

Assessment and Diagnostic Findings
- Sudden onset of symptoms and apparent source for the embolus is diagnostic.
- Two-dimensional transthoracic echocardiography or transesophageal echocardiography, chest x-ray, and electrocardiography may reveal underlying cardiac disease.
- Noninvasive duplex and Doppler ultrasonography can determine the presence and extent of underlying atherosclerosis, and arteriography may be performed.

Medical Management
- In cases of acute embolic occlusion, heparin therapy is initiated immediately, followed by minimally invasive

treatment such as emergency embolectomy. Embolectomy is the surgical procedure of choice only if the involved extremity is viable. Endovascular treatment for acute thrombosis uses percutaneous thrombectomy devices, which require inserting a catheter into the obstructed artery, and may also be used.

- When collateral circulation is adequate, IV anticoagulation with heparin is administered. Intra-arterial thrombolytic medications may be administered to dissolve the clot— such as a tissue plasminogen activator (e.g., reteplase) or a urokinase-type plasminogen activator. Contraindications to peripheral thrombolytic therapy include active internal bleeding, cerebrovascular hemorrhage, recent major surgery, uncontrolled hypertension, and pregnancy.

Nursing Management

- Maintain patient on bed rest with the affected extremity level or slightly dependent (15 degrees) before an intervention or surgery.
- Keep the affected part at room temperature and protected from trauma.
- Postoperatively assess for evidence of local (surgical incision) and systemic hemorrhage, including mental status changes.
- Encourage movement of patient's leg to stimulate circulation and prevent stasis.
- Continue anticoagulants to prevent thrombosis of the affected artery and to diminish development of subsequent thrombi.
- If treating with thrombolytic therapy, ensure weight-based dosing and continuous monitoring including vital signs; monitor for bleeding. Minimize punctures when inserting IV lines and obtaining blood samples; avoid IM injections; prevent any possible tissue trauma. Apply pressure at least twice as long as usual after any puncture is performed.
- Assess patient's pulses, Doppler signals, ankle brachial index (ABI), and motor and sensory function every hour for the first 24 hours, because significant changes may indicate re-occlusion.
- Assess patient for complications such as metabolic abnormalities, renal failure, and compartment syndrome.

For more information, see Chapter 30 in Hinkle, J. L., & Cheever, K. H. (2014). *Brunner and Suddarth's textbook of medical-surgical nursing* (13th ed.). Philadelphia: Lippincott Williams & Wilkins.

Arteriosclerosis and Atherosclerosis

Arteriosclerosis, or "hardening of the arteries," is the most common disease of the arteries. It is a diffuse process whereby the muscle fibers and the endothelial lining of the walls of small arteries and arterioles become thickened.

Atherosclerosis primarily affects the intima of the large and medium-sized arteries, causing changes that include the accumulation of lipids (atheromas), calcium, blood components, carbohydrates, and fibrous tissue on the intimal layer of the artery. Although the pathologic processes of arteriosclerosis and atherosclerosis differ, rarely does one occur without the other, and the terms often are used interchangeably. The most common direct results of atherosclerosis in the arteries include narrowing (stenosis) of the lumen and obstruction by thrombosis, aneurysm, ulceration, and rupture; ischemia and necrosis occur if the supply of blood, nutrients, and oxygen is severely and permanently disrupted.

Atherosclerosis can develop anywhere in the body but is most common in bifurcation or branch areas of blood vessels. Atherosclerotic lesions are of two types: fatty streaks (composed of lipids and elongated smooth muscle cells) and fibrous plaques (predominantly found in the abdominal aorta and coronary, popliteal, and internal carotid arteries).

Risk Factors

Many risk factors are associated with atherosclerosis; the greater the number of risk factors, the greater the likelihood of developing the disease.

- The use of tobacco products (strongest risk factor)
- High fat intake (suspected risk factor, along with high serum cholesterol and blood lipid levels)
- Hypertension
- Diabetes
- Obesity, stress, and lack of exercise
- Elevated C-reactive protein

Clinical Manifestations

Clinical features depend on the tissue or organ affected: heart (angina and myocardial infarction due to coronary atherosclerosis), brain (transient ischemic attacks and stroke due to cerebrovascular disease), and peripheral vessels (includes hypertension and symptoms of aneurysm of the aorta, renovascular disease, atherosclerotic lesions of the extremities). See specific condition for greater detail.

Medical Management

The management of atherosclerosis involves modification of risk factors, a controlled exercise program to improve circulation and its functioning capacity, medication therapy, and interventional or surgical graft procedures (inflow or outflow procedures).

Several radiologic techniques are important adjunctive therapies to surgical procedures. They include arteriography, percutaneous transluminal angioplasty, and stents and stent grafts.

For more information, see Chapter 30 in Hinkle, J. L., & Cheever, K. H. (2014). *Brunner and Suddarth's textbook of medical-surgical nursing* (13th ed.). Philadelphia: Lippincott Williams & Wilkins.

Arthritis, Rheumatoid

Rheumatoid arthritis (RA) is an autoimmune disorder that originates in the synovial membrane of the joints. Phagocytosis produces enzymes within the joint. The enzymes break down collagen, causing edema, proliferation of the synovial membrane, and ultimately pannus formation that destroys cartilage and erodes the bone. The consequence is loss of articular surfaces and joint motion. Muscle fibers undergo degenerative changes. Tendon and ligament elasticity and contractile power are lost. RA affects 1% of the population worldwide, affecting women two to four times more often than men.

Clinical Manifestations

Clinical features are determined by the stage and severity of the disease.

- Distal, symmetric joint pain, swelling, warmth, erythema, and lack of function are classic symptoms.
- Palpation of joints reveals spongy or boggy tissue.
- Fluid can usually be aspirated from the inflamed joint.

Characteristic Pattern of Joint Involvement

- RA begins with small joints in hands, wrists, and feet.
- It progressively involves knees, shoulders, hips, elbows, ankles, cervical spine, and temporomandibular joints.
- Symptoms are usually acute in onset, bilateral, and symmetric.
- Joints may be hot, swollen, and painful; joint stiffness often occurs in the morning.
- Deformities of the hands and feet can result from misalignment and immobilization.

Extraarticular Features

- Fever, weight loss, fatigue, anemia, sensory changes, and lymph node enlargement
- Raynaud's phenomenon (cold- and stress-induced vasospasm)
- Rheumatoid nodules, nontender and movable; found in subcutaneous tissue over bony prominences
- Arteritis, neuropathy, pericarditis, splenomegaly, and Sjögren syndrome (dry eyes and mucous membranes)

Assessment and Diagnostic Findings

- Several factors contribute to an RA diagnosis: rheumatoid nodules, joint inflammation detected on palpation, laboratory findings, extra-articular changes.
- Patient history and physical examination focus on manifestations such as bilateral and symmetric stiffness, tenderness, swelling, and temperature changes in the joints.
- Rheumatoid factor is present in about 80% of patients.
- Anti-cyclic citrullinated peptide (anti-CCP antibodies) have a specificity of approximately 95% at detecting rheumatoid arthritis
- Elevated erythrocyte sedimentation rate (ESR) occurs in the acute phases of RA.
- Red blood cell (RBC) count and C4 complement component are decreased.
- C-reactive protein (CRP) and antinuclear antibody (ANA) test results may be positive.
- Arthrocentesis and x-rays may be performed.

Medical Management

Treatment begins with education, a balance of rest and exercise, and referral to community agencies for support.

- Early RA: Medication management involves nonbiologic disease-modifying antirheumatic drugs (DMARDs; methotrexate [Rheumatrex], antimalarial agents, leflunomide [Arava], or sulfasalazine [Azulfidine]) to begin within 3 months of disease onset; research suggests methotrexate with low-dose prednisone has improved outcomes. Biologic DMARD agents include tumor necrosis factor-α (TNF-α), B-cell depleters, T-cell modulators, and interleukins IL-1 and IL-6. For pain and inflammation relief, NSAIDs such as ibuprofen and naproxen are low-cost analgesic medications that can be used, along with COX-2 enzyme blockers.

- Moderate, erosive RA: Use a formal program of occupational and physical therapy. An immunosuppressant such as cyclosporine may be added. Combination therapy involves one nonbiologic DMARD and one biologic DMARD.
- Persistent, erosive RA: Perform reconstructive surgery and low-dose corticosteroids.
- Advanced unremitting RA: Prescribe immunosuppressive agents such as high-dose methotrexate, cyclophosphamide, azathioprine, and leflunomide (highly toxic, can cause bone marrow suppression, anemia, GI tract disturbances, and rashes). Also promising for refractory RA is a Food and Drug Administration–approved apheresis device: a protein A immunoadsorption column (Prosorba) that binds circulating immune system complex (IgG).
- RA patients frequently experience anorexia, weight loss, and anemia, requiring careful dietary history to identify usual eating habits and food preferences. Corticosteroids may stimulate appetite and cause weight gain.
- Low-dose antidepressant medications (amitriptyline) are used to reestablish adequate sleep pattern and manage pain.

Nursing Management
The most common issues for the patient with RA include pain, sleep disturbance, fatigue, altered mood, and limited mobility. The patient with newly diagnosed RA needs information about the disease to make daily self-management decisions and to cope with having a chronic disease.

Relieving Pain and Discomfort
- Provide a variety of comfort measures (e.g., application of heat or cold; massage, position changes, rest; foam mattress, supportive pillow, splints; relaxation techniques, diversional activities).
- Administer anti-inflammatory, analgesic, and slow-acting antirheumatic medications as prescribed.
- Individualize medication schedule to meet patient's need for pain management.
- Encourage verbalization of feelings about pain and chronicity of disease.
- Educate patient in pathophysiology of pain and rheumatic disease, and assist patient to recognize that pain often leads to unproven treatment methods.
- Assist patient in identification of pain that leads to use of unproven methods of treatment.
- Assess for subjective changes in pain.

Reducing Fatigue

- Provide patient with instruction about fatigue: Describe relationship of disease activity to fatigue; describe comfort measures while providing them; develop and encourage a sleep routine (warm bath and relaxation techniques that promote sleep); explain importance of rest for relieving systematic, articular, and emotional stress.
- Explain to patient ways to use energy conservation techniques (pacing, delegating, setting priorities).
- Identify physical and emotional factors that can cause fatigue.
- Facilitate development of appropriate activity/rest schedule.
- Encourage patient's adherence to the treatment program.
- Refer to and encourage a conditioning program.
- Encourage adequate nutrition, including source of iron from food and supplements.

Increasing Mobility

- Encourage verbalization regarding limitations in mobility.
- Assess need for occupational or physical therapy consultation: emphasize range of motion of affected joints; promote use of assistive ambulatory devices; explain use of safe footwear; use individual appropriate positioning/posture.
- Assist patient in identifying environmental barriers.
- Encourage patient's independence in mobility and assist as needed: Allow ample time for activity; provide rest period after activity; reinforce principles of joint protection and work simplification.
- Initiate referral to a community health agency.

Facilitating Self-Care

- Assist patient in identifying self-care deficits and factors that interfere with ability to perform self-care activities.
- Develop a plan based on the patient's perceptions and priorities on ways to establish and achieve goals to meet self-care needs, incorporating joint protection, energy conservation, and work simplification concepts; provide appropriate assistive devices; reinforce correct and safe use of assistive devices; allow patient to control timing of self-care activities; explore with the patient different ways to perform difficult tasks or ways to enlist the help of someone else.
- Consult with community health care agencies when individuals have attained a maximum level of self-care yet still have some deficits, especially regarding safety.

Improving Body Image and Coping Skills

- Help patient identify elements of control over disease symptoms and treatment.
- Encourage patient's verbalization of feelings, perceptions, and fears; help patient to assess present situation and identify problems.
- Identify areas of life affected by disease. Answer questions and dispel possible myths.
- Assist patient in identifying past coping mechanisms. Assist patient in identifying effective coping mechanism.
- Develop a plan for managing symptoms and enlisting support of family and friends to promote daily function.

Monitoring and Managing Potential Complications

- Help patient recognize and deal with side effects from medications.
- Monitor for medication side effects, including GI tract bleeding or irritation, bone marrow suppression, kidney or liver toxicity, increased incidence of infection, mouth sores, rashes, and changes in vision. Other signs and symptoms include bruising, breathing problems, dizziness, jaundice, dark urine, black or bloody stools, diarrhea, nausea and vomiting, and headaches.
- Monitor closely for systemic and local infections, which often can be masked by high doses of corticosteroids.

Promoting Home- and Community-Based Care

Educating Patients About Self-Care

- Focus patient's education on the disease, possible changes related to it, the prescribed therapeutic regimen, side effects of medications, strategies to maintain independence and function, and safety in the home.
- Encourage patient and family to verbalize their concerns and ask questions.
- Address pain, fatigue, and depression before initiating an education program, because they can interfere with patient's ability to learn.
- Instruct patient about basic disease management and necessary adaptations in lifestyle.

Continuing Care

- Refer patient for home care as warranted (e.g., frail patient with significantly limited function).
- Assess patient's home environment and its adequacy for patient safety and management of the disorder.

- Identify any barriers to compliance, and make appropriate referrals.
- For patients at risk for impaired skin integrity, monitor skin status and also instruct, provide, or supervise the patient and family in preventive skin care measures.
- Assess patient's need for assistance in the home, and supervise home health aides.
- Make referrals to physical and occupational therapists as problems are identified and limitations increase.
- Alert patient and family to support services such as Meals on Wheels and local Arthritis Foundation chapters.
- Assess patient's physical and psychological status, adequacy of symptom management, and adherence to the management plan.
- Emphasize the importance of follow-up appointments to patient and family

For more information, see Chapter 39 in Hinkle, J. L., & Cheever, K. H. (2014). *Brunner and Suddarth's textbook of medical-surgical nursing* (13th ed.). Philadelphia: Lippincott Williams & Wilkins.

Asthma

Asthma is a chronic inflammatory disease of the airways causing hyperresponsiveness, mucosal edema, and mucus production. This inflammation ultimately leads to recurrent episodes of asthma symptoms: cough, chest tightness, wheezing, and dyspnea. Patients with asthma may experience symptom-free periods alternating with acute exacerbations that last from minutes to hours or days.

Asthma, the most common chronic disease of childhood, can occur at any age. Risk factors for asthma include family history, allergy (strongest factor), and chronic exposure to airway irritants or allergens (e.g., grass, tree, weed pollens, mold, dust, cockroaches, animal dander). Common triggers for asthma symptoms and exacerbations include airway irritants (e.g., air pollutants, cold, heat, weather changes, strong odors or perfumes, smoke, occupational exposure), foods (e.g., shellfish, nuts), exercise, stress, hormonal factors, medications, viral respiratory tract infections, and gastroesophageal reflux.

Pathophysiology

Asthma is a reversible diffuse airway inflammation that leads to long-term airway narrowing exacerbated by a variety of changes in the airway, including bronchoconstriction, airway edema, airway hyperresponsiveness, and airway remodeling. The interaction of these factors determines the clinical manifestations and severity of asthma. Mast cells, macrophages, T lymphocytes, neutrophils, and eosinophils all play a key role in the inflammation of asthma. When activated, mast cells release chemical mediators. including histamine, bradykinin, prostanoids, cytokines, and leukotrienes. that perpetuate the inflammatory response, causing increased blood flow, vasoconstriction, fluid leak from the vasculature, attraction of white blood cells to the area, mucus secretion, and bronchoconstriction.

Acute exacerbations of asthma cause bronchoconstriction in response due to allergens. An immunoglobulin E–dependent (IgE–dependent) release of mediators (histamine, tryptase, leukotrienes, and prostaglandins) from mast cells contracts the airway. Receptors of the sympathetic nervous system, alpha- and beta-2-adrenergic receptors, are controlled primarily by cyclic 3',5'-adenosine monophosphate (cAMP). The alpha-adrenergic receptors are stimulated, causing bronchoconstriction. The beta-2-adrenergic stimulation results in increased levels of cAMP, which inhibits the release of chemical mediators and causes bronchodilation.

As asthma becomes more persistent, the inflammation progresses, and other factors may be involved in airflow limitation. These include airway edema, mucus hypersecretion, and the formation of mucus plugs. Airway "remodeling" in response to chronic inflammation, causing further airway narrowing, may occur.

Clinical Manifestations

- Most common symptoms of asthma are cough (with or without mucus production), dyspnea, and wheezing (first on expiration, then possibly during inspiration as well).
- Asthma attacks frequently occur at night or in the early morning.
- Asthma exacerbation is frequently preceded by increasing symptoms over days, but it may begin abruptly.
- Chest tightness and dyspnea occur.
- Expiration requires effort and becomes prolonged.
- As exacerbation progresses, diaphoresis, tachycardia, and a widened pulse pressure and central cyanosis secondary to severe hypoxia may occur.

- Exercise-induced asthma symptoms are maximal during exercise, absent at night, and sometimes elicit only a description of a "choking" sensation during exercise.

Assessment and Diagnostic Findings
- Family history, environment, and occupation-related factors are essential.
- Comorbid conditions include gastroesophageal reflux disease, drug-induced asthma, and allergic bronchopulmonary aspergillosis.
- Eczema, rashes, and temporary edema are allergic reactions that may accompany asthma.
- During acute episodes, sputum and blood tests including eosinophil and IgE serum levels (both elevated), pulse oximetry, arterial blood gasses (ABGs) showing hypocapnia and respiratory alkalosis, and pulmonary function tests are performed. Forced expiratory volume in 1 second (FEV1) and forced vital capacity (FVC) are markedly decreased.

Prevention
Evaluation of impairment and testing for possible causes including workplace exposures are key methods to ensure control in patients with recurrent asthma. Work-related asthma should be part of the differential diagnosis of every case of adult-onset asthma. A detailed work history evaluation is key to identifying occupational asthma. Immediate treatment is aimed at removing or decreasing the exposure in the patient's environment and following up with the patient on an ongoing basis. Standard asthma medications may be prescribed to minimize bronchoconstriction and airway inflammation.

Complications
Complications of asthma may include status asthmaticus, respiratory failure, pneumonia, and atelectasis. Acute asthmatic episodes often result in hypoxemia from airway obstruction and dehydration from diaphoresis. Administration of oxygen and monitoring of pulse oximetry, ABGs, and fluids are required.

Medical Management
Immediate intervention may be necessary, because continuing and progressive dyspnea leads to increased anxiety, aggravating the situation. Recommendations are based on the concept of severity and control of asthma along with the domains of impairment and risk as keys to improving care. Primary treatment concerns are impairment of lung function and normal life

and risk of exacerbations, decline in lung function, and adverse effects from medications.

Pharmacologic Therapy

There are two general classes of asthma medications: quick-relief medications for immediate treatment of asthma symptoms and exacerbations and long-acting medications to achieve and maintain control of persistent asthma. Anti-inflammatory medications are regularly used to control persistent asthma and have systemic side effects when used over the long term. The route of choice for administration of these medications is a metered-dose inhaler or other type of inhaler, because it allows for topical administration.

Quick-Relief Medications

For relief of acute symptoms and prevention of exercise-induced asthma, *short-acting beta-2-adrenergic agonists* (albuterol [AccuNeb, Proventil, Ventolin], levalbuterol [Xopenex HFA], and pirbuterol [Maxair]) are used to relax smooth muscle.

Patients who do not tolerate short-acting beta-2-adrenergic agonists may use *anticholinergics* (e.g., ipratropium [Atrovent]) to inhibit muscarinic cholinergic receptors and reduce intrinsic vagal tone of the airway.

Long-Acting Control Medications

Currently, *corticosteroids* are the most potent anti-inflammatory medications effective in alleviating symptoms, improving airway function, and decreasing peak flow variability. Initially, an inhaled form is used with a spacer. Patients should rinse the mouth after administration to prevent thrush. A systemic preparation may be used to gain rapid control of the disease; to manage severe, persistent asthma; to treat moderate to severe exacerbations; to accelerate recovery; and to prevent recurrence.

Cromolyn sodium (Crolom, NasalCrom) and nedocromil (Alocril, Tilade) are mild to moderate anti-inflammatory agents and are considered alternative medications for treatment to stabilize mast cells. These medications prevent exercise-induced asthma and can be used in unavoidable exposure to known triggers on a prophylactic basis; however, they are contraindicated in acute asthma exacerbations.

Long-acting beta-2-adrenergic agonists (LABA) are used with anti-inflammatory medications to control asthma symptoms, especially at night. These agents are also effective in the prevention of exercise-induced asthma; however, they are not indicated for immediate relief of symptoms. Theophylline (Slo-Bid, Theo-Dur) is a mild to moderate bronchodilator used in combination therapy with inhaled corticosteroids for night-time asthma symptoms. For long-term control, Salmeterol (Serevent Diskus) and formoterol (Foradil Aerolizer) have a duration of at least 12 hours for bronchodilation.

Leukotriene modifiers (inhibitors), or *antileukotrienes,* include montelukast (Singulair), zafirlukast (Accolate), and zileuton (Zyflo). Leukotrienes, which are potent bronchoconstrictors that dilate blood vessels and alter permeability, are synthesized from membrane phospholipids through a cascade of enzymes. Leukotriene inhibitors interfere with leukotriene synthesis or block the receptors where leukotrienes exert their action. They are an alternative to inhaled corticosteroids for mild persistent asthma, or they may be added to a regimen of inhaled cortico-steroids in more severe asthma.

Immunomodulators prevent binding of IgE to the high-affinity receptors of basophils and mast cells. Omalizumab (Xolair) is a monoclonal antibody used for patients with allergies and severe persistent asthma.

Management of Exacerbations

The patient with moderate or severe persistent asthma or with a history of severe exacerbations requires education and early treatment with beta-2-adrenergic agonist medications for prompt relief of airflow obstruction. Systemic corticosteroids may be necessary to decrease airway inflammation in patients who fail to respond to inhaled beta-adrenergic medications. Oxygen supplementation may be required to relieve hypox-emia associated with moderate to severe exacerbations and treatment response monitored by serial measurements of lung function.

Antibiotics may be appropriate in the treatment of acute asthma exacerbations in patients with comorbid conditions (e.g., fever and purulent sputum, evidence of pneumonia, sus-pected bacterial sinusitis).

A written asthma action plan based on either symptoms or peak flow measurements helps to educate patients about self-management. The asthma action plan can focus on daily man-agement as well as the recognition and handling of worsening symptoms. Patient self-management and early recognition of problems lead to more efficient communication with health care providers about asthma exacerbations.

Peak Flow Monitoring

Peak flow meters measure the highest airflow during a forced expiration. Daily peak flow monitoring is considered an adjunct to asthma management for patients with moderate to severe persistent asthma. The patient is instructed in the proper technique using maximal PFV monitored for 2 or 3 weeks after receipt of optimal asthma therapy. Then the patient's "personal best" value is measured by zones (green: 80% to 100% of personal best; yellow: 60% to 80%; and red: <60%), with specific actions enabling the patient to monitor and manipulate his or her own therapy after careful instruction. Peak flow monitoring plans may enhance communication between the patient and health care providers and may increase the patient's awareness of disease status and control.

Nursing Management

The immediate nursing care of patients with asthma depends on the severity of symptoms. A calm approach is an important aspect of care for successful treatment both as an outpatient for mild symptoms and as a hospital patient for acute and severe symptoms. The nurse generally performs the following:

- Assesses the patient's respiratory status by monitoring the severity of symptoms, breath sounds, peak flow, pulse oximetry, and vital signs
- Obtains a history of allergic reactions to medications before administering medications
- Identifies medications the patient is currently taking
- Administers medications as prescribed and monitors the patient's responses to those medications, including any antibiotics if the patient has an underlying respiratory infection
- Administers fluids if the patient is dehydrated
- Assists with an intubation procedure, if required, while closely monitoring the patient and keeping the family informed

Promoting Home- and Community-Based Care

Educating Patients About Self-Care

Implementation of basic asthma management strategies includes education of health care providers, establishment of programs for asthma education (for patients and providers), use of outpatient follow-up care for patients, and a focus on chronic management versus acute episodic care. The patient with asthma is educated to formulate a self-care management plan. Nurses are pivotal to achievement of the daily therapy to perform as follows:

- Educate patient and family about asthma (chronic inflammatory), definitions of inflammation and bronchoconstriction, purpose and action of medications, triggers to avoid and ways to do so, and proper inhalation technique.
- Instruct patient and family about peak-flow monitoring.
- Educate patient how to implement an action plan, when to seek assistance, and how to do so.
- Obtain current educational materials for the patient based on the patient's diagnosis, causative factors, educational level, and cultural background and in an alternative format if the patient has a coexisting sensory impairment.

Continuing Care

Serious exacerbations may be prevented when having the nurse:

- Assess the patient's respiratory status and ability to manage self-care in the hospital, clinic, school, or office.
- Emphasize adherence to prescribed therapy, preventive measures, and need for follow-up appointments.
- Make home visits to assess for allergens, if indicated (with recurrent exacerbations).
- Refer patient to community support groups.
- Remind patients and families about the importance of health promotion strategies and recommended health screening.

For more information, see Chapter 24 in Hinkle, J. L., & Cheever, K. H. (2014). *Brunner and Suddarth's textbook of medical-surgical nursing* (13th ed.). Philadelphia: Lippincott Williams & Wilkins.

Asthma: Status Asthmaticus

Asthma exacerbation can range from mild to severe, with potential respiratory arrest. *Status asthmaticus* is used to describe rapid-onset, severe, and persistent asthma that does not respond to conventional therapy; attacks can occur with little or no warning and can progress rapidly to asphyxiation. Infection, anxiety, nebulizer abuse, dehydration, increased adrenergic blockage, and nonspecific irritants may contribute to these episodes. An acute episode may be precipitated by hypersensitivity to aspirin.

Pathophysiology

Status asthmaticus occurs when inflammation of bronchial mucosa, constriction of the bronchiolar smooth muscle, and thickened secretions cause a decrease in the diameter of the bronchi. Severe bronchospasm with mucus plugging leads to asphyxia and ventilation–perfusion abnormality. Initial respiratory alkalosis occurs with a reduced PaO_2, a decreased $PaCO_2$, and an increased pH. As status asthmaticus worsens, the $PaCO_2$ increases. and the pH decreases, reflecting respiratory acidosis.

Clinical Manifestations

- Status asthmaticus is the same as severe asthma: labored breathing, prolonged exhalation, engorged neck veins, and wheezing.
- Extent of wheezing does not indicate the severity of the attack.
- With greater obstruction, wheezing may disappear; this is a sign of impending respiratory failure.

Assessment and Diagnostic Findings

- Assessment includes degree of breathlessness, ability to talk, positioning of patient, level of alertness or cognitive function, respiratory rate, use of accessory muscles, presence of central cyanosis, auscultatory findings, pulse, and pulsus paradoxus.
- Laboratory evaluation includes pulmonary function studies, arterial blood gas (ABG) measurement, and pulse oximetry.
- Respiratory alkalosis is the most common finding

Medical Management

- Initial treatment includes short-acting beta-2-adrenergic agonists, corticosteroids, oxygen therapy, and IV fluids hydration. Sedatives are contraindicated.
- High-flow supplemental oxygen is best delivered using a partial or complete nonrebreathing mask.
- Magnesium sulfate, a calcium antagonist, may be administered to induce smooth-muscle relaxation.
- Hospitalization is required if patient does not respond to repeated treatments, blood gas levels deteriorate, pulmonary function test results are poor, or patient needs mechanical ventilation if in respiratory failure.
- Bronchial thermoplasty, a nondrug therapy, may be used in select patients with uncontrolled severe asthma.

Nursing Management

Nursing management focuses on actively assessing the airway, the patient's response to treatment, and the next intervention if the patient does not respond to treatment.

- Constantly monitor the patient for the first 12 to 24 hours or until severe exacerbation resolves. Blood pressure and cardiac rhythm should be monitored continuously during the acute phase and until the patient stabilizes and responds to therapy.
- Assess the patient's skin turgor for signs of dehydration; fluid intake is essential to combat dehydration, loosen secretions, and facilitate expectoration.
- Administer IV fluids as prescribed, up to 3 to 4 L per day, unless contraindicated.
- Encourage the patient to conserve energy.
- Ensure the patient's room is quiet and free of respiratory irritants (e.g., flowers, tobacco smoke, perfumes, or odors of cleaning agents); nonallergenic pillows should be used.
- Review the patient's medication plan.

For more information, see Chapter 24 in Hinkle, J. L., & Cheever, K. H. (2014). *Brunner and Suddarth's textbook of medical-surgical nursing* (13th ed.). Philadelphia: Lippincott Williams & Wilkins.

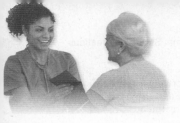

Back Pain, Low

Most low back pain is caused by one of many musculo-skeletal problems, including acute lumbosacral strain, unstable lumbosacral ligaments and weak muscles, intervertebral disk problems, and unequal leg length. Depression, obesity, and stress are frequent co-morbidities. In general, back pain due to musculoskeletal disorders usually is aggravated by activity, whereas pain due to other conditions is not.

🍁 Gerontologic Considerations

Older patients may experience back pain associated with osteo-porotic vertebral fractures, osteoarthritis of the spine, spinal stenosis, and spondylolisthesis, among other conditions.

Pathophysiology

The spinal column can be considered an elastic rod constructed of rigid units (vertebrae) and flexible units (inter-vertebral disks) held together by complex facet joints, multiple ligaments, and paravertebral muscles. Disuse weakens these supporting muscular structures. Intervertebral disks become more dense and irregularly shaped as a person ages, thereby decreasing the cushioning between vertebrae and associated nerve structures. Disk protrusion or facet joint changes can cause pressure on nerve roots as they leave the spinal canal, which results in pain that radiates along the nerve.

Clinical Manifestations

- Acute or chronic back pain (lasting more than 3 months without improvement) and fatigue are seen.
- Pain that radiates down the leg (radiculopathy, sciatica) may occur; presence of this symptom suggests nerve root involvement.
- Gait, spinal mobility, reflexes, leg length, leg motor strength, and sensory perception may be affected.
- Paravertebral muscle spasm (greatly increased muscle tone of back postural muscles) occurs, with loss of normal lumbar curve and possible spinal deformity.

- "Red flag" symptoms that may trigger additional diagnostic studies include suspected spinal infection, severe neurologic weakness, urinary or fecal incontinence, and a new onset of back pain in a patient with cancer.

Assessment and Diagnostic Findings
- Focused health history and physical examination (back examination, gait evaluation, neurologic testing)
- Spinal x-ray
- Bone scan and blood studies
- CT scan
- MRI scan
- Electromyogram (EMG) and nerve conduction studies
- Myelogram
- Ultrasound

Medical Management
Most back pain is self-limited and resolves within 4 weeks with analgesic medications, rest, and avoidance of strain. Management focuses on relief of pain and discomfort, activity modification, and patient education. Bed rest is no longer recommended; normal activities of daily living (ADLs) should be resumed as soon as possible. Other effective nonpharmacologic interventions include the application of superficial heat and spinal manipulation. Cognitive–behavioral therapy (e.g., biofeedback), exercise regimens, physical therapy, acupuncture, massage, and yoga are all effective nonpharmacologic interventions for treating chronic low back pain. Most patients need to alter their activity patterns to avoid aggravating the pain. They should avoid twisting, bending, lifting, and reaching, all of which stress the back; sitting should be limited to intervals of 20 to 50 minutes based on level of comfort. A quick return to normal activities and a program of low-stress aerobic exercise are recommended; conditioning exercises for both back and trunk muscles may begin after 2 weeks to prevent pain recurrence.

Pharmacologic Therapy
- Acute low back pain: nonprescription analgesic agents (e.g., acetaminophen [Tylenol]), nonsteroidal anti-inflammatory drugs (NSAIDs; e.g., ibuprofen [Motrin]), and short-term prescription muscle relaxants (e.g., cyclobenzaprine [Flexeril])
- Chronic low back pain: tricyclic antidepressant agents (e.g., amitriptyline [Elavil]), serotonin–norepinephrine reuptake

B

inhibitors (e.g., duloxetine [Cymbalta]), and atypical seizure medications (gabapentin [Neurontin])
• Opioids for short-term acute moderate to severe pain (e.g., morphine)

Nursing Management

Assessment

• Encourage patient to describe the discomfort (location, severity, duration, characteristics, radiation, weakness in the legs).
• Obtain history of pain origin and previous pain control; assess environmental variables, work situations, and family relationships.
• Observe patient's posture, position changes, and gait.
• Assess spinal curves, height of the iliac crests, leg length discrepancy, and shoulder symmetry.
• Palpate paraspinal muscles and note spasm and tenderness; spasms may resolve when the patient is in the prone position.
• Note discomfort and limitations in movement when patient bends forward and laterally; access the impact of these limitations on performing ADLs.
• Evaluate nerve involvement by assessing deep tendon reflexes, sensations, and muscle strength; back and leg pain on straight-leg raising (with the patient in supine position, the patient's leg is lifted upward with the knee extended) suggests nerve root involvement.
• Assess patient's response to analgesic agents; evaluate and note patient's response to various pain management modalities.

Interventions

• With severe pain, discourage extended periods of inactivity on bed rest.
• Advise patient to rest on a medium to firm, nonsagging mattress.
• Help patient to increase lumbar flexion by elevating the head and thorax 30 degrees using pillows or a foam wedge and slightly flexing the knees supported on a pillow; avoid prone position. Alternatively, the patient can assume a lateral position with knees and hips flexed (curled position) with a pillow between the knees and legs and a pillow supporting the head.
• Educate patient to get out of bed by rolling to one side and placing the legs down while pushing the torso up, keeping the back straight.

- As patient achieves comfort, help patient gradually resume activities and initiate an exercise program; begin with low-stress aerobic exercises. Begin conditioning exercises in coordination with physical therapist; each 30 minute daily exercise period should begin and end with relaxation.
- Encourage patient to adhere to the prescribed exercise program; alternating activities may facilitate adherence to regimen.
- Encourage patient to improve posture and use good body mechanics and to avoid excessive lumbar strain, twisting, or discomfort (e.g., avoid activities such as horseback riding and weight lifting).
- Educate patient regarding how to stand, sit, lie, and lift properly:
  - Shift weight frequently when standing and rest one foot on a low stool; wear low heels.
  - Sit with knees and hips flexed and knees level with hips or higher. Keep feet flat on the floor. Avoid sitting on stools or chairs that do not provide firm back support.
  - Sleep on side with knees and hips flexed or supine with knees flexed and supported; avoid sleeping prone.
  - Lift objects using thigh muscles, not back. Place feet hip-width apart for a wide base of support, bend the knees, tighten the abdominal muscles, and lift the object close to the body with a smooth motion. Avoid twisting and jarring motions.
- Assist patient to resume former role-related responsibilities when appropriate or develop modifications as needed.
- Refer patient to psychotherapy or counseling, if needed.
- If patient is obese, assist with weight reduction through diet modification; note achievement, and provide encouragement and positive reinforcement to facilitate adherence.

For more information, see Chapter 42 in Hinkle, J. L., & Cheever, K. H. (2014). *Brunner and Suddarth's textbook of medical-surgical nursing* (13th ed.). Philadelphia: Lippincott Williams & Wilkins.

Bell's Palsy

Bell's palsy (facial paralysis) is due to unilateral inflammation of the seventh cranial nerve, which results in weakness or paralysis of the facial muscles on the affected side. The cause is unknown, but possible causes may include vascular ischemia, viral disease (e.g., herpes simplex, herpes zoster), autoimmune disease, or a combination. Most patients recover completely, and Bell's palsy rarely recurs.

Pathophysiology

Bell's palsy may represent a type of pressure paralysis in which the inflamed, edematous nerve becomes compressed, resulting in ischemic necrosis of the facial nerve. Both motor and sensory components of the facial nerve may be affected.

Assessment and Diagnostic Findings

- Sudden onset of unilateral paralysis of the facial muscle, including the forehead and lower face
- Unilateral symptoms best assessed by careful examination of the cranial nerves
- Decreased lacrimation and inability to close eyelid properly
- Possibly, disturbances in taste
- Painful sensations in the face, behind the ear, and in the eye
- Possibly, speech difficulties, drooling, and difficulties in eating because of weakness or paralysis of the related facial muscles
- Absence of symptoms of other central nervous system, ear, or cerebellopontine diseases

Medical Management

The objectives of management are to maintain facial muscle tone and to prevent or minimize denervation. Corticosteroid therapy (prednisone) may be initiated to reduce inflammation and edema, which reduces vascular compression and permits restoration of blood circulation to the nerve. Early administration of corticosteroids appears to diminish severity, relieve pain, and minimize denervation. Facial pain is controlled with analgesic agents or heat applied to the involved side of the face. Additional modalities may include electrical stimulation applied to the face to prevent muscle atrophy, or surgical exploration of the facial nerve. Surgery may be performed if a tumor is suspected, for surgical decompression of the facial nerve, and for surgical rehabilitation of a paralyzed face.

Nursing Management

Patients need reassurance that a stroke has not occurred and that spontaneous recovery occurs within 3 to 5 weeks in most patients. Educating patients with Bell's palsy to care for themselves at home is an important nursing priority.

Educating Patients About Eye Care

Because the eye usually does not close completely, the blink reflex is diminished, so the eye is vulnerable to injury from dust and foreign particles. Corneal irritation and ulceration may occur. Distortion of the lower lid alters the proper drainage of tears. Key educational points include the following:

- Cover the eye with a protective shield at night.
- Apply moisturizing eye drops during the day and eye ointment at bedtime to keep eyelids closed during sleep.
- Close the paralyzed eyelid manually before going to sleep.
- Wear wraparound sunglasses or goggles to decrease normal evaporation from the eye.

Educating Patients About Maintaining Facial Muscle Tone

- After the nerve's sensitivity to touch has resolved, demonstrate to the patient how to perform facial massage with gentle upward motion several times daily when the patient can tolerate the massage.
- Demonstrate facial exercises, such as wrinkling the forehead, blowing out the cheeks, and whistling, in an effort to prevent muscle atrophy; encourage the patient to practice with a mirror.
- Instruct patient to avoid exposing the face to cold and drafts.

For more information, see Chapter 69 in Hinkle, J. L., & Cheever, K. H. (2014). *Brunner and Suddarth's textbook of medical-surgical nursing* (13th ed.). Philadelphia: Lippincott Williams & Wilkins.

Benign Prostatic Hyperplasia and Prostatectomy

Benign prostatic hyperplasia (BPH) is a noncancerous enlargement, or hypertrophy, of the prostate gland. It is one of the most common diseases in aging men (older than 40 years) and will affect as many as 90% of men by age 85 years; it is the second most common cause of surgical intervention in men older than 60 years. Smoking, heavy alcohol consumption, obesity, reduced activity level, hypertension, heart disease, diabetes, and a Western diet (high in animal fat and protein and refined carbohydrates, low in fiber) are risk factors for BPH.

B Pathophysiology

The prostate gland enlarges, extending upward into the bladder and obstructing the outflow of urine. Incomplete emptying of the bladder and urinary retention leading to urinary stasis may result in hydronephrosis, hydroureter, and urinary tract infections (UTIs). BPH develops over a prolonged period; changes in the urinary tract are slow and insidious. The cause is not well understood, but evidence suggests hormonal involvement.

Clinical Manifestations

- Symptoms vary, ranging from mild to severe; severity tends to increase with age.
- The prostate is large, rubbery, and nontender on digital rectal exam (DRE). Prostatism (obstructive and irritative symptom complex) is noted.
- Hesitancy in starting urination, increased frequency of urination, nocturia, urgency, and abdominal straining are seen.
- Decrease in volume and force of the urinary stream, interruption of the urinary stream, and dribbling may be present.
- Sensation of incomplete emptying of the bladder, acute urinary retention (more than 50 mL in middle-aged adults, more than 100 mL in older adults), and recurrent UTIs occur; ultimately, azotemia and renal failure result, with chronic urinary retention and large residual volumes.
- Fatigue, anorexia, nausea and vomiting, and pelvic discomfort are also reported.

Assessment and Diagnostic Findings

- Health history should focus on urinary tract, including previous surgical procedures, family history of prostate disease, and general health issues. Voiding diary may be helpful to assess frequency and related symptoms.
- Physical examination, including DRE, is performed.
- Urinalysis is used to screen for hematuria and UTI.
- Prostate-specific antigen (PSA) level is obtained if the patient has at least a 10-year life expectancy and knowledge of the presence of prostate cancer would change management.
- Urinary flow rate recording and the measurement of postvoid residual (PVR) urine are assessed.
- Urodynamic studies, urethrocystoscopy, and ultrasound may be performed.
- Complete blood studies, including clotting studies, are obtained.
- Cardiac status and respiratory function are assessed because of age group.

Medical Management

The treatment plan depends on the cause, severity of symptoms and obstruction, and condition of the patient. Treatment measures include the following:

- Immediate catheterization if patient cannot void (with consultation of a urologist if an ordinary catheter cannot be inserted); suprapubic cystostomy sometimes necessary
- "Watchful waiting" to monitor disease progression

Pharmacologic Management
- Alpha-adrenergic blockers (e.g., alfuzosin [Uroxatral], terazosin [Hytrin], doxazosin [Cardura], tamsulosin [Flomax]) relax the smooth muscle of the bladder neck and prostate.
- Hormonal manipulation with 5-alpha-reductase inhibitor that are antiandrogen agents (finasteride [Proscar] and dutasteride [Avodart]) prevents the conversion of testosterone to dihydrotestosterone (DHT) and decreases the size of the prostate.
- Use of phytotherapeutic agents and other dietary supplements (*Serenoa repens* [saw palmetto berry] and *Pygeum africanum* [African plum]) is not recommended, although they are commonly used. These should not be used with finasteride, dutasteride, or estrogen-containing medications.

Surgical Management
- Minimally invasive therapy: transurethral microwave heat treatment (TUMT; application of heat to prostatic tissue); transurethral needle ablation (TUNA; via thin needles placed in prostate gland); prostatic stents (but only for patients with urinary retention and in patients who are poor surgical risks)
- Surgical resection: transurethral resection of the prostate (TURP; benchmark for surgical treatment); transurethral incision of the prostate (TUIP); transurethral electrovaporization; laser therapy; and open prostatectomy

Nursing Management

See "Nursing Process: The Patient Undergoing Prostatectomy" under Cancer of the Prostate in Section C additional information.

For more information, see Chapter 59 in Hinkle, J. L., & Cheever, K. H. (2014). *Brunner and Suddarth's textbook of medical-surgical nursing* (13th ed.). Philadelphia: Lippincott Williams & Wilkins.

B Bone Tumors

Neoplasms of the musculoskeletal system are of various types, including osteogenic, chondrogenic, fibrogenic, muscle (rhabdomyogenic), and marrow (reticulum) cell tumors as well as nerve, vascular, and fatty cell tumors. They may be primary tumors or metastatic tumors from primary cancers elsewhere in the body (e.g., breast, lung, prostate, kidney). Metastatic bone tumors are more common than primary bone tumors.

Types

Benign Bone Tumors

Benign bone tumors are slow growing, well circumscribed, and encapsulated. They produce few symptoms and do not cause death. Benign primary neoplasms of the musculoskeletal system include osteochondroma, enchondroma, bone cyst (e.g., aneurysmal bone cyst), osteoid osteoma, rhabdomyoma, and fibroma. Benign tumors of the bone and soft tissue are more common than malignant primary bone tumors.

Osteochondroma, the most common benign bone tumor, may become malignant. Osteoid osteoma is a painful tumor that occurs in children and young adults. Enchondroma is a common tumor of the hyaline cartilage of the hand, femur, tibia, or humerus. Osteoclastomas (giant cell tumors) are benign for long periods but may invade local tissue and cause destruction. These tumors may undergo malignant transformation and metastasize. Bone cysts are expanding lesions within the bone (e.g., aneurysmal and unicameral).

Malignant Bone Tumors

Primary malignant musculoskeletal tumors are relatively rare and arise from connective and supportive tissue cells (sarcomas) or bone marrow elements (myelomas). Malignant primary musculoskeletal tumors include osteosarcoma, chondrosarcoma, Ewing's sarcoma, and fibrosarcoma. Soft tissue sarcomas include liposarcoma, fibrosarcoma, and rhabdomyosarcoma. Metastasis to the lungs is common.

- Osteosarcoma is the most common malignant bone tumor and is often fatal with metastasis to the lungs. It is most frequently seen in children, adolescents, and young adults (in bones that grow rapidly); in older people with Paget's disease of the bone; and in persons with a prior history of radiation exposure. Common sites are distal femur, the proximal tibia, and the proximal humerus.

- Chondrosarcoma, the second most common primary malignant bone tumor, is a large, bulky tumor that may grow and metastasize slowly or very rapidly, depending on the characteristics of the tumor cells involved. Tumor sites may include pelvis, femur, humerus, spine, scapula, and tibia. Tumors may recur after treatment.

Metastatic Bone Disease

Metastatic bone disease (secondary bone tumors) is more common than any primary malignant bone tumor. The most common primary sites of tumors that metastasize to bone are the kidney, prostate, lung, breast, ovary, and thyroid. Metastatic tumors most frequently attack the skull, spine, pelvis, femur, and humerus and often involve more than one bone.

Clinical Manifestations

Bone tumors present with a wide range of associated problems:

- Asymptomatic or pain (mild, occasional to constant, severe)
- Varying degrees of disability; at times, obvious bone growth
- Weight loss, malaise, and possible presence of fever
- Spinal metastasis resulting in cord compression and neurologic deficits (e.g., progressive pain, weakness, gait abnormality, paresthesia, paraplegia, urinary retention, loss of bowel or bladder control)

Assessment and Diagnostic Findings

- Assess history and perform a physical examination; may be diagnosed incidentally after pathologic fracture.
- Perform CT scan, bone scans, myelography, MRI, arteriography, and chest x-ray studies.
- Obtain biochemical assays of the blood and urine. (Alkaline phosphatase levels are frequently elevated with osteogenic sarcoma; serum acid phosphatase levels are elevated with metastatic carcinoma of the prostate; hypercalcemia is present with breast, lung, and kidney cancer bone metastases.)
- Perform surgical biopsy for histologic identification; staging based on tumor size, grade, location, and metastasis.

Medical Management

The goal of treatment is to destroy or remove the tumor, accomplished by surgical excision (ranging from local

B

excision to amputation and disarticulation), radiation, or chemotherapy.

- Limb-sparing (salvage) procedures are used to remove the tumor and adjacent tissue; surgical removal of the tumor may, however, require amputation of the affected extremity.
- Chemotherapy is started before and continued after surgery in an effort to eradicate micrometastatic lesions.
- Soft tissue sarcomas are treated with radiation, limb-sparing excision, and adjuvant chemotherapy.
- Advanced metastatic bone cancer treatment is palliative; the therapeutic goal is to relieve pain and discomfort as much as possible while promoting quality of life.
- Internal fixation of pathologic fractures, arthroplasty, or methylmethacrylate (bone cement) minimizes associated disability and pain in metastatic disease.

Nursing Management

- Assess patient's understanding of the disease process and clarify the treatment and prognosis to allay fears.
- Ask patient about the onset and course of symptoms and ways the patient has managed the pain; assess coping behaviors of the patient and family and encourage use of support systems.
- Gently palpate the mass and note its size and associated soft tissue swelling, pain, and tenderness.
- Assess patient's neurovascular status and range of motion of the extremity to provide baseline data for future comparisons; evaluate patient's mobility and ability to perform activities of daily living (ADLs).
- Provide nursing care similar to that of other patients who have had skeletal surgery: Monitor vital signs; assess blood loss; observe and assess for the development of complications such as venous thromboembolism (VTE), pulmonary emboli, infection, contracture, and disuse atrophy; elevate affected part to reduce edema; and assess the neurovascular status of the extremity.
- Educate patient and family about the disease process and diagnostic and management regimens; explain diagnostic tests, treatments (e.g., wound care), and expected results (e.g., decreased range of motion, numbness, change of body contours) to help patient deal with the procedures and changes and comply with the therapeutic regimen.

B

- Assess pain and provide pharmacologic and nonpharmacologic pain management techniques to relieve pain and increase comfort level; work with patient to design the most effective pain management regimen.
- Prepare patient and provide support during painful procedures.
- Administer prescribed IV or epidural analgesics to be used during the early postoperative period; later, oral or transdermal opioid or nonopioid analgesics are indicated to alleviate pain; external radiation or systemic radioisotopes may be prescribed.
- Support and handle the affected extremities gently; provide external supports (e.g., splints) for additional protection.
- Ensure that any prescribed weight-bearing restrictions are followed; with help of physical therapist, educate patient how to use assistive devices safely and how to strengthen unaffected extremities.
- Encourage patient and family to verbalize their fears, concerns, and feelings; refer to psychiatric advanced practice nurse, psychologist, counselor, or spiritual advisor if necessary.
- Assist patient in dealing with changes in body image due to surgery and possible amputation; provide realistic reassurance about the future and resumption of role-related activities and encourage self-care and socialization.
- Encourage patient to be as independent as possible.
- After surgery, frequently reposition patient to reduce skin breakdown and pressure ulcers and provide special therapeutic beds or mattresses to promote wound healing.
- Provide adequate nutrition and hydration to promote healing; administer antiemetics and instruct on relaxation techniques to reduce adverse chemotherapy gastrointestinal effects.
- Monitor for complications of hypercalcemia from bone breakdown. Symptoms include muscular weakness, uncoordination, anorexia, nausea and vomiting, constipation, electrocardiographic changes (e.g., shortened QT interval and ST segment, bradycardia, heart blocks), and altered mental states (e.g., confusion, lethargy, psychotic behavior).
- Emphasize continuing care with home health agency, need for follow-up visits and screening, and referral for hospice if appropriate.

For more information, see Chapter 42 in Hinkle, J. L., & Cheever, K. H. (2014). *Brunner and Suddarth's textbook of medical-surgical nursing* (13th ed.). Philadelphia: Lippincott Williams & Wilkins.

B Bowel Obstruction, Large

Intestinal obstruction (mechanical or functional) occurs when blockage prevents the flow of contents through the intestinal tract. Large bowel obstruction results in an accumulation of intestinal contents, fluid, and gas proximal to the obstruction. Obstruction in the colon can lead to severe distention and perforation unless gas and fluid can flow back through the ileal valve. Dehydration occurs more slowly than in small bowel obstruction. If the blood supply is cut off, intestinal strangulation and necrosis occur; this condition is life threatening. Adenocarcinoid tumors account for the majority of large bowel obstructions.

Clinical Manifestations
Symptoms develop and progress relatively slowly.

- Constipation may be the only symptom for months (obstruction in sigmoid colon or rectum).
- Blood loss may occur in the stool, which may result in iron deficiency anemia.
- The patient may experience weakness, weight loss, and anorexia.
- The abdomen eventually becomes markedly distended, loops of large bowel become visibly outlined through the abdominal wall, and the patient has crampy lower abdominal pain.
- Fecal vomiting develops; symptoms of shock may occur.

Assessment and Diagnostic Findings
Diagnosis is made based on symptoms plus imaging studies (abdominal x-ray and abdominal CT scan or MRI; barium studies are contraindicated). Occasionally, flexible sigmoidoscopy is used to confirm the diagnosis.

Medical Management
- Restoration of intravascular volume, correction of electrolyte abnormalities, and nasogastric aspiration and decompression are instituted immediately.
- Colonoscopy is performed to untwist and decompress the bowel, if obstruction is high in the colon.
- Cecostomy may be performed for patients who are poor surgical risks and who urgently need relief from the obstruction.
- Rectal tube is used to decompress an area that is lower in the bowel.
- Endoscopically placed stents may be used as a palliative intervention or bridge to definitive surgery.

- Usual treatment is surgical resection to remove the obstructing lesion; a temporary or permanent colostomy may be necessary; an ileoanal anastomosis may be performed if entire large bowel must be removed.

Nursing Management
- Monitor symptoms indicating worsening intestinal obstruction.
- Provide emotional support and comfort.
- Administer IV fluids and electrolyte replacement.
- Prepare patient for surgery if no response to medical treatment.
- Provide preoperative education as patient's condition indicates.
- After surgery, provide general abdominal wound care and routine postoperative nursing care.

For more information, see Chapter 48 in Hinkle, J. L., & Cheever, K. H. (2014). *Brunner and Suddarth's textbook of medical-surgical nursing* (13th ed.). Philadelphia: Lippincott Williams & Wilkins.

Bowel Obstruction, Small

Most bowel obstructions occur in the small intestine. Intestinal contents, fluid, and gas accumulate above the intestinal obstruction. Adhesions are the most common cause of small bowel obstruction, followed by hernias and neoplasms. The abdominal distention and retention of fluid reduce the absorption of fluids and stimulate more gastric secretion. With increasing distention, pressure within the intestinal lumen increases, causing a decrease in venous and arteriolar capillary pressure. This causes edema, congestion, necrosis, and eventual rupture or perforation of the intestinal wall, with resultant peritonitis.

Clinical Manifestations
- Initial symptom is usually crampy pain that is wavelike and colicky. Patient may pass blood and mucus but no fecal matter or flatus. Vomiting occurs.
- If the obstruction is complete, peristaltic waves become extremely vigorous and assume a reverse direction, propelling intestinal contents toward the mouth.
- If the obstruction is in the ileum, fecal vomiting takes place.
- Dehydration results in intense thirst, drowsiness, generalized malaise, aching, and a parched tongue and mucous membranes.

B

- Abdomen becomes distended (the lower the obstruction in the gastrointestinal tract, the more marked the distention); this may cause reflux vomiting.
- Vomiting results in loss of hydrogen ions and potassium from the stomach, leading to reduction of chlorides and potassium in the blood and to metabolic alkalosis.
- If uncorrected, hypovolemic shock occurs due to dehydration and loss of plasma volume; septic shock may also occur.

Assessment and Diagnostic Findings

Diagnosis is based on symptoms plus imaging studies (abdominal x-ray and abdominal CT scan revealing abnormal quantities of gas or fluid, or both, in intestines) and laboratory studies (electrolytes and complete blood cell count showing dehydration and possibly infection). The likelihood of strangulation must be assessed.

Medical Management

- Decompression of the bowel may be achieved through a nasogastric (NG) or small bowel tube.
- When the bowel is completely obstructed, the possibility of strangulation warrants surgical intervention.
- Surgical treatment depends on the cause of obstruction (e.g., hernia repair).
- Before surgery, IV therapy is instituted to replace water and correct electrolyte imbalances.

Nursing Management

- For the nonsurgical patient, maintain the function of the NG tube, assess and measure NG output, assess for fluid and electrolyte imbalance, monitor nutritional status, and assess improvement (e.g., return of normal bowel sounds, decreased abdominal distention, subjective improvement in abdominal pain and tenderness, passage of flatus or stool).
- Report discrepancies in intake and output, worsening of pain or abdominal distention, and increased NG output.

> ### Quality and Safety Nursing Alert
>
> Fluid and electrolyte balance are priority areas to monitor in a patient with a small bowel obstruction. The presence of the NG tube in conjunction with a "nothing by mouth" (NPO) status places the patient at substantial risk of imbalance in both these areas. Measures to promote fluid and electrolyte balance are critically important.

- If patient's condition does not improve, prepare him or her for surgery.
- Provide postoperative nursing care similar to that for other abdominal surgeries. (See Perioperative Nursing Management in Section P for additional information.)

For more information, see Chapter 48 in Hinkle, J. L., & Cheever, K. H. (2014). *Brunner and Suddarth's textbook of medical-surgical nursing* (13th ed.). Philadelphia: Lippincott Williams & Wilkins.

Brain Abscess

A brain abscess is a collection of infectious material within the tissue of the brain. Brain abscesses are rare in immunocompetent people; they are more frequently diagnosed in people who are immunosuppressed as a result of an underlying disease or use of immunosuppressive medications.

Pathophysiology

A brain abscess can result from intracranial surgery, penetrating head injury, or tongue piercing. Organisms causing brain abscess may reach the brain by hematologic spread from the lungs, gums, tongue, or heart or from a wound or intra-abdominal infection. The most common predisposing conditions in adults are otitis media and rhinitis.

Prevention

To prevent brain abscess, otitis media, mastoiditis, rhinosinusitis, dental infections, and systemic infections should be treated promptly.

Clinical Manifestations

- Generally, symptoms result from alterations in intracranial dynamics (edema, brain shift), infection, or the location of the abscess.
- Headache, usually worse in morning, is the most prevailing symptom.
- Fever may or may not be present.
- Vomiting and focal neurologic deficits (weakness and decreasing vision) occur as well.
- As the abscess expands, symptoms of increased intracranial pressure (ICP) such as decreasing level of consciousness and seizures are observed.

B

Assessment and Diagnostic Findings
- Complete blood count includes differential, platelet count, erythrocyte sedimentation rate (ESR), and C-reactive protein (CRP).
- Careful neurologic examination may identify changes in ICP.
- Neuroimaging studies such as MRI or CT scanning can identify the size and location of the abscess.
- Aspiration of the abscess is guided by CT or MRI to culture and identify the infectious organism.
- Blood cultures are used prior to antibiotic therapy, chest x-ray, and electroencephalogram (EEG).

Medical Management
The goal is to control ICP and provide targeted antimicrobial therapy to eliminate the abscess and primary source of infection. Treatment modalities include antimicrobial therapy based on culture and sensitivity results, surgical incision, or aspiration (CT-guided stereotactic needle). Corticosteroids may be used to reduce the inflammatory cerebral edema, and antiseizure medications may be prescribed for prophylaxis against seizures (phenytoin, phenobarbital). Abscess resolution is monitored with CT scans.

Nursing Management
Nursing interventions focus on monitoring the neurologic status, supporting the medical treatment, and providing patient education.

- Monitor ongoing neurologic status to assess for changes in ICP.
- Administer intravenous antimicrobial agent.
- Assess and document response to medications.
- Monitor blood laboratory tests (glucose and potassium) when corticosteroids are prescribed.
- Monitor environment to ensure patient safety and prevent falls in cases of decreased level of consciousness, motor weaknesses, or possible seizures.
- Assess needs for patient and family and inform them that neurologic deficits may remain after treatment (hemiparesis, seizures, visual deficits, and cranial nerve palsies).
- Assess the family's ability to express their distress at the patient's condition, cope with the patient's illness and deficits, and obtain support.

See "Nursing Management" under associated neurologic conditions (e.g., Epilepsies, Meningitis, or Increased Intracranial Pressure) for more information.

For more information, see Chapter 69 in Hinkle, J. L., & Cheever, K. H. (2014). *Brunner and Suddarth's textbook of medical-surgical nursing* (13th ed.). Philadelphia: Lippincott Williams & Wilkins.

Brain Tumors

A brain tumor is a localized intracranial lesion that occupies space within the skull. Primary brain tumors originate from cells and structures within the brain. Secondary, or metastatic, brain tumors develop from structures outside the brain (lung, breast, lower gastrointestinal tract, pancreas, kidney, and skin [melanomas]) and occur in 10% to 20% of all cancer patients. The highest incidence of brain tumors in adults occurs between the fifth and seventh decades. Brain tumors rarely metastasize outside the central nervous system but cause death by impairing vital functions (respiration) or by increasing the intracranial pressure (ICP). Brain tumors may be classified into several groups: those arising from the coverings of the brain (e.g., dural meningioma), those developing in or on the cranial nerves (e.g., acoustic neuroma), those originating within brain tissue (e.g., glioma), and metastatic lesions originating elsewhere in the body. Tumors of the pituitary and pineal glands and of cerebral blood vessels are also types of brain tumors. Tumors may be benign or malignant. A benign tumor may occur in a vital area and have effects as serious as a malignant tumor.

Types of Primary Brain Tumors

- Gliomas, the most common brain neoplasms, cannot be totally removed without causing damage, because they spread by infiltrating into the surrounding neural tissue.
- Meningiomas are common benign encapsulated tumors of arachnoid cells on the meninges. They are slow growing and occur most often in middle-aged women.
- An acoustic neuroma is a tumor of the eighth cranial nerve (hearing and balance). It may grow slowly and attain considerable size before it is correctly diagnosed.
- Pituitary adenomas may cause symptoms as a result of pressure on adjacent structures or hormonal changes such as hyperfunction or hypofunction of the pituitary.

B

- Angiomas are masses composed largely of abnormal blood vessels and are found in or on the surface of the brain; they may never cause symptoms, or they may give rise to symptoms of brain tumor. The walls of the blood vessels in angiomas are thin, increasing the risk for hemorrhagic stroke.

Clinical Manifestations

Increased Intracranial Pressure

- Headache, although not always present, is most common in the early morning and is made worse by coughing, straining, or sudden movement. Headaches are usually described as deep, expanding, or dull but unrelenting. Frontal tumors produce a bilateral frontal headache; pituitary gland tumors produce bitemporal pain; in cerebellar tumors, the headache may be located in the suboccipital region at the back of the head.
- Vomiting, seldom related to food intake, is usually due to irritation of the vagal centers in the medulla.
- Papilledema (edema of the optic nerve) is associated with visual disturbances such as diplopia.
- Seizures may be partial or generalized; tumors of the frontal, parietal and temporal lobes carry the greatest risk for seizures.
- Personality changes and a variety of focal deficits, including motor, sensory, and cranial nerve dysfunction, are common.

Localized Symptoms

The progression of the signs and symptoms is important because it indicates tumor growth and expansion. Many tumors can be localized by correlating the signs and symptoms to specific areas in the brain, as follows:

- Motor cortex tumor: hemiparesis and partial seizures on the opposite side of the body or generalized seizures
- Occipital lobe tumors: visual manifestations, such as contralateral homonymous hemianopsia (visual loss in half of the visual field on the opposite side of tumor) and visual hallucinations
- Cerebellar tumor: dizziness; an ataxic or staggering gait, with tendency to fall toward side of lesion; marked muscle incoordination; and nystagmus

B

- Frontal lobe tumor: changes in emotional state and behavior and an apathetic mental attitude. The patient often becomes extremely untidy and careless and may use obscene language
- Parietal lobe tumor: possibly decreased sensation on the opposite side of the body and sensory or generalized seizures
- Cerebellopontine angle tumor: usually originates in sheath of acoustic nerve; tinnitus and vertigo, then progressive nerve deafness (eighth cranial nerve dysfunction); staggering gait, numbness and tingling of the face and tongue, progressing to weakness and paralysis of the face; potential for abnormalities in motor function
- Brain stem tumors: may be associated with cranial nerve deficits and complex motor and sensory function

Assessment and Diagnostic Findings
- History of the illness and manner in which symptoms evolved
- Neurologic examination indicating areas involved
- CT, MRI, positron emission tomography (PET), computer-assisted stereotactic (three-dimensional) biopsy, cerebral angiography, electroencephalography (EEG), and cytologic studies of the cerebrospinal fluid

Medical Management
A variety of medical treatments, including chemotherapy and external-beam radiation therapy, are used alone or in combination with surgical resection.

Surgical Management
The objective of surgical management is to remove or destroy the entire tumor without increasing the neurologic deficit (paralysis, blindness) or to relieve symptoms by partial removal (decompression). A variety of surgical approaches may be used; the specific approach depends on the type of tumor, its location, and its accessibility. In many patients, combinations of these modalities are used.

Other Therapies
- Radiation therapy (the cornerstone of treatment for many brain tumors)
- Brachytherapy (the surgical implantation of radiation sources to deliver high doses at a short distance)
- Stereotactic procedures (linear accelerator or gamma knife to perform radiosurgery)

B

- Possibly, chemotherapy in conjunction with radiation or as the sole therapy
- IV autologous bone marrow transplantation for marrow toxicity associated with high doses of drugs and radiation
- Gene-transfer therapy (currently being tested)
- Pharmacologic therapy (corticosteroids, osmotic diuretics, antiseizure medications)

Nursing Management

- Assess for headache characteristics.
- Evaluate effectiveness of pain management interventions.
- Educate patient and family about the possibility of seizure and the need to adhere to prophylactic seizure medications if prescribed.
- Consider providing medications to alleviate nausea and prevent vomiting.
- Evaluate gag reflex and ability to swallow preoperatively.
- Educate patient to direct food and fluids toward the unaffected side. Assist patient to an upright position to eat, offer a semisoft diet, and have suction readily available if gag response is diminished.
- Administer corticosteroids to control headache and neurologic symptoms. Assess for corticosteroid adverse effects, including hyperglycemia, electrolyte abnormalities, and muscle weakness.
- Perform neurologic checks, monitor vital signs, and maintain a neurologic flowchart. Space nursing interventions to prevent rapid increase in ICP.
- Reorient patient when necessary to person, time, and place. Use orienting devices (personal possessions, photographs, lists, clock).
- Supervise and assist with self-care. Monitor and intervene to prevent injury.
- Monitor patients with seizures.
- Check motor function at intervals; assess sensory disturbances.
- Evaluate speech and educate patients with speech deficits to use alternative forms of communication
- Assess eye movement, pupil size, and reaction.
- Educate patient regarding ways to conserve energy and promote rest.

For more information, see Chapter 70 in Hinkle, J. L., & Cheever, K. H. (2014). *Brunner and Suddarth's textbook of medical-surgical nursing* (13th ed.). Philadelphia: Lippincott Williams & Wilkins.

Bronchiectasis

Bronchiectasis is a chronic, irreversible dilation of the bronchi and bronchioles and is considered a disease process separate from chronic obstructive pulmonary disease (COPD). The result is retention of secretions, obstruction, and eventual alveolar collapse. Bronchiectasis may be caused by a variety of conditions, including airway obstruction, diffuse airway injury, pulmonary infections and obstruction of the bronchus or complications of long-term pulmonary infections, genetic disorders (e.g., cystic fibrosis), abnormal host defense (e.g., ciliary dyskinesia or humoral immunodeficiency), and idiopathic causes. Bronchiectasis is usually localized, affecting a segment or lobe of a lung, most frequently the lower lobes. People may be predisposed to bronchiectasis as a result of recurrent respiratory infections in early childhood, measles, influenza, tuberculosis, or immunodeficiency disorders. Average age at death is approximately 55 years.

Clinical Manifestations
- Chronic cough and production of copious purulent sputum
- Hemoptysis, clubbing of the fingers, and repeated episodes of pulmonary infection

Assessment and Diagnostic Findings
- A definite diagnostic clue is prolonged history of productive cough, with sputum consistently negative for tubercle bacilli.
- Diagnosis is established by bronchial dilatation on CT scan.

Medical Management
- Treatment objectives are to promote bronchial drainage to clear excessive secretions from the affected portion of the lungs and to prevent or control infection.
- The treatment plan includes chest physiotherapy with percussion, postural drainage, expectorants, or bronchoscopy to remove bronchial secretions.
- Antimicrobial therapy is guided by sputum sensitivity studies.
- Antimicrobial therapy may be a year-round regimen of antibiotics, alternating types of drugs or intermittent regimens (e.g., during winter or when upper respiratory infections are present).
- Vaccination against influenza and pneumococcal pneumonia are highly recommended.
- Bronchodilators may be required.
- Smoking cessation is essential.

Surgical Management
- Surgical intervention (segmental resection of lobe or lung removal) is used infrequently.
- In preparation for surgery, ensure vigorous postural drainage, suction through bronchoscope, and administer antibacterial therapy.

Nursing Management
See "Nursing Management" under Chronic Obstructive Pulmonary Disease in Section C, as well as Perioperative Nursing Management in Section P, for additional information.

For more information, see Chapter 24 in Hinkle, J. L., & Cheever, K. H. (2014). *Brunner and Suddarth's textbook of medical-surgical nursing* (13th ed.). Philadelphia: Lippincott Williams & Wilkins.

Burn Injury

Burn injury is caused by heat transfer from a heat source to the body, exposure to a chemical, or radiation exposure.

Pathophysiology
The depth of the burn injury depends on the physical or chemical characteristics of the burning agent and the duration of contact with it. The burn wound is not homogenous; rather, tissue necrosis occurs at the center of the injury with regions of tissue viability toward the periphery. The skin and the mucosa of the upper airways are the most common sites of tissue destruction. Burns disrupt the skin, which leads to increased fluid loss; infection; hypothermia; scarring; compromised immunity; and changes in function, appearance, and body image. Young children and older adults continue to have increased morbidity and mortality as compared to individuals in other age groups with similar injuries. Inhalation injuries in addition to cutaneous burns worsen the prognosis. Burns are categorized by severity (e.g., major, minor), type (e.g., thermal, chemical, radiation), depth of tissue destruction (degree), and breadth (extent of body surface area burned).

Burn Depth and Breadth

Depth
The depth of a burn injury depends on the type of injury, causative agent, temperature of the burn agent, duration of contact

with the agent, and the skin thickness. Burns are classified according to the depth of tissue destruction:

- Superficial partial-thickness burns (similar to first-degree), such as sunburn: The epidermis and possibly a portion of the dermis are destroyed.
- Deep partial-thickness burns (similar to second-degree), such as a scald: The epidermis and upper to deeper portions of the dermis are injured.
- Full-thickness burns (third-degree), such as a burn from a flame or electric current: The epidermis, entire dermis, and sometimes the underlying tissue, muscle, and bone are destroyed.

Breadth: Extent of Body Surface Area Burned

How much total body surface area is burned is determined by one of the following methods:

- Rule of nines: an estimation of the total body surface area burned by assigning percentages in multiples of nine to major body surfaces
- Lund and Browder method: a more precise method of estimating the extent of the burn; takes into account that the percentage of the surface area represented by various anatomic parts (head and legs) changes with growth
- Palm method: used to estimate percentage of scattered burns, using the size of the patient's palm (about 1% of body surface area) to assess the extent of burn injury

🍂 Gerontologic Considerations

Older adults are at higher risk for burn injury because of reduced coordination and declines in cognitive ability, strength, sensation, and vision. Fire or flame is the most common etiology of burns in the older adult; mortality increases between the ages of 60 and 80 years as compared to younger adults. Predisposing factors and the health history in the older adult influence the complexity of care for the patient. Pulmonary function is limited in the older adult and therefore airway exchange, lung elasticity, and ventilation can be affected. This can be further affected by a history of smoking. Decreased cardiac function and coronary artery disease increase the risk of complications in older patients with burn injuries; decreases in renal and hepatic function can impact metabolism of medications. Malnutrition and presence of diabetes or other

B

endocrine disorders present nutritional challenges and require close monitoring. Varying degrees of orientation may present themselves on admission or through the course of care, making assessment of pain and anxiety a challenge for the burn team. The skin of the older adult is thinner and less elastic, which affects the depth of injury and its ability to heal.

> **Quality and Safety Nursing Alert**

Education on the prevention of burn injury is especially important among older adults. Assess an older patient's ability to safely perform activities of daily living (ADLs), assist older patients and families to modify their environment to ensure safety, and make referrals as needed.

Clinical Manifestations
The clinical manifestations vary with the depth, degree, location, and mechanism of the injury.

- First-degree (superficial) burns: tingling, hyperesthesia, pain soothed by cooling, erythematous areas that blanche with pressure, minimal or no edema, possible blisters, peeling, itching
- Second-degree (partial-thickness) burns: pain; hyperesthesia; sensitive to air currents; blistered, mottled red base; disrupted epidermis; weeping surface; edema
- Third-degree (full-thickness) burns: numbness (insensate); shock; myoglobinuria; possible hemolysis; possible contact points may be visible (e.g., entrance or exit wounds in electrical burns); skin that is pale white, red brown, leathery or charred; coagulated vessels may be visible; edema
- Fourth-degree (full-thickness that includes fat, fascia, muscle and/or bone) burns: shock, myoglobinuria, possible hemolysis, charred skin

Other symptoms associated with a major burn include:

- Hemodynamic instability from loss of capillary integrity
- Subsequent shift of protein and sodium from intravascular space to interstitial space, leading to hypovolemic shock
- Impaired organ perfusion
- Sepsis, acute respiratory distress syndrome, ileus, and renal failure
- Coagulation abnormalities

Inhalation injury may be recognized by the following symptoms and signs:

- Presence of burns to face and neck, singed nasal hair, or soot around the external nares
- Hoarseness, high-pitched voice change, stridor
- Soot in sputum, dyspnea or tachypnea
- Erythema of oral or pharyngeal mucosa
- Pulse oximetry readings possibly inaccurate with high levels of carboxyhemoglobin from carbon monoxide poisoning associated with the fire.

Prevention
Nurses in community and home settings can provide education on the prevention of burn injury, especially among older adults and children.

For Older Adults
- Alcohol significantly impairs judgment and ability; smoking in bed while intoxicated is a common cause of fires.
- Cognitive and sensory impairments may decrease reaction time in recognizing fire and may delay escape; limitations in mobility may also delay escape from a fire.

For Children
- Advise that matches and lighters be kept out of the reach of children.
- Emphasize the importance of never leaving children unattended around fire.
- Recommend the development and practice of a home exit fire drill with all members of the household.
- Advise that hot irons and curling irons be kept out of the reach of children.
- Recommend caution in situations where children have access to very hot water, such as in bathtubs and faucets; the temperature of a hot water heater should be set lower than 120 degrees.
- Warn that pots or tea kettles should never be left unattended on the stove.

Medical Management
The major goals relating to burn management are prevention, rapid assessment of severity of burn, institution of life-saving measures for the severely burned person, prevention of disability and disfigurement, and rehabilitation.

B NURSING PROCESS

The Emergent or Resuscitative Phase

Assessment

- Focus on the major priorities of any trauma patient (airway, breathing, and circulation); the burn wound is a secondary consideration, although aseptic management of the burn wounds and invasive lines continues.
- Assess circumstances surrounding the injury: time of injury, mechanism of burn, whether the burn occurred in a closed space, the possibility of inhalation of noxious chemicals, and any related trauma.
- Monitor vital signs frequently, including temperature; evaluate apical, carotid, and femoral pulses, particularly in areas of circumferential burn injury to an extremity.
- Assess breath sounds and respiratory rate, rhythm, depth, and symmetry; monitor for hypoxia.
- Observe for signs of inhalation injury: blistering of lips or buccal mucosa; singed nostrils; burns of face, neck, or chest; increasing hoarseness; or soot in sputum or respiratory secretions.
- Assess cardiac rhythm if indicated (e.g., initially and if there is a history of cardiac or respiratory problems, electrical injury).
- Check peripheral pulses on burned extremities hourly; use Doppler as needed.
- Assess adequacy of fluid intake (IV fluids) based on degree of body surface burned and output (urinary catheter) and measure hourly. Note amount of urine obtained when catheter is inserted (indicates preburn renal function and fluid status).
- Assess body temperature, body weight, history of preburn weight, allergies, tetanus immunization, past medical-surgical problems, current illnesses, and use of medications.
- Arrange for patients with facial burns to be assessed for corneal injury and possible airway injury.
- Continue to assess the extent of the burn; assess depth of wound and identify areas of full- and partial-thickness injury.
- Assess neurologic status: consciousness, psychological status, pain and anxiety levels, and behavior.
- Assess the patient's and family's understanding of injury and treatment. Assess patient's support system and coping skills.

Diagnosis

NURSING DIAGNOSES

- Impaired gas exchange related to carbon monoxide poisoning, smoke inhalation, and upper airway obstruction
- Ineffective airway clearance related to edema and effects of smoke inhalation
- Impaired hemodynamic function due to edema and fluid shifts
- Deficient fluid volume related to increased capillary permeability and evaporative losses from the burn wound
- Hypothermia related to loss of skin microcirculation and open wounds
- Increased risk of infection due to disruption of skin integrity
- Acute pain related to tissue and nerve injury
- Anxiety related to fear and the emotional impact of burn injury

COLLABORATIVE PROBLEMS/POTENTIAL COMPLICATIONS

Other possible complications include acute respiratory failure, distributive shock, acute renal failure, compartment syndrome, paralytic ileus, and Curling's ulcer.

Nursing Interventions

PROMOTING GAS EXCHANGE AND AIRWAY CLEARANCE

- Provide humidified oxygen, and monitor arterial blood gases (ABGs), pulse oximetry, and carboxyhemoglobin levels.

> **Quality and Safety Nursing Alert**
>
> Standard pulse oximetry monitors are not reliable to assess hypoxia when significant levels of carboxyhemoglobin are present in the blood, owing to carbon monoxide (CO) toxicity. CO toxicity is a common finding in patients burned in a fire.

- Report labored respirations, decreased depth of respirations, or signs of hypoxia to physician immediately; prepare to assist with intubation.
- Monitor mechanically ventilated patient closely.
- Institute aggressive pulmonary care measures: turning, coughing, deep breathing, periodic forceful inspiration using spirometry, and tracheal suctioning.

B

- Maintain proper positioning to promote removal of secretions and patent airway and to promote optimal chest expansion; use artificial airway as needed.
- Elevate the head of the bed to improve ventilation and lessen the effects of edema.

PROMOTING ADEQUATE HEMODYNAMIC FUNCTION
- Institute electrocardiographic monitoring based on results of initial assessment
- Provide frequent assessments of hemodynamic indices (e.g., pulmonary artery wedge pressure [PAWP], central venous pressure [CVP], arterial pressure) if invasive monitoring is indicated.
- Apply clean dressing underneath blood pressure cuff to protect burned area from contamination; remove cuff after each reading.
- A Doppler (ultrasound) device or a noninvasive electronic blood pressure device may be helpful if blood pressure cannot be obtained owing to edema.
- Assess peripheral pulse distal to the burn frequently.
- Elevate the burned extremity above the level of the heart to decrease edema.

RESTORING FLUID AND ELECTROLYTE BALANCE
- Monitor vital signs and urinary output (hourly), CVP, pulmonary artery pressure, and cardiac output. Note and report signs of hypovolemia or fluid overload.
- Maintain IV lines and regular fluids at appropriate rates, as prescribed. Document intake and output and daily weight.
- Elevate the head of bed and burned extremities.
- Monitor serum electrolyte levels (e.g., sodium, potassium, calcium, phosphorus, bicarbonate); recognize developing electrolyte imbalances.
- Notify physician immediately of decreased urine output; blood pressure; CVP or PAWP; or increased pulse rate.

MAINTAINING NORMAL BODY TEMPERATURE
- Provide warm environment: use heat shield, space blanket, heat lights, or blankets.
- Assess core body temperature frequently.
- Work quickly when wounds must be exposed, to minimize heat loss from the wound.

PREVENTING INFECTION

- Place clean sheets under and over patient to protect wound from contamination, maintain body temperature, and reduce pain on burned tissue caused by air currents.
- Maintain strict aseptic technique to prevent introducing pathogens via invasive procedures; use clean technique for wound care procedures.

MINIMIZING PAIN AND ANXIETY

- Use a pain scale to assess pain level (i.e., 1 to 10); differentiate between restlessness due to pain and restlessness due to hypoxia.
- Administer IV opioid analgesics as prescribed, and assess response to medication; observe for respiratory depression in patients who are not mechanically ventilated.
- Provide emotional support, reassurance, and simple explanations about procedures.
- Assess patient and family understanding of burn injury, coping strategies, family dynamics, and anxiety levels. Provide individualized responses to support patient and family coping; explain all procedures in clear, simple terms.
- Provide pain relief, and give antianxiety medications if patient remains highly anxious and agitated after psychological interventions.

MONITORING AND MANAGING POTENTIAL COMPLICATIONS

- Acute respiratory failure: Assess for increasing dyspnea, stridor, changes in respiratory patterns; monitor pulse oximetry and ABG values to detect problematic oxygen saturation and increasing CO_2; monitor chest x-rays; assess for cerebral hypoxia (e.g., restlessness, confusion); report deteriorating respiratory status immediately to physician; and assist as needed with intubation or escharotomy.
- Distributive shock: Monitor for early signs of shock (decreased urine output, cardiac output, pulmonary artery pressure, pulmonary capillary wedge pressure, blood pressure, or increasing pulse) or progressive edema. Administer fluid resuscitation as ordered in response to physical findings; continue monitoring fluid status.
- Acute renal failure: Monitor and report abnormal urine output and quality and blood urea nitrogen (BUN) and creatinine levels; assess for urine hemoglobin or myoglobin; administer increased fluids as prescribed.

B

- Compartment syndrome: Assess peripheral pulses hourly with Doppler; assess neurovascular status of extremities hourly (warmth, capillary refill, sensation, and movement); remove blood pressure cuff after each reading; elevate burned extremities; report any extremity pain and loss of peripheral pulses or sensation; prepare to assist with escharotomies.
- Paralytic ileus: Maintain nasogastric tube on low intermittent suction until bowel sounds resume; auscultate abdomen regularly for distention and bowel sounds.
- Curling's ulcer: Assess gastric aspirate for blood and pH; assess stools for occult blood; administer antacid medications and histamine blockers (e.g., ranitidine [Zantac]) as prescribed.

NURSING PROCESS

The Acute or Intermediate Phase

The acute or intermediate phase begins 48 to 72 hours after the burn injury. Infection prevention, burn wound care, pain management, nutritional support, and early positioning and mobility are priorities at this stage.

Assessment

- Focus on hemodynamic alterations, wound healing, pain and psychosocial responses, and early detection of complications.
- Measure vital signs frequently; respiratory and fluid status remain highest priority.
- For first few days after the burn, assess peripheral pulses frequently for restricted blood flow.
- Closely observe hourly fluid intake and urinary output, as well as blood pressure and cardiac rhythm; changes should be reported to the burn surgeon promptly.
- For patients with inhalation injury, regularly monitor level of consciousness, pulmonary function, and ability to ventilate; if patient is intubated and placed on a ventilator, frequent suctioning and assessment of the airway are priorities.
- Monitor ABGs and carboxyhemoglobin levels.

Diagnosis

NURSING DIAGNOSES

Refer to the Nursing Diagnoses section above in Nursing Process: The Emergent or Resuscitative Phase.

Nursing Interventions

RESTORING NORMAL FLUID BALANCE

- Monitor IV and oral fluid intake; use IV infusion pumps.
- Measure intake and output and daily weight.
- Report changes (e.g., blood pressure, pulse rate) to physician.

PROMOTING GAS EXCHANGE AND AIRWAY CLEARANCE

- Monitor respiratory rate and effort.
- Elevate the head of the bed to improve ventilation and lessen the effects of edema.
- If patient is intubated due to an inhalation injury, implement strategies to prevent ventilator-associated pneumonia.

PREVENTING INFECTION

- Provide a clean and safe environment; protect patient from sources of cross-contamination (e.g., visitors, other patients, staff, equipment).
- Closely scrutinize wound to detect early signs of infection. Monitor culture results and white blood cell counts.
- Practice clean technique for wound care procedures and aseptic technique for any invasive procedures. Use meticulous hand hygiene before and after contact with patient.
- Caution patient to avoid touching wounds or dressings; wash unburned areas and change linens regularly.
- Assess temperature regularly. Hyperthermia is common in severe burns; however, increases in core temperature may also be due to bacteremia or septicemia.

MAINTAINING ADEQUATE NUTRITION

- Initiate oral fluids slowly when bowel sounds resume: Record tolerance; if vomiting and distention do not occur, fluids may be increased gradually and the patient may be advanced to a normal diet or to tube feedings.
- Collaborate with dietitian to plan a protein- and calorie-rich diet acceptable to patient. Encourage family to bring the patient's favorite nutritious foods. Provide nutritional and vitamin and mineral supplements if prescribed.
- Document caloric intake. Insert feeding tube if caloric goals cannot be met by oral feeding (for continuous or bolus feedings); note residual volumes.
- Weigh patient daily and graph weights.

PROMOTING SKIN INTEGRITY

- Assess wound status.
- Support patient during distressing and painful wound care.

B

- Coordinate complex aspects of wound care and dressing changes.
- Assess burn for size, color, odor, eschar, exudate, epithelial buds (small pearllike clusters of cells on the wound surface), bleeding, granulation tissue, the status of graft take, healing of the donor site, and the condition of the surrounding skin; report any significant changes to the physician.
- Inform all members of the health care team of latest wound care procedures in use for the patient.
- Assist, instruct, support, and encourage patient and family to take part in dressing changes and wound care.
- Early on, assess strengths of patient and family in preparing for discharge and home care.

RELIEVING PAIN AND DISCOMFORT

- Frequently assess pain and discomfort; administer analgesic and anxiolytic medications, as prescribed, before the pain becomes severe. Assess and document the patient's response to medication and any other interventions.
- Encourage patient to use analgesic medications prior to painful procedures.
- Educate patient regarding relaxation techniques. Give some control over wound care and analgesia. Provide frequent reassurance.
- Use guided imagery and distraction to alter patient's perceptions and responses to pain; hypnosis, music therapy, and virtual reality are also useful.
- Assess the patient's sleep patterns daily; administer sedatives, if prescribed.
- Work quickly to complete treatments and dressing changes.
- Promote comfort during healing phase with the following: oral antipruritic agents, a cool environment, frequent lubrication of the skin with water or a silica-based lotion, exercise and splinting to prevent skin contracture, and diversional activities.

PROMOTING PHYSICAL MOBILITY

- Prevent complications of immobility (e.g., atelectasis, pneumonia, edema, pressure ulcers, and contractures) by deep breathing, turning, and proper repositioning.
- Modify interventions to meet patient's needs. Encourage early sitting and ambulation. When legs are involved, apply elastic pressure bandages before assisting patient to upright position.

- Make aggressive efforts to prevent contractures and hypertrophic scarring of the wound area after wound closure for a year or more.
- Initiate passive and active range of motion exercises from admission until after grafting, within prescribed limitations.
- Encourage active range of motion during bathing.
- Apply splints or functional devices to extremities for contracture control; monitor for signs of vascular insufficiency, nerve compression, and skin breakdown.
- Anticipate the necessity of venous thromboembolism (VTE) prophylaxis.

STRENGTHENING COPING STRATEGIES
- Assist patient to develop effective coping strategies: Set specific expectations for behavior, promote truthful communication to build trust, help patient practice coping strategies, and give positive reinforcement when appropriate.
- Demonstrate acceptance of patient. Enlist a noninvolved person to whom patient can vent feelings without fear of retaliation.
- Include patient in decisions regarding care. Encourage patient to assert individuality and preferences. Set realistic expectations for self-care.

SUPPORTING PATIENT AND FAMILY PROCESSES
- Support and address the verbal and nonverbal concerns of the patient and family.
- Instruct family in ways to support patient.
- Make psychological or social work referrals as needed.
- Provide information about burn care and expected course of treatment.
- Initiate patient and family education during burn management. Assess and consider preferred learning styles; assess ability to grasp and cope with the information; determine barriers to learning when planning and executing education.
- Remain sensitive to the possibility of changing family dynamics.

MONITORING AND MANAGING POTENTIAL COMPLICATIONS
- Heart failure: Assess for fluid overload, decreased cardiac output, oliguria, jugular vein distention, edema, or onset of S_3 or S_4 heart sounds.

B

- Pulmonary edema: Assess for increasing CVP, pulmonary artery and wedge pressures, and crackles; report promptly. Position comfortably with the head of bed elevated unless contraindicated. Administer medications and oxygen as prescribed and assess response.
- Sepsis: Assess for increased temperature, increased pulse, widened pulse pressure, and flushed, dry skin in unburned areas (early signs), and note trends in the data. Perform wound and blood cultures as prescribed. Give scheduled antibiotic agents on time.
- Acute respiratory failure and acute respiratory distress syndrome (ARDS): Monitor respiratory status for dyspnea, change in respiratory pattern, and onset of adventitious sounds. Assess for decrease in tidal volume and lung compliance in patients on mechanical ventilation. The hallmark of onset of ARDS is hypoxemia on 100% oxygen, decreased lung compliance, and significant shunting; notify physician of deteriorating respiratory status.
- Visceral damage (from electrical burns): Monitor ECG and report dysrhythmias; pay attention to pain related to deep muscle ischemia and report. Early detection may minimize severity of this complication. Fasciotomies may be necessary to relieve swelling and ischemia in the muscles and fascia; monitor patient for excessive blood loss and hypovolemia after fasciotomy.

NURSING PROCESS

The Rehabilitation Phase

Rehabilitation should begin immediately after the burn has occurred. Wound healing, psychosocial support, and restoring maximum functional activity remain priorities. Maintaining fluid and electrolyte balance and improving nutrition status continue to be important.

Assessment

- In early assessment, obtain information about patient's educational level, occupation, leisure activities, cultural background, religion, and family interactions.
- Assess self-concept, mental status, emotional response to the injury and hospitalization, level of intellectual functioning,

previous hospitalizations, response to pain and pain relief measures, and sleep pattern.

- Perform ongoing assessments relative to rehabilitation goals, including range of motion of affected joints, functional abilities in ADLs, early signs of skin breakdown from splints or positioning devices, evidence of neuropathies (neurologic damage), activity tolerance, and quality or condition of healing skin.
- Document participation and self-care abilities in ambulation, eating, wound cleaning, and applying pressure wraps.
- Maintain comprehensive and continuous assessment for early detection of complications, with specific assessments as needed for specific treatments, such as postoperative assessment of patient undergoing primary excision.

Diagnosis

NURSING DIAGNOSES

- Activity intolerance related to pain on exercise, limited joint mobility, muscle wasting, and limited endurance
- Disturbed body image related to altered appearance and self-concept
- Impaired physical mobility due to contractures or hypertrophic scarring
- Deficient knowledge of postdischarge home care and recovery needs

COLLABORATIVE PROBLEMS/POTENTIAL COMPLICATIONS

- Contractures
- Inadequate psychological adaptation to burn injury

Planning and Goals

Goals include increased mobility and participation in ADLs; increased understanding of the injury, treatment, and planned follow-up care; adaptation and adjustment to alterations in body image, self-concept, and lifestyle; and absence of complications.

Nursing Interventions

PROMOTING ACTIVITY TOLERANCE

- Schedule care to allow periods of uninterrupted sleep. Administer hypnotic agents, as prescribed, to promote sleep.
- Communicate plan of care to family and other caregivers.
- Reduce metabolic stress by relieving pain, preventing chilling or fever, and promoting integrity of all body systems to

B

help conserve energy. Monitor fatigue, pain, and fever to determine amount of activity to be encouraged daily.

- Incorporate physical therapy exercises to prevent muscular atrophy and maintain mobility required for daily activities.
- Support positive outlook, and increase tolerance for activity by scheduling diversion activities in periods of increasing duration.

Gerontologic Considerations for Promoting Activity

In older adult patients and those with chronic illnesses and disabilities, rehabilitation must take into account preexisting functional abilities and limitations.

IMPROVING BODY IMAGE AND SELF-CONCEPT

- Take time to listen to patient's concerns and provide realistic support; refer patient to a support group to develop coping strategies to deal with losses.
- Assess patient's psychosocial reactions; provide support and develop a plan to help the patient handle feelings. Promote a healthy body image and self-concept by helping patient practice responses to people who stare or ask about the injury.
- Support patient through small gestures such as providing a birthday cake, combing patient's hair before visitors, and sharing information on cosmetic resources to enhance appearance.
- Educate patient about the different ways to direct attention away from a disfigured body to the self within.
- Coordinate communications of consultants, such as psychologists, social workers, vocational counselors, and teachers, during rehabilitation.

MONITORING AND MANAGING POTENTIAL COMPLICATIONS

- Contractures: Provide early and aggressive physical and occupational therapy; support patient if surgery is needed to achieve full range of motion.
- Impaired psychological adaptation to the burn injury: Obtain psychological or psychiatric referral as soon as evidence of major coping problems appears.

PROMOTING HOME- AND COMMUNITY-BASED CARE

Educating Patients About Self-Care

- Throughout the phases of burn care, make efforts to prepare patient and family for the care they will perform at home. Provide them with information about measures and procedures.

- Provide verbal and written instructions about wound care, prevention of complications, pain management, and nutrition.
- Inform and review with patient specific exercises and use of elastic pressure garments and splints; provide written instructions.
- Educate patient and family to recognize abnormal signs and report them to the physician.
- Assist the patient and family in planning for the patient's continued care by identifying and acquiring supplies and equipment that are needed at home.
- Encourage and support follow-up wound care.
- Refer patient with inadequate support system to home care resources for assistance with wound care and exercises.
- Evaluate patient status periodically for modification of home care instructions or planning for reconstructive surgery or both.

Evaluation

EXPECTED PATIENT OUTCOMES
- Demonstrates physical mobility and activity tolerance required for desired daily activities
- Adapts to altered body image
- Demonstrates knowledge of required self-care and follow-up care
- Exhibits no complications

For more information, see Chapter 62 in Hinkle, J. L., & Cheever, K. H. (2014). *Brunner and Suddarth's textbook of medical-surgical nursing* (13th ed.). Philadelphia: Lippincott Williams & Wilkins.

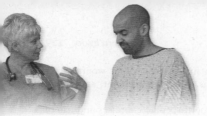

Cancer

Cancer is not a single disease with a single cause; rather, it is a group of distinct diseases with different causes, manifestations, treatments, and prognoses. Cancer can involve any organ system, with treatment approaches having multisystem effects. Cancer nursing practice, known as *oncology nursing,* covers all age groups and includes a variety of settings including acute care institutions, outpatient centers, rehabilitation facilities, the home, and long-term care facilities.

Nurses need to identify their own perception of cancer to meet realistic goals in caring for patients with cancer, because most people still associate cancer with pain and death. In addition, nurses caring for patients with cancer must be prepared to support patients and families through a wide range of physical, emotional, social, cultural, financial, and spiritual challenges.

Epidemiology

Cancer is second only to cardiovascular disease as a cause of death in the United States, with more than 1.5 million cases of cancer diagnosed in Americans in 2011. The leading causes of cancer death in the United States, in order of frequency and location, are lung, prostate, and colorectal cancer in men and lung, breast, and colorectal cancer in women. Most cancer occurs in people older than 65 years, with higher incidence in men than in women and a higher incidence in industrialized than nonindustrialized nations.

Overall cancer death rates have declined; however, cancer death rates in African American men remain substantially higher than those among Caucasian men and twice those of Hispanic men. Disparities in treatment, morbidity, and mortality are related to patient, physician, and system factors such as attitudes, knowledge, cultural beliefs, socioeconomic issues, level of education, insurance coverage, lifestyle choices (e.g., use of tobacco), misconceptions, communication skills, and other epidemiologic factors that exist within the health care system and community.

Pathophysiology of the Malignant Process

Cancer is a disease process that begins when an abnormal cell is transformed by the genetic mutation of the cellular DNA. Genetic mutations may result from inherited or acquired mutations that lead to abnormal cell behavior. The initial genetically altered cell forms a clone and begins to proliferate abnormally, evading normal intracellular and extracellular growth-regulating processes or signals as well as other defense mechanisms of the body. The cells acquire invasive character-istics, and changes occur in surrounding tissues. The cells infil-trate these tissues and gain access to lymph and blood vessels, which carry the cells to other areas of the body.

Proliferative Patterns

Various body tissues normally undergo periods of rapid or pro-liferative growth that must be distinguished from malignant growth activity. Several patterns of cell growth exist: hyperpla-sia, metaplasia, dysplasia, anaplasia, and neoplasia. Cancerous cells are described as malignant neoplasms and are classified and named by tissue of origin. Both benign and malignant growths are classified and named by tissue of origin. The International Classification of Diseases for Oncology (2011) is used by scientists and clinicians around the world as the nomenclature for malignant disease.

The failure of the immune system to promptly destroy abnormal cells permits these cells to grow too large to be man-aged by normal immune mechanisms. Agents or factors impli-cated in carcinogenesis include viruses and bacteria, physical agents, chemical agents, genetic and familial factors, dietary factors, and hormonal agents.

Clinical Manifestations

- Cancerous cells spread from one organ or body part to another by invasion and metastasis; therefore, manifestations are related to the system affected and degree of disruption (see the specific type of cancer).
- Generally, cancer causes anemia, weakness, weight loss (dys-phagia, anorexia, blockage), and pain (often in late stages).
- Symptoms are from tissue destruction and replacement with nonfunctional cancer tissue or overproductive cancer tissue (e.g., bone marrow disruption and anemia or excess adre-nal steroid production); pressure on surrounding structures; increased metabolic demands; and disruption of production of blood cells.

C

Assessment and Diagnostic Findings

Screening to detect cancer early usually focuses on cancers with the highest incidence or those that have improved survival rates if diagnosed early. Examples of these cancers include breast, colorectal, cervical, endometrial, testicular, skin, and oropharyngeal cancers. Patients with suspected cancer undergo extensive testing to

- Determine the presence and extent of tumors.
- Identify possible spread (metastasis) of disease or invasion of other body tissues.
- Evaluate the function of involved and uninvolved body systems and organs.
- Obtain tissue and cells for analysis, including evaluation of tumor stage and grade.

Diagnostic tests may include tumor marker identification, genetic profiling, imaging studies (mammography, MRI, CT, fluoroscopy, ultrasonography, endoscopy, nuclear medicine imaging, positron emission tomography [PET], PET fusion, radioimmunoconjugates), and biopsy.

Detection and Prevention of Cancer

- Educate community about cancer risks (avoid carcinogens).
- Encourage individuals to make dietary and lifestyle changes (smoking cessation, decreased caloric and alcohol intake, increased physical activity).
- Encourage individuals to achieve and maintain a healthy weight throughout life with physically active lifestyle.
- Screen women for breast cancer, cervix, and endometrial cancer and men for prostate cancer as indicated.

Tumor Staging and Grading

Staging

Staging determines the size of the tumor and the existence of local invasion and distant metastasis (see the Stages of Tumors box). Several systems exist for classifying the anatomic extent of disease. The TNM (tumor, nodes, and metastases) system is one system used to describe many solid tumors.

Grading

Grading is the pathologic classification of the tumor cells. Grading systems seek to define the type of tissue from which the tumor originated and the degree to which the tumor cells

C

Stages of Tumors

Stage I   Tumor <2 cm, negative lymph node involvement, no detectable metastases

Stage II   Tumor >2 cm but <5 cm, negative or positive unfixed lymph node involvement, no detectable metastases

Stage III   Large tumor >5 cm, or a tumor of any size with invasion of the skin or chest wall or positive fixed lymph node involvement in the clavicular area without evidence of metastases

Stage IV   Tumor of any size, positive or negative lymph node involvement, and distant metastases

retain the functional and histologic characteristics of the tissue of origin. Samples of cells to be used to establish the grade of a tumor may be obtained from tissue scrapings, body fluids, secretions, washings, biopsy, or surgical excision. This information helps providers predict the behavior and prognosis of various tumors. The tumor grade is assigned a numeric value ranging from I (well differentiated) to IV (poorly differentiated or undifferentiated).

Medical Management

The range of possible treatment goals may include complete eradication of malignant disease (cure), prolonged survival and containment of cancer cell growth (control), or relief of symptoms associated with the disease (palliation). Treatment approaches are initiated after diagnosis of cancer along with staging and grading are completed. Treatment options include the following:

- Surgery (e.g., local or wide excisions, video-assisted endoscopic surgery including use of robotics, salvage surgery, electrosurgery, cryosurgery, chemosurgery, or laser surgery) may be the primary method of treatment or may be prophylactic, palliative, or reconstructive. The goal of surgery is to remove the tumor or as much of the tumor as is feasible.
- Radiation therapy and chemotherapy may be used individually or in combination with other treatment options.
- Hematopoietic stem cell transplantation is another treatment option.

- Thermal therapy (hyperthermia) may be useful.
- Other targeted therapies (e.g., biologic response modifiers [BRMs], growth factors and cytokines, gene therapy, and complementary and alternative medicine [CAM]) are possible treatment modalities.

Nursing Management

Maintaining Tissue Integrity

Some of the most frequently encountered disturbances of tissue integrity include stomatitis, skin and tissue reactions to radiation therapy, cutaneous toxicities associated with targeted therapy, alopecia, and metastatic skin lesions.

Managing Mucositis and Stomatitis

- Assess oral cavity daily and instruct patient to report changes in sensation, mild erythema, edema, painful ulcerations, and bleeding.
- Assess for risk factors and comorbidities associated with stomatitis that include poor oral hygiene, general debilitation, existing dental disease, prior irradiation to the head and neck region, impaired salivary gland function, use of other medications that dry mucous membranes, myelosuppression, advanced age, tobacco use, previous stomatoxic chemotherapy, diminished renal function, and impaired nutritional status.
- Instruct patient to use normal saline mouth rinses and a soft toothbrush or toothette, remove dentures except during meals (ensure dentures fit properly), apply water-soluble lip lubricant, and take in a liquid or pureed diet. Advise patient to avoid irritants such as commercial mouthwashes, foods that are spicy or hard to chew and those with extremes of temperature, alcoholic beverages, and tobacco.
- Help patient minimize discomfort by using prescribed topical anesthetic, administering prescribed systemic analgesic agents, and performing appropriate mouth care.

Managing Radiation-Associated Skin Impairment

- Maintain skin integrity, cleansing, promotion of comfort, pain reduction, prevention of additional trauma, prevention and management of infection, and promotion of a moist wound healing environment.
- Provide careful skin care by avoiding the use of soaps, cosmetics, perfumes, powders, lotions and ointments, and deodorants.

- Educate patient about using only lukewarm water to bathe the area and to avoid constricting and irritating clothing; applying hot-water bottles, heating pads, or ice; shaving; or using adhesive tape on affected area.
- Instruct the patient to avoid rubbing or scratching the area or exposing the area to sunlight or cold weather. Also instruct the patient to apply vitamin A and D ointment to decrease itching.
- If moist desquamation occurs, apply calendula cream and some formulations of hyaluronic acid. If wet desquamation occurs, do not disrupt any blisters that have formed, report blistering, and use prescribed creams or ointments. If the area weeps, apply a nonadhesive absorbent dressing. If the area is without drainage, use moisture and vapor permeable dressings such as hydrocolloids and hydrogels on noninfected areas to promote comfort.

Addressing Alopecia

- Discuss potential hair loss and regrowth with patient and family; advise that hair loss may occur on body parts other than the head.
- Explore potential impact of hair loss resulting in challenges to self-esteem, interpersonal relationships, and sexuality and feelings of anger, rejection, isolation, helplessness, reluctance, fear, and depression.
- Prevent or minimize hair loss. Use scalp hypothermia and scalp tourniquets, if appropriate; cut long hair before treatment; use mild shampoo, gently pat dry, and avoid excessive shampooing and any hair processing; and avoid excessive combing or brushing.
- Suggest ways to assist in coping with hair loss (e.g., purchase wig or hairpiece before hair loss).
- Instruct patient to limit sun exposure, wear sunscreen, and wear a hat or scarf.
- Explain that hair growth usually begins again once therapy is completed.

Managing Malignant Skin Lesions

- Carefully assess and cleanse the skin, reducing superficial bacteria, controlling bleeding, reducing odor, protecting skin from pain and further trauma, and relieving pain.
- Assist and guide the patient and family regarding care for these skin lesions at home; refer for home care as indicated.

C

Promoting Nutrition

Most patients with cancer experience some weight loss during their illness. Anorexia, malabsorption, and cachexia are common examples of nutritional problems.

- Educate the patient to avoid unpleasant sights, odors, and sounds in the environment during mealtime.
- Suggest foods that are preferred and well tolerated by the patient, preferably high-calorie and high-protein foods. Respect ethnic and cultural food preferences.
- Encourage adequate fluid intake, but limit fluids at mealtime.
- Instruct patient to adjust diet before and after drug administration; suggest smaller, more frequent meals.
- Promote relaxed, quiet environment during mealtime with increased social interaction as desired.
- Encourage nutritional supplements and high-protein foods between meals.
- Encourage frequent oral hygiene and provide pain relief measures to make meals more pleasant.
- Administer antiemetic agents, sedatives, and corticosteroids and provide use of alternative therapies to help control nausea and vomiting before and after chemotherapy.
- Decrease anxiety by encouraging verbalization of fears and concerns, use of relaxation techniques, and imagery at mealtime.
- For collaborative management, provide enteral tube feedings of commercial liquid diets, elemental diets, or blenderized foods as prescribed.
- Administer appetite stimulants as prescribed by physician.
- Encourage family and friends not to nag or cajole patient about eating.
- Assess and address other contributing factors to nausea, vomiting, and anorexia, such as other symptoms, constipation, gastrointestinal (GI) irritation, electrolyte imbalance, radiation therapy, medications, and central nervous system metastasis.

Relieving Pain and Discomfort

- Instruct patient to report pain using pain scale and include location, quality, frequency, and duration.
- Collaborate with patient and health care team to determine optimal management of pain for optimal quality of life.
- Assure patient that you know that pain is real and will assist him or her in reducing it.

- Provide patient and family education regarding importance of prescribed analgesic regimen and address any misconceptions about opioid analgesic agents due to lack of knowledge about use.
- Encourage strategies of pain relief that patient has used successfully in previous pain experience.
- Educate patient about nonpharmacologic strategies to relieve pain and discomfort: distraction, imagery, relaxation, cutaneous stimulation, and the like.

Decreasing Fatigue

- Help patient and family to understand that fatigue is usually an expected and temporary side effect of the cancer process and treatments.
- Encourage patient to rearrange daily schedule and organize activities to conserve energy expenditure; promote normal sleep habits; encourage patient to alternate rest and activity.
- Encourage patient and family to plan to reallocate responsibilities, such as child care, housework, shopping, and cooking. Encourage patient to reduce the number of hours worked per week.
- Encourage adequate protein and calorie intake; assess for fluid and electrolyte disturbances.
- Encourage a planned exercise program to help increase endurance and stamina and lower fatigue.
- Encourage use of relaxation techniques and guided imagery.
- Address factors that contribute to fatigue and implement pharmacologic and nonpharmacologic strategies to manage pain.
- Administer blood products as prescribed to increase oxygen availability.
- Collaborate with physical and occupational therapy to facilitate mobility and increase energy.
- Administer erythropoietin (EPO), which stimulates red blood cell production, thus decreasing the symptoms of treatment-induced chronic anemia and reducing the need for blood transfusions.

Improving Body Image and Self-Esteem

- Assess patient's feelings about body image and level of self-esteem. Encourage patient to verbalize concerns and participate in activities and decision making.
- Identify potential threats to patient's self-esteem (e.g., altered appearance, decreased sexual function, hair loss, decreased energy, role changes). Validate concerns with patient.

- Assist patient in self-care when fatigue, lethargy, nausea, vomiting, and other symptoms prevent independence.
- Promote positive body image by assisting patient in selecting and using cosmetics, scarves, hairpieces, and clothing that increase his or her sense of attractiveness.
- Encourage patient and partner to share concerns about altered sexuality and sexual function and to explore alternatives to their usual sexual expression.
- Refer patient to collaborating specialists as needed.

Assisting in Grieving Process

- Encourage verbalization of fears, concerns, negative feelings, and questions regarding disease, treatment, and future implications. Explore previous successful coping strategies.
- Encourage active participation of patient or family in care and treatment decisions.
- Visit family frequently to establish and maintain relationships and physical closeness.
- Involve spiritual advisor as desired by the patient and family.
- Allow for progression through the grieving process at the individual pace of the patient and family, allowing for periods of crying and expression of sadness.
- Advise professional counseling as indicated for patient or family to alleviate pathologic or nonadaptive grieving.
- If patient enters the terminal phase of disease, assist patient and family to acknowledge and cope with their reactions and feelings.
- Maintain contact with the surviving family members after death of the patient. This may help them to work through their feelings of loss and grief.

Monitoring and Managing Potential Complications

Managing Infection

- Assess patient for evidence of infection: Check vital signs every 4 hours, monitor white blood cell (WBC) count and differential each day and inspect all sites that may serve as entry ports for pathogens (e.g., IV sites, wounds, skin folds, bony prominences, perineum, and oral cavity).
- Report fever (38.3°C [101°F] or higher, or 38°C [100.4°F] or higher for longer than 1 hour), chills, diaphoresis, swelling, heat, pain, erythema, and exudate on any body surfaces. Also report change in respiratory or mental status, urinary frequency or burning, malaise, myalgias, arthralgias, rash, or diarrhea.

- Discuss with patient and family the placement of patient in private room if absolute WBC count is less than 1,000/mm³ and the importance of patient avoiding contact with people who have known or recent infection or recent vaccination; encourage avoidance of crowds.
- Instruct all personnel in careful hand hygiene before and after entering room.
- Avoid rectal or vaginal procedures (rectal temperatures, examinations, suppositories, vaginal tampons) and intramuscular injections. Avoid insertion of urinary catheters; if catheters are necessary, use strict aseptic technique.
- Educate patient and family about food hygiene and safe food handling; instruct them to change water pitcher, denture cleaning fluids, and respiratory equipment containing water each day and to practice meticulous personal hygiene.

Managing Septic Shock
- Assess frequently for infection and inflammation throughout the course of the disease.
- Prevent septicemia and septic shock, or detect and report for prompt treatment.
- Monitor for signs and symptoms of septic shock (altered mental status, either subnormal or elevated temperature, cool and clammy skin, decreased urine output, hypotension, tachycardia, other dysrhythmias, electrolyte imbalances, tachypnea, and abnormal arterial blood gas [ABG] values).
- Instruct patient and family about signs of septicemia, methods for preventing infection, and actions to take if infection or septicemia occurs.

Managing Risk of Bleeding
- Monitor platelet count and assess for bleeding (e.g., petechiae or ecchymosis; decrease in hemoglobin or hematocrit; prolonged bleeding from invasive procedures, venipunctures, minor cuts, or scratches; frank or occult blood in any body excretion, emesis, or sputum; bleeding from any body orifice; altered mental status).
- Instruct patient and family about ways to minimize bleeding (e.g., use soft toothbrush or toothette for mouth care, avoid commercial mouthwashes, use electric razor for shaving, use emery board for nail care, avoid foods that are difficult to chew).
- Initiate measures to minimize bleeding (e.g., draw blood for all laboratory work with one daily venipuncture; avoid taking

temperature rectally or administering suppositories and enemas; avoid intramuscular injections, but use smallest needle
possible if necessary; lubricate lips with water-based lubricant; avoid bladder catheterizations, but use smallest catheter
if necessary; maintain fluid intake of at least 3 L per 24 hours
unless contraindicated; use stool softeners or increase bulk in
diet; avoid medications that will interfere with clotting, such
as aspirin; recommend use of water-based lubricant before
sexual intercourse).
- When platelet count is less than 20,000/mm^3, institute bed
  rest with padded side rails, avoidance of strenuous activity,
  and platelet transfusions as prescribed.
- Monitor, educate, and assist patient about ways to participate
  in self-protection.

Promoting Home- and Community-Based Care

Educating Patients About Self-Care
- Provide information needed by patient and family to address the
  most immediate care needs likely to be encountered at home.
- Verbally review, and reinforce with written information, the
  side effects of treatments and changes in the patient's status
  that should be reported.
- Discuss with patient and family strategies to deal with side
  effects of treatment or symptom management.
- Identify learning needs on the basis of the priorities identified
  by patient and family as well as on the complexity of home care.
- Provide ongoing support that allows the patient and family
  to feel comfortable and proficient in managing treatments at
  home.
- Refer for home care nursing to provide care and support for
  patients receiving advanced technical care, including home
  administration of chemotherapy, enteral or parenteral nutrition,
  blood products, parenteral antibiotics, and analgesics, as well as
  management of symptoms and care of vascular access devices.
- Assess and monitor for risk of venous thromboembolism on
  an ongoing basis.
- Provide follow-up visits and telephone calls to patient and
  family and evaluate the patient's progress and ongoing needs
  of the patient and family.

Continuing Care
- Refer patient for home care (assessment of the home environment, suggestions for modifications in home or in care

to help the patient and family address patient's physical needs and physical care, and assessment of the psychological and emotional impact of the illness on patient and family).

- Assess changes in the patient's physical status and report relevant changes to all involved health care providers to ensure that appropriate and timely modifications in therapy are made.
- Assess adequacy of pain management and the effectiveness of other strategies to prevent or manage side effects of treatment modalities and disease progression.
- Assess patient's and family's understanding of the treatment plan and management strategies and reinforce previous education.
- Make referrals and coordinate available community resources (e.g., local office of the American Cancer Society, home aides, church groups, faith community nurses, and support groups) to assist patients and caregivers.

Nursing Management Related to Treatment

Cancer Surgery
- Complete a thorough preoperative assessment for all factors that may affect patients undergoing surgery, individualized according to age, organ impairment, specific deficits, comorbidities, and cultural implications.
- Assist patient and family in dealing with the possible changes and outcomes resulting from surgery; provide education and emotional support by assessing patient and family needs and exploring with them their fears and coping mechanisms. Encourage them to take an active role in decision making when possible.
- Explain and clarify information the physician has provided about the results of diagnostic testing and surgical procedures, if asked.
- Communicate frequently with members of the health care team to ensure that the information provided is consistent.
- Postoperatively, assess patient's responses to the surgery and monitor for complications such as infection, bleeding, thrombophlebitis, wound dehiscence, fluid and electrolyte imbalance, and organ dysfunction.
- Provide postoperative education that addresses wound care, pain management and comfort, activity, nutrition, and medication information.

- Initiate plans for discharge, follow-up, home care, and treatment as early as possible to ensure continuity of care.
- Encourage patient and family to use community resources such as the American Cancer Society for support and information.

Radiation Therapy

- Explain and allow for questions related to the procedure, equipment, duration, and possible need for immobilizing the patient during the procedure, and the absence of new sensations, including pain, during the procedure.
- Assist the patient and family to discuss fears about the effects of radiation on others, on the tumor, and on normal tissues and organs.
- Assess patient's skin and oropharyngeal mucosa, nutritional status, and general feeling of well-being.
- Reassure the patient that systemic symptoms (e.g., weakness, fatigue) are a result of the treatment and do not represent deterioration or progression of the disease.
- If a radioactive implant is used, inform patient about the restrictions placed on visitors and health care personnel and other radiation precautions as well as the patient's own role before, during, and after the procedure.
- Maintain bed rest for patient with an intracavitary delivery device. Use the log-roll maneuver when positioning patient to prevent displacing the intracavitary device. Provide a low-residue diet and antidiarrheal agents to prevent bowel movements during therapy so that the radioisotopes are not displaced. Maintain an indwelling urinary catheter to ensure that the bladder empties.
- Assist the weak or fatigued patient with activities of daily living and personal hygiene, including gentle oral hygiene to remove debris, prevent irritation, and promote healing.
- Follow the instructions provided by the radiation safety officer from the radiology department, which specify the maximum time a health care provider can spend safely in the patient's room, the shielding equipment to be used, and special precautions and actions to be taken if the implant is dislodged. Explain the rationale for these precautions to patient.

> ### ◤ Quality And Safety Nursing Alert
>
> For safety in brachytherapy, assign the patient to a private room and post appropriate notices about radiation safety precautions. Have staff members wear dosimeter badges. Make sure that pregnant staff members are not assigned to this patient's care. Prohibit visits by children or pregnant women and limit visits from others to 30 minutes daily. Instruct and monitor visitors to ensure they maintain a 6-ft distance from the radiation source.

Chemotherapy

- Evaluate laboratory and physical assessments of metabolic indices; the hematologic, hepatic, renal, cardiovascular, neurologic, and pulmonary systems are critical in evaluating the body's response to chemotherapy.
- Assess patient's nutritional and fluid and electrolyte status frequently. Use creative ways to encourage adequate fluid and dietary intake.
- Because of increased risk of anemia, infection, and bleeding disorders, nursing assessment and care focuses on identifying and modifying factors that further increase the risk and on monitoring laboratory blood cell counts.
- Use aseptic technique and gentle handling to prevent infection and trauma.
- Educate patient and family on prescribed self-administered premedication before presenting to the infusion center, recognizing and reporting the signs and symptoms after infusion has started, and signs and symptoms that may occur at home which may warrant medication administration or transportation to the emergency department.
- Carefully select peripheral veins and perform venipuncture and carefully administer drugs. Monitor for indications of extravasation during drug administration (e.g., absence of blood return from the IV catheter; resistance to flow of IV fluid; or burning or pain, swelling, or redness at the site).

> ### ◤ Quality and Safety Nursing Alert
>
> If extravasation is suspected, stop the drug administration immediately and apply ice to the site (unless the extravasated vesicant is a vinca alkaloid).

C

- Assist patient with delayed nausea and vomiting (occurring later than 48 to 72 hours after chemotherapy) by instructing the patient to take antiemetic medications as necessary for the first week at home after chemotherapy and by educating about relaxation techniques and imagery, which can help to decrease stimuli contributing to symptoms.
- Advise patient to eat small frequent meals, bland foods, and comfort foods, which may reduce the frequency or severity of symptoms.
- Monitor blood cell counts frequently, note and report neutropenia, and protect the patient from infection and injury, particularly when blood cell counts are depressed.
- Monitor blood urea nitrogen (BUN), serum creatinine, creatinine clearance, and serum electrolyte levels, and report any findings that indicate decreasing renal function.
- Provide adequate hydration, diuresis, and alkalinization of the urine to prevent formation of uric acid crystals; administer allopurinol to prevent these side effects.
- Monitor closely for signs of heart failure, cardiac ejection fraction, and pulmonary fibrosis (e.g., pulmonary function test results).
- Inform patient and partner about potential changes in reproductive ability resulting from chemotherapy, in addition to their options moving forward. (Banking of sperm is recommended for men before treatments.) Advise patient and partner to use reliable birth control measures while receiving chemotherapy because sterility is not certain.
- Inform patient that the taxanes and plant alkaloids, especially vincristine, can cause peripheral neurologic damage with sensory alterations in the feet and hands; these side effects are usually reversible after completion of chemotherapy, but they may take months to resolve.
- Help patient and family to plan strategies to combat fatigue.
- Use precautions developed by the Occupational Safety and Health Administration (OSHA), Oncology Nursing Society (ONS), hospitals, and other health care agencies to protect health care personnel who handle chemotherapeutic agents.

Hematopoietic Stem Cell Transplantation
- Before hematopoietic stem cell transplantation (HSCT), perform nutritional assessments and extensive physical examinations, organ function tests, and psychological evaluations.

C

- Obtain blood work, including assessment of past infectious antigen exposure (e.g., hepatitis virus, cytomegalovirus, herpes simplex virus, HIV, and syphilis).
- Ensure that patient's social support systems and financial and insurance resources are evaluated.
- Reinforce HSCT information for informed consent.
- Provide patient education about the procedure and pretransplantation and posttransplantation care.
- During the treatment phase, closely monitor for signs of acute toxicities (e.g., nausea, diarrhea, mucositis, and hemorrhagic cystitis) and give constant attention to patient.
- During the HSCT, monitor vital signs with oxygen saturation, assess for adverse effects (e.g., fever, chills, shortness of breath, chest pain, cutaneous reactions, nausea, vomiting, hypotension or hypertension, tachycardia, anxiety, and taste changes), and provide ongoing education to patient, families, and caregivers.
- Support patient with blood products and hemopoietic growth factors and protect from infection owing to high risk of bleeding and sepsis.
- Assess for early graft-versus-host disease (GVHD) effects on the skin, liver, and GI tract. GVHD may be acute or chronic. Acute manifestations include rash, blistering, diarrhea, abdominal pain, hepatomegaly, nausea, vomiting, and mucositits. Some complications that occur are encephalopathy, hemolytic uremia syndrome, hemolytic anemia, and thrombotic thrombocytopenic purpura.
- Monitor for pulmonary complications, such as pulmonary edema and pneumonias, which often complicate recovery after HSCT.
- Provide follow-up visits to detect late effects (100 days or later) after HSCT, such as infections (e.g., varicella zoster), restrictive pulmonary abnormalities, and recurrent pneumonias, as well as chronic GVHD involving the skin, liver, intestine, esophagus, eye, lungs, joints, and vaginal mucosa. Cataracts may develop after total body irradiation.
- Assess and address the psychosocial needs of donors and family members and educate and support to reduce anxiety and promote coping. Assist family members to maintain realistic expectations of themselves as well as of the patients.

Hyperthermia
- Explain to patient and family about the procedure, its goals, and its effects.
- Assess the patient to reduce occurrence and severity of side effects, which include burns, fatigue, hypotension, peripheral neuropathies, thrombophlebitis, nausea, vomiting, diarrhea, and electrolyte imbalances.
- Provide local skin care at the site of the implanted hyperthermic probes.

Targeted Biological Therapies
- Targeted biological therapies include biological response modifiers (BRM) such as monoclonal antibodies (MoAb), growth factors and gene therapies.
- Assess the need for education, support, and guidance for both patient and family (often the same needs as patients having other treatment approaches, but BRMs may be perceived as a last-chance effort by patients who have not responded to standard treatments).
- Monitor therapeutic and adverse effects (e.g., fever, myalgia, nausea, and vomiting, as seen with interferon [IFN] or mild to severe hypersensitivity reactions as seen with MoAb infusions) and life-threatening side effects (e.g., capillary leak syndrome, pulmonary edema, and hypotension).
- Educate patient about self-care, including self-administered oral agents and such symptoms of toxicities as dose-limiting papulopustular rashes, pruritis, purulent nail changes, nail fissures, and skin flaking.
- Promote comfort and improving patient quality of life in hope of maximizing adherence to treatment and avoiding treatment delays or discontinuation. Educate patients and families, as needed, regarding how to administer BRM agents through subcutaneous injections.
- Provide instructions about side effects and identify strategies for the patient and family to manage many of the common side effects of BRM therapy (e.g., fatigue, anorexia, flulike symptoms).
- Arrange for home care nurses to monitor patient's responses to treatment, and provide education and continued care.
- Educate patients and families about cancer screening and prophylactic and therapeutic vaccines.

For more information, see Chapter 15 in Hinkle, J. L., & Cheever, K. H. (2014). *Brunner and Suddarth's textbook of medical-surgical nursing* (13th ed.). Philadelphia: Lippincott Williams & Wilkins.

Cancer of the Bladder

Cancer of the urinary bladder is more common in people older than 55 years, affects men more often than women (4:1), and is more common in Caucasians than in African Americans. Tobacco use continues to be a leading risk factor for all urinary tract cancers. People who smoke develop bladder cancer twice as often as those who do not smoke.

Pathophysiology

Bladder tumors usually arise at the base of the bladder and involve the ureteral orifices and bladder neck. Cancers arising from the prostate, colon, and rectum in males and from the lower gynecologic tract in females may metastasize to the bladder. Transitional cell carcinomas and carcinomas in situ shed recognizable cancer cells, which assist in diagnosis.

Clinical Manifestations

- Visible, painless hematuria is the most common symptom.
- Infection of the urinary tract is common and produces frequency and urgency.
- Any alteration in voiding or change in the urine is indicative.
- Pelvic or back pain may occur with metastasis.

Assessment and Diagnostic Findings

Biopsies of the tumor and adjacent mucosa are definitive, but the following procedures are also used:

- Cystoscopy (the mainstay of diagnosis)
- Excretory urography
- CT scan
- Ultrasonography
- Bimanual examination under anesthesia
- Cytologic examination of fresh urine and saline bladder washings
- Newer diagnostic tools being studied, such as bladder tumor antigens, nuclear matrix proteins, adhesion molecules, cytoskeletal proteins, and growth factors

Medical Management

Treatment of bladder cancer depends on the grade of tumor, the stage of tumor growth, and the multicentricity of the tumor. Age and physical, mental, and emotional status are considered in determining treatment.

C

Surgical Management
- Transurethral resection (TUR) or fulguration for simple papillomas with intravesical bacille Calmette–Guérin (BCG) is the treatment of choice.
- Monitoring of benign papillomas with cytology and cystoscopy is used periodically for the rest of patient's life.
- Simple cystectomy or radical cystectomy is useful for invasive or multifocal bladder cancer.
- Trimodal therapy (TUR, radiation, and chemotherapy) to avoid cystectomy remains investigational in the United States.

Pharmacologic Therapy
- Intravenous chemotherapy with a combination of methotrexate (Rheumatrex), 5-fluorouracil (5-FU), vinblastine (Velban), doxorubicin (Adriamycin), and cisplatin (Platinol) has been effective in producing partial remission of transitional cell carcinoma of the bladder in some patients; topical chemotherapy (intravesical chemotherapy) or instillation of antineoplastic agents into the bladder may be considered where there is a high risk of recurrence, cancer in situ, or incomplete tumor resection.
- Intravesical BCG is effective with superficial transitional cell carcinoma.

Radiation Therapy
- Radiation of tumor preoperatively to reduce microextension and viability and in combination with surgery to control inoperable tumors
- Hydrostatic therapy: for advanced bladder cancer or patients with intractable hematuria (after radiation therapy)
- Formalin, phenol, or silver nitrate instillations to achieve relief of hematuria and strangury (slow and painful discharge of urine) in some patients

Investigational Therapy
Chemoprevention and the use of photodynamic techniques in treating superficial bladder cancer are under investigation.

Nursing Management
For additional information, see "Nursing Management" under Cancer for the patient undergoing cancer surgery, radiation therapy, and chemotherapy.

For more information, see Chapter 55 in Hinkle, J. L., & Cheever, K. H. (2014). *Brunner and Suddarth's textbook of medical-surgical nursing* (13th ed.). Philadelphia: Lippincott Williams & Wilkins.

Cancer of the Breast

Cancer of the breast is categorized by the type of breast tissue involved: ductal (carcinoma in situ [DCIS] or infiltrating), lobular, medullary, mucinous, tubular ductal, or inflammatory. Breast cancer can be localized (e.g., DCIS) or become metastatic. Risk of developing breast cancer increases with age; approximately two of three invasive breast cancers are found in women age 55 years or older. Only about 5% to 10% of breast cancer cases are thought to be hereditary, resulting directly from gene defects (cell mutations) inherited from a biological parent.

Pathophysiology

Cancer of the breast is a pathologic entity that starts with a genetic alteration in a single cell and may take several years to become palpable. The most common histologic type of breast cancer is infiltrating ductal carcinoma (80% of cases), whereby tumors arise from the duct system and invade the surrounding tissues. Infiltrating lobular carcinoma accounts for 10% to 15% of cases. These tumors arise from the lobular epithelium and typically occur as an area of ill-defined thickening in the breast. Infiltrating ductal and lobular carcinomas usually spread to bone, lung, liver, adrenals, pleura, skin, or brain. Several less common invasive cancers, such as medullary carcinoma (5% of cases), mucinous carcinoma (3% of cases), and tubular ductal carcinoma (2% of cases), have very favorable prognoses. Inflammatory carcinoma and Paget's disease are less common forms of breast cancer. DCIS is a noninvasive form of cancer (also called *intraductal carcinoma*) but, if left untreated, there is an increased likelihood that it will progress to invasive cancer. There is no one specific cause of breast cancer; rather, a combination of genetic, hormonal, and possibly environmental events may contribute to its development. If lymph nodes are unaffected, the prognosis is better. The key to improved cure rates is early diagnosis, before metastasis.

Risk Factors

- Gender (female) and increasing age are primary factors.
- Previous breast cancer: The risk of developing cancer in the same or opposite breast is significantly increased.
- Family history: Having a first-degree relative with breast cancer (mother, sister, daughter) increases the risk

twofold; having two first-degree relatives increases the risk fivefold.

- Genetic mutations (*BRCA1* or *BRCA2*) account for majority of inherited breast cancers; however, 80% of breast cancer patients have no family history of the disease.
- Hormonal factors include early menarche (before 12 years of age), nulliparity, first birth after 30 years of age, late menopause (after 55 years of age), and hormone therapy (formerly referred to as *hormone replacement therapy*).
- Other factors may include exposure to ionizing radiation during adolescence, a history of benign proliferative breast disease, early adulthood obesity, alcohol intake (beer, wine, or liquor), and a high-fat diet (controversial; more research is needed).

Protective Factors

Protective factors may include regular vigorous exercise (decreased body fat), pregnancy before age 30 years, and breast-feeding. Management of stress through the use of meditation or prayer or involvement in support groups may also be protective.

Prevention Strategies

Patients at high risk for breast cancer may consult with specialists regarding possible or appropriate prevention strategies such as the following:

- Long-term surveillance consists of twice-yearly clinical breast examinations starting at age 25 years, yearly mammography, and possibly MRI (in *BRCA1* and *BRCA2* carriers); ultrasonography may be useful.
- Chemoprevention can be used to prevent disease before it starts, using tamoxifen (Nolvadex) and possibly raloxifene (Evista).
- Also possible are prophylactic mastectomy ("risk-reducing" mastectomy) for patients with a strong family history of breast cancer, a diagnosis of lobular carcinoma in situ (LCIS) or atypical hyperplasia, a *BRCA* gene mutation, an extreme fear of cancer ("cancer phobia"), or previous cancer in one breast; the procedure does not confer 100% protection against the development of breast cancer.

Clinical Manifestations

- Generally, lesions are nontender, fixed, and hard with irregular borders; most occur in the upper outer quadrant. Breast may change in shape, or nipple discharge may occur.

- Some women have no symptoms and no palpable lump but have an abnormal mammogram.
- Advanced signs may include skin dimpling, nipple retraction, or skin ulceration.

Assessment and Diagnostic Findings

- Biopsy (e.g., percutaneous, surgical) and histologic examination of cancer cells
- Tumor staging and analysis of additional prognostic factors to determine the prognosis and optimal treatment regimen
- Chest x-rays, CT, MRI, positron emission tomography (PET) scan, bone scans, and blood work (complete blood cell count, comprehensive metabolic panel, tumor markers [i.e., carcinoembryonic antigen (CEA), CA15-3]).

Staging of Breast Cancer

Classifying tumors as stage 0, I, or IV is fairly straightforward. Stage II and III tumors represent a wide spectrum of breast cancers and are subdivided into stages IIA, IIB, IIIA, IIIB, and IIIC. Factors determining stages include number and characteristics of axillary lymph nodes, status of other regional lymph nodes, and involvement of the skin or underlying muscle. See "Staging" under Cancer.

Medical Management

Various management options are available. The patient and physician may decide on surgery, radiation therapy, chemotherapy, hormonal therapy, or a combination of therapies.

Surgical Management

- Modified radical mastectomy involves removal of the entire breast tissue, including the nipple–areola complex and a portion of the axillary lymph nodes via axillary lymph node dissection (ALND).
- Total mastectomy involves removal of the breast and nipple–areola complex but not ALND.
- Breast-conserving surgery includes lumpectomy, wide excision, partial or segmental mastectomy, or quadrantectomy followed by lymph node removal for invasive breast cancer.
- Sentinel lymph node biopsy is considered a standard of care for the treatment of early-stage breast cancer.
- Breast reconstruction may be used.

Radiation Therapy

External-beam radiation therapy: Typically whole-breast radiation, but partial-breast radiation (radiation to the lumpectomy site alone) is now being evaluated at some institutions in carefully selected patients.

Pharmacologic Therapy

- Chemotherapy is often given in combinations to eradicate micrometastatic spread of the disease: cyclophosphamide (Cytoxan), methotrexate, fluorouracil, anthracycline-based regimens (e.g., doxorubicin [Adriamycin], epirubicin [Ellence]), taxanes (paclitaxel [Taxol], docetaxel [Taxotere]).
- Hormonal therapy is based on the index of estrogen and progesterone receptors: Tamoxifen (Soltamox) is the primary hormonal agent used to suppress hormonal-dependent tumors; others are inhibitors, anastrazole (Arimidex), letrozole (Femara), and exemestane (Aromasin).
- Targeted therapy involves trastuzumab (Herceptin) and bevacizumab (Avastin).

NURSING PROCESS

The Patient Undergoing Surgery for Breast Cancer

See "Nursing Management" under Cancer for additional information.

Assessment

- Perform a health history.
- Assess patient's reaction to the diagnosis and ability to cope with it.
- Ask about coping skills, support systems, knowledge deficit, and presence of discomfort.

Diagnosis

PREOPERATIVE NURSING DIAGNOSES

- Deficient knowledge about the planned surgical treatments
- Anxiety related to cancer diagnosis
- Fear related to specific treatments and body image changes
- Risk for ineffective coping (individual or family) related to the diagnosis of breast cancer and treatment options
- Decisional conflict related to treatment options

POSTOPERATIVE NURSING DIAGNOSES
- Pain and discomfort related to surgical procedure
- Disturbed sensory perception related to nerve irritation in affected arm, breast, or chest wall
- Disturbed body image related to loss or alteration of the breast
- Risk for impaired coping related to the diagnosis of cancer and surgical treatment
- Self-care deficit related to partial immobility of upper extremity on operative side
- Risk for sexual dysfunction related to loss of body part, change in self-image, and fear of partner's responses
- Deficient knowledge: drain management after breast surgery
- Deficient knowledge: arm exercises to regain mobility of affected extremity
- Deficient knowledge: hand and arm care after an ALND

COLLABORATIVE PROBLEMS/POTENTIAL COMPLICATIONS
- Lymphedema
- Hematoma or seroma formation
- Infection

Planning and Goals

The major goals may include increased knowledge about the disease and its treatment; reduction of preoperative and postoperative fear, anxiety, and emotional stress; improvement of decision-making ability; pain management; improvement in coping abilities; improvement in sexual function; and the absence of complications.

Preoperative Nursing Interventions

PROVIDING EDUCATION AND PREPARATION ABOUT
SURGICAL TREATMENTS
- Review treatment options by reinforcing information provided to the patient and answer any questions.
- Fully prepare the patient for what to expect before, during, and after surgery.
- Inform patient that she will often have decreased arm and shoulder mobility after an ALND; demonstrate range-of-motion exercises prior to discharge.
- Reassure patient that appropriate analgesia and comfort measures will be provided.

C

REDUCING FEAR AND ANXIETY AND IMPROVING COPING ABILITY

- Help patient cope with the physical and emotional effects of surgery.
- Provide patient with realistic expectations about the healing process and expected recovery to help alleviate fears (e.g., fear of pain, concern about inability to care for oneself and one's family, concern about time off work, coping with an uncertain future).
- Inform patient about available resources at the treatment facility and in the breast cancer community (e.g., social workers, psychiatrists, and support groups); patient may find it helpful to talk to a breast cancer survivor who has undergone similar treatments.

PROMOTING DECISION-MAKING ABILITY

- Help patient and family weigh the risks and benefits of each option.
- Ask patient questions about specific treatment options to help her focus on choosing an appropriate treatment (e.g., How would you feel about losing your breast? Are you considering breast reconstruction? If you choose to retain your breast, would you consider undergoing radiation treatments 5 days a week for 5 to 6 weeks?).
- Support whatever decision the patient makes.

Postoperative Nursing Interventions

RELIEVING PAIN AND DISCOMFORT

- Carefully assess patient for pain; individual pain varies.
- Encourage patient to use analgesic agents.
- Prepare patient for a possible slight increase in pain after the first few days of surgery; this may occur as patients regain sensation around the surgical site and become more active.
- Evaluate patients who complain of excruciating pain to rule out any potential complications such as infection or a hematoma.
- Suggest alternative methods of pain management (e.g., taking warm showers, using distraction methods such as guided imagery).

MANAGING POSTOPERATIVE SENSATIONS

Reassure patients that postoperative sensations (e.g., tenderness, soreness, numbness, tightness, pulling, and twinges; phantom sensations after a mastectomy) are a normal part of healing and that these sensations are not indicative of a problem.

PROMOTING POSITIVE BODY IMAGE
- Assess the patient's readiness to see the incision for the first time and provide gentle encouragement; ideally, the patient will be with the nurse or another health care provider for support.
- Maintain the patient's privacy.
- Ask the patient what she perceives, acknowledge her feelings, and allow her to express her emotions; reassure patient that her feelings are normal.
- If desired, provide patient who has not had immediate reconstruction with a temporary breast form to place in her bra.

PROMOTING POSITIVE ADJUSTMENT AND COPING
- Provide ongoing assessment of how the patient is coping with her diagnosis and treatment.
- Assist patient in identifying and mobilizing her support systems; the patient's spouse or partner may also need guidance, support, and education; provide resources (e.g., Reach to Recovery program of the American Cancer Society [ACS], advocacy groups, or a spiritual advisor).
- Encourage the patient to discuss issues and concerns with other patients who have had breast cancer.
- Provide patient with information about the plan of care after treatment.
- If patient displays ineffective coping, consultation with a mental health practitioner may be indicated.

IMPROVING SEXUAL FUNCTION
- Encourage the patient to discuss how she feels about herself and about possible reasons for a decrease in libido (e.g., fatigue, anxiety, self-consciousness).
- Suggest that the patient vary the time of day for sexual activity (when the patient is less tired), assume positions that are more comfortable, and express affection using alternative measures (e.g., hugging, kissing, manual stimulation).
- If sexual issues cannot be resolved, a referral for counseling (e.g., psychologist, psychiatrist, psychiatric clinical nurse specialist, social worker, sex therapist) may be helpful.

MONITORING AND MANAGING POTENTIAL COMPLICATIONS
- Promote collateral or auxiliary lymph drainage by encouraging movement and exercise (e.g., hand pumps) through postoperative education.

C

- Elevate arm above the heart.
- Obtain referral for patient to therapist for compression sleeve or glove, exercises, manual lymph drainage, and a discussion of ways to modify daily activities.
- Educate patient regarding proper incision care and signs and symptoms of infection and the time to contact surgeon or nurse.
- Monitor surgical site for gross swelling or drainage output and notify surgeon promptly.
- If ordered, apply compression wrap to the incision.

PROMOTING HOME- AND COMMUNITY-BASED CARE
Educating Patients About Self-Care
- Assess patient's readiness to assume self-care and identify any gaps in knowledge. Focus on educating about incision care, signs to report (infection, hematoma/seroma, arm swelling), pain management, arm exercises, hand and arm care, drainage management, and activity restriction. Include family members in educational plans.
- Provide follow-up with telephone calls to discuss concerns about incision, pain management, and patient and family adjustment.

Continuing Care
- Reinforce earlier education as needed.
- Encourage patient to call with any questions or concerns.
- Refer patient for home care as indicated or desired by patient.
- Remind patient of the importance of participating in routine health screening.
- Reinforce need for follow-up visits to the physician (every 3 to 6 months for the first several years).

Evaluation

EXPECTED PATIENT OUTCOMES
- Exhibits knowledge about diagnosis and treatment options
- Verbalizes willingness to deal with anxiety and fears related to diagnosis and the effects of surgery on self-image and sexual functioning
- Demonstrates ability to cope with diagnosis and treatment
- Makes decisions regarding treatment options in a timely manner

- Reports pain has decreased and states pain and discomfort management strategies are effective
- Identifies postoperative sensations and recognizes that they are a normal part of healing
- Exhibits clean, dry, and intact surgical incision without signs of inflammation or infection
- Lists signs and symptoms of infection to be reported
- Verbalizes feelings regarding change in body image
- Discusses meaning of diagnosis, surgical treatment, and fears appropriately
- Participates actively in self-care measures
- Discusses issues of sexuality and resumption of sexual relations
- Demonstrates knowledge of postdischarge recommendations and restrictions
- Experiences no complications

For more information, see Chapter 58 in Hinkle, J. L., & Cheever, K. H. (2014). *Brunner and Suddarth's textbook of medical-surgical nursing* (13th ed.). Philadelphia: Lippincott Williams & Wilkins.

Cancer of the Cervix

Cancer of the cervix is predominantly squamous cell cancer and also includes adenocarcinomas. It is less common than it once was because of early detection by the Pap smear, but it remains the third most common reproductive cancer in women and is estimated to affect more than 12,000 women in the United States every year. Risk factors vary from multiple sex partners, early sexual debut (younger than 20 years), smoking, and family history of cervical cancer to chronic cervical infection (exposure to human papillomavirus [HPV]).

Clinical Manifestations
- Cervical cancer is most often asymptomatic. When discharge, irregular bleeding, or pain or bleeding after sexual intercourse occurs, the disease may be advanced.
- Vaginal discharge gradually increases in amount, becomes watery, and finally is dark and foul-smelling because of necrosis and infection of the tumor.

C

- Bleeding occurs at irregular intervals between periods or after menopause, may be slight (enough to spot undergarments), and is usually noted after mild trauma (intercourse, douching, or defecation). As disease continues, bleeding may persist and increase.
- Leg pain, dysuria, rectal bleeding, and edema of the extremities signal advanced disease.
- Nerve involvement, producing excruciating pain in the back and legs, occurs as cancer advances and tissues outside the cervix are invaded, including the fundus and lymph glands anterior to the sacrum.
- Extreme emaciation and anemia, often with fever due to secondary infection and abscesses in the ulcerating mass, and fistula formation may occur in the final stage.

Assessment and Diagnostic Findings

- Screening should begin within 3 years of initiation of sexual intercourse or at 21 years of age.
- Pap smear and biopsy results may show severe dysplasia, high-grade epithelial lesion (HGSIL), or carcinoma in situ.
- Other tests may include x-rays, laboratory tests, special examinations (e.g., punch biopsy and colposcopy), dilation and curettage (D&C), CT scan, MRI, IV urography, cystography, positron emission tomography (PET), and barium x-ray studies.

Medical Management

Disease may be staged (usually the tumor, nodes, and metastases [TNM] system) to estimate the extent of the disease so that treatment can be planned more specifically and prognosis.

- Conservative treatments include monitoring, cryotherapy (freezing with nitrous oxide), laser therapy, loop electrosurgical excision procedure (LEEP), or conization (removing a cone-shaped portion of cervix).
- Simple hysterectomy is performed if preinvasive cervical cancer (carcinoma in situ) occurs when a woman has completed childbearing. Radical trachelectomy is an alternative to hysterectomy for women of childbearing age.
- For invasive cancer, surgery, radiation (external beam or brachytherapy), platinum-based agents, or a combination of these approaches may be used.
- For recurrent cancer, pelvic exenteration is considered.

NURSING PROCESS

The Patient Undergoing Hysterectomy

C

See "Nursing Management" under Cancer for additional care measures and nursing care of patients with varied treatment regimens.

Assessment

- Obtain a health history.
- Perform a physical and pelvic examination and laboratory studies.
- Gather data about the patient's psychosocial supports and responses.

Diagnosis

NURSING DIAGNOSES

- Anxiety related to the diagnosis of cancer, fear of pain, perceived loss of femininity, or childbearing potential
- Disturbed body image related to altered fertility, fears about sexuality, and relationships with partner and family
- Pain related to surgery and other adjuvant therapy
- Deficient knowledge of perioperative aspects of hysterectomy and self-care

COLLABORATIVE PROBLEMS/POTENTIAL COMPLICATIONS

- Hemorrhage
- Deep vein thrombosis
- Bladder dysfunction
- Infection

Planning and Goals

The major goals may include relief of anxiety, acceptance of loss of the uterus, absence of pain or discomfort, increased knowledge of self-care requirements, and absence of complications.

Nursing Interventions

RELIEVING ANXIETY

- Determine how this experience affects the patient and allow the patient to verbalize feelings and identify strengths.
- Explain all pre- and postoperative and recovery period preparations and procedures.

IMPROVING BODY IMAGE

- Assess how patient feels about undergoing a hysterectomy related to the nature of diagnosis, significant others, religious beliefs, and prognosis.
- Acknowledge patient's concerns about ability to have children, loss of femininity, and impact on sexual relations.
- Educate patient about sexual relations: sexual satisfaction, orgasm arising from clitoral stimulation, sexual feeling, or comfort related to shortened vagina.
- Explain that depression and heightened emotional sensitivity are expected because of upset hormonal balances.
- Exhibit interest, concern, and willingness to listen to fears.

RELIEVING PAIN

- Assess the intensity of the patient's pain and administer analgesics.
- Encourage patient to resume intake of food and fluids gradually when peristalsis is auscultated (1 to 2 days). Encourage early ambulation.
- Apply heat to abdomen or insert a rectal tube if prescribed for abdominal distention.

MONITORING AND MANAGING COMPLICATIONS

- Hemorrhage: Count perineal pads used and assess extent of saturation, monitor vital signs, check abdominal dressings for drainage, and provide guidelines for restricting activity to promote healing and prevent bleeding.
- Deep vein thrombosis: Apply elastic compression stockings; encourage and assist in changing positions frequently; assist with early ambulation and leg exercises; monitor leg pain; instruct patient to avoid prolonged pressure at the knees (sitting) and immobility.
- Bladder dysfunction: Monitor urinary output and assess for abdominal distention after catheter is removed; initiate measures to encourage voiding.

PROMOTING HOME- AND COMMUNITY-BASED CARE

Educating Patients About Self-Care

- Tailor information according to patient's needs: no menstrual cycles, need for hormones.
- Instruct patient to check surgical incision daily and report redness, purulent drainage, or discharge.
- Stress the importance of adequate oral intake and maintaining bowel and urinary tract function.

- Instruct patient to resume activities gradually; no sitting for long periods; postoperative fatigue should gradually decrease.
- Inform that showers are preferable to tub baths to reduce risk for infection and injury getting in and out of tub.
- Encourage patient to avoid lifting, straining, sexual intercourse, or driving until advised by physician.
- Educate patient about reporting vaginal discharge, foul odor, excessive bleeding, leg redness or pain, or elevated temperature to health care professional promptly.

Continuing Care
- Make follow-up telephone contact with patient to address concerns and determine progress; remind patient about postoperative follow-up appointments.
- Remind patient to discuss hormone therapy with primary physician, if ovaries were removed.

Evaluation

EXPECTED PATIENT OUTCOMES
- Reports decreased anxiety
- Has improved body image
- Reports minimal pain and discomfort
- Verbalizes knowledge and understanding of self-care
- Experiences no complications

For more information, see Chapter 57 in Hinkle, J. L., & Cheever, K. H. (2014). *Brunner and Suddarth's textbook of medical-surgical nursing* (13th ed.). Philadelphia: Lippincott Williams & Wilkins.

Cancer of the Colon and Rectum
(Colorectal Cancer)

Colorectal cancer is predominantly (95%) adenocarcinoma, with colon cancer affecting more than twice as many people as rectal cancer. It may start as a benign polyp but may become malignant, invade and destroy normal tissues, and extend into surrounding structures. Cancer cells may migrate away from the primary tumor and spread to other parts of the body (most often to the liver, peritoneum, and lungs). Incidence increases with age (the incidence is highest in people older than 85 years) and is higher in people with a family history of colon cancer and those with inflammatory bowel disease (IBD) or polyps. A hereditary colorectal cancer, Lynch syndrome (also known as *hereditary nonpolyposis colorectal cancer* [HNPCC]), is characterized by early age onset and can include cancers of the colorectum, uterus, ovaries, urinary epithelium, and small bowel. Patients with familial adenomatous polyposis (FAP) are at higher risk for colorectal cancer. If the disease is detected and treated at an early stage before the disease spreads, the 5-year survival rate is 90%; however, only 39% of colorectal cancers are detected at an early stage. Survival rates after late diagnosis are very low. Stage at presentation is the single consistent variable affecting prognosis.

Clinical Manifestations
- Changes in bowel habits (most common presenting symptom), passage of blood in or on the stools (second most common symptom)
- Unexplained anemia, anorexia, weight loss, and fatigue
- Right-sided lesions possibly accompanied by dull abdominal pain and melena (black tarry stools)
- Left-sided lesions associated with obstruction (abdominal pain and cramping, narrowing stools, constipation, and distention) and bright red blood in stool
- Rectal lesions associated with tenesmus (ineffective painful straining at stool), rectal pain, feeling of incomplete evacuation after a bowel movement, alternating constipation and diarrhea, and bloody stool
- Signs of complications: partial or complete bowel obstruction, tumor extension and ulceration into the surrounding blood vessels (perforation, abscess formation, peritonitis, sepsis, or shock)
- In many instances, no symptoms until colorectal cancer is at an advanced stage

Assessment and Diagnostic Findings
- Abdominal and rectal examination; fecal occult blood testing; double-contrast barium enema; proctosigmoidoscopy; and colonoscopy, biopsy, or cytology smears are performed.
- Carcinoembryonic antigen (CEA) is a tumor marker to assess progression or recurrence of gastrointestinal cancers; CEA values should return to normal within 48 hours

of tumor excision (reliable in predicting prognosis and recurrence).

🦠 Gerontologic Considerations

Carcinomas of the colon and rectum are common malignancies in advanced age. In men, only the incidence of prostate cancer and lung cancer exceeds that of colorectal cancer. In women, only the incidence of breast cancer exceeds that of colorectal cancer. Symptoms are often insidious. Patients with colorectal cancer usually report fatigue, which is caused primarily by iron deficiency anemia. In early stages, minor changes in bowel patterns and occasional bleeding may occur. The later symptoms most commonly reported by older adult patients are abdominal pain, obstruction, tenesmus, and rectal bleeding.

Colon cancer in the older adult has been closely associated with dietary carcinogens. Lack of fiber is a major causative factor because the passage of feces through the intestinal tract is prolonged, which extends exposure to possible carcinogens. Excess dietary fat, high alcohol consumption, and smoking all increase the incidence of colorectal tumors. Physical activity and dietary folate have protective effects.

Medical Management

Treatment of cancer depends on the stage of disease and consists of surgery to remove the tumor, supportive therapy, and adjuvant therapy (i.e., chemotherapy, radiation therapy, immunotherapy, or multimodal therapy). Obstruction is treated with IV fluids and nasogastric suction and with blood therapy if bleeding is significant.

Surgical Management

- Surgery is the primary treatment for most colon and rectal cancers; the type of surgery depends on the location and size of tumor, and it may be curative or palliative.
- Cancers limited to one site can be removed through a colonoscope.
- Laparoscopic colotomy with polypectomy minimizes the extent of surgery needed in some cases.
- Laparoscopic colectomy has been shown to have surgical outcomes equivalent to those of open colectomy with decreased length of hospital stay and use of pain medications as well as improved quality of life.

C

- Neodymium: yttrium-aluminum-garnet (Nd: YAG) laser is effective with some lesions.
- Bowel resection with anastomosis and possible temporary or permanent colostomy or ileostomy (less than one third of patients) or coloanal reservoir (colonic J pouch).
- Insertion of a stent in cases of acute malignant colorectal cancer obstruction may be an option for decompression prior to elective surgical intervention.

🐾 Gerontologic Considerations

Older adults are at increased risk of postoperative complications. Decreased vision and hearing and difficulty with fine motor control make mastery of ostomy self-care tasks more challenging. Skin care is a major concern with a colostomy because of age-related skin changes (i.e., epithelial and subcutaneous fatty layers are thinned and skin is irritated easily). Some patients have delayed elimination after irrigation because of decreased peristalsis and mucus production.

NURSING PROCESS

The Patient With Colorectal Cancer

Assessment

- Obtain a health history about the presence of fatigue, abdominal or rectal pain, past and present elimination patterns, and characteristics of stool.
- Obtain a history of IBD or colorectal polyps, a family history of colorectal disease, and current medication therapy.
- Assess dietary patterns, including fat and fiber intake, amounts of alcohol consumed, and history of smoking; describe and document a history of weight loss and feelings of weakness and fatigue.
- Auscultate abdomen for bowel sounds; palpate for areas of tenderness, distention, and solid masses; inspect stool for blood.

Diagnosis

NURSING DIAGNOSES

- Imbalanced nutrition: less than body requirements, related to nausea and anorexia
- Risk for deficient fluid volume and electrolyte imbalance related to vomiting and dehydration

- Anxiety related to impending surgery and diagnosis of cancer
- Risk for ineffective self-care management related to deficient knowledge concerning the diagnosis, surgical procedure, and self-care after discharge
- Impaired skin integrity related to surgical incisions, stoma, and fecal contamination of peristomal skin
- Disturbed body image related to colostomy
- Ineffective sexuality patterns related to ostomy and changes in body image and self-concept

COLLABORATIVE PROBLEMS/POTENTIAL COMPLICATIONS
- Intraperitoneal infection
- Complete large bowel obstruction
- Gastrointestinal bleeding and hemorrhage
- Bowel perforation
- Peritonitis, abscess, or sepsis

Planning and Goals

The major goals may include attainment of optimal level of nutrition; maintenance of fluid and electrolyte balance; reduction of anxiety; attainment of knowledge about the diagnosis, surgical procedure, and self-care after discharge; maintenance of optimal tissue healing; protection of peristomal skin; gained knowledge about how to irrigate the colostomy (sigmoid colostomies) and change the appliance; ability to express feelings and concerns about the colostomy and the impact on self; and avoidance of complications.

Nursing Interventions

PREPARING PATIENT FOR SURGERY
- Physically prepare patient for surgery (diet high in calories, protein, and carbohydrates and low in residue; full or clear liquid diet 24 to 48 hours before surgery or parenteral nutrition, if prescribed).
- Administer antibiotics, laxatives, enemas, or colonic irrigations as prescribed.
- Perform intake and output measurements including vomitus, nasogastric tube outputs, and IV fluids; assess electrolytes.
- Observe for signs of hypovolemia (e.g., tachycardia, hypotension, decreased pulse volume); monitor hydration status (e.g., skin turgor, mucous membranes).

C

- Monitor for signs of obstruction or perforation (increased abdominal distention, loss of bowel sounds, pain, or rigidity).
- Reinforce and supplement patient's knowledge about diagnosis, prognosis, surgical procedure, and expected level of function postoperatively. Include information about postoperative wound and ostomy care, dietary restrictions, pain control, and medical management.

See "Nursing Management" under Cancer for additional information.

PROVIDING EMOTIONAL SUPPORT

- Assess patient's level of anxiety and coping mechanisms and suggest methods for reducing anxiety, such as deep breathing exercises and visualizing a successful recovery from surgery and cancer.
- Arrange meetings with a spiritual advisor, if desired.
- Provide meetings for patient and family with physicians and nurses to discuss treatment and prognosis; a meeting with a wound-ostomy-continence (WOC) nurse and a person who has successfully managed with a colostomy may be useful.
- Help reduce fear by presenting facts about the surgical procedure and the creation and management of the ostomy.
- Promote patient comfort by projecting a relaxed, professional, and empathetic attitude.
- Provide patient and family with additional resources about living with an ostomy (i.e., United Ostomy Association of America).

PROVIDING POSTOPERATIVE CARE

- Care for patients undergoing colon resection or colostomy is similar to nursing care for any abdominal surgery patient, including pain management during the immediate postoperative period.
- Monitor for complications.
- Assess and document return of peristalsis and initial stool characteristics.

MAINTAINING OPTIMAL NUTRITION

- Educate patient and family about the health benefits of a healthy diet; diet is individualized as long as it is nutritionally sound and does not cause diarrhea or constipation. Return to normal diet is rapid.

- Advise patient to avoid foods that cause excessive odor and gas, including foods in the cabbage family, eggs, asparagus, fish, beans, and high-cellulose products such as peanuts; non-irritating foods are substituted for those that are restricted so that deficiencies are corrected.
- Suggest fluid intake of at least 2 L per day; constipation may be managed with prune or apple juices or mild laxatives.

MAINTAINING FLUID AND ELECTROLYTE BALANCE

- Administer antiemetics and restrict fluids and food to prevent vomiting; monitor abdomen for distention, loss of bowel sounds, or pain or rigidity (signs of obstruction or perforation).
- Record intake and output, and restrict fluids and oral food to prevent vomiting.
- Monitor serum electrolytes to detect hypokalemia and hyponatremia.
- Assess vital signs to detect signs of hypovolemia: tachycardia, hypotension, and decreased pulse volume.
- Assess hydration status and report decreased skin turgor, dry mucous membranes, and concentrated urine.

PROVIDING WOUND CARE

- Provide information about signs and symptoms of skin irritation or inflammation.
- Demonstrate for patient how to gently cleanse peristomal skin.
- Demonstrate correct techniques for applying skin barrier and removing pouch.

SUPPORTING A POSITIVE BODY IMAGE

- Encourage patient to verbalize feelings and concerns.
- Provide a supportive environment and attitude to promote adaptation to lifestyle changes related to stoma care.
- Listen to the patient's concerns about sexuality and function (e.g., mutilation, fear of impotence, leakage during sex). Offer support and, if appropriate, refer to a WOC nurse, sex counselor or therapist, or advanced practice nurse.

MONITORING AND MANAGING COMPLICATIONS

- Before and after surgery, observe for symptoms of complications; report and institute necessary care.
- Administer antibiotics as prescribed to reduce intestinal bacteria in preparation for bowel surgery.

- Postoperatively, examine wound dressing frequently during first 24 hours, checking for infection, dehiscence, hemorrhage, and excessive edema. Rectal bleeding must be reported immediately.
- Assess abdomen including bowel sounds and abdominal girth.
- Frequent activity (i.e., turning every 2 hours, coughing and deep breathing, and early ambulation) can reduce risk of pulmonary complications of atelectasis and pneumonia.

PROMOTING HOME- AND COMMUNITY-BASED CARE

Educating Patients About Self-Care
- Assess patient's need and desire for information, and provide information to patient and family (see "Providing Emotional Support" earlier under "Nursing Interventions").
- Provide patients being discharged with specific information relevant to their needs.
- If patient has an ostomy, include information about ostomy care and complications to observe for, including obstruction, infection, stoma stenosis, retraction or prolapse, and peristomal skin irritation.
- Provide dietary instructions to help patient identify and eliminate foods that can cause diarrhea or constipation.
- Provide patient with a list of prescribed medications, with information on action, purpose, and possible side effects.
- Demonstrate and review treatments and dressing changes, stoma care, and ostomy irrigations, and encourage family to participate.
- Provide patient with specific directions about when to call his or her primary care provider and what complications require prompt attention (e.g., bleeding, abdominal distention and rigidity, diarrhea, fever, wound drainage, and disruption of suture line).
- Review side effects of radiation therapy (anorexia, vomiting, diarrhea, and exhaustion) if necessary.

Continuing Care
- Refer patient for home nursing care and WOC nurse as indicated.
- Provide patient and family with local resources for additional support (i.e., ostomy support group).

Evaluation

EXPECTED PATIENT OUTCOMES

- Consumes a healthy diet and maintains fluid balance
- Experiences reduced anxiety
- Acquires information about diagnosis, surgical procedure, preoperative preparation, and self-care after discharge
- Maintains clean incision, stoma, and perineal wound
- Verbalizes feelings and concerns about self
- Recovers without complications

For more information, see Chapter 48 in Hinkle, J. L., & Cheever, K. H. (2014). *Brunner and Suddarth's textbook of medical-surgical nursing* (13th ed.). Philadelphia: Lippincott Williams & Wilkins.

Cancer of the Endometrium

Cancer of the uterine endometrium (fundus or corpus) is the fourth most common cancer in women, with more than 42,100 new cases of uterine cancer diagnosed each year. The disease occurs twice as often in Caucasian women as compared to African American women; however, African American women have a less favorable prognosis. Cumulative exposure to estrogen (without the use of progestin) is considered the major risk factor. Other risk factors include age above 55 years, obesity, early menarche, late menopause, nulliparity, anovulation, infertility, and diabetes as well as use of tamoxifen.

Pathophysiology

Most uterine cancers are endometrioid (i.e., originating in the lining of the uterus). Type 1, which accounts for 80% of cases, is estrogen related and occurs in younger, obese, and perimenopausal women; it is usually low grade with a favorable outcome. Type 2, which occurs in about 10% of cases, is high grade and usually serous cell or clear cell; older women and African American women are at higher risk for type 2. Type 3, which also occurs in about 10% of cases, is the hereditary or genetic type, some of which cases are related to the Lynch II syndrome (also known as *hereditary non-polyposis colorectal cancer* and associated with the occurrence of breast, ovarian, colon, endometrial, and other cancers throughout a family).

C

Clinical Manifestations

Irregular bleeding and postmenopausal bleeding raise suspicion of endometrial cancer.

Assessment and Diagnostic Findings

- Perform annual checkups and gynecologic examination.
- Endometrial aspiration or biopsy is performed with peri-menopausal or menopausal bleeding.
- Transvaginal ultrasonography is useful.

Medical Management

Treatment consists of surgical staging, total or radical hysterectomy, and bilateral salpingo-oophorectomy and node sampling. Cancer antigen 125 (CA125) levels must be monitored, because elevated levels are a significant predictor of extrauterine disease or metastasis. Adjuvant radiation may be used in a patient who is considered high risk. Recurrent lesions in the vagina are treated with surgery and radiation. Recurrent lesions beyond the vagina are treated with hormonal therapy or chemotherapy. Progestin therapy is used frequently.

Nursing Management

See "Nursing Process" under Cancer of the Cervix for additional information.

For more information, see Chapter 57 in Hinkle, J. L., & Cheever, K. H. (2014). *Brunner and Suddarth's textbook of medical-surgical nursing* (13th ed.). Philadelphia: Lippincott Williams & Wilkins.

Cancer of the Esophagus

Carcinoma of the esophagus is usually of the squamous cell epidermoid type; the incidence of adenocarcinoma of the esophagus is increasing in the United States. Tumor cells may involve the esophageal mucosa and muscle layers and can spread to the lymphatics; in later stages, they may obstruct the esophagus, perforate the mediastinum, or erode into the great vessels.

Risk Factors

- Gender (male)
- Race (African American)
- Age (greater risk in fifth decade of life)
- Geographic locale (much higher incidence in China and northern Iran)
- Chronic esophageal irritation

- Use of alcohol and tobacco
- Gastroesophageal reflux disease (GERD)
- Other possible factors: chronic ingestion of hot liquids or foods, nutritional deficiencies, poor oral hygiene, and exposure to nitrosamines in the environment or food

Clinical Manifestations
- Usual presentation: advanced ulcerated lesion of the esophagus
- Dysphagia present, first with solid foods and eventually liquids
- Sensation of a mass in the throat and painful swallowing
- Substernal pain or fullness; regurgitation of undigested food with halitosis and hiccups later
- Hemorrhage; progressive loss of weight and strength from inadequate nutrition

Assessment and Diagnostic Findings
Esophagogastroduodenoscopy (EGD) with biopsy and brushings confirms the diagnosis most often. Other studies include CT of chest and abdomen, position emission tomography, endoscopic ultrasound, and exploratory laparoscopy.

Medical Management
Treatment of esophageal cancer is directed toward cure if cancer is in early stage; in late stages, palliation is the goal of therapy. Each patient is approached in a way that appears best for him or her.

- Surgery (e.g., esophagectomy), radiation, chemotherapy, or a combination of these modalities, depending on extent of disease
- Palliative treatment to maintain esophageal patency: dilation of the esophagus, laser therapy, placement of an endoprosthesis (stent), radiation, and chemotherapy

Nursing Management
See "Nursing Management" under Cancer for additional information. Intervention for esophageal cancer is directed toward improving the patient's nutritional and physical status in preparation for surgery, radiation therapy, or chemotherapy.

- Promote weight gain based on a high-calorie and high-protein diet, in liquid or soft form, if adequate food can be taken by mouth; if this is not possible, initiate parenteral or enteral nutrition.

- Monitor nutritional status throughout treatment.
- Inform patient about postoperative equipment that will be used, including closed chest drainage, nasogastric suction, parenteral fluid therapy, and gastric intubation.
- Place patient in a low Fowler's position after recovery from anesthesia and later in a Fowler's position.
- Observe patient carefully for regurgitation and dyspnea.
- Implement vigorous pulmonary plan of care to include incentive spirometry, sitting up in a chair and, if necessary, nebulizer treatments; avoid chest physiotherapy due to the risk of aspiration.
- Monitor drainage from cervical neck wound and patient's temperature to detect any elevation that may indicate an esophageal leak.
- Maintain nothing by mouth; parenteral or enteral support is warranted.
- Monitor for and treat cardiac complications, especially atrial fibrillation.
- Encourage patient to swallow small sips of water once feeding begins. Eventually, the diet is advanced as tolerated to a soft, mechanical diet; discontinue parenteral fluids when appropriate.
- Maintain patient in upright position for at least 2 hours after eating to allow the food to move through the GI tract.
- Involve family to prepare home-cooked favorite foods to help the patient eat; antacids may help patients with gastric distress; metoclopramide (Reglan) is useful in promoting gastric motility.
- Provide liquid supplements if esophagitis occurs; may be more easily tolerated. (Avoid supplements such as Boost and Ensure because they promote vagotomy syndrome [dumping syndrome].)
- Provide oral suction if patient cannot handle oral secretions or place a wick-type gauze at the corner of the mouth to direct secretions to a dressing or emesis basin.
- Instruct the family about ways to promote nutrition, what observations to make, what measures to take if complications occur, how to keep patient comfortable, and how to obtain needed physical and emotional support.

For more information, see Chapter 46 in Hinkle, J. L., & Cheever, K. H. (2014). *Brunner and Suddarth's textbook of medical-surgical nursing* (13th ed.). Philadelphia: Lippincott Williams & Wilkins.

Cancer of the Kidneys (Renal Tumors)

According to the American Cancer Society (2012), renal cancer accounts for about 5% of all cancers in the United States. The most common type of renal carcinoma arises from the renal epithelium and accounts for more than 85% of all kidney tumors. These tumors may metastasize early to the lungs, bone, liver, brain, and contralateral kidney. One-fourth of patients have metastatic disease at the time of diagnosis. Risk factors include gender (male), tobacco use, occupational exposure to industrial chemicals, obesity, unopposed estrogen therapy, and polycystic kidney disease.

Clinical Manifestations

- Many tumors produce no symptoms and are discovered as a palpable abdominal mass on routine examination.
- The classic triad, occurring in only 10% of patients, is hematuria, pain, and a mass in the flank.
- The sign that usually first calls attention to the tumor is painless hematuria, either intermittent and microscopic or continuous and gross.
- Dull pain occurs in the back from pressure due to compression of the ureter, extension of the tumor, or hemorrhage into the kidney tissue.
- Colicky pains occur if a clot or mass of tumor cells passes down the ureter.
- Symptoms from metastasis may be the first manifestation of renal tumor, including unexplained weight loss, increasing weakness, and anemia.

Assessment and Diagnostic Findings

- IV urography
- Cystoscopic examination
- Renal angiograms
- Ultrasonography
- CT scan

Medical Management

The goal of management is to detect the tumor early and to eradicate these slow-growing tumors before metastasis occurs.

- Radical nephrectomy is the preferred treatment, including removal of the kidney (and tumor), adrenal gland, surrounding fat and Gerota's fascia, and lymph nodes.
- Laparoscopic nephrectomy can be performed for removal of the kidney with a small tumor.

C

- Radiation therapy, hormonal therapy, or chemotherapy may be used with surgery.
- Immunotherapy may be helpful; allogeneic stem cell transplantation may be indicated if no response to immunotherapy.
- Nephron-sparing surgery (partial nephrectomy) may be used for patients with small local tumors or solid renal lesions.
- Laparoscopic nephroureterectomy may be performed for patients with upper tract transitional cell carcinoma.
- Renal artery embolization may be used in patients with metastatic renal carcinoma to impede the blood supply to the tumor and kill the tumor cells. Postinfarction syndrome occurs, lasting 2 to 3 days (flank and abdominal pain, elevated temperature, and GI complaints).
- Biological response modifiers such as interleukin-2 (IL-2) or interferon may be used.

Nursing Management

See "Nursing Management" under Cancer for additional information.

- Monitor for infection at surgical incision from use of immunosuppressant agents and maintain a patent urinary catheter.
- Monitor urine output and adequate measurement.
- After surgery, provide frequent analgesia for pain and muscle soreness.
- If postinfarction syndrome occurs, treat pain with parenteral analgesic agents and administer acetaminophen (Tylenol) to control fever; provide antiemetic medications, restrict oral intake, and provide IV fluids to treat the GI symptoms.
- Assist patient with turning, coughing, use of incentive spirometry, and deep breathing to prevent atelectasis and other pulmonary complications.
- Support patient and family in coping with diagnosis and uncertainties about outcome and uncertain prognosis.
- Educate patient to inspect and care for the incision and perform other general postoperative care.
- Inform patient of limitations on activities, lifting, and driving.
- Educate patient about correct use of pain medications.
- Provide instructions about follow-up care and need to notify physician about fever, breathing difficulty, wound drainage, blood in urine, pain, or swelling of the legs.

- Encourage patient to eat a healthy diet and to drink adequate liquids to avoid constipation and to maintain an adequate urine volume.
- Educate patient and family in need for follow-up care to detect signs of metastases; evaluate all subsequent symptoms with possible metastases in mind.
- Reinforce need for yearly physical examination and chest x-ray throughout life, which are required for patients who have had surgery for renal carcinoma.
- With follow-up chemotherapy, educate patient and family thoroughly, including treatment plan or chemotherapy protocol, what to expect with visits, and how to notify the physician. Explain the need for periodic evaluation of renal function (creatinine clearance, blood urea nitrogen, and creatinine).
- Refer to home care nurse as needed to monitor and support patient and coordinate services and resources needed.

For more information, see Chapter 54 in Hinkle, J. L., & Cheever, K. H. (2014). *Brunner and Suddarth's textbook of medical-surgical nursing* (13th ed.). Philadelphia: Lippincott Williams & Wilkins.

Cancer of the Larynx

Cancer of the larynx accounts for approximately half of all head and neck cancers. Almost all malignant tumors of the larynx arise from the surface epithelium and are classified as squamous cell carcinoma. Risk factors include male gender, age ≥65 years, tobacco use (including smokeless), alcohol use, vocal straining, chronic laryngitis, occupational exposure to carcinogens, nutritional deficiencies (riboflavin), and family predisposition.

Clinical Manifestations
- Hoarseness of >2 weeks' duration, noted early with cancer in glottic area; harsh, raspy, low-pitched voice
- Persistent cough; pain and burning in the throat when drinking hot liquids or citrus juices
- Lump felt in the neck
- Late symptoms: dysphagia, dyspnea, unilateral nasal obstruction or discharge, persistent hoarseness or ulceration, and foul breath
- Enlarged cervical nodes, unintentional weight loss, general debility, and pain radiating to the ear with possible metastasis

C

Assessment and Diagnostic Findings
- Complete history to identify risk factors, family history, and underlying medical conditions
- Physical examination of head and neck
- Indirect laryngoscopy
- Endoscopy, virtual endoscopy, barium swallow, optical imaging, CT, MRI, (to assess regional adenopathy, soft tissue involvement, and tumor staging), and a positron emission tomography scan (to detect recurrence of tumor after treatment)
- Direct laryngoscopic examination under local or general anesthesia
- Fine-needle aspiration biopsy of suspicious tissue

Medical Management
- The goals of treatment of laryngeal cancer include cure, preservation of safe effective swallowing, preservation of useful voice, and avoidance of permanent tracheostoma.
- Treatment options include surgery, radiation therapy, and adjuvant chemoradiation, or combinations.
- Before treatment begins, a complete dental examination is performed to rule out oral disease. Dental problems should be resolved before surgery and after radiation therapy.
- Radiation therapy provides excellent results in early-stage glottic tumors and lesions without lymph node involvement, when only one cord is affected and mobile; may be used preoperatively to reduce tumor size, combined with surgery and adjuvant chemotherapy in advanced laryngeal cancer (stages III and IV), or as a palliative measure.

Surgical Management
- Surgical procedures for early-stage tumors may include transoral endoscopic laser resection, classic open vertical hemilaryngectomy for glottic tumors, or classic horizontal supraglottic laryngectomy.
- Other surgical options include the following:
  - Vocal cord stripping: used to treat dysplasia, hyperkeratosis, and leukoplakia; often curative for these lesions
  - Cordectomy: for lesions limited to the middle third of the vocal cord
  - Laser surgery: for treatment of early glottic cancers
  - Partial laryngectomy: recommended in early stages of glottic cancer with only one vocal cord involved; high cure rate

- Total laryngectomy: can provide the desired cure in most advanced stage IV laryngeal cancers, when the tumor extends beyond the vocal cords, or for cancer that recurs or persists after radiation therapy; results in total loss of voice and permanent tracheostomy
- Speech therapy should be undertaken when indicated: esophageal speech, artificial larynx (electrolarynx), or tracheo-esophageal puncture.

NURSING PROCESS

The Patient Undergoing Laryngectomy

Assessment

- Obtain a health history and assess patient's physical, psycho-social, and spiritual domains including assessment of general state of nutrition and pattern of alcohol intake.
- Assess for hoarseness, sore throat, dyspnea, dysphagia, or pain and burning in the throat.
- Perform a thorough head and neck examination; palpate the neck and thyroid for swelling, nodularity, or adenopathy.
- Assess patient's ability to hear, see, read, and write and obtain evaluation by speech therapist if indicated.
- Determine the nature of surgery; assess patient's psycho-logical status; evaluate patient's and family's coping methods preoperatively and postoperatively; and provide effective support.

Diagnosis

NURSING DIAGNOSES
Based on all the assessment data, major nursing diagnoses may include the following:

- Deficient knowledge about the surgical procedure and post-operative course
- Anxiety and depression related to the diagnosis of cancer and impending surgery
- Ineffective airway clearance related to excess mucus production secondary to surgical alterations in the airway
- Impaired verbal communication related to anatomic deficit secondary to removal of the larynx and to edema

C

- Imbalanced nutrition: less than body requirements, related to inability to ingest food secondary to swallowing difficulties
- Disturbed body image and low self-esteem secondary to major neck surgery, change in appearance, and altered structure and function
- Self-care deficit related to pain, weakness, and fatigue and musculoskeletal impairment related to surgical procedure and postoperative course

COLLABORATIVE PROBLEMS/POTENTIAL COMPLICATIONS

Based on assessment data, potential complications that may develop include the following:

- Respiratory distress (hypoxia, airway obstruction, tracheal edema)
- Hemorrhage, infection, wound breakdown
- Aspiration
- Tracheostomal stenosis

Planning and Goals

The major goals for the patient may include knowledge about treatment, reduced anxiety, maintenance of a patent airway, effective use of alternative means of communication, optimal levels of nutrition and hydration, improvement in body image and self-esteem, improved self-care management, and absence of complications.

Nursing Interventions

PROVIDING PREOPERATIVE PATIENT EDUCATION

- Clarify any misconceptions and give patient and family educational materials about surgery (written and audiovisual) for review and reinforcement.
- Explain to patient that natural voice will be lost if complete laryngectomy is planned.
- Assure patient that much can be done through training in a rehabilitation program.
- Review equipment and treatments that will be part of postoperative care.
- Teach coughing and deep-breathing exercises and provide for return demonstration.

REDUCING ANXIETY

- Assess patient's psychological preparation and give patient and family opportunity to verbalize feelings and share

perceptions; give patient and family complete, concise answers to questions.
- Arrange a visit from a postlaryngectomy patient to help patient cope with the situation and know that rehabilitation is possible.
- Learn from patient what activities promote feelings of comfort and assist patient in such activities (e.g., listening to music, reading); relaxation techniques such as guided imagery and meditation are often helpful.

MAINTAINING A PATENT AIRWAY
- Position patient in semi-Fowler's or Fowler's position after recovery from anesthesia.
- Observe patient for restlessness, labored breathing, apprehension, and increased pulse rate, which may indicate possible respiratory or circulatory problems; assess lung sounds and report changes that may indicate impending complications.
- Use medications, particularly opioids, which depress respirations with caution; however, adequate use of analgesic medications is essential, as postoperative pain can result in shallow breathing and ineffective cough.
- Encourage patient to turn, cough, and deep breathe; suction if necessary; encourage early ambulation.
- Care for the laryngectomy tube in the same way as for a tracheostomy tube; humidification and suctioning are essential if there is no inner cannula.
- Keep stoma clean by cleansing daily as prescribed, and wipe opening clean as needed after coughing.
- Ensure adequate humidification of the environment to decrease cough, mucus production, and crusting around stoma.

PROMOTING ALTERNATIVE COMMUNICATION METHODS
- Work with patient, speech therapist, and family to encourage use of alternative communication methods; these methods must be used consistently postoperatively.
- Provide patient with a call or hand bell; a Magic Slate may be used for communication.
- Use nonwriting arm for IV infusions.
- If patient cannot write, a picture–word–phrase board, hand-held electronic device, or hand signals can be used.
- Provide adequate time for patient to communicate his or her needs.

C

Promoting Adequate Nutrition and Hydration

- Maintain patient *non per os* (nothing by mouth) for at least 7 days and provide alternative sources of nutrition as ordered: IV fluids, enteral feedings, and parenteral nutrition; explain nutritional plan to patient and family.
- Once patient is cleared to begin oral feedings, start oral feedings with thick fluids for easy swallowing; instruct patient to avoid sweet foods, which increase salivation and suppress appetite; introduce solid foods as tolerated.
- Instruct patient to rinse mouth with warm water or mouthwash and brush teeth frequently.
- Observe patient for difficulty in swallowing (particularly with eating); report occurrence to physician.
- Monitor patient's weight and laboratory data to ensure nutritional and fluid intake are adequate; monitor skin turgor and vital signs for signs of decreased fluid volume.

Improving Self-Concept and Promoting
Self-Care Management

- Encourage patient to express feelings about changes from surgery (e.g., fear, anger, depression, and isolation); encourage use of previous effective coping strategies; be a good listener and support the family.
- Refer patient to a support group, such as the International Association of Laryngectomees, WebWhispers, and I Can Cope.
- Use a positive approach; promote participation in self-care activities as soon as possible.

Monitoring and Managing Potential Postoperative
Complications

Potential complications after laryngectomy include respiratory distress and hypoxia, hemorrhage, infection, wound breakdown, aspiration, and tracheostomal stenosis.

- Monitor patient for signs and symptoms of respiratory distress and hypoxia, particularly restlessness, irritation, agitation, confusion, tachypnea, use of accessory muscles, and decreased oxygen saturation on pulse oximetry (SpO_2); always be prepared for possible intubation and mechanical ventilation.
- Monitor patient's vital signs for changes: increase in pulse, decrease in blood pressure, or rapid, deep respirations.

C

- Cold, clammy, pale skin may indicate active bleeding; notify surgeon promptly of any active bleeding.
- Observe patient for early signs and symptoms of infection: increase in temperature or pulse, change in type of wound drainage, increased areas of redness or tenderness at surgical site, purulent drainage, odor, and increase in wound drainage; monitor white blood cell (WBC) count.
- Observe the stoma area for wound breakdown, hematoma, and bleeding and report significant changes to the surgeon.
- Monitor patient carefully, particularly for carotid hemorrhage.
- Elevate the head of the bed at least 30 degrees during oral and tube feedings and for 30 to 45 minutes afterward.
- Monitor patient for possible reflux and aspiration; keep suction equipment available.
- Perform tracheostomy care routinely.

 Gerontologic Considerations

In older adult patients, infection can be present without an increase in the patient's WBC count; therefore, the nurse must monitor the patient for more subtle signs, such as lethargy, weakness, and decreased appetite.

> **Quality and Safety Nursing Alert**
>
> Postoperatively, be alert for the possible serious complications of rupture of the carotid artery. Should this occur, apply direct pressure over the artery, summon assistance, and provide psychological support until the vessel can be ligated.

PROMOTING HOME- AND COMMUNITY-BASED CARE
Educating Patients About Self-Care
- Provide discharge instructions as soon as patient is able to participate; assess readiness to learn.
- Assess patient's knowledge about self-care management; reassure patient and family that strategies can be mastered.
- Give patient specific information about tracheostomy and stomal care, wound care, and oral hygiene, including suctioning and emergency measures; instruct the patient about the need for adequate dietary intake, safe hygiene, and recreational activities.
- Instruct patient to provide adequate humidification of the environment, minimize air-conditioning, and drink fluids.

C

- Educate patient to take precautions when showering to prevent water from getting into the stoma.
- Discourage swimming, because the patient with a laryngectomy can drown.
- Recommend that patient avoid getting hair spray, loose hair, and powder into stoma.
- Educate patient and caregiver regarding the signs and symptoms of infection and identify indications that require contacting the physician after discharge.
- Stress that activity should be undertaken in moderation; when tired, the patient will have more difficulty in speaking with the new voice.
- Instruct patient to wear or carry medical identification, such as a bracelet or card, to alert medical personnel to the special requirements for resuscitation should this need arise.

Continuing Care
- Refer to a home care agency for patient and family assistance, follow-up assessment, and teaching.
- Encourage patient to visit physician regularly for physical examinations and advice.
- Remind patient to participate in health promotion activities and health screening.

Evaluation

EXPECTED PATIENT OUTCOMES
- Demonstrates an adequate level of knowledge, verbalizing an understanding of the surgical procedure, and performing self-care adequately
- Demonstrates less anxiety and is aware of community resources to provide support
- Maintains a clear airway and handles own secretions
- Demonstrates practical, safe, and correct technique for cleaning and changing the tracheostomy or laryngectomy tube
- Acquires effective communication techniques
- Maintains adequate nutrition and fluid intake
- Exhibits improved body image, self-esteem, and self-concept
- Exhibits no complications
- Adheres to rehabilitation and home care program

For more information, see Chapter 22 in Hinkle, J. L., & Cheever, K. H. (2014). *Brunner and Suddarth's textbook of medical-surgical nursing* (13th ed.). Philadelphia: Lippincott Williams & Wilkins.

Cancer of the Liver

C

Hepatic tumors may be malignant or benign. Benign liver tumors were uncommon until oral contraceptives were in widespread use. Now benign liver tumors such as hepatic adenomas occur most frequently in women who are in their reproductive years and taking oral contraceptives. Few cancers originate in the liver. Primary liver tumors usually are associated with chronic liver disease, hepatitis B and C, and cirrhosis. Hepatocellular carcinoma (HCC), the most common type of primary liver tumor, usually cannot be resected because of rapid growth and metastasis elsewhere. Other types include cholangiocellular carcinoma and combined hepatocellular and cholangiocellular carcinoma. If found early, resection may be possible; however, early detection is unlikely.

Cirrhosis, chronic infection with hepatitis B and C, and exposure to certain chemical toxins have been implicated as causes of HCC. Cigarette smoking, especially when combined with alcohol use, has also been identified as a risk factor. Other substances that have been implicated include aflatoxins and other similar toxic molds that can contaminate food such as ground nuts and grains and may act as co-carcinogens with hepatitis B. Metastases from other primary sites, particularly the digestive system, breast, and lung, are found in the liver 2.5 times more frequently than tumors due to primary liver cancers.

Clinical Manifestations
- Early manifestations include pain (dull ache in upper right quadrant, epigastrium, or back), weight loss, loss of strength, anorexia, and anemia.
- Liver enlargement and irregular surface may be noted on palpation.
- Jaundice is present only if larger bile ducts are occluded.
- Ascites develops if such nodules obstruct the portal veins or if tumor tissue is seeded in the peritoneal cavity.

Assessment and Diagnostic Findings
Diagnosis is made on the basis of clinical signs and symptoms, history and physical examination, and results of laboratory and x-ray studies, PET scans, liver scans, CT scans, ultrasound, MRI, arteriography, laparoscopy, or biopsy. Leukocytosis, erythrocytosis, hypercalcemia, hypoglycemia, and hypocholesterolemia also be seen on laboratory assessment. Elevated levels of

serum alpha-fetoprotein (AFP) and carcinoembryonic antigen (CEA) may be found.

Medical Management

Radiation Therapy

- IV or intra-arterial injection of antibodies tagged with radioactive isotopes that specifically attack tumor-associated antigens
- Percutaneous placement of a high-intensity source for interstitial radiation therapy

Chemotherapy

- Systemic chemotherapy; embolization of tumor vessels with chemotherapy
- An implantable pump to deliver high-concentration chemotherapy to the liver through the hepatic artery in cases of metastatic disease

Percutaneous Biliary Drainage

- Percutaneous biliary or transhepatic drainage is used to bypass biliary ducts obstructed by the liver, pancreatic, or bile ducts in patients with inoperable tumors or those who are poor surgical risks.
- Complications include sepsis, leakage of bile, hemorrhage, and reobstruction of the biliary system.
- Observe patient for fever and chills, bile drainage around the catheter, changes in vital signs, and evidence of biliary obstruction, including increased pain or pressure, pruritus, and recurrence of jaundice.

Other Nonsurgical Treatments

- Laser hyperthermia has been used to treat hepatic metastases.
- Heat has been directed to tumors to cause necrosis of the tumors while sparing normal tissue through several methods: radiofrequency thermal ablation inserted into the liver tumor and radiofrequency energy, which causes tumor cell death from coagulation necrosis.
- Immunotherapy may be used: Lymphocytes with antitumor reactivity are administered.
- Transcatheter arterial embolization results in ischemia and necrosis of the tumor.
- For multiple small lesions, ultrasound-guided injection of alcohol promotes dehydration of tumor cells and tumor necrosis.

Surgical Management

Hepatic resection can be performed when the primary hepatic tumor is localized or when the primary site can be completely excised and the metastasis is limited. Capitalizing on the regenerative capacity of the liver cells, surgeons have successfully removed 90% of the liver. The presence of cirrhosis limits the ability of the liver to regenerate. In preparation for surgery, the patient's nutritional, fluid, and general physical status are assessed, and efforts are undertaken to ensure the best physical condition possible.

- Lobectomy: Removal of a lobe of the liver is the most common surgical procedure for excising a liver tumor.
- Local ablation: For patients who are not candidates for resection or transplantation, ablation of HCC may be accomplished by chemicals such as ethanol or by physical means such as radiofrequency ablation or microwave coagulation.
- Immunotherapy: Interferon may be used after surgical resection for HCC to prevent recurrence of the lesion related to hepatitis B or C.
- Liver transplantation: Removing the liver and replacing it with a healthy donor organ is another way to treat liver cancer.

Nursing Management: Postoperative

See "Nursing Management" under Cancer for additional information.

- Provide close monitoring and care for the first 2 or 3 days.
- Assess for problems related to cardiopulmonary involvement, vascular complications, and respiratory and liver dysfunction.
- Monitor metabolic abnormalities (glucose, protein, and lipids).
- Instruct patient and family about care of the biliary catheter and the potential complications and side effects of hepatic artery chemotherapy.
- Educate patient about the importance of follow-up visits to permit frequent checks on the response of patient and tumor to chemotherapy, condition of the implanted pump site, and any toxic effects.
- Refer patient for home care.
- Encourage patient to resume routine activities as soon as possible, while cautioning about activities that may damage the pump or site.

C

- Provide reassurance and instruction to patient and family to reduce fear that the percutaneous biliary drainage catheter will fall out.
- Provide verbal and written instructions as well as demonstration of biliary catheter care to patient and family; instruct in techniques to keep catheter site clean and dry, to assess the catheter and its insertion site, and to irrigate the catheter to prevent debris and promote patency.
- Collaborate with the health care team, patient, and family to identify and implement pain management strategies and approaches to management of other problems: weakness, pruritus, inadequate dietary intake, jaundice, and symptoms associated with metastasis.
- Assist patient and family in making decisions about hospice care and initiate referrals. Encourage patient to discuss end-of-life care preferences with family and health care providers.

For more information, see Chapter 49 in Hinkle, J. L., & Cheever, K. H. (2014). *Brunner and Suddarth's textbook of medical-surgical nursing* (13th ed.). Philadelphia: Lippincott Williams & Wilkins.

Cancer of the Lung
(Bronchogenic Carcinoma)

Lung cancers arise from a single transformed epithelial cell in the tracheobronchial airways. The most common cause of lung cancer is inhaled carcinogens. A carcinogen (e.g., cigarette smoke, radon gas, other occupational and environmental agents) damages the cell, causing abnormal growth and development into a malignant tumor. Most lung cancers are classified into one of two major categories: small cell lung cancer (SCLC; 10% to 20% of tumors) and non–small cell lung cancer (NSCLC; approximately 85% to 90% of tumors). NSCLC cell types include squamous cell carcinoma (25% to 30%), which is usually more centrally located; large cell carcinoma (10% to 15%), which is fast-growing and tends to arise peripherally; and adenocarcinoma (40%), which presents as peripheral masses, often metastasizes, and includes bronchoalveolar carcinoma. Most small cell cancers arise in the major bronchi and spread by infiltration along the bronchial wall. In SCLC, the two general cell types include small cell and combined small cell. In addition to classification according to cell type, lung cancers are staged based on size, location, lymph node involvement, and whether cancer has spread.

Environmental risk factors include tobacco smoke, second-hand (passive) smoke, and environmental and occupational exposures. Other risk factors include male gender, genetic predisposition, dietary deficits, and underlying respiratory disease (e.g., chronic obstructive pulmonary disease and tuberculosis). The American Cancer Society (ACS) reports that smoking is responsible for approximately 78% of lung cancer in men and 44% in women. Smokers who use smokeless tobacco products increase their risk of lung cancer. Almost all cases of SCLC are due to cigarette smoking; however, passive smoking has been identified as a cause of lung cancer in nonsmokers.

Clinical Manifestations
- Lung cancer often develops insidiously and is asymptomatic until late in its course.
- Signs and symptoms depend on location, tumor size, degree of obstruction, and existence of metastases to regional or distant sites.
- The most common symptom is cough or change in a chronic cough.

> ### Quality and Safety Nursing Alert
>
> A cough that changes in character should arouse suspicion of lung cancer.

- Dyspnea is prominent early in the disease.
- Hemoptysis or blood-tinged sputum may be expectorated.
- Chest pain or shoulder pain may indicate chest wall or pleural involvement. Pain is a late symptom and may be related to bone metastasis.
- Recurring fever may be an early symptom.
- Chest pain, tightness, hoarseness, dysphagia, head and neck edema, and symptoms of pleural or pericardial infusion exist if the tumor spreads to adjacent structures and lymph nodes.
- Common sites of metastases are lymph nodes, bone, brain, contralateral lung, adrenal glands, and liver.
- Weakness, anorexia, and weight loss may be present.

Assessment and Diagnostic Findings

- Assess history of smoking (past and current) and presence of relevant risk factors.
- Obtain chest x-ray, CT scans, bone scans, abdominal scans, MRI or PET scans, and liver ultrasound.
- Perform sputum examinations, fiberoptic bronchoscopy, transthoracic fine-needle aspiration, endoscopy with esophageal ultrasound, mediastinoscopy or mediastinotomy, and endobronchial ultrasound biopsy.
- Conduct pulmonary function tests, arterial blood gas (ABG) analysis, ventilation–perfusion (V̇/Q̇) scans, and exercise testing.
- Staging of the tumor refers to the size of the tumor, its location, whether lymph nodes are involved, and whether the cancer has spread. (See "Tumor Staging and Grading" under Cancer for additional information.)

Medical Management

See "Medical Management" under Cancer for additional information.

- The objective of management is to provide a cure if possible. Treatment depends on cell type, stage of the disease, and patient's physiologic status.
- Treatment may involve surgery (preferred), radiation therapy, or chemotherapy—or a combination of these. Newer and more specific therapies to modulate the immune system (e.g., gene therapy, therapy with defined tumor antigens or growth factor receptor inhibitors) are under study and show promise.

Surgical Management

- Surgery is the preferred method for treating localized NSCLC without metastasis in the face of adequate cardiopulmonary function. The cure rate depends on type and stage of cancer.
- The most common surgical procedure for a small tumor is lobectomy; in some cases, an entire lung may be removed (pneumonectomy).

Radiation Therapy

- Radiation therapy may offer a cure for a small percentage of patients; it is also used to reduce tumor size, relieve symptoms and, sometimes, as a prophylaxis to treat microscopic metastases to the brain.
- Radiation treatment is toxic to normal tissue within the radiation field; complications include esophagitis, pneumonitis, and radiation lung fibrosis.

Chemotherapy
Chemotherapy is used to alter tumor growth patterns, to treat distant metastases or as an adjunct to surgery and radiation.

Palliative Therapy
Palliative care, concurrent with standard oncologic care for lung cancer, should be considered early in the course of illness for any patient with metastatic cancer or high symptom burden.

Nursing Management
See "Nursing Management" under Cancer for additional information.

Managing Symptoms
Educate patient and family about the side effects of specific treatments and strategies to manage them.

Relieving Breathing Problems
- Maintain airway patency; remove secretions through deep-breathing exercises, chest physiotherapy, directed cough, suctioning and, in some instances, bronchoscopy.
- Administer bronchodilator medications; supplemental oxygen will probably be necessary.
- Encourage patient to assume positions that promote lung expansion and to perform breathing exercises.
- Educate patient about energy conservation and airway clearance techniques.
- Refer for pulmonary rehabilitation as indicated.

Reducing Fatigue
- Assess level of fatigue; identify potentially treatable causes.
- Educate the patient in energy conservation techniques and guided exercise as appropriate.
- Refer patient to physical or occupational therapist as indicated.

Providing Psychological Support
- Help patient and family deal with poor prognosis and relatively rapid progression of the disease (when indicated).
- Assist patient and family with informed decision making regarding treatment options.
- Suggest methods to maintain the patient's quality of life during the course of this disease.
- Support patient and family in end-of-life decisions and treatment options.
- Help to identify potential resources for the patient and family.

C

Gerontologic Considerations

- At time of diagnosis, most patients are older than 65 years and have advanced disease (Stage III or IV).
- Age is not a significant prognostic factor for overall survival for NSCLC or SCLC; however, adjustments to treatments may need to be made based on the presence of comorbidities and the patient's cognitive, functional, nutritional, and social status.

For more information, see Chapter 23 in Hinkle, J. L., & Cheever, K. H. (2014). *Brunner and Suddarth's textbook of medical-surgical nursing* (13th ed.). Philadelphia: Lippincott Williams & Wilkins.

Cancer of the Oral Cavity and Pharynx

Cancer of the oral cavity and pharynx can occur in any part of the mouth (lips, lateral tongue, floor of mouth [most common]) or throat and is highly curable if discovered early. Risk factors for cancer of the oral cavity and pharynx include cigarette, cigar, and pipe smoking; use of smokeless tobacco; excessive use of alcohol; and infection with the human papilloma virus (HPV). Oral cancers are often associated with the combined use of alcohol and tobacco. Other factors include gender (male), age (older than 50 years), and African American descent. Malignancies of the oral cavity are usually squamous cell cancers.

Clinical Manifestations

- Few or no symptoms; most commonly a painless sore or mass that will not heal
- May bleed easily and present as a red or white patch that persists
- Typical lesion: a painful indurated ulcer with raised edges
- As the cancer progresses, possible patient complaint of tenderness; difficulty in chewing, swallowing, or speaking; coughing of blood-tinged sputum; or enlarged cervical lymph nodes

Assessment and Diagnostic Findings

Oral examination, assessment of cervical lymph nodes, and biopsies of suspicious lesions (not healed within 2 weeks).

Medical Management

Management varies with the nature of the lesion, preference of the physician, and patient choice. Surgical resection, radiation therapy, chemotherapy, or a combination may be effective.

- For lip cancer, small lesions are excised liberally; larger lesions may be treated by radiation therapy.
- Tongue cancer is treated aggressively; recurrence rate is high. Radiation therapy and chemotherapy; surgical procedures include total glossectomy or hemiglossectomy.
- Radical neck dissection is used for metastases of oral cancer to lymphatic channel in the neck region with reconstructive surgery.

Nursing Management

Preoperative
- Assess patient's nutritional status; a dietary consultation may be necessary.
- Implement enteral (through the GI tract) or parenteral (IV) feedings as needed to maintain adequate nutrition.
- If a radial graft is needed, perform an Allen test on the donor arm to ensure that the ulnar artery is patent and can provide blood flow to the hand after removal of the radial artery.
- Assess patient's ability to communicate in writing as verbal communication may be impaired by radical surgery for oral cancer (provide a pen and paper after surgery to patients who can use them to communicate).
- Obtain a communication board with commonly used words or pictures (given after surgery to patients who cannot write so that they may point to needed items).
- Consult a speech therapist.

Postoperative
- Assess for a patent airway.
- Perform suctioning if patient is unable to manage oral secretions; if grafting was part of the surgery, suctioning must be performed with care to prevent damage to the graft.
- Assess the graft for viability; assess color (white may indicate arterial occlusion, and blue mottling may indicate venous congestion), although it can be difficult to assess the graft by looking into the mouth.
- A Doppler ultrasound device may be used to locate the radial pulse at the graft site and to assess graft perfusion.

For more information, see Chapter 46 in Hinkle, J. L., & Cheever, K. H. (2014). *Brunner and Suddarth's textbook of medical-surgical nursing* (13th ed.). Philadelphia: Lippincott Williams & Wilkins.

Cancer of the Ovary

Ovarian cancer is the leading cause of gynecological cancer deaths in the United States. Despite careful physical examination, ovarian tumors are often difficult to detect because they are usually deep in the pelvis. No definitive causative factors have been determined, but pregnancy and oral contraceptives appear to provide a protective effect. The incidence increases after 40 years of age, with the frequency highest in industrialized countries; it affects women of all races and ethnic backgrounds. A family history in a first-degree relative, older age, early menarche, late menopause, and obesity may increase the risk; however, the majority of patients have no known risk factors. In 5% to 10% of cases, ovarian cancer is familial and of these, most are associated with mutations in the BRCA1 gene (most commonly) and BRCA2 (less commonly).

Pathophysiology

Most ovarian cancers (90%) are epithelial in origin; other tumors include germ cell tumors and stromal tumors (10%). Ovarian tumors are classified as benign if there is no proliferation or invasion, borderline if there is proliferation but no invasion, and malignant if there is invasion.

Clinical Manifestations

- Increased abdominal girth, pelvic pressure, bloating, back pain, constipation, abdominal pain, urinary urgency, indigestion, flatulence, increased waist size, leg pain, and pelvic pain
- Vague gastrointestinal (GI) symptoms without a known cause
- Palpable ovary in a postmenopausal woman

Assessment and Diagnostic Findings

- No screening mechanism exists; tumor markers are being explored. Biannual pelvic examinations are recommended for at-risk women.
- Any enlarged ovary must be investigated; pelvic examination does not detect early ovarian cancer, and pelvic imaging techniques are not always definitive.
- Transvaginal and pelvic ultrasound, abdominal MRI, chest x-rays, and CA-125 antigen testing are helpful for high-risk women.

Medical Management

- Surgical removal is the treatment of choice.

C

- Preoperative workup can include a barium enema or colonoscopy, upper GI series, MRI, ultrasound, chest x-rays, IV urography, and CT scan.
- Staging of the tumor is performed using the tumor, nodes, and metastases (TNM) system to direct treatment.
- Likely treatment involves a total abdominal hysterectomy with removal of the fallopian tubes and ovaries and, possibly, the omentum (bilateral salpingo-oophorectomy and omentectomy); tumor debulking; para-aortic and pelvic lymph node sampling; diaphragmatic biopsies; random peritoneal biopsies; and cytologic washings.
- Chemotherapy uses a combination of taxane and platinum agents. The most common treatments are paclitaxel (Taxol) and carboplatin (Paraplatin).
- Newer treatments used in the case of recurrence are liposomal preparations, intraperitoneal drug administration, anticancer vaccines, monoclonal antibodies directed against cancer antigens, gene therapy, and antiangiogenic treatments.

Nursing Management
- Perform nursing measures, including treatments related to surgery, radiation, chemotherapy, and palliation. See "Nursing Management" under Cancer, and see Perioperative Nursing Management in Section P.
- Monitor for complications of therapy and abdominal surgery; report manifestations of complications to physician.
- Determine patient's emotional needs, including desire for childbearing. Provide emotional support by giving comfort, showing attentiveness, and caring. Allow patient to express feelings about condition and risk for death.

For more information, see Chapter 57 in Hinkle, J. L., & Cheever, K. H. (2014). *Brunner and Suddarth's textbook of medical-surgical nursing* (13th ed.). Philadelphia: Lippincott Williams & Wilkins.

Cancer of the Pancreas

Cancer may develop in the head, body, or tail of the pancreas. Symptoms vary depending on the location of the lesion and whether functioning insulin-secreting pancreatic islet cells are involved. Cancer of the pancreas is the fourth and fifth leading cause of cancer death in men and women, respectively. It is very rare before the age of 45 years, and most patients present in or beyond the sixth decade of life. Risk factors include cigarette smoking; exposure to industrial chemicals or toxins in the environment; and a diet high in fat, meat, or both. Pancreatic cancer is also associated with diabetes, chronic pancreatitis, and hereditary pancreatitis. Tumors that originate in the head of the pancreas are the most common and obstruct the common bile duct; functioning islet cell tumors are responsible for the syndrome of hyperinsulinism, particularly in islet cell tumors. The pancreas can also be the site of metastasis from other tumors. Pancreatic carcinoma has a 5% survival rate at 5 years, regardless of the stage of disease at diagnosis.

Clinical Manifestations

- Classic signs of pancreatic carcinoma are pain, jaundice, or both, which are present in more than 80% of patients and, along with weight loss, often do not appear until the disease is far advanced.
- Rapid, profound, and progressive weight loss occur.
- Vague upper or mid-abdominal pain or discomfort unrelated to any GI function; radiates as a boring pain in the midback and is more severe at night and when lying in the supine position; pain is often progressive and severe. Ascites is common.
- Symptoms of insulin deficiency (diabetes: glucosuria, hyperglycemia, and abnormal glucose tolerance) may be an early sign of carcinoma.
- Meals often aggravate epigastric pain; jaundice and pruritus.
- Malabsorption of nutrients and fat-soluble vitamins, anorexia and malaise, and clay-colored stools and dark urine are common with tumors in the head of the pancreas.
- Gastrointestinal x-rays may show deformities in adjacent viscera related to pancreatic mass.

Assessment and Diagnostic Findings

- Spiral (helical) CT is more than 85% to 90% accurate in the diagnosis and staging of pancreatic cancer and is currently the most useful preoperative imaging technique.
- MRI, endoscopic retrograde cholangiopancreatography (ERCP), endoscopic ultrasound (EUS), GI x-rays, percutaneous fine-needle biopsy, percutaneous transhepatic cholangiography, angiography, laparoscopy, or intraoperative ultrasonography may be useful.

- A glucose tolerance test can be used to diagnose a pancreatic islet tumor or neuroectodermal tumor.
- Tumor markers such as cancer antigen (CA) 19-9, carcino-embryonic antigen (CEA), and DU-PAN-2 are useful indicators of disease progression.

Medical Management

- Surgical procedure is extensive to remove resectable localized tumors (e.g., pancreatectomy, Whipple resection).
- Radiation and chemotherapy may be used; intraoperative radiation therapy (IORT) or interstitial implantation of radioactive sources may be used for pain relief.
- Diet high in protein with pancreatic enzymes, adequate hydration, vitamin K, and treatment of anemia with blood components and total parenteral nutrition may be instituted before surgery when indicated.
- Treatment is often limited to palliative measures owing to widespread metastases, especially to liver, lungs, and bones.
- A biliary stent may be used to relieve jaundice.

Nursing Management

See Perioperative Nursing Management in Section P for additional information.

- Provide preoperative patient and family education related to extent of surgery and alterations in pancreatic function.
- Provide pain management and attention to nutrition.
- Assist patient to explore all aspects and effects of radiation therapy, chemotherapy, or surgery on an individual basis.
- Provide skin care and measures to relieve pain and discomfort associated with jaundice, anorexia, and profound weight loss.
- Monitor patient postoperatively: vital signs, arterial blood gasses and pressures, pulse oximetry, laboratory values, and urine output.
- Provide emotional support to patient and family before, during, and after treatment.
- Discuss patient-controlled analgesia (PCA) for severe, escalating pain.
- If chemotherapy is elected, focus education on prevention of side effects and complications of agents used.
- If surgery was performed, educate patient about managing the drainage system and monitoring for complications.

- Educate patient and family about strategies to prevent skin breakdown and relieve pain, pruritus, and anorexia, including instruction about PCA, total parenteral nutrition, and diet modification with pancreatic enzymes if indicated because of malabsorption and hyperglycemia.
- Monitor serum glucose levels. Be alert for hypoglycemia in patient with pancreatic islet tumor. Administer glucose as prescribed.
- Discuss palliative care with patient and family to relieve discomfort, assist with care, and comply with end-of-life decisions.
- Educate family about changes in patient's status that should be reported to the health care provider.
- Refer patient for home care for help dealing with problems, discomforts, and psychological effects. Discharge to a long-term care setting with communication to staff about prior education.

For more information, see Chapter 50 in Hinkle, J. L., & Cheever, K. H. (2014). *Brunner and Suddarth's textbook of medical-surgical nursing* (13th ed.). Philadelphia: Lippincott Williams & Wilkins.

Cancer of the Prostate

Cancer of the prostate is the most common cancer in men (other than nonmelanoma skin cancer) and is the second most common cause of cancer deaths in American men. African American men are twice as likely than men of any other racial or ethnic group to die of prostate cancer. Risk factors include increasing age (older than 50 years), a family history of prostate cancer or *BRCA1* and *BRCA2* mutations and, possibly, a diet consisting of excessive red meat and dairy products that are high in fat. Endogenous hormones, such as androgens and estrogens, also may be associated with the development of prostate cancer. The rate of cure with early detection is high.

Pathophysiology

Prostate cancer develops when rates of cell division exceed that of cell growth resulting in uncontrolled growth in the prostate. Most prostate cancers (95%) are adenocarcinomas and are multifocal (e.g., arise from different tissues within the prostate). Prostate cancers may be locally invasive or metastatic to lymph nodes and bones.

Clinical Manifestations
- Usually asymptomatic in early stage; variable course
- Nodule felt within the substance of the gland or extensive hardening in the posterior lobe
- Sexual dysfunction common before diagnosis

Advanced Stage
- Lesion is stony hard and fixed.
- If large enough to encroach on bladder neck, obstructive symptoms (difficulty and frequency of urination, urinary retention, decreased size and force of urinary stream) will be seen.
- Blood in urine or semen and painful ejaculation occur.
- Symptoms of metastases include backache, hip pain, perineal and rectal discomfort, anemia, weight loss, weakness, nausea, oliguria, and spontaneous pathologic fractures; hematuria may result from urethral or bladder invasion.

Assessment and Diagnostic Findings
- Digital rectal examination (DRE; preferably by the same examiner) and prostate-specific antigen (PSA) level are used for screening.
- Transrectal ultrasound (TRUS); bone scans, skeletal x-rays, and MRI; pelvic CT scans; or radiolabeled monoclonal antibody-based imaging may also be used.
- The diagnosis is confirmed by a histologic examination of tissue removed surgically by transurethral resection of the prostate (TURP), open prostatectomy, ultrasound-guided transrectal needle biopsy, or fine-needle aspiration.
- Tumor cell types are graded using the Gleason score; an increase in Gleason score reflects increased tumor aggressiveness.

Medical Management
Treatment is based on the patient's life expectancy, symptoms, risk of recurrence after definitive treatment, size of the tumor, Gleason score, PSA level, likelihood of complications, and patient preference. Management can range from nonsurgical methods that involve "watchful waiting" to surgery (e.g., prostatectomy).

Surgical Management
- Surgical management includes TURP; prostatectomy via suprapubic, perineal, or retropubic approaches; transurethral incision of the prostate (TUIP); laparoscopic radical prostatectomy (including robotic-assisted laparoscopic

techniques); and pelvic node dissection (for staging or micro-scopic metastasis).

- Radical prostatectomy is considered first-line treatment for tumors confined to the prostate; this includes removal of the prostate, seminal vesicles, tips of the vas deferens, and often the surrounding fat, nerves, and blood vessels.
- Sexual impotency and various degrees of urinary inconti-nence commonly follow radical prostatectomy; lower mor-bidity and improved outcomes are noted with laparoscopic approaches.

Radiation Therapy

- Teletherapy (external-beam radiation therapy [EBRT]) is a treatment option for patients with low-risk prostate can-cer. A computer-controlled robotic radiosurgery system (CyberKnife®) is being evaluated in clinical trials for pros-tate cancer.
- Brachytherapy (internal implants) is a commonly used monotherapy treatment option for early, clinically organ-confined prostate cancer.
- Combination therapies (brachytherapy and EBRT) with or without adjuvant hormone therapy may be used for interme-diate risk.
- Side effects include inflammation of the rectum, bowel, and bladder (proctitis, enteritis, and cystitis); acute urinary dys-function; pain with urination and ejaculation; rectal urgency, diarrhea, and tenesmus; rectal proctitis, bleeding, and rectal fistula; painless hematuria; chronic interstitial cystitis; ure-thral stricture erectile dysfunction; and rarely, secondary can-cers of the rectum and bladder.

Hormone Therapy

- Androgen deprivation therapy (ADT) is accomplished either by surgical castration (bilateral orchiectomy, removal of the testes) or by medical castration with the administration of medications, such as luteinizing hormone–releasing hor-mone (LHRH) agonists (lueprolide [Lupton] and goserelin [Zoladex]). Antiandrogen receptor antagonists, including flu-tamide (Eulexin), bicalutamide (Casodex), and nilutamide (Nilandron), may be added.
- Hypogonadism is responsible for the adverse effects of ADT, which include vasomotor flushing, loss of libido, decreased bone density (resulting in osteoporosis and fractures),

anemia, fatigue, increased fat mass, lipid alterations, decreased muscle mass, gynecomastia (increased breast tissue), mastodynia (breast and nipple tenderness), increased risk of diabetes, metabolic syndrome, and cardiovascular disease.

Other Therapies

- Chemotherapy (docetaxel-based regimens)
- Cryosurgery for those who cannot physically tolerate surgery or for recurrence
- Repeated TURPs to keep urethra patent; suprapubic or transurethral catheter drainage when repeated TURP is impractical
- Opioid or nonopioid medications to control pain with metastasis to bone
- Blood transfusions to maintain adequate hemoglobin levels
- For metastatic prostate cancer nonresponsive to hormone therapy, possible benefit from a therapeutic cancer vaccine, Sipuleucel-T (Provenge; Dendreon Corp)
- Antiangiogenic and gene-based therapies emerging as adjuvant treatment options
- Various forms of complementary and alternative medicine, though data regarding efficacy are lacking

NURSING PROCESS

The Patient Undergoing Prostatectomy

Assessment

- Take a complete history, with emphasis on urinary function and the effect of the underlying disorder on patient's lifestyle.
- Note reports of urgency, frequency, nocturia, dysuria, urinary retention, hematuria, or decreased ability to initiate voiding.
- Note family history of cancer, heart disease, or kidney disease, including hypertension.

Diagnosis

PREOPERATIVE NURSING DIAGNOSES

- Anxiety related to inability to void
- Acute pain related to bladder distention
- Deficient knowledge of factors related to the disorder and treatment protocol

POSTOPERATIVE NURSING DIAGNOSES
• Acute pain related to surgical incision, catheter placement, and bladder spasms
• Deficient knowledge about postoperative care

COLLABORATIVE PROBLEMS/POTENTIAL COMPLICATIONS
• Hemorrhage and shock
• Infection
• Venous thromboembolism (VTE)
• Catheter obstruction
• Fluid volume imbalance
• Sexual dysfunction

Planning and Goals

The major preoperative goals for the patient may include reduced anxiety and learning about his prostate disorder and the perioperative experience. The major postoperative goals may include maintenance of fluid volume balance, relief of pain and discomfort, ability to perform self-care activities, and absence of complications.

Preoperative Nursing Interventions

REDUCING ANXIETY
• Clarify the nature of the surgery and expected postoperative outcomes.
• Provide privacy, and establish a trusting and professional relationship.
• Encourage patient to discuss feelings and concerns.

RELIEVING DISCOMFORT
• While patient is on bed rest, administer analgesic agents; initiate measures to relieve anxiety.
• Monitor voiding patterns; watch for bladder distention.
• Insert indwelling catheter if urinary retention is present or if laboratory test results indicate azotemia.
• Prepare patient for a cystostomy if urinary catheter is not tolerated.

See Perioperative Nursing Management under Section P for additional information.

PROVIDING EDUCATION
• Review with the patient the anatomy of the affected structures and their function in relation to the urinary and reproductive systems, using diagrams and other educational aids if indicated.

- Explain what will take place while the patient is prepared for diagnostic tests and then for surgery (depending on the type of prostatectomy planned).
- Reinforce information given by the surgeon.
- Explain procedures expected to occur during the immediate perioperative period, answer questions the patient or family may have, and provide emotional support.
- Provide information about postoperative pain management.

PREPARING PATIENT FOR TREATMENT
- Apply graduated compression stockings.
- Administer enema, if ordered.

Postoperative Nursing Interventions

MAINTAINING FLUID BALANCE
- Closely monitor urine output and the amount of fluid used for irrigation; maintain intake and output record.
- Monitor for electrolyte imbalances (e.g., hyponatremia), increasing blood pressure, confusion, and respiratory distress.

🍁 Gerontologic Considerations
The risk of fluid and electrolyte imbalances is greater in older patients with preexisting cardiovascular or respiratory disease.

RELIEVING PAIN
- Distinguish cause and location of pain, including bladder spasms.
- Give analgesic agents for incisional pain and smooth muscle relaxants for bladder spasm.
- Monitor drainage tubing and irrigate drainage system to correct any obstruction.
- Secure catheter to leg or abdomen.
- Monitor dressings, and adjust to ensure they are not too snug or not too saturated or are improperly placed.
- Provide stool softener and prune juice to ease bowel movements and to prevent straining.

MONITORING AND MANAGING COMPLICATIONS
- Hemorrhage: Observe catheter drainage; note bright red bleeding with increased viscosity and clots; closely monitor vital signs; administer medications, IV fluids, and blood component therapy as prescribed; maintain accurate record

C

of intake and output; and carefully monitor drainage to ensure adequate urine flow and patency of the drainage system. Provide explanations and reassurance to patient and family.

- Infection: Use aseptic technique with dressing changes; avoid rectal thermometers, tubes, and enemas; provide sitz bath and heat lamps to promote healing after sutures are removed; assess for urinary tract infection (UTI) and epididymitis; administer antibiotic medications as prescribed. Educate patient and family to recognize signs and symptoms of infection.

- Venous thromboembolism: Assess for VTE and pulmonary embolism; apply compression stockings. Assist patient to progress from leg dangling on the day of surgery to ambulating the next morning; encourage patient to walk but not sit for long periods of time. Monitor the patient receiving heparin for excessive bleeding.

- Obstructed catheter: Observe lower abdomen for bladder distention; examine drainage bag, dressings, and surgical incision for bleeding; monitor vital signs to detect hypotension; observe patient for restlessness, diaphoresis, pallor, any drop in blood pressure, and an increasing pulse rate. Provide for patent drainage system; perform gentle irrigation as prescribed to remove blood clots. Note that the amount drained must equal the amount instilled.

- Urinary incontinence: Encourage patient to take steps to prevent incontinence, improve continence, anticipate leakage, and cope with lack of complete control.

- Sexual dysfunction: Erectile dysfunction, decreased libido, and fatigue may be a concern soon or months after surgery. Medications, surgically placed implants, or negative pressure devices may help restore function. Reassurance that libido usually returns and fatigue diminishes after recuperation may help. Providing privacy, confidentiality, and time to discuss issues of sexuality is important. Referral to a sex therapist may be indicated.

▶ *Quality and Safety Nursing Alert*

Urine leakage around the wound may be noted after catheter removal.

Promoting Home- and Community-Based Care

Educating Patients About Self-Care

- Instruct patient and family about how to manage drainage system, monitor urinary output, perform wound care, and use strategies to prevent complications.
- Inform patient about signs and symptoms that should be reported to the physician (e.g., blood in the urine, decreased urine output, fever, change in wound drainage, or calf tenderness).
- Discuss perineal exercises to help regain urinary control.
- As indicated, discuss possible sexual dysfunction (provide a private environment) and refer for counseling.
- Instruct patient not to perform Valsalva maneuver for 6 to 8 weeks because it increases venous pressure and may produce hematuria.
- Urge patient to avoid long car trips and strenuous exercise, which increases tendency to bleed.
- Inform patient that spicy foods, alcohol, and coffee can cause bladder discomfort.
- Encourage fluids to avoid dehydration and clot formation.

Continuing Care

- Refer for home care as indicated.
- Remind patient that return of bladder control may take time.

Evaluation

Expected Preoperative Patient Outcomes

- Demonstrates reduced anxiety
- States pain and discomfort are decreased
- Relates understanding of surgical procedure and postoperative care (perineal muscle exercises and bladder control techniques)

Expected Postoperative Patient Outcomes

- Relates relief of discomfort
- Exhibits fluid and electrolyte balance
- Performs self-care measures
- Is free of complications
- Reports understanding of changes in sexual function

For more information, see Chapter 59 in Hinkle, J. L., & Cheever, K. H. (2014). *Brunner and Suddarth's textbook of medical-surgical nursing* (13th ed.). Philadelphia: Lippincott Williams & Wilkins.

Cancer of the Skin (Malignant Melanoma)

A malignant melanoma is a cancerous neoplasm in which atypical melanocytes are present in both the epidermis and the dermis (and sometimes the subcutaneous cells). It is the most lethal of all skin cancers. Malignant melanoma can occur in one of several forms: superficial spreading melanoma, lentigo-maligna melanoma, nodular melanoma, and acral-lentiginous melanoma.

Most melanomas are derived from cutaneous epidermal melanocytes; some appear in preexisting nevi (moles) in the skin or develop in the uveal tract of the eye. Melanomas occasionally appear simultaneously with cancer of other organs. The incidence and mortality rates of malignant melanoma are increasing, probably related to increased recreational sun exposure and better early detection. Prognosis is related to the depth of dermal invasion and the thickness of the lesion. Malignant melanoma can spread through both the bloodstream and the lymphatic system and can metastasize to the bones, liver, lungs, spleen, central nervous system (CNS), and lymph nodes.

Risk Factors

The cause of malignant melanoma is unknown, but ultraviolet rays are strongly suspected. Risk factors include the following:

- Fair-skinned or freckled, blue-eyed, light-haired
- Celtic or Scandinavian origin
- Tendency to burn and not tan; significant history of severe sunburn
- Environmental exposure to intense sunlight (older Americans retiring to the southwestern United States and countries near the equator)
- Family or personal history of melanoma, the absence of a gene on chromosome 9P, presence of giant congenital nevi
- Dysplastic nevus syndrome

Clinical Manifestations

Superficial Spreading Melanoma
- Most common form; usually affects middle-aged people, occurs most frequently on trunk and lower extremities
- Circular lesions with irregular outer portions
- Margins of lesion flat or elevated and palpable

- May appear in combination of colors, with hues of tan, brown, and black mixed with gray, blue-black, or white; sometimes a dull, pink-rose color noted in a small area within the lesion

Lentigo-Maligna Melanoma
- Slowly evolving pigmented lesion
- Occurs on exposed skin areas; hand, head, and neck in older people
- First appears as tan, flat lesion, which in time undergoes changes in size and color

Nodular Melanoma
- Spherical, blueberrylike nodule with relatively smooth surface and uniform blue-black color
- May be dome-shaped with a smooth surface or have other shadings of red, gray, or purple
- May appear as irregularly shaped plaques
- May be described as a blood blister that fails to resolve
- Directly invades the adjacent dermis (vertical growth); poor prognosis

Acral-Lentiginous Melanoma
- Occurs in areas not excessively exposed to sunlight and where hair follicles are absent
- Found on the palms of the hands, soles, in nail beds, and mucous membranes in dark-skinned people
- Appears as an irregular pigmented macule that develops nodules
- Becomes invasive early

Assessment and Diagnostic Findings
- Thorough history and physical examination include a meticulous skin examination and palpation of regional lymph nodes that drain the lesional area.
- Excisional biopsy specimen is obtained; incisional biopsy is performed when the suspicious lesion is too large to be removed safely without extensive scarring.
- Chest x-ray, complete blood cell count, liver function tests, and radionuclide or CT scans are usually performed to stage the extent of disease.

Medical Management
Treatment depends on the level of invasion and the depth of the lesion. In addition to surgery, chemotherapy and

induced hyperthermia may be used to enhance treatment. Investigators are exploring the potential for the use of lipid-lowering medications and vaccine therapy to prevent melanoma.

Surgical Management

- Surgical excision is the treatment of choice for small superficial lesions.
- Deeper lesions require wide local excision and skin graft.
- A regional lymph node dissection may be performed to rule out metastasis, although newer approaches call for sentinel node biopsy to avoid problems from extensive lymph node removal.
- Debulking the tumor or other palliative procedures may be performed.

NURSING PROCESS

Care of the Patient With Malignant Melanoma

Assessment

Question the patient with a lesion specifically about pruritus, tenderness, and pain, which are not features of a benign nevus. Also investigate changes in preexisting moles or development of new pigmented lesions. Assess people at risk carefully, focusing on the skin.

- Use a magnifying lens to examine for irregularity and changes in the mole.
- Signs that suggest malignant changes include asymmetry (irregular surface), irregular border, variegated color, and large diameter; referred to as the *ABCDs of moles*.
- Pay particular attention to common sites of melanomas (e.g., back, legs, between toes, face, feet, scalp, fingernails, and backs of hands).

Diagnosis

NURSING DIAGNOSES

- Acute pain related to surgical excision and grafting
- Anxiety and depression related to possible life-threatening consequences of melanoma and disfigurement
- Deficient knowledge about early signs of melanoma

C

COLLABORATIVE PROBLEMS/POTENTIAL COMPLICATIONS
- Metastasis
- Infection of surgical site

Planning and Goals

The major goals for the patient may include relief of pain and discomfort, reduced anxiety and depression, increased knowledge of early signs of melanoma, and absence of complications.

Nursing Interventions

RELIEVING PAIN AND DISCOMFORT
Promote comfort and anticipate need for and administer appropriate analgesic agents.

REDUCING ANXIETY AND DEPRESSION
- Provide support, and allow patient to express feelings (e.g., anxiety, depression).
- Convey understanding of feelings.
- Answer questions, and clarify information during the diagnostic workup and staging of the tumor.
- Point out resources, past effective coping mechanisms, and support systems to help the patient cope with diagnosis and treatment.
- Include family members in all discussions to clarify information and provide emotional support.

MONITORING AND MANAGING POTENTIAL COMPLICATIONS:
METASTASIS
- Educate patient about treatment and deliver supportive care, provide and clarify information about the therapy and the rationale for its use, identify potential side effects of therapy and ways to manage them, and instruct the patient and family about the expected outcomes of treatment.
- Monitor and document symptoms that may indicate metastasis: lung (e.g., difficulty breathing, shortness of breath, increasing cough), bone (e.g., pain, decreased mobility and function, pathologic fractures), and liver (e.g., change in liver enzyme levels, pain, jaundice).
- Encourage patient to have hope in the therapy while being realistic.
- Provide time for patient to express fears and concerns about the future.
- Offer information about support groups and contact people.

• Arrange for hospice and palliative care services.

See "Nursing Management" under Cancer for additional nursing care measures.

PROMOTING HOME- AND COMMUNITY-BASED CARE

• Educate patient about the early signs; include education on the way to examine the skin and scalp monthly in a systematic manner and on seeking prompt medical attention if changes are detected.
• Promote sun-avoiding measures.
• Advise on importance of annual assessment by a health care provider.

Evaluation

EXPECTED PATIENT OUTCOMES

• Experiences relief of pain and discomfort
• Achieves reduced anxiety
• Demonstrates understanding of the means for detecting and preventing melanoma
• Experiences absence of complications

For more information, see Chapter 61 in Hinkle, J. L., & Cheever, K. H. (2014). *Brunner and Suddarth's textbook of medical-surgical nursing* (13th ed.). Philadelphia: Lippincott Williams & Wilkins.

Cancer of the Stomach (Gastric Cancer)

Most gastric cancers are adenocarcinomas; they can occur anywhere in the stomach. Gastric cancer typically occurs in males and individuals older than 40 years (occasionally in younger people). Asian Americans, Native Americans, Hispanic Americans, and African Americans are twice as likely as Caucasian Americans to develop gastric cancer; the incidence of gastric cancer is much greater in Japan. Diet appears to be a significant factor (i.e., high in smoked foods and lacking in fruits and vegetables). Other factors related to the incidence of gastric cancer include chronic inflammation of the stomach, *Helicobacter pylori* (*H. pylori*) infection, pernicious anemia, smoking, achlorhydria, gastric ulcers, previous subtotal gastrectomy (more than 20 years ago), and genetics. Prognosis is generally poor because most patients have metastases (liver, pancreas, and esophagus or duodenum) at the time of diagnosis.

Pathophysiology

Most gastric cancers are adenocarcinomas; the majority occur either in the lower part (40%) or middle part of the stomach (40%) and, to a lesser degree, in the upper part (15%) or in multiple sites (10%). The tumor infiltrates the surrounding mucosa, penetrating the wall of the stomach and adjacent organs. The liver, pancreas, esophagus, and duodenum are often already affected at the time of diagnosis; metastasis via the lymphatic system to the peritoneal cavity occurs later in the disease.

Clinical Manifestations

- Early stages: Symptoms may be absent or may resemble those of patients with benign ulcers (e.g., pain relieved with antacids).
- Progressive disease: Symptoms include dyspepsia (indigestion), early satiety, weight loss, abdominal pain just above the umbilicus, loss or decrease in appetite, bloating after meals, nausea and vomiting, and symptoms similar to those of peptic ulcer disease.

Assessment and Diagnostic Findings

- Esophagogastroduodenoscopy (EGD) for biopsy and cytologic washings is the diagnostic study of choice.
- Barium x-ray examination of the upper gastrointestinal (GI) tract, endoscopic ultrasound (EUS), and CT may be used.
- Advanced gastric cancer may be palpable as a mass; ascites and hepatosplenomegaly may be apparent if there is metastasis to the liver.
- Palpable lymph nodes around the umbilicus are a sign of GI cancer.

Medical Management

- Diagnostic laparoscopy may be performed to evaluate tumor and obtain tissue sample for pathological diagnosis and to detect metastasis.
- Removal of gastric carcinoma is curative if tumor can be removed while still localized to the stomach.
- Effective palliation (to prevent symptoms such as obstruction) can occur by resection of the tumor, total gastrectomy, radical subtotal gastrectomy, proximal subtotal gastrectomy, or esophagogastrectomy.
- Reconstruction of the GI tract via esophagojejunostomy may be performed.

- Complications of advanced gastric cancer may require surgery including gastric outlet obstruction, bleeding, and gastric perforation. Palliative surgical procedures may be used for severe pain.
- Chemotherapy can be used for further disease control or for palliation (5-fluorouracil, cisplatin, doxorubicin, etoposide, and mitomycin-C) as single or combination therapies.
- Newer therapies include treatment with recombinant anti-HER-2 monoclonal antibodies in combination with cisplatin, and antiangiogenesis agents.
- Radiation may be used for palliation.
- Tumor marker assessments indirectly determine treatment effectiveness.

🍂 Gerontologic Considerations

The number of older patients (75 years and older) with gastric cancer is increasing; 60% of cancer-related deaths occur in people 65 and older. Confusion, agitation, and restlessness may be the only symptoms seen in older adult patients, who may have no gastric symptoms until their tumors are well advanced. Patients may present with reduced functional ability and other signs and symptoms of malignancy.

Surgery is more hazardous for the older adult, and the risk increases proportionately with increasing age. Nonetheless, gastric cancer should be treated with traditional surgery in older patients. Patient education is important to prepare older patients with cancer for treatment, to help them manage adverse effects, and to face the challenges that cancer and aging present.

NURSING PROCESS

The Patient With Stomach Cancer

Assessment

- Elicit detailed history of dietary intake.
- Identify weight loss, including time frame and amount; assess appetite, satiety, and eating habits; include pain assessment.
- Obtain smoking and alcohol history and family history (e.g., any first- or second-degree relatives with gastric or other cancer); inquire about history of *H. pylori* infection.

- Assess psychosocial support (marital status, coping skills, emotional and financial resources).
- Perform complete physical examination (palpate and percuss abdomen for tenderness, masses, or ascites).

Diagnosis

Nursing Diagnoses

- Anxiety related to disease and anticipated treatment
- Imbalanced nutrition, less than body requirements, related to early satiety or anorexia
- Pain related to tumor mass
- Grieving related to diagnosis of cancer
- Deficient knowledge regarding self-care activities

Planning and Goals

The major goals for the patient may include reduced anxiety, optimal nutrition, relief of pain, and adjustment to the diagnosis and anticipated lifestyle changes.

Nursing Interventions

Reducing Anxiety

- Provide a relaxed, nonthreatening atmosphere (helps patient express fears, concerns, and anger).
- Encourage family or significant other in efforts to support the patient, offering assurance, and supporting positive coping measures.
- Advise about any procedures and treatments.

Promoting Optimal Nutrition

- Encourage small, frequent feedings of nonirritating foods to decrease gastric irritation; encourage fluid consumption between meals rather than with meals.
- Facilitate tissue repair by ensuring food supplements are high in calories and vitamins A and C and iron.
- Administer parenteral vitamin B_{12} indefinitely if a total gastrectomy is performed.
- Monitor rate and frequency of IV therapy.
- Record intake, output, and daily weights.
- Assess signs of dehydration (thirst, dry mucous membranes, poor skin turgor, tachycardia, decreased urine output).

- Review results of daily laboratory studies to note any metabolic abnormalities (sodium, potassium, glucose, blood urea nitrogen).
- Administer antiemetic agents as prescribed.

RELIEVING PAIN
- Administer analgesic agents as prescribed (continuous infusion of an opioid or patient-controlled analgesia [PCA] pump).
- Assess frequency, intensity, and duration of pain to determine effectiveness of analgesic agent.
- Work with patient to help manage pain by suggesting nonpharmacologic methods for pain relief, such as position changes, imagery, distraction, relaxation exercises (using relaxation audiotapes), back rubs, massage, and periods of rest and relaxation.

PROVIDING PSYCHOSOCIAL SUPPORT
- Help patient express fears, concerns, and grief about diagnosis.
- Answer patient's questions honestly.
- Encourage patient to participate in treatment decisions and self-care activities if possible.
- Support patient's disbelief and time needed to accept diagnosis.
- Offer emotional support and involve family members and significant others whenever possible; reassure that emotional responses are normal and expected.
- Be aware of mood swings and defense mechanisms (denial, rationalization, displacement, regression).
- Provide professional services as necessary (e.g., clergy, psychiatric clinical nurse specialists, psychologists, social workers, and psychiatrists).
- Assist with decisions regarding end-of-life care and make referrals as warranted.

PROMOTING HOME- AND COMMUNITY-BASED CARE
See "Nursing Management" under Cancer for additional information.

EDUCATING PATIENTS ABOUT SELF-CARE
- Educate about self-care activities specific to treatment regimen.
- Include information about diet and nutrition, treatment regimens, activity and lifestyle changes, pain management, and complications.

- Explain that the possibility of dumping syndrome exists with any enteral feeding and educate patient about ways to manage it.
- Explain need for daily rest periods and frequent visits to physician after discharge.
- Refer for home care; nurse can supervise any enteral or parenteral feeding and instruct patient and family members in ways to use equipment and formulas as well as ways to detect complications.
- Instruct patient to record daily intake and output and weight.
- Educate patient about how to cope with pain, nausea, vomiting, and bloating.
- Educate patient to recognize and report complications that require medical attention, such as bleeding (overt or covert hematemesis, melena), obstruction, perforation, or any symptoms that become consistently worse.
- Explain chemotherapy or radiation regimen and the care needed during and after treatment.

Continuing Care
- Plans for care should be individualized to the patient and coordinated with patient and caregivers.
- Reinforce nutritional counseling and assess competence of caregivers in enteral or parenteral feedings.
- Educate patient and family to assess daily intake and output, strategies to manage symptoms (e.g., pain, nausea, and vomiting) and recognition of complications (e.g., bleeding, obstruction, perforation).
- Review treatment regimen to ensure patient and family understand home care related to treatments.
- Assist patient, family and significant other with decisions regarding end-of-life care and make referrals as warranted.

Evaluation

EXPECTED PATIENT OUTCOMES
- Reports less anxiety and has decreased pain
- Attains optimal nutrition
- Performs self-care activities and adjusts to lifestyle changes
- Verbalizes knowledge of disease management

For more information, see Chapter 47 in Hinkle, J. L., & Cheever, K. H. (2014). *Brunner and Suddarth's textbook of medical-surgical nursing* (13th ed.). Philadelphia: Lippincott Williams & Wilkins.

Cancer of the Testis

C

Testicular cancer is the most common cancer in men ages 15 to 35 years and the second most common cancer in men ages 35 to 39 years. It is highly treatable and usually curable; the 5-year survival rates for all testicular cancers are 95% and 99%, respectively, if the cancer has not metastasized. Risk factors for testicular cancer include undescended testicles (cryptorchidism), family history of testicular cancer, and personal history of testicular cancer. Other risk factors include race and ethnicity, HIV infection, and occupational hazards (e.g., exposure to chemicals).

Pathophysiology

Testicular cancer is classified as germinal or nongerminal (stromal). Germinal tumors make up approximately 90% of all cancers of the testis and may be further classified as seminomas (slow-growing, remain localized, most commonly found in ages 30 to 40 years) and nonseminomas (fast-growing, more common). Nonseminomas are further differentiated according to the type of cell including choriocarcinomas (rare), embryonal carcinomas, teratomas, and yolk sac tumors. Differences between seminomas and nonseminomas affect treatment and prognosis. Nongerminal tumors (Leydig cell tumors and Sertoli cell tumors) account for less than 10% of tumors and may develop in the supportive and hormone-producing tissues, or stroma, of the testicles. Some testicular tumors tend to metastasize early, spreading from the testis to the lymph nodes in the retroperitoneum and to the lungs. Secondary testicular tumors (lymphoma) metastasize from other organs.

Clinical Manifestations

- Symptoms appear gradually, with a mass or lump on the testicle.
- Painless enlargement of the testis occurs; patient may complain of heaviness in the scrotum, inguinal area, or lower abdomen.
- Backache, pain in the abdomen, weight loss, and general weakness may result from metastasis.

Assessment and Diagnostic Findings

- Monthly testicular self-examination (TSE) is an effective early detection method.

- Elevated alpha-fetoprotein (AFP) and beta-human chorionic gonadotropin levels are used as tumor markers as well as for diagnosis, staging, and monitoring the response to treatment.
- Blood chemistry, including lactate dehydrogenase (LDH), is useful.
- Chest x-ray is used to assess for metastasis in the lungs, and transscrotal testicular ultrasound is performed.
- Inguinal orchiectomy, abdominal or pelvic CT, and chest CT (if the abdominal CT or chest x-ray is abnormal), brain MRI, and bone scan can stage and assess extent of disease.

Medical Management

The goals of management are to eradicate the disease and achieve a cure. Therapy is based on the cell type, the stage of the disease, and risk classification tables (determined as good, intermediate, and poor risks). National Comprehensive Cancer Network (NCCN) Practice consensus guidelines are used for diagnosis, treatment, and follow-up.

- Orchiectomy of affected testis and retroperitoneal lymph node dissection (RPLND) are performed; alternatives to more invasive open RPLND include nerve-sparing and laparoscopic RPLND.
- Sperm banking before surgery, chemotherapy, or radiation therapy is suggested.
- Good results may be obtained by combining different types of treatments, including surgery, radiation therapy, and chemotherapy.

Nursing Management

See "Nursing Management" under Cancer for additional information.

- Assess the patient's physical and psychological status and monitor for response to and possible effects of surgery, chemotherapy, and radiation therapy.
- Address issues related to body image and sexuality.
- Encourage patient to maintain a positive attitude during therapy.
- Encourage follow-up evaluation studies for recurrence or late side effects of treatment and continual TSE. (A patient with a history of one tumor of the testis has a greater chance of developing subsequent tumors.)

- Encourage healthy behaviors, including smoking cessation, healthy diet, minimization of alcohol intake, and cancer screening activities.

For more information, see Chapter 59 in Hinkle, J. L., & Cheever, K. H. (2014). *Brunner and Suddarth's textbook of medical-surgical nursing* (13th ed.). Philadelphia: Lippincott Williams & Wilkins.

Cancer of the Thyroid

Cancer of the thyroid is less prevalent than other forms of cancer, with 80% of new cases in patients younger than age 65. It accounts for 90% of endocrine malignancies. The most common type, papillary adenocarcinoma, accounts for 70% of endocrine malignancies; it starts in childhood or early adult life, remains localized, and eventually metastasizes. When papillary adenocarcinoma occurs in an older patient, it is more aggressive. Risk factors include female gender and external irradiation of the head, neck, or chest in infancy and childhood. Other types of thyroid cancer include follicular adenocarcinoma, medullary, anaplastic, and thyroid lymphoma.

Clinical Manifestations
- Lesions that are single, hard, and fixed on palpation or associated with cervical lymphadenopathy suggest malignancy.
- Recurrence of nodules or masses in the neck and signs of hoarseness, dysphagia, or dyspnea are evident.

Assessment and Diagnostic Findings
- Needle biopsy or aspiration biopsy of thyroid gland
- Thyroid function tests (free T_4, thyroid-stimulating hormone [TSH]), and serum calcium and phosphorus levels
- Ultrasound, MRI, CT scan, skeletal x-rays, thyroid scans, radioactive iodine uptake studies, and thyroid suppression tests

Medical Management
- Treatment of choice is surgical removal (total or near-total thyroidectomy).
- Modified or extensive radical neck dissection is done if lymph nodes are involved.
- Reduce risk of postoperative hypocalcemia and tetany by sparing parathyroid tissue.

- Ablation procedures with radioactive iodine are used to eradicate residual thyroid tissue and thyroid cancer with metastasis.
- Thyroid hormone is administered in suppressive doses after surgery to lower the levels of TSH to a euthyroid state.
- Lifelong thyroxine is required if remaining thyroid tissue is inadequate to produce sufficient hormone.
- Radiation therapy is administered orally or externally.
- Chemotherapy is used infrequently.

Nursing Management

- Inform patient about the purpose of any preoperative tests and explain what preoperative preparations to expect; education includes demonstrating to the patient how to support the neck with the hands after surgery to prevent stress on the incision.
- Provide postoperative care (e.g., assess and reinforce surgical dressings, observe for bleeding, monitor pulse and blood pressure for signs of internal bleeding, assess respiratory status, assess intensity of pain, and administer analgesic medications as prescribed).
- Monitor and observe patient for potential complications such as hemorrhage, hematoma formation, edema of the glottis, and injury to the recurrent laryngeal nerve.
- Educate patient and family about signs and symptoms of possible complications and those that should be reported; suggest strategies for managing postoperative pain at home and for increasing humidification.
- Explain to the patient and family the need for rest, relaxation, and nutrition; patient can resume former activities and responsibilities once recovered from surgery.
- Administer thyroxine if remaining thyroid tissue is inadequate to produce sufficient thyroid hormone.
- Emphasize importance of taking prescribed medications and following recommendations for follow-up monitoring after radiation therapy.
- Educate patient receiving radiation therapy to assess and manage side effects of treatment.
- Refer for home care, if indicated.

See "Nursing Management" under Cancer for additional information.

For more information, see Chapter 52 in Hinkle, J. L., & Cheever, K. H. (2014). *Brunner and Suddarth's textbook of medical-surgical nursing* (13th ed.). Philadelphia: Lippincott Williams & Wilkins.

Cancer of the Vagina

C

Cancer of the vagina is rare and usually takes years to develop. Primary cancer of the vagina is usually squamous in origin. Malignant melanoma and sarcomas can occur. Risk factors include previous cervical cancer, in utero exposure to diethylstilbestrol (DES), previous vaginal or vulvar cancer, previous radiation therapy, history of human papillomavirus (HPV) infection, or pessary use. Any patient with previous cervical cancer should be examined regularly for vaginal lesions. Improper use of a vaginal pessary has been associated with vaginal cancer due to resulting chronic irritation.

Clinical Manifestations
- Disease is often asymptomatic, but slight bleeding after intercourse may be reported.
- Spontaneous bleeding, vaginal discharge, pain, and urinary or rectal symptoms may occur.

Assessment and Diagnostic Findings
- Colposcopy for women exposed to DES in utero
- Pap smear of the vagina

Medical Management
- Treatment of early lesions may include local excision, topical chemotherapy, or laser.
- Surgery is used for more advanced lesions (depends on the size and the stage of the cancer) followed by reconstructive surgery, if needed, and radiation (via external-beam or intracavity methods).

Nursing Management
- Encourage close follow-up by health care providers.
- Provide emotional support.
- Inform women who have had vaginal reconstructive surgery that regular intercourse may be helpful in preventing vaginal stenosis.
- Inform patient that water-soluble lubricants are helpful in reducing dyspareunia.

For more information, see Chapter 57 in Hinkle, J. L., & Cheever, K. H. (2014). *Brunner and Suddarth's textbook of medical-surgical nursing* (13th ed.). Philadelphia: Lippincott Williams & Wilkins.

Cancer of the Vulva

Primary cancer of the vulva is seen mostly in postmenopausal women, but its incidence in younger women is rising. The median age for cancer limited to the vulva is 50 years; the median age for invasive vulvar cancer is 70 years. Possible risk factors include smoking, human papillomavirus (HPV) infection, HIV infection, and immunosuppression; chronic vulvar irritation may increase risk.

Pathophysiology
Squamous cell carcinoma accounts for most primary vulvar tumors; less common are Bartholin's gland cancer, vulvar sarcoma, and malignant melanoma. Vulvar intraepithelial lesions are preinvasive and are also called *vulvar carcinoma in situ*. Morbidity with recurrence of the disease is high, and patterns of recurrence vary.

Clinical Manifestations
- Long-standing pruritus and soreness are the most common symptoms; itching occurs in half of all patients.
- Bleeding, foul-smelling discharge, and pain are signs of advanced disease.
- Early lesions appear as chronic dermatitis; later, lesions appear as a lump that continues to grow and becomes a hard, ulcerated, cauliflowerlike growth.

Assessment and Diagnostic Findings
- Regular pelvic examinations, Pap smears, and vulvar self-examination are helpful in early detection.
- Biopsy is performed.

Medical Management
- For preinvasive (vulvar carcinoma in situ), local excision, laser ablation, chemotherapeutic creams (fluorouracil), or cryosurgery can be performed.
- For invasive cancer, wide excision or vulvectomy, external-beam radiation, laser therapy, or chemotherapy may be used.
- If a widespread area is involved or the disease is advanced, a radical vulvectomy with bilateral groin dissection may be performed; antibiotic and heparin prophylaxis may be continued postoperatively; sequential compression stockings can be applied.

Nursing Management

Assessment

- Obtain a health history; tactfully elicit the reason why a delay, if any, occurred in seeking health care.
- Assess health habits and lifestyle; evaluate receptivity to learning.
- Assess psychosocial factors; provide preoperative preparation and psychological support.

Preoperative Nursing Interventions

Relieving Anxiety

- Allow patient time to talk and ask questions.
- Advise patient that the possibility of having sexual relations is good and that pregnancy is possible after a wide excision.
- Reinforce information about the surgery and address patient's questions and concerns.

Preparing Skin for Surgery

Skin preparation may include cleansing the lower abdomen, inguinal areas, upper thighs, and vulva with a detergent germicide for several days before the surgical procedure. The patient may be instructed to do this at home.

Postoperative Nursing Interventions

Relieving Pain and Discomfort

- Administer analgesic agents preventively; patient-controlled analgesia may be indicated.
- Position patient to relieve tension on incision (pillow under knees or low Fowler's position), and give soothing back rubs.

Improving Skin Integrity

- Provide pressure-reducing mattress.
- Install over-bed trapeze.
- Protect intact skin from drainage and moisture.
- Change dressings as needed to ensure patient comfort, to perform wound care and irrigation (if prescribed), and to permit observation of the surgical site.
- Always protect patient from exposure when visitors arrive or someone else enters the room.

Supporting Positive Sexuality and Sexual Function

- Establish a trusting relationship with patient.
- Encourage patient to share and discuss concerns with sexual partner.

- Consult with surgeon to clarify expected changes.
- Refer patient and partner to a sex counselor, as indicated.

Monitoring and Managing Potential Complications
- Monitor closely for local and systemic signs and symptoms of infection: purulent drainage, redness, increased pain, fever, increased white blood cell (WBC) count.
- Assist in obtaining tissue specimens for culture.
- Administer antibiotic agents as prescribed.
- Avoid cross-contamination; carefully handle catheters, drains, and dressings; hand hygiene is crucial.
- Provide a low-residue diet to prevent straining on defecation and wound contamination.
- Assess for signs and symptoms of deep vein thrombosis and pulmonary embolism; apply elastic compression stockings; encourage ankle exercises.
- Encourage and assist in frequent position changes, avoiding pressure behind the knees.
- Encourage fluid intake to prevent dehydration.
- Monitor closely for signs of hemorrhage and hypovolemic shock.

Promoting Home- and Community-Based Care

Educating Patients About Self-Care
- Encourage patient to share concerns as she recovers.
- Encourage participation in dressing changes and self-care.
- Give complete instructions to family members or others who will provide posthospital care regarding wound care, urinary catheterization, and possible complications.

Continuing Care
- Encourage communication with home care nurse to ensure continuity of care.
- Reinforce education with follow-up call between home visits.

For more information, see Chapter 57 in Hinkle, J. L., & Cheever, K. H. (2014). *Brunner and Suddarth's textbook of medical-surgical nursing* (13th ed.). Philadelphia: Lippincott Williams & Wilkins.

Cardiac Arrest

In cardiac arrest, the heart is unable to pump and circulate blood to the body's organs and tissues. It may be caused by a dysrhythmia such as ventricular fibrillation, progressive bradycardia, or asystole. Cardiac arrest can also occur when electrical activity is present but there is ineffective cardiac contraction or circulating volume, which is called *pulseless electrical activity* (PEA). PEA can be caused by hypovolemia (e.g., hemorrhage), hypoxia, hypothermia, hyperkalemia, massive pulmonary embolism, myocardial infarction, or medication overdose. Rapid identification of these problems and prompt intervention can restore circulation in some patients.

Clinical Manifestations
In cardiac arrest, consciousness, pulse, and blood pressure are lost immediately. Ineffective respiratory gasping may occur. The pupils of the eyes begin dilating in less than a minute, and seizures may occur. Pallor and cyanosis are seen in the skin and mucous membranes. The risk of organ damage, irreversible brain damage, and death increases with every minute that circulation ceases. The interval varies with the age and underlying condition of the patient. During this period, the diagnosis of cardiac arrest must be made and measures must be taken immediately to restore circulation.

Emergency Assessment and Management: Cardiopulmonary Resuscitation
- On recognition of sudden cardiac arrest, the patient is checked for responsiveness and breathing.
- The Emergency Response System (ERS; "Code Blue" or 911) is activated.
- Cardiopulmonary resuscitation (CPR) is initiated immediately.
- Cardiac rhythm is analyzed and defibrillation provided as soon as possible with automated external defibrillator (AED) or defibrillator.
- Placement of an advanced airway such as an endotracheal (ET) tube may be performed during resuscitation to ensure a patent airway and adequate ventilation.
- Medications are administered to reverse cardiopulmonary arrest according to Advanced Cardiac Life Support guidelines for advanced support interventions.
- Follow-up monitoring is instituted once patient is resuscitated, including continuous electrocardiographic (ECG) monitoring, frequent blood pressure assessments until hemodynamic stability is attained, and identification and treatment of factors that precipitated the arrest, such as dysrhythmias or electrolyte or metabolic imbalances.

- Patient is assessed after resuscitation and return of spontaneous circulation; patients who are comatose may benefit from therapeutic hypothermia protocols.

For more information, see Chapter 30 in Hinkle, J. L., & Cheever, K. H. (2014). *Brunner and Suddarth's textbook of medical-surgical nursing* (13th ed.). Philadelphia: Lippincott Williams & Wilkins.

Cardiomyopathies

Cardiomyopathy is a heart muscle disease associated with cardiac dysfunction. It is classified according to the structural and functional abnormalities of the heart muscle: dilated cardiomyopathy (DCM; most common), restrictive cardiomyopathy (RCM; previously known as *constrictive cardiomyopathy*), hypertrophic cardiomyopathy (HCM; rare autosomal dominant condition), arrhythmogenic right ventricular cardiomyopathy (ARVC), and unclassified cardiomyopathies. *Ischemic cardiomyopathy* is a term frequently used to describe an enlarged heart caused by coronary artery disease, which is usually accompanied by heart failure. The 2006 American Heart Association *Contemporary Classifications* system for cardiomyopathies is divided into two major groups based on predominant organ involvement. These include *primary* cardiomyopathies (genetic, nongenetic, and acquired), which are focused primarily on the heart muscle, and *secondary* cardiomyopathies, which show myocardial involvement secondary to the influence of a vast list of disease processes.

Pathophysiology
The pathophysiology of all cardiomyopathies is a series of events that culminate in impaired cardiac output. Decreased stroke volume stimulates the sympathetic nervous system and the renin–angiotensin–aldosterone response, resulting in increased systemic vascular resistance and increased sodium and fluid retention, which places an increased workload on the heart. These alterations can lead to heart failure.

Dilated Cardiomyopathy
DCM is the most common form of cardiomyopathy, with an incidence of 5 to 8 cases per 100,000 people per year. DCM involves significant dilation of the ventricles without simultaneous hypertrophy and systolic dysfunction. The ventricles

demonstrate elevated systolic and diastolic volumes but a decreased ejection fraction.

DCM is caused by multiple conditions and diseases, including pregnancy, heavy alcohol intake, viral infection, chemotherapeutic medications, and Chagas disease. When the causative factor cannot be identified, the diagnosis is idiopathic DCM, which accounts for the largest subset of patients with DCM. Approximately 20% to 30% of all idiopathic DCM can be linked to familial genetics, and an echocardiography and ECG should be used to screen all first-degree blood relatives. Early diagnosis and treatment can prevent or delay significant symptoms and sudden death.

Restrictive Cardiomyopathy

RCM is characterized by diastolic dysfunction caused by rigid ventricular walls that impair diastolic filling and ventricular stretch. Systolic function is usually normal. RCM may be associated with amyloidosis and other such infiltrative diseases. However, the cause is unknown in most cases. Signs and symptoms are similar to constrictive pericarditis and include dyspnea, nonproductive cough, and chest pain. Echocardiography, as well as measurement of pulmonary artery systolic pressure (PASP), pulmonary artery wedge pressure (PAWP), and central venous pressure (CVP), are used to differentiate the two conditions.

Hypertrophic Cardiomyopathy

HCM is a rare autosomal dominant condition that is often detected after puberty, with an estimated prevalence rate of 0.05% to 0.2% of the population in the United States. Echocardiograms may be performed every year from 12 to 18 years of age and then every 5 years from 18 to 70 years of age, especially in those with a family history of HCM. Doppler echocardiography may also be used to detect HCM and blood flow alterations. HCM also may be idiopathic.

In HCM, the heart muscle asymmetrically increases in size and mass, especially along the septum. The increased thickness of the heart muscle reduces the size of the ventricular cavities and causes the ventricles to take a longer time to relax after systole. During the first part of diastole, it is more difficult for the ventricles to fill with blood. The atrial contraction at the end of diastole becomes critical for ventricular filling and systolic contraction. Also, the coronary arteriole walls thicken, which decreases the internal diameter of the arterioles. The narrow arterioles restrict the blood supply to the myocardium, causing numerous small areas of ischemia and necrosis. The necrotic areas of the myocardium ultimately fibrose and scar, further impeding ventricular contraction.

Arrhythmogenic Right Ventricular Cardiomyopathy

ARVC occurs when the myocardium of the right ventricle is progressively infiltrated and replaced by fibrous scar and adipose tissue. Initially, only localized areas of the right ventricle are affected but, as the disease progresses, the entire heart is affected. Eventually, the right ventricle dilates and develops poor contractility, right ventricular wall abnormalities, and dysrhythmias. ARVC is an uncommon form of inherited heart muscle disease and often is not recognized. Therefore, the prevalence is largely unknown, though it is estimated to be about 1:5000. Palpitations or syncope may develop between 15 and 40 years of age. ARVC should be considered in patients with ventricular tachycardia or left bundle branch block originating in the right ventricle, or in patients who suffer sudden death, especially among young athletes. ARVC is an autosomal dominant gene so first-degree blood relatives should be screened for the disease with a 12-lead ECG, Holter monitor, and echocardiography.

Unclassified Cardiomyopathies

Unclassified cardiomyopathies are different from or have characteristics of more than one of the previously described types and are caused by fibroelastosis, noncompacted myocardium, systolic dysfunction with minimal dilation, and mitochondrial diseases. Examples of unclassified cardiomyopathies are left ventricular noncompaction and stress-induced (Takotsubo) cardiomyopathy.

Clinical Manifestations

- Patient presents initially with signs and symptoms of heart failure (e.g., dyspnea on exertion [DOE], fatigue), which may become severe (lethal dysrhythmias and death).
- Patient may also report paroxysmal nocturnal dyspnea [PND], cough with exertion, and orthopnea.
- Other symptoms include fluid retention, peripheral edema, nausea, chest pain, palpitations, dizziness, and syncope with exertion.
- With HCM, cardiac arrest (i.e., sudden cardiac death) may be the initial manifestation in young people.

C

Assessment and Diagnostic Findings

- Tachycardia, extra heart sounds, crackles on pulmonary auscultation, jugular vein distention, pitting edema of dependent body parts, and enlarged liver on physical examination
- Patient history; other causes of heart failure ruled out
- Echocardiogram, cardiovascular magnetic resonance imaging (CMR), ECG, chest x-ray, cardiac catheterization and, possibly, an endomyocardial biopsy

Medical Management

Medical management is directed toward identifying and managing possible underlying or precipitating causes and correcting the heart failure. Treatment includes beta-blockers, a low-sodium diet with fluid restriction to 2 L each day, and an exercise–rest regimen. Dysrhythmias can be controlled with antiarrhythmic medications such as amiodarone and, possibly, with an implanted electronic device, such as an implantable cardioverter defibrillator.

Surgical Management

Surgical intervention is considered when heart failure has progressed and medical treatment is no longer effective. Surgical management may include the following:

- Left ventricular outflow tract surgery: When patients with HCM become symptomatic despite medical therapy and a 50 mm Hg or more pressure difference exists between the left ventricle and the aorta, a septal myectomy, myotomy–myectomy, or mitral valvuloplasty is considered. The primary complication of these procedures is dysrhythmia, and postoperative surgical complications include pain, ineffective airway clearance, deep vein thrombosis, risk of infection, and delayed surgical recovery.
- Heart transplantation: Typical candidates have severe symptoms uncontrolled by medical therapy, no other surgical options, and a prognosis of less than 2 years to live. Rejection of the donor heart is the most significant risk; however, the risk of infection is increased due to immunosuppressant drugs that prevent rejection, so patients must adhere to a complex regimen of diet, medications, activity, follow-up laboratory studies, biopsies of the transplanted heart (to diagnose rejection), and clinic visits.
- In some cases, a mechanical assist device or total artificial heart is implanted.

NURSING PROCESS

The Patient With a Cardiomyopathy

C

Assessment

- Obtain a history of presenting signs and symptoms as well as possible etiologic factors, such as heavy alcohol intake, recent illness or pregnancy, or history of the disease in immediate family members.
- Review systems, including reports of chest pain with precipitating factors, the presence of orthopnea with number of pillows needed to sleep, PND, syncope or dyspnea with exertion, usual weight along with any weight change, and limitations on activities of daily living. Evaluate usual diet to determine sodium intake, optimize nutrition, or supplement with vitamins. Determine New York Heart Association Classification for heart failure.
- Perform psychosocial assessment focused on patient's role within family and community, patient's support system, identification of stressors, and emotional status.
- Perform physical assessment focused on signs and symptoms of heart failure. Evaluate vital signs, pulse pressure, pulsus paradoxus, weight and any gain or loss, palpation for a shift to the left of the point of maximum impulse, auscultation for a systolic murmur and S_3 and S_4 heart sounds, pulmonary auscultation for crackles, measurement of jugular vein distention, and edema.

Diagnosis

NURSING DIAGNOSES

- Decreased cardiac output related to structural disorders caused by cardiomyopathy or dysrhythmia from the disease process and medical treatments
- Risk for ineffective cardiopulmonary, cerebral, peripheral, and renal tissue perfusion related to decreased peripheral blood flow
- Impaired gas exchange related to pulmonary congestion secondary to myocardial failure
- Activity intolerance related to decreased cardiac output or excessive fluid volume, or both
- Anxiety related to the change in health status and in role functioning

C

- Powerlessness related to disease process
- Noncompliance with medication and diet therapies

COLLABORATIVE PROBLEMS/POTENTIAL COMPLICATIONS
- Heart failure
- Ventricular and atrial dysrhythmias
- Cardiac conduction defects
- Pulmonary or cerebral embolism
- Valvular dysfunction

Planning and Goals

Patient goals include improvement or maintenance of cardiac output, increased activity tolerance, reduction of anxiety, adherence to the self-care program, increased sense of power with decision making, and absence of complications.

Nursing Interventions

IMPROVING CARDIAC OUTPUT AND PERIPHERAL BLOOD FLOW
- Assist patient into a resting position (usually sitting with legs down) during a symptomatic episode.
- Administer oxygen if indicated.
- Administer prescribed medications on time.
- Assist patient with medication planning schedule.
- Ensure low-sodium diet and adequate fluid intake.
- Monitor daily weight, noting any significant change.
- Keep patient warm, and change position frequently to stimulate circulation and reduce skin breakdown.

INCREASING ACTIVITY TOLERANCE AND
IMPROVING GAS EXCHANGE
- Plan patient's activities to occur in cycles, alternating rest and activity.
- Ensure the patient recognizes the symptoms indicating the need for rest and actions to take when the symptoms occur.

REDUCING ANXIETY
- Spiritual, psychological, and emotional support may be indicated for patients, families, and significant others.
- Provide patient with appropriate information about cardiomyopathy and self-management activities.
- Provide an atmosphere in which the patient feels free to verbalize concerns and receive assurance that his or her concerns are legitimate.

- Provide time for the patient to discuss concerns if facing death or awaiting transplantation; provide realistic hope.
- Help the patient, family, and significant others with anticipatory grieving.

Decreasing the Sense of Powerlessness
- Assist patient in identifying things he or she has lost (e.g., foods enjoyed, ability to engage in active lifestyle).
- Assist patient in identifying emotional responses to the loss (e.g., anger and feelings of sadness).
- Assist patient in identifying the amount of control that he or she still has (e.g., selecting food choices, managing medications).

Promoting Home- and Community-Based Care
Educating Patients About Self-Care
- Educate patients about the medication regimen, symptom monitoring, and symptom management.
- Help patient balance lifestyle and work while accomplishing therapeutic activities.
- Help patient cope with disease status; help patient adjust lifestyle and implement a self-care program at home.
- Promote patient's sense of well-being.

Continuing Care
- Reinforce previous education and perform ongoing assessment of the patient's symptoms and progress.
- Assist patient and family to adjust to lifestyle changes; instruct patient to read nutrition labels, record daily weights and symptoms, and organize daily activities.
- Assess patient's response to diet, fluid intake, and medication regimen.
- Stress the signs and symptoms that should be reported to the physician; educate the patient's family about cardiopulmonary resuscitation (CPR) and use of an automated external defibrillator (AED).
- Assess the psychosocial needs of the patient and family on an ongoing basis.
- Establish trust with patient and patient's family, and provide support during end-of-life decisions.
- Refer patient for home care and support if necessary.

Evaluation

EXPECTED PATIENT OUTCOMES
- Maintains or improves cardiac function
- Maintains or increases activity tolerance
- Feels less anxious
- Decreases sense of powerlessness
- Adheres to self-care program

For more information, see Chapter 28 in Hinkle, J. L., & Cheever, K. H. (2014). *Brunner and Suddarth's textbook of medical-surgical nursing* (13th ed.). Philadelphia: Lippincott Williams & Wilkins.

Cataract

A cataract is a lens opacity or cloudiness. More than half of all Americans have cataracts by 80 years of age; cataracts are the leading cause of blindness in the world.

Pathophysiology

Cataracts can develop in one or both eyes and at any age. Cigarette smoking; long-term use of corticosteroids, especially at high doses; sunlight and ionizing radiation; diabetes; obesity; and eye injuries can increase the risk of cataracts. The three most common types of senile (age-related) cataracts are defined by their location in the lens: nuclear, cortical, and posterior subcapsular. The extent of visual impairment depends on the size, density, and location in the lens; more than one type can be present in one eye.

Clinical Manifestations

- Painless, blurry vision
- Perception that surroundings are dimmer (as if glasses need cleaning)
- Light scattering; reduced contrast sensitivity, sensitivity to glare, and reduced visual acuity
- Other possible effects: myopic shift (return of ability to do close work [e.g., reading fine print] without eyeglasses), astigmatism (refractive error due to an irregularity in the curvature of the cornea), monocular diplopia (double vision), and color changes as the lens becomes more brown in color

Assessment and Diagnostic Findings
- Decrease in visual acuity that is directly proportionate to density of the cataract
- Snellen visual acuity test
- Ophthalmoscopy
- Slit-lamp biomicroscopic examination

Medical Management
No nonsurgical treatment (medications, eye drops, eyeglasses) cures cataracts or prevents age-related cataracts. Optimal medical treatment is prevention, including patient education regarding risk reduction strategies such as smoking cessation and wearing sunglasses outdoors.

Surgical Management
In general, if reduced vision from cataract does not interfere with normal activities, surgery may not be needed. The decision regarding when cataract surgery is to be performed should include the patient's functional and visual status as a primary consideration. Surgical options include phacoemulsification (method of extracapsular cataract surgery) and lens replacement (intraocular lens [IOL] implants [most common], contact lenses, and aphakic eyeglasses [used in conjunction with contacts, rarely used alone]). Cataracts are removed under local anesthesia on an outpatient basis. When both eyes have cataracts, one eye is treated first, with at least several weeks (preferably months) separating the two procedures. IOL implants are contraindicated in patients with recurrent uveitis, proliferative diabetic retinopathy, neovascular glaucoma, or rubeosis iridis.

Nursing Management

Providing Preoperative Care
- Provide the usual preoperative care for ambulatory surgical procedures, with specific preoperative testing indicated by patient's medical history.
- Obtain a careful medication history, including the use of alpha-agonists (particularly tamsulosin [Flomax] used for treatment for an enlarged prostate).
- Administer dilating eye drops prior to surgery.
- Educate patient regarding use of postoperative eye medications (antibiotic, corticosteroid, and anti-inflammatory drops) that will need to be self-administered to prevent infection and inflammation.

Providing Postoperative Care

- Provide patient with verbal and written instructions regarding eye protection, administration of eye drop medications, recognition of complications, activities to avoid, and obtaining emergency care.
- Educate the patient about the expectation of minimal discomfort and availability of mild analgesic agents (e.g., acetaminophen) as needed.
- Review medications prescribed including antibiotic medications and anti-inflammatory and corticosteroid eye drops or ointments.

Promoting Home- and Community-Based Care

Educating Patients About Self-Care

- Educate the patient about postoperative care, including wearing a protective eye patch for the first 24 hours after surgery, followed by eyeglasses during the day and an eye shield at night. Sunglasses should be worn at all times outdoors owing to the eyes' increased sensitivity to light.
- Slight amount of discharge in the morning, some redness, and a scratchy feeling in the operated eye is to be expected in the first few days; gently wiping with a damp washcloth to remove discharge may be suggested.
- Educate patient to notify surgeon if new floaters, flashing lights, decreased visual acuity, pain, or increased redness occur.

Continuing Care

- If an eye patch is worn, it is removed at the first follow-up visit, usually 48 hours after surgery.
- Educate patient regarding the importance of keeping follow-up appointments, monitoring visual status, and seeking prompt intervention for postoperative complications to enhance a good visual outcome.
- Visual acuity will stabilize after eye is completely healed, usually 6 to 12 weeks, when the final visual correction will be assessed for any remaining refractive errors.
- Advise patients with multifocal IOL implants that there may be an increased night glare and contrast sensitivity.

For more information, see Chapter 63 in Hinkle, J. L., & Cheever, K. H. (2014). *Brunner and Suddarth's textbook of medical-surgical nursing* (13th ed.). Philadelphia: Lippincott Williams & Wilkins.

Cholelithiasis (and Cholecystitis)

In cholelithiasis, calculi (gallstones) usually form in the gallbladder from solid constituents of bile and vary greatly in size, shape, and composition. There are two major types of gallstones: pigment stones, which contain an excess of unconjugated pigments in the bile, and cholesterol stones (the more common form), which result from bile supersaturated with cholesterol due to increased synthesis of cholesterol and decreased synthesis of bile acids that dissolve cholesterol. Risk factors for pigment stones include cirrhosis, hemolysis, and infections of the biliary tract. These stones cannot be dissolved and must be removed surgically. Risk factors for cholesterol stones include gender (women are two to three times more likely to develop cholesterol stones); use of oral contraceptives, estrogens, and clofibrate; age (usually older than 40 years); multiparous status; and obesity. There is also an increased risk related to diabetes, GI tract disease, T-tube fistula, and ileal resection or bypass.

Acute cholecystitis, a complication of cholelithiasis, is an acute infection of the gallbladder. Most patients with cholecystitis have gallstones (calculous cholecystitis). A gallstone obstructs bile outflow, and bile in the gallbladder initiates a chemical reaction, resulting in edema, compromise of the vascular supply, and gangrene. In the absence of gallstones, cholecystitis (acalculous) may occur after surgery, severe trauma, or burns, or with torsion, cystic duct obstruction, multiple blood transfusions, and primary bacterial infections of the gallbladder. Infection causes pain, tenderness, and rigidity of the upper right abdomen and is associated with nausea and vomiting and the usual signs of inflammation. Purulent fluid inside the gallbladder indicates an empyema of the gallbladder. See "Nursing Process" for additional information.

Clinical Manifestations

- It may be silent, producing no pain and only mild GI symptoms.
- It may be acute or chronic with epigastric distress (fullness, abdominal distention, and vague upper right quadrant pain); may follow a meal rich in fried or fatty foods.
- If the cystic duct is obstructed, the gallbladder becomes distended, inflamed, and eventually infected, possibly

producing fever and palpable abdominal mass; biliary colic with excruciating upper right abdominal pain, radiating to back or right shoulder with nausea and vomiting several hours after a heavy meal; restlessness; and constant or colicky pain.

- Jaundice may be accompanied by marked pruritis, with obstruction of the common bile duct, in a small few patients.
- Very dark urine and grayish or clay-colored stool are seen.
- Deficiencies of vitamins A, D, E, and K (fat-soluble vitamins) may occur.

Assessment and Diagnostic Findings

Stones may be detected incidentally during surgery or evaluation for unrelated problems.

- Abdominal x-ray
- Radionuclide imaging or cholescintigraphy
- Cholecystogram, cholangiogram; celiac axis arteriography
- Laparoscopy
- Ultrasonography; endoscopic ultrasound (EUS)
- Helical CT scans and MRI; endoscopic retrograde cholangiopancreatography (ERCP) with fluoroscopy; percutaneous transhepatic cholangiography (PTC)
- Serum alkaline phosphatase; gamma-glutamyl (GGT), gamma-glutamyl transpeptidase (GGTP), and lactate dehydrogenase (LDH)
- Cholesterol levels

Medical Management

Major objectives of medical therapy are to reduce the incidence of acute episodes of gallbladder pain and cholecystitis by supportive and dietary management and, if possible, to remove the cause by pharmacotherapy, endoscopic procedures, or surgical intervention (laparoscopic cholecystectomy).

Nutritional and Supportive Therapy

- Achieve remission with rest, IV fluids, nasogastric suction, analgesia, and antibiotics.
- Diet immediately after an episode is usually low-fat liquids with high protein and carbohydrates followed by solid soft foods as tolerated; avoid eggs, cream, pork, fried foods, cheese, rich dressings, gas-forming vegetables, and alcohol.

Pharmacologic Therapy

- Ursodeoxycholic acid (UDCA [Urso, Actigall]) and cheno-deoxycholic acid (chenodiol or CDCA [Chenix]) are effective in dissolving primarily cholesterol stones.
- Patients with significant, frequent symptoms, cystic duct occlusion, or pigment stones are not candidates for therapy with UDCA.

Nonsurgical Removal of Gallstones

In addition to dissolving gallstones by infusion of a solvent (mono-octanoin or methyl tertiary butyl ether [MTBE]) into the gallbladder, stones can be removed by other instrumentation (e.g., catheter and instrument with a basket attached threaded through the T-tube tract or fistula formed at the time of T-tube insertion, ERCP endoscope), intracorporeal lithotripsy (laser pulse), or extracorporeal shock wave therapy (lithotripsy or extracorporeal shock wave lithotripsy [ESWL]).

Surgical Management

Goal of surgery is to relieve persistent symptoms, to remove the cause of biliary colic, and to treat acute cholecystitis.

- Laparoscopic cholecystectomy: Procedure is performed through a small incision or puncture made through the abdominal wall in the umbilicus.
- Cholecystectomy: Gallbladder is removed through an abdominal incision (usually right subcostal) after ligation of the cystic duct and artery.
- Small-incision cholecystectomy: Gallbladder is removed through a small incision.
- Choledochostomy: Incision is into the common duct for stone removal.
- Cholecystostomy (surgical or percutaneous): Gallbladder is opened, and the stone, bile, or purulent drainage is removed.

Gerontologic Considerations

- Surgical intervention for disease of the biliary tract is the most common operation performed in older adults.
- Biliary disease may be accompanied or preceded by symptoms of septic shock: oliguria, hypotension, changes in mental status, tachycardia, and tachypnea.
- Cholecystectomy is usually well tolerated and carries a low risk if expert assessment and care are provided before, during, and after surgery.

- Higher mortality results from serious complications and pre-existing associated diseases; shorter hospital stays make it essential that older patients and their family members receive specific information about signs and symptoms of complications and measures to prevent them.

NURSING PROCESS

The Patient Undergoing Surgery for Gallbladder Disease

Assessment

- Complete preadmission testing a week or longer before admission.
- Assess health history: Note history of smoking or prior respiratory problems.
- Assess respiratory status: Note shallow respirations, persistent cough, or ineffective or adventitious breath sounds.
- Evaluate nutritional status (dietary history, general examination, and laboratory study results).

Diagnosis

NURSING DIAGNOSES
- Acute pain and discomfort related to surgical incision
- Impaired gas exchange related to high abdominal surgical incision
- Impaired skin integrity related to altered biliary drainage after surgical incision
- Imbalanced nutrition, less than body requirements, related to inadequate bile secretion
- Deficient knowledge about self-care activities related to incisional care, dietary modifications (if needed), medications, reportable signs or symptoms (fever, bleeding, vomiting)

COLLABORATIVE PROBLEMS/POTENTIAL COMPLICATIONS
- Bleeding
- GI symptoms (possibly related to biliary leak or injury to the bowel)

Planning and Goals

Goals include relief of pain, adequate ventilation, intact skin and improved biliary drainage, optimal nutritional intake, absence of complications, and understanding of self-care routines.

Nursing Interventions

- Place patient in low Fowler's position.
- Provide IV fluids and nasogastric suction.
- Provide water and other fluids and soft diet, after bowel sounds return.

RELIEVING PAIN

- Administer analgesic agents as prescribed.
- Help patient turn, cough, breathe deeply, and ambulate as indicated.
- Educate patient to use a pillow or binder to splint incision.

IMPROVING RESPIRATORY STATUS

- Encourage patient to take deep breaths and cough every hour.
- Educate patient on use of incentive spirometry to expand the lungs fully and prevent atelectasis; promote early ambulation.
- Monitor older and obese patients and those with preexisting pulmonary disease most closely for respiratory problems.

MAINTAINING SKIN INTEGRITY AND PROMOTING BILIARY DRAINAGE

- Connect tubes to drainage receptacle and secure tubing to avoid kinking (elevate above abdomen).
- Place drainage bag in patient's pocket or fasten below waist when ambulating.
- Observe for indications of infection, leakage of bile, and obstruction of bile drainage.
- Change dressing frequently, using ointment to protect skin from irritation.
- Observe for jaundice (check the sclera).
- Note and report right upper quadrant abdominal pain, nausea and vomiting, bile drainage around any drainage tube, clay-colored stools, and a change in vital signs.
- Measure bile collected every 24 hours; document amount, color, and character of drainage.
- Keep careful record of intake and output.

IMPROVING NUTRITIONAL STATUS

- Encourage patient to eat a diet low in fats and high in carbohydrates and proteins immediately after surgery.

- Educate patient at discharge to maintain a healthy diet and avoid excessive fats; fat restriction is usually lifted in 4 to 6 weeks.

MONITORING AND MANAGING COMPLICATIONS
- Bleeding: Assess periodically for increased tenderness and rigidity of abdomen and report; instruct patient and family to report change in color of stools. Monitor vital signs closely. Inspect incision for bleeding.
- Gastrointestinal symptoms: Assess for loss of appetite, vomiting, pain, distention of abdomen, and temperature elevation; report promptly and instruct patient and family to report symptoms promptly; provide written reinforcement of verbal instructions.

PROMOTING HOME- AND COMMUNITY-BASED CARE

Educating Patients about Self-Care
- Educate patient about medications and their actions.
- Inform patient to report to primary provider symptoms of jaundice, dark urine, pale stools, pruritus, or signs of inflammation and infection (e.g., pain or fever).
- Educate patient, verbally and in writing, about proper care of drainage tubes and importance of reporting promptly any changes in amount or characteristics of drainage to primary provider.
- Refer for home care if necessary.
- Emphasize importance of keeping follow-up appointments and importance of participating in health screenings.

Evaluation

EXPECTED PATIENT OUTCOMES
- Reports decrease in pain
- Demonstrates appropriate respiratory function
- Exhibits normal skin integrity around biliary drainage sites
- Obtains relief from dietary intolerance
- Absence of complications

For more information, see Chapter 50 in Hinkle, J. L., & Cheever, K. H. (2014). *Brunner and Suddarth's textbook of medical-surgical nursing* (13th ed.). Philadelphia: Lippincott Williams & Wilkins.

Chronic Obstructive Pulmonary Disease

Chronic obstructive pulmonary disease (COPD) is a preventable and treatable disease with some significant extrapulmonary effects. COPD is characterized by airflow limitation that is not fully reversible, usually progressive, and associated with an abnormal inflammatory response to noxious particles or gases. The airflow limitation results in narrowing of airways, hypersecretion of mucus, and changes in the pulmonary vasculature. Other diseases such as cystic fibrosis, bronchiectasis, and asthma that were previously classified as types of COPD are now classified as chronic pulmonary disorders, although symptoms may overlap with those of COPD. Cigarette smoking, air pollution, and occupational exposure (e.g., to coal, cotton, grain) are important risk factors that contribute to COPD development, which may occur over a 20- to 30-year span. Complications of COPD vary but include respiratory insufficiency and failure (major complications) and pneumonia, atelectasis, and pneumothorax. COPD and associated conditions (chronic lower respiratory diseases) are the fourth leading cause of death in the United States.

Pathophysiology

Chronic Bronchitis

Chronic bronchitis, a disease of the airways, is defined as the presence of cough and sputum production for at least 3 months in each of 2 consecutive years. Constant irritation from smoke or environmental irritants causes the mucus-secreting glands and goblet cells to increase in number, leading to increased mucus production. Mucus plugging of the airway reduces ciliary function, and the bronchial walls become thickened, with narrowing of the bronchial lumen. Alveoli adjacent to the bronchioles may become damaged and fibrosed, resulting in altered function of the alveolar macrophages; as a result, the patient becomes more susceptible to respiratory infection.

Emphysema

In emphysema, impaired oxygen and carbon dioxide exchange results from destruction of the walls of overdistended alveoli beyond the terminal bronchioles and destruction of the walls of the alveoli. As the walls of the alveoli are destroyed (a

C

process accelerated by recurrent infections), the alveolar surface area in direct contact with the pulmonary capillaries continually decreases. This causes an increase in dead space (lung area where no gas exchange can occur) and impaired oxygen diffusion, which leads to hypoxemia. In the later stages of disease, carbon dioxide elimination is impaired, resulting in increased carbon dioxide tension in arterial blood (hypercapnia), leading to respiratory acidosis. As the alveolar walls continue to break down, the pulmonary capillary bed is reduced in size, thereby increasing the resistance to pulmonary blood flow, forcing the right ventricle to maintain a higher blood pressure in the pulmonary artery. For this reason, right-sided heart failure (cor pulmonale) is one of the complications of emphysema. There are two main types of emphysema: the panlobular (panacinar) type (destruction of the respiratory bronchiole, alveolar duct, and alveolus) and the centrilobular (centroacinar) type, (pathologic changes mainly in the center of the secondary lobule, preserving the peripheral portions of the acinus). Both may be present in an individual patient.

Risk Factors

- Environmental factors (e.g., active and passive smoking) and prolonged, intense exposure to occupational dusts and chemicals, and indoor or outdoor air pollution
- Host factors involving a gene-environment interaction (e.g., alpha$_1$-antitrypsin deficiency predisposing young people to develop rapid lobular emphysema in the absence of smoking)

Clinical Manifestations

- COPD is characterized by chronic cough, sputum production, and dyspnea on exertion and often worsens over time.
- COPD is classified stage I to IV depending on the severity as measured by pulmonary function tests (FEV$_1$/FVC ratio and FEV$_1$ ratio of patient versus predicted value) and severity of symptoms.
- Weight loss is common.
- Chronic hyperinflation seen with emphysema may develop a "barrel chest" thorax configuration; use of accessory muscles during inspiration may be seen.
- Symptoms are specific to the disease. See "Clinical Manifestations" under Asthma in Section A and under Bronchiectasis in Section B.

🌾 Gerontologic Considerations

COPD accentuates many of the physiologic changes associated with aging and is manifested in airway obstruction (in bronchitis) and excessive loss of elastic lung recoil (in emphysema). Additional changes in ventilation–perfusion ratios occur. Vaccination (including pneumococcal and annual influenza) is recommended in all patients 65 years or older and having COPD.

Medical Management

- Smoking cessation, if appropriate
- Bronchodilators, corticosteroids, and other drugs (e.g., alpha$_1$-antitrypsin augmentation therapy, antibiotic agents, mucolytic agents, antitussive agents, vasodilators, narcotics); vaccines possibly effective in reducing serious morbidity due to influenza and pneumonia
- Oxygen therapy, including nighttime oxygen

> ▶ *Quality and Safety Nursing Alert*
>
> Oxygen therapy is variable in COPD patients; its aim in COPD is to achieve an acceptable oxygen level without a fall in the pH (increasing hypercapnia).

- Varied treatments are specific to disease. See "Medical Management" under Asthma in Section A and under Bronchiectasis in Section B.

Surgical Management

- Bullectomy to reduce dyspnea; lung volume reduction to improve lobar elasticity and function
- Lung volume reduction surgery, a palliative surgical option in a selected subset of patients (e.g., stage IV with homogenous disease or disease that is focused in one area and not widespread throughout the lungs); not curative, providing only symptomatic relief
- Lung transplantation

Nursing Management

Assessment

- Obtain information about current symptoms and previous disease manifestations, particularly smoking exposure and history. Review the results of available diagnostic tests.
- Assess patient's understanding of normal anatomy and physiology of the lung, pathophysiology of COPD, and expected changes.

- Assess for informational deficits in components of pulmonary rehabilitation (e.g., medications and home oxygen therapy, nutrition, respiratory therapy treatments, symptom alleviation). Emphasize importance of smoking cessation.
- Assess patient's need to discuss quality of life issues, such as sexuality and COPD and coping with chronic disease. Emphasize the importance of communicating with the health care team.
- Address patient's need to plan for the future (advance directives, living wills, informed decision making about health care alternatives).

Achieving Airway Clearance

- Monitor patient for wheezing, diminished breath sounds, dyspnea, and hypoxemia.
- If bronchodilators or corticosteroids are prescribed, administer the medications properly and be alert for potential side effects.
- Confirm relief of bronchospasm by measuring improvement in expiratory flow rates and volumes (the force of expiration, how long it takes to exhale, and the amount of air exhaled) as well as by assessing the dyspnea and making sure that it has lessened.
- Encourage patient to eliminate or reduce all pulmonary irritants, particularly cigarette smoking.
- Instruct patient in directed or controlled coughing.
- Chest physiotherapy with postural drainage, intermittent positive pressure breathing, increased fluid intake, and bland aerosol mists (with normal saline solution or water) may be useful for some patients with COPD.

Improving Breathing Patterns

- Inspiratory muscle training and breathing retraining may help to improve ineffective breathing patterns.
- Training in diaphragmatic breathing reduces the respiratory rate, increases alveolar ventilation, and sometimes helps to expel as much air as possible during expiration.
- Pursed-lip breathing helps to slow expiration, prevents collapse of small airways, and controls the rate and depth of respiration; it also promotes relaxation.

Improving Activity Tolerance

- Evaluate patient's activity tolerance and limitations and use teaching strategies to promote independent activities of daily living and ways to decrease energy expenditure.

C

- Determine whether patient is a candidate for exercise training to strengthen the muscles of the upper and lower extremities and to improve exercise tolerance and endurance.
- Recommend use of walking aids, if appropriate, to improve activity levels and ambulation.
- Consult with other health care professionals (e.g., rehabilitation therapist, occupational therapist, physical therapist) as needed.

Monitoring and Managing Complications

- Assess patient for complications (respiratory insufficiency and failure, respiratory infection, and chronic atelectasis).
- Monitor for cognitive changes, increasing dyspnea, tachypnea, and tachycardia.
- Monitor pulse oximetry values and administer oxygen as prescribed.
- Instruct patient and family about signs and symptoms of infection or other complications and to report changes in physical or cognitive status.
- Encourage patient to be immunized against influenza and *Streptococcus pneumonia*.
- Caution patient to avoid going outdoors if the pollen count is high or if there is significant air pollution and to avoid exposure to high outdoor temperatures with high humidity.
- If a rapid onset of shortness of breath occurs, quickly evaluate patient for potential pneumothorax by assessing the symmetry of chest movement, differences in breath sounds, and pulse oximetry.

Promoting Home- and Community-Based Care

Educating Patients About Self-Care

- Provide instructions about self-management and assess the knowledge of patient and family members about self-care and the therapeutic regimen.
- Educate patient and family members about the early signs and symptoms of infection and other complications so that they seek appropriate health care promptly.

> ### ▶ Quality and Safety Nursing Alert
>
> Education is essential and should be tailored to the stage of COPD.

- Assist patient in setting and accepting realistic short-term and long-term goals based on the severity of COPD.
- Instruct patient to avoid extremes of heat and cold and air pollutants (e.g., fumes, smoke, dust, talcum, lint, and aerosol sprays). High altitudes aggravate hypoxemia.

- Encourage patient to adopt a lifestyle of moderate activity, ideally in a climate with minimal shifts in temperature and humidity; patient should avoid emotional disturbances and stressful situations and should be encouraged to stop smoking.
- Review educational information and have patient demonstrate correct metered-dose inhaler use before discharge, during follow-up visits, and during home visits.

Continuing Care
- Refer patient for home care if necessary.
- Direct patient to community resources (e.g., pulmonary rehabilitation programs and smoking cessation programs) and remind patient and family about the importance of participating in general health promotion activities and health screening.
- Address quality of life and issues surrounding the end of life for patients with end-stage COPD (e.g., symptom management, quality of life, satisfaction with care, information/communication, use of care professionals, use of care facilities, hospital admission, and place of death).

For more information, see Chapter 24 in Hinkle, J. L., & Cheever, K. H. (2014). *Brunner and Suddarth's textbook of medical-surgical nursing* (13th ed.). Philadelphia: Lippincott Williams & Wilkins.

Cirrhosis, Hepatic

Cirrhosis is a chronic disease characterized by replacement of normal liver tissue with diffuse fibrosis that disrupts the structure and function of the liver. Cirrhosis, or scarring of the liver, is divided into three types:

- Alcoholic cirrhosis, most frequently due to chronic alcoholism and the most common type of cirrhosis
- Postnecrotic cirrhosis, a late result of a previous acute viral hepatitis
- Biliary cirrhosis, a result of chronic biliary obstruction and infection (least common type of cirrhosis)

Major causative factors include nutritional deficiency with reduced protein intake and excessive alcohol intake. Other factors may play a role, including exposure to certain chemicals (carbon tetrachloride, chlorinated naphthalene, arsenic, or phosphorus) or infectious schistosomiasis. Most patients are between ages 40 and 60, with twice as many men as women affected.

Clinical Manifestations
- Compensated cirrhosis: usually found secondary to routine physical examination; vague symptoms including intermittent mild fever, vascular spider, palmar erythema, unexplained epistaxis, ankle edema, vague morning indigestion, flatulent dyspepsia, abdominal pain, splenomegaly and firm, enlarged liver
- Decompensated cirrhosis: symptoms of decreased proteins, clotting factors, and other substances and manifestations of portal hypertension
- Liver enlargement early in the course (fatty liver); later in course, liver size decreased from scar tissue, ascites, jaundice, weakness, muscle wasting, weight loss, continuous mild fever, finger clubbing with white nails, purpura, spontaneous bruising, epistaxis, hypotention, sparse body hair and gonadal atrophy
- Portal obstruction and ascites: late sign where organs become congested, causing indigestion, altered bowel function, and ascites
- Infection and peritonitis: Clinical signs may be absent, spontaneous bacterial peritonitis or abscess necessitating paracentesis for diagnosis and may cause hepatorenal failure
- Gastrointestinal varices: prominent, distended abdominal blood vessels; distended blood vessels throughout the GI tract; varices or hemorrhoids; hemorrhage from the stomach
- Generalized edema, often affecting the lower extremities, the upper extremities, and the presacral area
- Vitamin deficiency (A, C, and K) and anemia
- Mental deterioration with impending hepatic encephalopathy and hepatic coma

Assessment and Diagnostic Findings
- Liver function tests (e.g., serum alkaline phosphatase, aspartate aminotransferase [AST], alanine aminotransferase [ALT], gamma-glutamyl transferase [GGT], serum cholinesterase, and bilirubin), prothrombin time, arterial blood gases (ABGs), biopsy

C

- Ultrasound scans
- CT scan
- MRI
- Radioisotopic liver scans

Medical Management

Medical management is based on presenting symptoms, since the only definitive test to confirm hepatic cirrhosis is biopsy.

- Treatment includes antacids, vitamins and nutritional supplements, adequate diet, potassium-sparing diuretics (for ascites), and avoidance of alcohol.
- Colchicine, angiotensin system inhibitors, statins, diuretics including spironalactone (Aldactone), immunosuppressants, and glitazones possess antifibrotic activity for treatment.
- Patients with end-stage liver disease (ESLD) with cirrhosis can use the herb milk thistle (*Silybum marianum*) to treat jaundice and other symptoms.
- Primary biliary cirrhosis has been treated with ursodeoxycholic acid (Actigall, URSO) to improve liver function.

Nursing Management

Promoting Rest

- Position bed for maximal respiratory efficiency; provide oxygen if needed.
- Initiate efforts to prevent respiratory, circulatory, and vascular disturbances.
- Encourage patient to increase activity gradually and plan rest with activity and mild exercise.

Improving Nutritional Status

- Provide a nutritious, high-protein diet supplemented by vitamins B complex, A, C, and K.
- Encourage patient to eat: Provide small, frequent meals, consider patient preferences, and provide protein supplements, if indicated.
- Provide nutrients by feeding tube or total parenteral nutrition if needed.
- Provide patients who have fatty stools (steatorrhea) with water-soluble forms of fat-soluble vitamins A, D, and E and provide folic acid and iron to prevent anemia.
- Provide a low-protein diet temporarily if patient shows signs of impending or advancing coma; restrict sodium if necessary.

C

Providing Skin Care
- Change patient's position frequently.
- Avoid using irritating soaps and adhesive tape.
- Provide lotion to soothe irritated skin; take measures to prevent patient from scratching the skin.

Reducing Risk of Injury
- Use padded side rails if patient becomes agitated or restless.
- Orient to time, place, and procedures to minimize agitation.
- Instruct patient to ask for assistance to get out of bed.
- Evaluate any injury because of the possibility of internal bleeding.
- Provide safety measures to prevent injury or cuts (electric razor, soft toothbrush).
- Apply pressure to venipuncture sites to minimize bleeding.

Monitoring and Managing Potential Complications
- Monitor for bleeding and hemorrhage.
- Monitor patient's mental status closely and report changes so that treatment of hepatic encephalopathy can be initiated promptly.
- Monitor serum electrolyte levels and correct if abnormal.
- Administer oxygen if oxygen desaturation occurs; monitor for fever or abdominal pain, which may signal the onset of bacterial peritonitis or other infection.

Fluid Volume Excess
- Assess cardiovascular and respiratory status; administer diuretics, implement fluid restrictions, and enhance patient positioning, if needed.
- Monitor input and output and daily weight changes.
- Assess changes in abdominal girth and edema formation.
- Monitor for nocturia and, later, for oliguria, because these states indicate increasing severity of liver dysfunction.

See "Nursing Management" under Hepatic Encephalopathy and Hepatic Coma in Section H for additional information.

Promoting Home- and Community-Based Care
- Prepare for discharge by providing dietary instruction, including exclusion of alcohol.
- Refer to Alcoholics Anonymous, psychiatric care, counseling, or spiritual advisor if indicated.
- Continue sodium restriction; stress avoidance of raw shellfish.

C

- Educate patient and family using written instructions, reinforcement, and support.
- Encourage rest and probably a change in lifestyle (adequate dietary intake and elimination of alcohol).
- Instruct family about symptoms of impending encephalopathy and possible bleeding tendencies and susceptibility to infection.
- Offer support and encouragement to the patient and provide positive feedback when the patient experiences success.
- Refer patient to home care nurse, and assist in transition from hospital to home.

For more information, see Chapter 49 in Hinkle, J. L., & Cheever, K. H. (2014). *Brunner and Suddarth's textbook of medical-surgical nursing* (13th ed.). Philadelphia: Lippincott Williams & Wilkins.

Constipation

Constipation refers to an abnormal infrequency or irregularity of defecation, abnormal hardening of stool that makes passage difficult and sometimes painful, decrease in stool volume, prolonged retention of stool in the rectum, or persistent sensation of abdominal fullness. It can be caused by certain medications; rectal or anal disorders; obstruction; metabolic, neurologic, and neuromuscular conditions; endocrine disorders; lead poisoning; connective tissue disorders; and a variety of disease conditions. Other causes may include weakness, immobility, debility, fatigue, inadequate dietary intake of fiber and fluids, and inability to increase intra-abdominal pressure to pass stools. Constipation develops when people do not take the time or ignore the urge to defecate or as the result of dietary habits (low consumption of fiber and inadequate fluid intake), lack of regular exercise, and a stress-filled life. Perceived constipation is a subjective problem that occurs when an individual's bowel elimination pattern is not consistent with what he or she perceives as normal; however, constipation can indicate an underlying disease or motility disorder of the gastrointestinal (GI) tract. Chronic laxative use contributes to this problem.

Pathophysiology

The pathophysiology of constipation is poorly understood, but it is thought to include interference with one of three major functions of the colon: mucosal transport (i.e., mucosal secretions facilitate the movement of colon contents), myoelectric activity (i.e., mixing of the rectal mass and propulsive actions), or the processes of defecation (e.g., pelvic floor dysfunction). Any of the causative factors previously identified can interfere with any of these three processes. If all organic causes are eliminated, idiopathic or functional constipation is diagnosed.

Clinical Manifestations

- Fewer than three bowel movements per week, abdominal distention, and pain and pressure
- Decreased appetite, headache, fatigue, indigestion, sensation of incomplete emptying
- Straining at stool; elimination of small volume of hard, dry stool
- Complications such as hypertension, hemorrhoids and fissures, fecal impaction, and megacolon
- True chronic constipation: presence of symptoms noted above for at least 12 weeks of the preceding 12 months

Assessment and Diagnostic Findings

Diagnosis is based on history, physical examination, possibly a barium enema or sigmoidoscopy, stool for occult blood, anorectal manometry (pressure studies), defecography, and colonic transit studies. The Rome Diagnostic Criteria are used to categorize the symptoms of constipation based on specific characteristics related to defecation. Tests such as pelvic floor MRI may identify occult pelvic floor defects.

Gerontologic Considerations

Visits to primary providers for treatment of constipation are common in people 65 years and older; a common complaint is the need to strain when passing a stool. The aging process generates changes in the colon; but the extent and physiologic implications for defecation remain unclear. Contributing factors to constipation in older adults include preference for soft, processed, and low-fiber foods due to dental or chewing difficulties, decreased food intake, reduced mobility, overuse of laxatives, and weak abdominal muscles. Chronic illnesses and resulting polypharmacy, depression, weakness, and prolonged bed rest may also be contributing factors. Chronic constipation impairs quality of life in degrees comparable to changes in quality of life in such other chronic illnesses as diabetes, rheumatoid arthritis, and osteoarthritis.

C

Medical Management

- Treatment should target the underlying cause of constipation and aim to prevent recurrence, including education, exercise, bowel habit training, increased fiber and fluid intake, and judicious use of laxatives.
- Educate the patient to sit on the toilet with legs supported following a meal that includes a warm drink to support the gastrocolic reflex that facilitates defecation.
- Increase fluid intake; include fiber in diet; try biofeedback and an exercise routine to strengthen abdominal muscles.
- Discontinue laxative abuse; if a laxative is necessary, use bulk-forming agents, saline and osmotic agents, lubricants, stimulants, or fecal softeners.
- Specific medication therapy may be used to increase intrinsic motor function (e.g., cholinergic agents, cholinesterase inhibitors, or prokinetic agents); medical probiotics may help some by creating improved bacterial balance.
- Alternative or complementary therapies include abdominal massage, aromatherapy, acupuncture, and the use of Chinese herbal medications; these should be used only with unremitting constipation.

Nursing Management

- Use tact and respect with patient when talking about bowel habits and obtaining health history. Note the following:
  - Onset and duration of constipation, current and past elimination patterns, patient's expectation of normal bowel elimination, and lifestyle information (e.g., exercise and activity level, occupation, food and fluid intake, and stress level)
  - Medical and surgical history, current medications, history of laxative or enema use
- Report any of the following: rectal pressure or fullness, abdominal pain, straining at defecation, and flatulence.
- Set specific goals for education; goals for the patient include restoring or maintaining a regular pattern of elimination by responding to the urge to defecate, ensuring adequate intake of fluids and high-fiber foods, learning about methods to avoid constipation, relieving anxiety about bowel elimination patterns, and avoiding complications.

For more information, see Chapter 48 in Hinkle, J. L., & Cheever, K. H. (2014). *Brunner and Suddarth's textbook of medical-surgical nursing* (13th ed.). Philadelphia: Lippincott Williams & Wilkins.

Coronary Atherosclerosis

Coronary atherosclerosis is the most common cause of cardio-vascular disease in the United States and is characterized by an abnormal accumulation of lipid or fatty substances and fibrous tissue in the vessel wall. These substances block or narrow the vessel, reducing blood flow to the myocardium. Atherosclerosis involves a repetitious inflammatory response to injury of the artery wall and subsequent alteration in the structural and biochemical properties of the arterial walls.

Risk Factors

Modifiable
- Elevated low-density lipoprotein (LDL) and total blood cholesterol (hyperlipidemia)
- Cigarette smoking, tobacco use
- Elevated blood pressure
- Hyperglycemia (diabetes)
- Metabolic syndrome including insulin resistance, central obesity, dyslipidemia, elevated blood pressure, proinflammatory state (increased levels of high-sensitivity C-reactive protein [hs-CRP]), prothrombotic state (high fibrinogen levels)
- Obesity
- Physical inactivity

Not Modifiable
- Positive family history (a first-degree relative with cardiovascular disease at age 55 years or younger for men and at age 65 years or younger for women)
- Age (older than 45 years for men, older than 55 years for women)
- Gender, cardiovascular disease developing at an earlier age in men than in women
- Race (higher incidence in African Americans than in Caucasians)

Clinical Manifestations

Symptoms and complications develop according to the location and degree of narrowing of the arterial lumen, thrombus formation, and obstruction of blood flow to the myocardium.

Symptoms include the following:

- Ischemia
- Chest pain: angina pectoris
- Atypical symptoms of myocardial ischemia (shortness of breath, nausea, weakness, epigastric distress, pain radiating to the jaw or left arm)
- Myocardial infarction
- Dysrhythmias, sudden death

Assessment and Diagnostic Findings
Identification of risk factors for coronary heart disease (CHD) primarily involves taking a thorough history, including family history, physical examination (note blood pressure and weight), and laboratory work (e.g., total cholesterol levels, LDL, high-density lipoprotein [HDL], hs-CRP levels, and glucose).

Prevention
The major management goal is prevention of CHD. Modifiable risk factors—including cholesterol abnormalities, tobacco use, hypertension, diabetes, metabolic syndrome, and physical inactivity—have been cited as major risk factors for coronary artery disease and its complications. As a result, they receive much attention in health promotion programs.

Medical Management
See "Medical Management" in Section A and under Acute Coronary Syndrome and Myocardial Infarction in Section A for additional information.

Nursing Management
See "Nursing Process" in Section A and under Acute Coronary Syndrome and Myocardial Infarction in Section A for additional information.

For more information, see Chapter 27 in Hinkle, J. L., & Cheever, K. H. (2014). *Brunner and Suddarth's textbook of medical-surgical nursing* (13th ed.). Philadelphia: Lippincott Williams & Wilkins.

Crohn's Disease (Regional Enteritis)

Regional enteritis (known as *Crohn's disease*) is a subacute and chronic inflammation of the gastrointestinal (GI) tract wall that extends through all layers.

Pathophysiology

Crohn's disease (CD) is usually first diagnosed in adolescents or young adults but can appear at any time of life. The clinical course and symptoms vary. In some patients, periods of remission and exacerbation occur but, in others, the disease follows a fulminating course. Although the most common areas in which it is found are the distal ileum and colon, it can occur anywhere along the GI tract. One theory suggests that CD is the result of defects in the immune system in genetically predisposed individuals that allow bacteria to invade the gastric mucosa, resulting in an overactive immune response. Fistulas, fissures, and abscesses form as the inflammation extends into the peritoneum. In advanced cases, the intestinal mucosa has a cobblestonelike appearance. As the disease advances, the bowel wall thickens and becomes fibrotic and the intestinal lumen narrows. Diseased bowel loops sometimes adhere to other loops surrounding the diseased loop.

Clinical Manifestations

- Onset of symptoms is usually insidious, with prominent right lower quadrant abdominal pain and diarrhea unrelieved by defecation.
- Abdominal tenderness and spasm are seen.
- Crampy pains occur after meals; the patient tends to limit intake, causing weight loss, malnutrition, and secondary anemia.
- Chronic diarrhea may occur, resulting in a patient who is uncomfortable and is thin and emaciated from inadequate food intake and constant fluid loss. The inflamed intestine may perforate and form intra-abdominal and anal abscesses.
- Fever and leukocytosis occur.
- Abscesses, fistulas, and fissures are common.
- Symptoms extend beyond the GI tract to include joint disorders (e.g., arthritis), skin lesions (e.g., erythema nodosum), ocular disorders (e.g., conjunctivitis), and oral ulcers.

Assessment and Diagnostic Findings

- Barium study of the upper GI tract is the most conclusive diagnostic aid; it shows the classic "string sign" of the terminal ileum (constriction of a segment of intestine) as well as cobblestone appearance, fistulas, and fissures.
- Endoscopy, colonoscopy, and intestinal biopsies may be used to confirm the diagnosis.

- Video capsule endoscopy can provide extensive evaluation of the small intestine.
- Proctosigmoidoscopic examination and CT scan are helpful.
- Stool examination should be performed for occult blood and steatorrhea.
- Complete blood cell count (decreased Hgb and Hct), erythrocyte sedimentation rate (elevated), albumin, and protein levels (usually decreased owing to malnutrition) should be obtained.

Medical Management

See "Medical Management" under Ulcerative Colitis in Section U for additional information.

Nursing Management

See "Nursing Process: The Patient With Inflammatory Bowel Disease" under Ulcerative Colitis in Section U for additional information.

For more information, see Chapter 48 in Hinkle, J. L., & Cheever, K. H. (2014). *Brunner and Suddarth's textbook of medical-surgical nursing* (13th ed.). Philadelphia: Lippincott Williams & Wilkins.

Cushing Syndrome

Cushing syndrome results from excessive, rather than deficient, adrenocortical activity. It is commonly caused by use of corticosteroid medications and is infrequently the result of excessive corticosteroid production secondary to hyperplasia of the adrenal cortex. It may be caused by several mechanisms, including a tumor of the pituitary gland or less commonly, an ectopic malignancy that produces adrenocorticotropic hormone (ACTH) referred to as Cushing disease. Regardless of the cause, the normal feedback mechanisms that control the function of the adrenal cortex become ineffective, resulting in oversecretion of glucocorticoids, androgens, and possibly mineralocorticoid. Cushing syndrome occurs five times more often in women ages 20 to 40 years than in men.

Clinical Manifestations

- Classic features include central-type obesity, with a fatty "buffalo hump" in the neck and supraclavicular areas, a heavy trunk, and relatively thin extremities; skin is thin, fragile, easily traumatized, with ecchymoses and striae.

- Weakness and lassitude occur; sleep is disturbed because of altered diurnal secretion of cortisol.
- Excessive protein catabolism with muscle wasting and osteoporosis are seen; kyphosis, backache, and compression fractures of the vertebrae may result.
- Retention of sodium and water produces hypertension and heart failure.
- "Moon-faced" appearance, oiliness of skin, and acne are evident.
- Increased susceptibility to infection and slow healing of minor cuts and bruises occurs.
- Hyperglycemia or overt diabetes may develop.
- Virilization occurs in females (due to excess androgens) with appearance of masculine traits and recession of feminine traits (e.g., excessive hair on face, breast atrophy, cessation of menses, enlarged clitoris, and deepening voice); libido is lost in males and females.
- Changes occur in mood and mental activity; psychosis may develop, and distress and depression are common.
- If Cushing syndrome is the result of a pituitary tumor, visual disturbances are possible because of pressure on the optic chiasm.

Assessment and Diagnostic Findings

The three tests used to diagnose Cushing syndrome are serum cortisol, urinary cortisol, and low-dose dexamethasone (Decadron) suppression tests, with results of at least two of these three tests being unequivocally abnormal to diagnose Cushing syndrome.

- Dexamethasone suppression test overnight to measure plasma cortisol level (stress, obesity, depression, and medications may falsely elevate results).
- Laboratory studies (e.g., blood eosinophil count, serum sodium, blood glucose, serum potassium, plasma, urinary); 24-hour urinary free cortisol level
- CT, ultrasound, or MRI scan to aid in localizing adrenal tissue and detect adrenal tumors

Medical Management

Treatment is usually directed at the pituitary gland because most cases are due to pituitary tumors rather than tumors of the adrenal cortex.

- Surgical removal of the tumor by transsphenoidal hypophysectomy is the treatment of choice (80% success rate).

C

- Radiation of the pituitary gland is successful but takes several months for symptom control.
- Adrenalectomy is performed in patients with primary adrenal hypertrophy.
- Postoperatively, temporary replacement therapy with hydro-cortisone may be necessary for several months, until the adrenal glands begin to respond normally.
- If bilateral adrenalectomy was performed, lifetime replacement of adrenal cortex hormones is necessary.
- Adrenal enzyme inhibitors (e.g., metyrapone, amino-glutethimide, mitotane, ketoconazole) may be used with ectopic ACTH-secreting tumors that cannot be totally removed; monitor closely for inadequate adrenal function and side effects.
- If Cushing syndrome results from exogenous corticosteroids, taper the drug to the minimum level or use alternate-day therapy to treat the underlying disease.

NURSING PROCESS

The Patient With Cushing Syndrome

Assessment

- Focus on the effects on the body of high concentrations of adrenal cortex hormones.
- Assess patient's level of activity and ability to carry out routine and self-care activities.
- Observe skin for trauma, infection, breakdown, bruising, and edema.
- Note changes in appearance and patient's responses to these changes; family is a good source of information about patient's emotional status and changes in appearance.
- Assess patient's mental function, including mood, response to questions, depression, and awareness of environment.

Diagnosis

NURSING DIAGNOSES

- Risk for injury related to weakness
- Risk for infection related to altered protein metabolism and inflammatory response
- Self-care deficits related to weakness, fatigue, muscle wasting, and altered sleep patterns

- Impaired skin integrity related to edema, impaired healing, and thin and fragile skin
- Disturbed body image related to altered appearance, impaired sexual functioning, and decreased activity level
- Ineffective coping related to mood swings, irritability, and depression

COLLABORATIVE PROBLEMS/POTENTIAL COMPLICATIONS
- Addisonian crisis
- Adverse effects of adrenocortical activity

Planning and Goals

Major goals include decreased risk of injury, decreased risk of infection, increased ability to carry out self-care activities, improved skin integrity, improved body image, improved mental function, and absence of complications.

Nursing Interventions

DECREASING RISK OF INJURY
- Provide a protective environment to prevent falls, fractures, and other injuries to bones and soft tissues.
- Assist patient who is weak in ambulating to avoid falling or bumping into furniture.
- Recommend foods high in protein, calcium, and vitamin D to minimize muscle wasting and osteoporosis; refer to dietitian for assistance.

DECREASING RISK OF INFECTION
- Avoid unnecessary exposure to others with infections.
- Assess frequently for subtle signs of infections (corticosteroids mask signs of inflammation and infection).

PREPARING PATIENT FOR SURGERY
Monitor blood glucose levels and assess stools for blood because diabetes and peptic ulcer are common problems (see also "Nursing Process: The Preoperative Patient" under Perioperative Nursing Management in Section P).

ENCOURAGING REST AND ACTIVITY
- Encourage moderate activity to prevent complications of immobility and promote self-esteem.
- Plan rest periods throughout the day and promote a relaxing, quiet environment for rest and sleep.

C

PROMOTING SKIN INTEGRITY
- Use meticulous skin care to avoid traumatizing fragile skin.
- Avoid adhesive tape, which can tear and irritate the skin.
- Assess skin and bony prominences frequently.
- Encourage and assist patient to change positions frequently.

IMPROVING BODY IMAGE
- Discuss the impact that changes have had on patient's self-concept and relationships with others. Major physical changes will disappear in time if the cause of Cushing syndrome can be treated.
- Weight gain and edema may be modified by a low-carbohydrate, low-sodium diet; a high-protein intake can reduce some bothersome symptoms.

IMPROVING COPING
- Explain to patient and family the cause of emotional instability and help them cope with mood swings, irritability, and depression.
- Report any psychotic behavior.
- Encourage patient and family members to verbalize feelings and concerns.

MONITORING AND MANAGING COMPLICATIONS
- Regarding adrenal hypofunction and addisonian crisis, monitor for hypotension; rapid, weak pulse; rapid respiratory rate; pallor; and extreme weakness. Note factors that may have led to crisis (e.g., stress, trauma, surgery).
- Administer IV fluids and electrolytes and corticosteroids before, during, and after surgery or treatment as indicated.
- Monitor for circulatory collapse and shock present in addisonian crisis; treat promptly.
- Assess fluid and electrolyte status by monitoring laboratory values and daily weight.
- Monitor blood glucose level and report elevations to primary provider.

EDUCATING PATIENTS ABOUT SELF-CARE
- Present verbal and written information about Cushing syndrome to patient and family.
- Reinforce to patient and family that stopping corticosteroid use abruptly and without medical supervision can result in adrenal insufficiency and reappearance of symptoms.

C

- Emphasize the need to keep an adequate supply of the corticosteroid to prevent running out or skipping a dose, because this could result in addisonian crisis.
- Ensure dietary modifications include adequate calcium intake without increasing risk for hypertension, hyperglycemia, and weight gain.
- Educate patient and family to monitor blood pressure, blood glucose levels, and weight.
- Advise patient to wear a medical alert bracelet and notify other health professionals (e.g., dentist) that he or she has Cushing syndrome.
- Refer for home care as indicated to ensure safe environment with minimal stress and risk for falls and other side effects.
- Emphasize importance of regular medical follow-up and ensure patient is aware of side and toxic effects of medications.
- Remind patient and family about the importance of health promotion activities and recommended health screening, including bone mineral density testing.

Evaluation

EXPECTED PATIENT OUTCOMES
- Decreases risk of injury
- Decreases risk of infection
- Increases participation in self-care activities
- Attains or maintains skin integrity
- Achieves improved body image
- Exhibits improved mental functioning
- Exhibits absence of complications

For more information, see Chapter 52 in Hinkle, J. L., & Cheever, K. H. (2014). *Brunner and Suddarth's textbook of medical-surgical nursing* (13th ed.). Philadelphia: Lippincott Williams & Wilkins.

Cystitis (Lower Urinary Tract Infection)

Cystitis is an inflammation of the urinary bladder. Cystitis occurs more often in women, particularly sexually active women. Cystitis in men is secondary to other factors (e.g., infected prostate, epididymitis, or bladder stones).

Pathophysiology

For infection to occur, bacteria must gain access to the bladder, attach to and colonize the epithelium of the urinary tract to avoid being washed out with voiding, evade host defense mechanisms, and initiate inflammation. Bacteria may enter the urinary tract in three ways: by the transurethral route (ascending infection), through the bloodstream (hematogenous spread), or by means of a fistula from the intestine (direct extension). The most common route of infection is transurethral, often from fecal contamination, ureterovesical reflux, or the use of a catheter or cystoscope. In women, sexual intercourse forces bacteria from the urethra into the bladder.

Clinical Manifestations

- Urgency, frequency, burning, and pain on urination
- Nocturia; incontinence; and back, suprapubic, or pelvic pain
- Hematuria
- With complicated urinary tract infections (UTIs; e.g., patients with indwelling catheters), range of symptoms from asymptomatic bacteriuria to a gram-negative sepsis with shock

🍁 Gerotontologic Considerations

The incidence of bacteriuria in older adults differs from that in younger adults. Bacteriuria increases with age and disability, and women are affected more frequently than men. UTI is the most common cause of acute bacterial sepsis in patients older than 65 years, in whom gram-negative sepsis carries a mortality rate exceeding 50%. In older patients who reside in nursing homes, 25% to 50% of women and 15% to 40% of men have chronic bacteriuria. Older adults are at increased risk for UTI owing to structural abnormalities related to aging (e.g., decreased bladder tone, neurogenic bladder, urethral strictures), use of indwelling catheters, incomplete emptying of the bladder, prostatic hyperplasia, and colonization and increased adherence of bacteria to the vagina and urethra in postmenopausal women. The most common subjective presenting symptom of UTI in older adults is generalized fatigue.

 Quality and Safety Nursing Alert

Older patients often lack the typical symptoms of UTI and sepsis. Although frequency and urgency may occur, such non-specific symptoms as altered sensorium, lethargy, anorexia, new incontinence, hyperventilation, and low-grade fever may be the only clues.

Assessment and Diagnostic Findings

- Urine cultures, colony counts, and cellular studies are indicated.
- Leukocyte esterase test and nitrite testing may be performed.
- Tests for sexually transmitted infections (STIs) should be obtained
- CT scans and transrectal ultrasonography (to assess prostate and bladder) are helpful; cystourethroscopy may be indicated to visualize the ureters or to detect strictures, calculi, or tumors.

Medical Management

Management of UTIs typically involves pharmacologic therapy and patient education. The nurse educates the patient about prescribed medication regimens and infection prevention measures.

Acute Pharmacologic Therapy

- Ideal treatment is an antibacterial agent that eradicates bacteria from the urinary tract with minimal effects on fecal and vaginal flora.
- Medications may include cephalexin (Keflex), cotrimoxazole (TMP-SMZ, Bactrim, Septra), cefadroxil (Duricef, Unicef), nitrofurantoin (Macrodantin, Furadantin), ciprofloxacin (Cipro), levofloxacin (Levaquin), and phenazopyridine (Pyridium).
- Occasionally, ampicillin or amoxicillin is prescribed (but *Escherichia coli* has developed resistance to these agents).

Long-Term Pharmacologic Therapy

- About 20% of women treated for uncomplicated UTIs experience a recurrence; 90% of recurrences represent infection with new bacteria.
- Recurrence in men is usually due to persistence of the same organism; further evaluation and treatment are indicated.
- If diagnostic evaluation reveals no structural abnormalities, patient may be instructed to begin treatment on own, testing urine with a dipstick whenever symptoms occur, and to contact health care provider only with persistence of symptoms, at the occurrence of fever, or if the number of treatment episodes exceeds four in a 6-month period.
- Long-term use of antimicrobial agents decreases risk of reinfection.

NURSING PROCESS

C

The Patient With Cystitis

Assessment

- Take careful history of urinary signs and symptoms.
- Assess for pain and urinary frequency, urgency, and hesitancy and changes in urine; document and report findings.
- Determine usual pattern of voiding to detect factors that may predispose patient to infection.
- Assess for infrequent emptying of the bladder, association of symptoms of UTIs with sexual intercourse, contraceptive practices, and personal hygiene.
- Assess patient's knowledge about prescribed medication and preventive health measures.
- Check urine for volume, color, concentration, cloudiness, and odor.

Diagnosis

NURSING DIAGNOSES
- Acute pain related to infection within the urinary tract
- Deficient knowledge related to factors predisposing to infection and recurrence, detection and prevention of recurrence, and pharmacologic therapy

COLLABORATIVE PROBLEMS/POTENTIAL COMPLICATIONS
- Sepsis (urosepsis)
- Renal failure, which may occur as the long-term result of an extensive infective or inflammatory process

Planning and Goals

Goals of the patient may include relief of pain and discomfort, increased knowledge of preventive measures and treatment modalities, and absence of complications.

Nursing Interventions

RELIEVING PAIN
- Use antispasmodic drugs to relieve bladder irritability and pain.
- Relieve pain and spasm with analgesic agents and heat to the perineum.
- Encourage patient to drink liberal amounts of fluid (water is best).

- Instruct patient to avoid urinary tract irritants (e.g., coffee, tea, citrus, spices, colas, alcohol).
- Encourage frequent voiding (every 2 to 3 hours).

MONITORING AND MANAGING COMPLICATIONS
- Recognize and educate patient to recognize the signs and symptoms of UTIs early; initiate prompt treatment.
- Manage UTIs with appropriate antimicrobial therapy, liberal fluids, frequent voiding, and hygiene measures.
- Instruct patient to notify physician if fatigue, nausea, vomiting, or pruritus occurs.
- Provide for periodic monitoring of renal function and evaluation for strictures, obstructions, or stones.
- Avoid indwelling catheters if possible; use smallest size possible and remove at earliest opportunity. Use strict aseptic technique if an indwelling catheter is necessary; maintain a closed system and meticulous daily perineal care.
- Check vital signs and level of consciousness for impending sepsis.
- Report positive blood cultures and elevated white blood cell (WBC) counts.

PROMOTING HOME- AND COMMUNITY-BASED CARE
Educating Patients About Self-Care
- Educate patient regarding health-related behaviors that help prevent recurrent UTIs, including practicing careful personal hygiene, increasing fluid intake to promote voiding and dilution of urine, urinating regularly and more frequently, and adhering to the therapeutic regimen.
- Educational goals should meet the patient's individual needs.

Evaluation

EXPECTED PATIENT OUTCOMES
- Experiences relief of pain
- Explains UTIs and their treatment
- Experiences no complications

For more information, see Chapter 55 in Hinkle, J. L., & Cheever, K. H. (2014). *Brunner and Suddarth's textbook of medical-surgical nursing* (13th ed.). Philadelphia: Lippincott Williams & Wilkins.

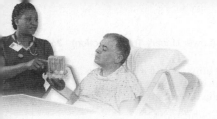

Dermatitis, Contact

Contact dermatitis (also called *eczema*) is an inflammatory reaction of the skin to physical, chemical, or biologic agents. It may be of the primary irritant type, or it may be allergic. The epidermis is damaged by repeated physical and chemical irritation. Common causes of irritant dermatitis are soaps, detergents, scouring compounds, and industrial chemicals. Predisposing factors include extremes of heat and cold, frequent use of soap and water, and a preexisting skin disease. Women tend to be affected more commonly than men.

Clinical Manifestations
- Eruptions occur when the causative agent contacts the skin.
- Pruritus, burning, and erythema are followed by edema, papules, vesicles, and oozing or weeping as first reactions.
- In the subacute phase, the vesicular changes are less marked and alternate with crusting, drying, fissuring, and peeling.
- If repeated reactions occur or the patient continually scratches the skin, lichenification and pigmentation occur; secondary bacterial invasion may follow.

Medical Management
- The goal of management is to soothe and heal the involved skin and protect it from further damage.
- The distribution pattern of the reaction needs to be determined to differentiate between allergic type and irritant type.
- The offending irritant should be identified and removed; soap is generally not used on the site until healed.
- Barrier cream that contains ceramide (e.g., Impruv, Cerave) or dimethicone (e.g., Cetaphil) can be used for small patches of erythema; cool, wet dressings can be applied over small areas of vesicular dermatitis; a corticosteroid ointment may be used.
- Medicated baths at room temperature are prescribed for larger areas of dermatitis.
- In severe, widespread conditions, a short course of systemic steroids may be prescribed.

Nursing Management

- Assess detailed history and have patient think about what may have caused the problem.
- Instruct patient to adhere to the following instructions for at least 4 months, until the skin appears completely healed:
  - Avoid contact with known irritants, or wash skin thoroughly immediately after exposure to them.
  - Avoid heat, soap, and rubbing the skin.
  - Choose bath soaps, detergents, and cosmetics that do not contain fragrance; avoid using a fabric softener dryer sheet.
  - Avoid topical medications, lotions, or ointments, except when prescribed.
  - When wearing gloves (e.g., for washing dishes, cleaning), make sure they are cotton-lined; do not wear for more than 15 to 20 minutes at a time.
- Educate patient on ways to treat and prevent further bouts of irritant dermatitis.

For more information, see Chapter 61 in Hinkle, J. L., & Cheever, K. H. (2014). *Brunner and Suddarth's textbook of medical-surgical nursing* (13th ed.). Philadelphia: Lippincott Williams & Wilkins.

Dermatitis, Exfoliative

Exfoliative dermatitis, also called *erythroderma,* is a serious condition characterized by scaling erythematous dermatitis that may involve more than 90% of the skin. This condition starts acutely as either a patchy or a generalized erythematous eruption. Exfoliative dermatitis has a variety of causes. It is considered to be a process secondary or reactive to an underlying skin or systemic disease. It may appear as a part of the lymphoma group of diseases and may precede the appearance of lymphoma. Preexisting skin disorders implicated as a cause include psoriasis, atopic dermatitis, and contact dermatitis. It also appears as a severe medication reaction to penicillin and phenylbutazone. The cause is idiopathic (i.e., unknown) in approximately 30% of cases; idiopathic generalized exfoliative dermatitis is also called *red man syndrome*.

Clinical Manifestations

- Patchy or generalized erythematous eruption accompanied by chills, fever, malaise, prostration, severe toxicity, a pruritic scaling of the skin, and occasionally gastrointestinal symptoms

D

- Profound loss of stratum corneum (outermost layer of the skin), causing capillary leakage, hypoproteinemia, and negative nitrogen balance
- Widespread dilation of cutaneous vessels, resulting in large amounts of body heat loss
- Skin color change from pink to dark red; after a week, exfoliation (scaling) beginning in the form of thin flakes that leave the underlying skin smooth and red, with new scales forming as the older ones come off
- Possible hair loss
- Relapse common
- Systemic effects: high-output heart failure, other gastrointestinal disturbances, breast enlargement, hyperuricemia, temperature disturbances

Assessment and Diagnostic Findings

- Presence of scaling, erythematous dermatitis, particularly when this occurs in tandem with a known skin disease or a new prescription medication, increasing the suspicion that generalized exfoliative dermatitis may be diagnosed
- Hypoalbuminemia, negative nitrogen balance, and increased erythrocyte sedimentation rate (ESR)
- Skin biopsy indicated, as it may confirm the underlying cause and diagnosis

Medical Management

- The goals of management are to prevent infection and support the patient through individualized treatment, which should be started as soon as the condition is diagnosed.
- The patient should be hospitalized and placed on bed rest.
- All medications that may be implicated should be discontinued.
- A comfortable room temperature should be maintained because of patient's abnormal thermoregulatory control.
- Fluid and electrolyte balance must be properly maintained because of considerable water and protein loss from skin surface.
- Plasma expanders may be administered.

 Quality and Safety Nursing Alert

Observe for signs and symptoms of high-output heart failure due to hyperemia and increased blood flow.

Nursing Management

- Provide continual nursing assessment to detect infection.
- Administer prescribed antibiotics on the basis of culture and sensitivity test results.
- Assess for hypothermia because of increased skin blood flow coupled with increased heat and water loss through the skin leads to heat loss by radiation, conduction, and evaporation.
- Closely monitor and report changes in vital signs.
- Use topical therapy for symptomatic relief.
- Recommend soothing baths, compresses, and lubrication with emollients to treat extensive dermatitis.
- Administer sedating antihistamine medications before bedtime as prescribed to relieve the itching and promote sleep.
- Administer prescribed oral or topical corticosteroids when disease is not controlled by more conservative therapy.
- Advise patient to avoid all irritants, particularly medications.

For more information, see Chapter 61 in Hinkle, J. L., & Cheever, K. H. (2014). *Brunner and Suddarth's textbook of medical-surgical nursing* (13th ed.). Philadelphia: Lippincott Williams & Wilkins.

Diabetes

Diabetes mellitus, commonly referred to as *diabetes*, is a group of metabolic disorders characterized by elevated levels of blood glucose (hyperglycemia) resulting from defects in insulin secretion, insulin action, or both. The major classifications of diabetes are type 1 diabetes, type 2 diabetes, gestational diabetes, and diabetes associated with other conditions or syndromes. Prediabetes is classified as impaired glucose tolerance (IGT) or impaired fasting glucose (IFG) and refers to a condition in which blood glucose concentrations fall between normal levels and those considered diagnostic for diabetes. Three major acute complications of diabetes related to short-term imbalances in blood glucose levels are hypoglycemia, diabetic ketoacidosis (DKA), and hyperglycemic hyperosmolar syndrome (HHS). Long-term hyperglycemia may contribute to chronic microvascular complications (kidney and eye disease) and neuropathic complications. Diabetes is also associated with an increased occurrence of macrovascular diseases, including coronary artery disease (myocardial infarction), cerebrovascular disease (stroke), and peripheral vascular disease. Diabetes is prevalent in older adults; minority populations including patients of African American, Native American, and Hispanic descent are disproportionately affected as compared to Caucasians.

Pathophysiology

Insulin is a hormone secreted by beta cells in the pancreas and moves glucose from the blood into muscle, liver, and fat cells. In those cells, insulin has a number of anabolic functions including transporting and metabolizing glucose for energy, stimulating storage of glucose in the liver as glycogen, enhancing storage of dietary fat in adipose tissue, and accelerating transport of amino acids into cells. During fasting periods (between meals and overnight), the pancreas continuously releases a small amount of insulin (basal insulin) and, in conjunction with another pancreatic hormone called *glucagon*, stimulates the liver to release stored glucose. The insulin and the glucagon together maintain a constant level of glucose in the blood. DKA is a metabolic derangement that occurs most commonly in people with type 1 diabetes. An insulin deficiency or deficit causes the breakdown of fat (lipolysis) into free fatty acids and glycerol. The free fatty acids are converted into ketone bodies by the liver. These highly acidic ketone bodies accumulate and, subsequently, metabolic acidosis occurs. The three major metabolic derangements in DKA are hyperglycemia, ketosis, and metabolic acidosis.

Types of Diabetes

Type 1 (Formerly *Insulin-Dependent Diabetes Mellitus*)

- About 5% to 10% of patients with diabetes have type 1 diabetes. It is characterized by destruction of the pancreatic beta cells due to genetic, immunologic, and possibly environmental (e.g., viral) factors. Insulin injections are needed to control the blood glucose levels.
- DKA is most common in individuals with type 1 diabetes.
- Type 1 diabetes has a sudden onset, usually before the age of 30 years.

Type 2 (Formerly *Non–Insulin-Dependent Diabetes Mellitus*)

- About 90% to 95% of patients with diabetes have type 2 diabetes. It results from a decreased sensitivity to insulin (insulin resistance) or from a decreased amount of insulin secretion.

- Insulin resistance may also lead to metabolic syndrome, a constellation of symptoms including hypertension, hypercholesterolemia, abdominal obesity, and other abnormalities.
- Type 2 diabetes is first treated with diet and exercise and then with oral antidiabetic agents as needed.
- Type 2 diabetes has a slow, progressive onset and occurs most frequently in patients older than 30 years and in patients with obesity.

Gestational Diabetes

- Gestational diabetes is characterized by any degree of glucose intolerance with onset during pregnancy (second or third trimester).
- Risks for gestational diabetes include marked obesity, a personal history of gestational diabetes or abnormal oral glucose tolerance test (OGTT), glycosuria, or a strong family history of diabetes. Other risk factors include patient age greater than 25 years, a previous pregnancy resulting in a baby heavier than 9 pounds, and previous unexplained stillbirth.
- High-risk ethnic groups include Hispanic Americans, Native Americans, Asian Americans, African Americans, and Pacific Islanders. Patients who are members of these ethnic groups have an increased risk for hypertensive disorders of pregnancy.

Clinical Manifestations

- Polyuria, polydipsia, and polyphagia
- Fatigue and weakness, sudden vision changes, tingling or numbness in hands or feet, dry skin, skin lesions or wounds that are slow to heal, and recurrent infections
- Onset of type 1 diabetes possibly associated with sudden weight loss or nausea, vomiting, or stomach pains
- Type 2 diabetes resulting from a slow (over years), progressive glucose intolerance and resulting in long-term complications if diabetes goes undetected for many years (e.g., eye disease, peripheral neuropathy, peripheral vascular disease); complications possibly developing before the actual diagnosis is made
- Signs and symptoms of DKA including abdominal pain, nausea, vomiting, hyperventilation, and a fruity breath odor; untreated DKA possibly resulting in altered level of consciousness, coma, and death

Assessment and Diagnostic Findings

- Physical examination and complete history focusing on relevant risk factors for and symptoms of diabetes

D

- High blood glucose levels (diagnostic for diabetes): fasting plasma glucose levels of 126 mg/dL or more, or random plasma glucose or 2 hour postload glucose levels of more than 200 mg/dL
- Fasting lipid profile, serum creatinine
- Urinalysis including microalbuminuria
- Glycosylated hemoglobin (hemoglobin A_1C) used as measure of glucose control over time as an ongoing assessment for patients with known diabetes
- Electrocardiogram
- Evaluation for complications

Prevention

For patients who are obese (especially those with type 2 diabetes), weight loss and moderate intensity exercise are the keys to treatment and the major preventive factor for the development of diabetes.

Complications of Diabetes

Complications associated with diabetes are classified as acute and chronic. Acute complications occur from short-term imbalances in blood glucose and include the following:

- Hypoglycemia
- DKA
- HHS

Chronic complications generally occur 10 to 15 years after the onset of diabetes. The complications include the following:

- Macrovascular (large vessel) disease affects coronary, peripheral vascular, and cerebral vascular circulations.
- Microvascular (small vessel) disease affects the eyes (retinopathy) and kidneys (nephropathy); control blood glucose levels to delay or avoid onset of both microvascular and macrovascular complications.
- Neuropathic disease affects sensory motor and autonomic nerves and contributes to such problems as impotence and foot ulcers.

🍂 Gerontologic Considerations

Type 2 diabetes is the seventh leading cause of death and affects approximately 20% of older adults. There is a high prevalence among African Americans and older patients ages 65 to 74. Early detection is important, but symptoms may be absent or nonspecific. A glucose tolerance test is more effective in diagnosis than urine testing for glucose in older patients, owing to the higher renal threshold for glucose.

Medical Management

The main goal of treatment is to normalize insulin activity and blood glucose levels to reduce the development of vascular and neuropathic complications. The therapeutic goal within each type of diabetes is to achieve normal blood glucose levels (euglycemia) without hypoglycemia and without seriously disrupting the patient's usual activities. There are five components of management for diabetes: nutrition, exercise, monitoring glucose levels and ketones, pharmacologic therapy, and education.

- Primary treatment of type 1 diabetes is insulin.
- Primary treatments of type 2 diabetes are weight reduction and dietary changes.
- Exercise is important in enhancing the effectiveness of insulin.
- Use oral antidiabetic agents if diet and exercise are not successful in controlling blood glucose levels; insulin injections may be used in acute situations.
- Because treatment varies throughout the course due to changes in lifestyle and physical and emotional status and advances in therapy, continuously assess and modify the treatment plan and daily adjustments in therapy; education is needed for both patient and family.

Nutritional Management

- Most important objectives in diabetes nutritional management are control of total caloric intake to attain or maintain a reasonable body weight, control of blood glucose levels, and normalization of lipids and blood pressure to prevent heart disease.
- Meal plan should consider the patient's food preferences, lifestyle, usual eating times, and ethnic and cultural background. Plans should maintain the pleasure of eating by limiting food choices only when indicated by scientific evidence.
- For patients who require insulin to help control blood glucose levels, maintaining as much consistency as possible in the amount of calories and carbohydrates ingested at each meal is essential; consistency in time intervals between meals helps prevent hypoglycemic reactions and maintain overall blood glucose control.
- Initial education addresses the importance of consistent eating habits, the relationship of food and insulin, and the

provision of an individualized meal plan. In-depth follow-up education then focuses on management skills, such as eating at restaurants; reading food labels; and adjusting the meal plan for exercise, illness, and special occasions.

Caloric Requirements
- Determine basic caloric requirements, taking into consideration age, gender, body weight, and height and factoring in degree of activity.
- Long-term weight reduction can be achieved (1- to 2-lb loss per week) by reducing daily caloric intake by 500 to 1,000 cal from calculated daily caloric requirements.
- The American Diabetes and American Dietetic Associations recommend that for all levels of caloric intake, 50% to 60% of calories be derived from carbohydrates, 20% to 30% from fat, and the remaining 10% to 20% from protein. Using food combinations to lower the glycemic response (glycemic index) can be useful. Carbohydrate counting via food labels and the MyPlateFood Guide can be useful tools.

Other Dietary Concerns
Alcohol consumption may be allowed in moderation; however, it should be consumed with food to slow absorption; the major danger of alcohol consumption by the patient with diabetes is hypoglycemia, especially for patients who take insulin or insulin secretagogues (medications that increase the secretion of insulin by the pancreas).

Exercise
- Exercise lowers blood glucose, improves insulin utilization, and improves circulation and muscle tone.
- Exercise helps patients lose weight, ease stress, and maintain a feeling of well-being, and it alters blood lipid concentrations, specifically, increasing levels of high-density lipoproteins and decreasing total cholesterol and triglyceride levels.
- A slow, gradual increase in exercise is encouraged for beginning an exercise program; regular exercise is the goal.
- Patients who are older than 30 years and who have two or more risk factors for heart disease should have an exercise stress test prior to beginning an exercise program.
- Insulin dosages may need to be modified, and additional snacks may need to be added during exercise.

Nursing Management

Nursing management of patients with diabetes can involve treatment of a wide variety of physiologic disorders, depending on the patient's health status and whether the patient is newly diagnosed or seeking care for an unrelated health problem. Because all patients with diabetes must master the concepts and skills necessary for long-term management and avoidance of potential complications of diabetes, a solid educational foundation is necessary for competent self-care and is an ongoing focus of nursing care.

Managing Glucose Control in the Hospital Setting

As hyperglycemia can prolong lengths of stay and increase infection rates and mortality, nurses need to address glucose management in all hospital patients and include the following principles:

- Blood glucose targets are 140 to 180 mg/dL.
- Insulin (SQ or IV) is preferred to oral antidiabetic agents to manage hyperglycemia.
- Hospital insulin protocols or order sets should minimize complexity, ensure adequate staff training, include standardized hypoglycemic treatment, and make guidelines available for glycemic goals and insulin dosing.
- Appropriate timing of blood glucose checks, meal consumption, and insulin dose are all crucial for glucose control and to avoid hypoglycemia.

Providing Patient Education

Diabetes is a chronic illness that requires a lifetime of special self-management behaviors. Nurses play a vital role in identifying patients with diabetes, assessing self-care skills, providing basic education, reinforcing the education provided by the specialist, and referring patients for follow-up care after discharge.

Developing a Diabetic Education Plan

- Determine how to organize and prioritize the vast amount of information that must be provided to patients with diabetes. Many hospitals and outpatient diabetes centers have devised written guidelines, care plans, and documentation forms that may be used to document and evaluate the education provided.
- The American Association of Diabetes Educators recommends organizing educational material using the following seven tips for managing diabetes: healthy eating, being

active, monitoring, taking medication, problem solving, healthy coping, and reducing risks.
- Another general approach is to organize information and skills into two main categories: basic, initial ("survival") skills and information, and in-depth (advanced) or continuing education.
- Basic information is what patients must know to survive (e.g., to avoid severe hypoglycemic or acute hyperglycemic complications after discharge) and includes simple pathophysiology; treatment modalities; recognition, treatment, and prevention of acute complications; and other pragmatic information (e.g., where to buy and store insulin, how to contact physician).
- In-depth and continuing education involves providing more detailed information related to survival skills and educating the patient regarding preventive measures for avoiding long-term diabetic complications, such as foot care, eye care, general hygiene, and risk factor management (e.g., blood pressure control and blood glucose normalization). More advanced continuing education may include alternative methods for insulin delivery, for example.

Assessing Readiness to Learn
- Assess the patient's (and family's) readiness to learn; assess the patient's coping strategies; reassure the patient and family that feelings of depression and shock are normal.
- Ask the patient and family about their major concerns or fears to learn about any misinformation that may be contributing to anxiety; provide simple, direct information to dispel misconceptions.
- Evaluate the patient's social situation for factors that may influence the diabetes treatment and education plan (e.g., low literacy level, limited financial resources or lack of health insurance, presence or absence of family support, typical daily schedule, any neurologic deficits).

Educating Experienced Patients
- Continue to assess the skills and self-care behaviors of patients who have had diabetes for many years, including direct observation of skills, not just the patient's self-report of self-care behaviors.
- Ensure these patients are fully aware of preventive measures related to foot care, eye care, and risk factor management.
- Encourage patient to discuss feelings and fears related to complications; provide appropriate information regarding diabetic complications.

Determining Educational Methods
- Maintain flexibility with regard to educational approaches; a method that worked for one patient might not work for another.
- If desired, use various tools to complement education (e.g., booklets, video tapes).
- Written handouts should match the patient's learning needs (including different languages, low-literacy information, and large print) and reading level.
- Encourage patients to continue learning about diabetes care by participating in activities sponsored by local hospitals and diabetes organizations; inform patient that magazines and Web sites with information on diabetes management are available.

Educating Patients to Self-Administer Insulin
Insulin injections are self-administered into the subcutaneous tissue with the use of special insulin syringes. Basic information includes explanations of the equipment, types of insulins and syringes, and how to mix insulin (if necessary).

- Storing insulin: Vials or pens not in use, including spare vials or pens, should be refrigerated; extremes of temperature should be avoided; insulin should not be allowed to freeze and should not be kept in direct sunlight or in a hot car; insulin vials in use should be kept at room temperature (for up to 1 month). Instruct patient to always have a spare vial of the type or types of insulin needed. Also instruct patient to thoroughly mix any cloudy insulins by gently inverting the vial or rolling it between the hands before drawing the solution into a syringe or a pen and to discard any bottles of intermediate-acting insulin showing evidence of flocculation (a frosted, whitish coating inside the bottle). Encourage patients to note the expiration date on the insulin container to verify that it is current.
- Selecting syringes: Syringes must be matched with the insulin concentration (U-100 is standard in the United States); currently, three sizes of U-100 insulin syringes are available (1-mL syringes that hold 100 units capacity, 0.5-mL syringes that hold 50 units capacity, and 0.3-mL syringes that hold 30 units capacity). Small syringes allow patients who require small amounts of insulin to measure and draw up the amount of insulin accurately. Patients who require large amounts of insulin use larger syringes. Smaller syringes (marked in 1-unit

increments) may be easier to use for patients with visual deficits. Very thin patients and children may require smaller needles (e.g., 31 gauge, 8 mm long).

- Mixing insulins: The most important issues are (1) that patients are consistent in technique, so as not to draw up the wrong dose in error or the wrong type of insulin, and (2) that patients do not inject one type of insulin into the bottle containing a different type of insulin. Patients who have difficulty mixing insulins may use a premixed insulin, have prefilled syringes prepared, or take two injections.

- Withdrawing insulin: Most (if not all) of the printed materials available on insulin dose preparation instruct patients to inject air into the bottle of insulin equivalent to the number of units of insulin to be withdrawn; this is to prevent the formation of a vacuum inside the bottle, which would make it difficult to withdraw the proper amount of insulin.

- Selecting and rotating the injection site: The four main areas for injection are the abdomen (fastest absorption), upper arms (posterior surface), thighs (anterior surface), and hips (slowest absorption). Systematic rotation of injection sites within an anatomic area is recommended; encourage the patient to use all available injection sites within one area rather than randomly rotating sites from area to area. The patient should try not to use the same site more than once in 2 to 3 weeks.

- Preparing the skin: Use of alcohol to cleanse the skin is not recommended, but patients who have learned this technique often continue to use it; caution these patients to allow the skin to dry after cleansing with alcohol to avoid carrying it into the tissues, which can result in a localized reddened area and a burning sensation.

- Inserting the needle: The correct technique is based on the need for the insulin to be injected into the subcutaneous tissue; injection that is too deep or too shallow may affect the rate of absorption; a 90-degree insertion angle is best for most patients. Aspiration is generally not recommended with self-injection of insulin.

- Disposing of syringes and needles: Insulin syringes and pens, needles, and lancets should be disposed of according to local regulations. If community disposal programs are unavailable, used sharps should be placed in a puncture-resistant container. Instruct patient to contact local trash authorities for instructions about proper disposal of filled containers.

Promoting Home- and Community-Based Care

Educating the Patient About Self-Care

- If poor glucose control or preventable complications occur, the nurse needs to assess the reasons for the patient's ineffective management of the treatment regimen; do not assume that problems with diabetes management are related to the patient's willful decision to ignore self-management; problem may be correctable simply through providing complete information and ensuring that the patient understands the information or there may be cultural or religious beliefs that interfere with adherence.
- Assess for certain physical (e.g., decreased visual acuity) or emotional factors (e.g., denial, depression) that may be impairing the patient's ability to perform self-care skills.
- Help the patient to establish priorities if family, personal, or work problems may be of higher priority than self-care.
- Assess the patient for infection or emotional stress, which may lead to elevated blood glucose levels despite adherence to the treatment regimen.
- Promote self-care management skills by addressing any underlying factors that may affect diabetic control, simplifying and/or adjusting the treatment regimen, establishing a specific plan or contract with the patient, providing positive reinforcement, helping patient identify personal motivating factors, and encouraging the patient to pursue life goals and interests.

Continuing Care

- Age, socioeconomic status, existing complications, type of diabetes, and comorbid conditions all may dictate the frequency of follow-up visits.
- In addition to individualized follow-up appointments, remind the patient to participate in recommended health promotion activities (e.g., immunizations) and age-appropriate health screenings (e.g., pelvic examinations, mammograms).
- Encourage all patients with diabetes to participate in support groups.

For more information, see Chapter 51 in Hinkle, J. L., & Cheever, K. H. (2014). *Brunner and Suddarth's textbook of medical-surgical nursing* (13th ed.). Philadelphia: Lippincott Williams & Wilkins.

Diabetes Insipidus

D

Diabetes insipidus (DI) is the most common disorder of the posterior lobe of the pituitary gland and is characterized by a deficiency of antidiuretic hormone (ADH) also called *vasopressin*.

Pathophysiology

Lack of ADH causes excessive thirst (polydipsia) and large volumes of dilute urine (polyuria), which characterize the disorder. It may occur secondary to head trauma, brain tumor, or surgical ablation or irradiation of the pituitary gland. It may also occur with infections of the central nervous system (meningitis, encephalitis, tuberculosis), conditions that increase intracranial pressure, surgery near to (or that causes edema to) the pituitary gland or hypothalamus, or with tumors (e.g., metastatic disease, lymphoma of the breast or lung). Manipulation of the pituitary gland during surgery may cause transient DI lasting several days. Another cause of DI is failure of the renal tubules to respond to ADH; this nephrogenic form may be related to hypokalemia, hypercalcemia, and a variety of medications (e.g., lithium, demeclocycline [Declomycin]).

The disease cannot be controlled by limiting fluid intake, because the high-volume loss of urine continues even without fluid replacement. Attempts to restrict fluids cause the patient to experience an insatiable craving for fluid and to develop hypernatremia and severe dehydration.

Clinical Manifestations

- Polyuria: enormous daily output of very dilute urine (specific gravity 1.001 to 1.005)
- Polydipsia: patient experiencing intense thirst, drinking 2 to 20 L of fluid daily, with a special craving for cold water
- Polyuria continuing even without fluid replacement
- In inherited DI, primary symptoms possibly beginning at birth; in adults, onset possibly insidious or abrupt

Assessment and Diagnostic Findings

- Urine specific gravity
- Fluid deprivation test: fluids withheld for 8 to 12 hours until 3% to 5% of the body weight is lost; inability to increase specific gravity and osmolality of the urine during test characteristic of DI
- Other diagnostic procedures: concurrent measurements of plasma levels of ADH and plasma and urine osmolality and a trial of desmopressin (synthetic vasopressin) therapy and IV infusion of hypertonic saline solution

Medical Management

The objectives of therapy are (1) to replace ADH (which is usually a long-term therapeutic program), (2) to ensure adequate fluid replacement, and (3) to identify and correct the underlying intracranial pathology. Nephrogenic causes require different management approaches.

Pharmacologic Therapy

- Desmopressin (DDAVP) is a synthetic vasopressin administered intranasally, one or two administrations daily to control symptoms.
- Chlorpropamide (Diabinese) and thiazide diuretics are also used in mild forms of the disease because they potentiate the action of vasopressin.
- Thiazide diuretic agents, mild salt depletion, and prostaglandin inhibitors (ibuprofen [Advil, Motrin], indomethacin [Indocin], and aspirin) are used to treat the nephrogenic form of DI.

Nursing Management

- Educate patient and family members about follow-up care, prevention of complications, and emergency measures.
- Provide specific verbal and written instructions, including the dose, actions, and adverse effects of all medications; demonstrate correct medication administration and observe return demonstrations. Educate the patient and family to recognize the signs and symptoms of hyponatremia.
- Advise patient to wear a medical identification bracelet and to carry medication information about this disorder at all times.

For more information, see Chapters 52 and 66 in Hinkle, J. L., & Cheever, K. H. (2014). *Brunner and Suddarth's textbook of medical-surgical nursing* (13th ed.). Philadelphia: Lippincott Williams & Wilkins.

Diabetic Ketoacidosis

Diabetic ketoacidosis (DKA) is a metabolic derangement seen in patients with type 1 diabetes. The deficiency of insulin in diabetes causes elevations in blood glucose, resulting in the formation of highly acidic ketone bodies, which ultimately causes acidosis.

Pathophysiology

Without insulin, the amount of glucose entering the cells is reduced. The three main clinical features of DKA are (1) hyperglycemia, due to decreased use of glucose by the cells and increased production of glucose by the liver; (2) dehydration and electrolyte loss, resulting from an osmotic diuresis characterized by polyuria, with a loss of up to 6.5 L of water and up to 400 to 500 mEq each of sodium, potassium, and chloride over 24 hours; and (3) acidosis, due to an excess breakdown of fat to fatty acids and production of ketone bodies, which are also acids. Three main causes of DKA are decreased, insufficient or missed dose of insulin, illness or infection, and initial manifestation of undiagnosed or untreated diabetes.

Clinical Manifestations

- Polyuria, polydipsia (increased thirst), and marked fatigue
- Blurred vision, weakness, and headache
- Orthostatic hypotension in patients with volume depletion
- Frank hypotension with weak, rapid pulse
- Gastrointestinal symptoms, such as anorexia, nausea and vomiting, and abdominal pain (possibly severe)
- Acetone breath (fruity odor)
- Kussmaul respirations: hyperventilation with very deep, but not labored, respirations
- Widely varied mental status from patient to patient (alert to lethargic or comatose)

Assessment and Diagnostic Findings

- Blood glucose level: 300 to 800 mg/dL (possibly lower or higher)
- Low serum bicarbonate level: 0 to 15 mEq/L
- Low pH: 6.8 to 7.3
- Low PCO_2: 10 to 30 mm Hg
- Ketone bodies in blood and urine
- Low, normal, or high sodium and potassium levels depending on amount of water loss (dehydration)
- Elevated creatinine, blood urea nitrogen (BUN), and hematocrit values possible with dehydration; after rehydration, continued elevation in the serum creatinine and BUN levels suggesting underlying renal insufficiency

Medical Management

In addition to treating hyperglycemia, management of DKA is aimed at correcting dehydration, electrolyte loss, and acidosis before correcting the hyperglycemia with insulin.

Rehydration

Patients need as much as 6 to 10 L of normal saline IV fluid (0.9% NaCl) administered at a high rate of 0.5 to 1 L/h for 2 to 3 hours) to replace fluid loss caused by polyuria, hyperventilation, diarrhea, and vomiting. Hypotonic NS (0.45% NaCl) solution may be used for hypertension or hypernatremia and for those at risk for heart failure. This is the fluid of choice (200 to 500 mL/h for several additional hours) after the first few hours, provided that blood pressure is stable and sodium level is not low. When the blood glucose level reaches 300 mg/dL (16.6 mmol/L) or less, the IV solution may be changed to dextrose 5% in water (D_5W) to prevent a precipitous decline in the blood glucose level. Plasma expanders may be used to correct severe hypotension that does not respond to IV fluid treatment.

Restoring Electrolytes

Potassium is the main electrolyte of concern in treating DKA. Frequent monitoring and cautious but timely replacement of potassium is vital for avoiding severe cardiac dysrhythmias that occur with hypokalemia.

 Quality and Safety Nursing Alert

Because a patient's serum potassium level may drop quickly as a result of rehydration and insulin treatment, potassium replacement must begin once potassium levels drop to normal in the patient with DKA.

Reversing Acidosis

Acidosis of DKA is reversed with insulin, which inhibits the breakdown of fat. Insulin (only regular insulin) is infused at a slow, continuous rate (e.g., 5 units per hour). Hourly blood glucose must be measured. The IV fluid solutions with higher concentrations of glucose, such as NS solution (e.g., D_5NS, D_5 0.45% NaCl), are administered when blood glucose levels reach 250 to 300 mg/dL (13.8 to 16.6 mmol/L), to avoid too rapid a drop in the blood glucose level. IV insulin must be infused continuously until subcutaneous administration of insulin can be resumed. However, IV insulin must be continued until the serum bicarbonate level improves and patient can eat.

> **Quality and Safety Nursing Alert**

When hanging the insulin drip, the nurse must flush the insulin solution through the entire IV infusion set and discard the first 50 mL of the fluid. Insulin molecules adhere to the inner surface of the plastic infusion set; therefore, the initial fluid may contain a decreased concentration of insulin.

NURSING PROCESS

The Patient With DKA

Assessment

- Monitor the electrocardiogram (ECG) for dysrhythmias indicating abnormal potassium levels.
- Assess vital signs (especially blood pressure and pulse), arterial blood gases, breath sounds, and mental status every hour and record on a flow sheet.
- Include neurologic status checks as part of the hourly assessment as cerebral edema can be a severe and sometimes fatal outcome.
- Check blood glucose hourly.

Diagnosis

NURSING DIAGNOSES
- Risk for deficient fluid volume related to polyuria and dehydration
- Risk for fluid and electrolyte imbalance related to fluid loss or shifts
- Deficient knowledge about diabetes self-care skills and information
- Anxiety related to loss of control, fear of inability to manage diabetes, misinformation related to diabetes, fear of diabetes complications

COLLABORATIVE PROBLEMS/POTENTIAL COMPLICATIONS
- Fluid overload, pulmonary edema, and heart failure
- Hypokalemia
- Hyperglycemia and ketoacidosis
- Hypoglycemia
- Cerebral edema

Planning and Goals

The major goals for the patient may include maintenance of fluid and electrolyte balance, optimal control of blood glucose levels, increased knowledge about diabetes survival skills and self-care, decreased anxiety, and absence of complications.

Nursing Interventions

MAINTAINING FLUID AND ELECTROLYTE BALANCE

- Measure intake and output.
- Administer IV fluids and electrolytes as prescribed; encourage oral fluid intake when permitted.
- Monitor laboratory values of serum electrolytes (especially sodium and potassium).
- Monitor vital signs hourly for signs of dehydration (tachycardia, orthostatic hypotension) along with assessment of breath sounds, level of consciousness, presence of edema, and cardiac status (ECG rhythm strips).

INCREASING KNOWLEDGE ABOUT DIABETES MANAGEMENT

- Carefully assess the patient's understanding of and adherence to the diabetes management plan.
- Explore with the patient and family factors that may have led to the development of DKA.
- If the patient's self-management differs from those identified in the diabetes management plan, discuss their relationship to the development of DKA, along with early manifestations of DKA.
- If other factors (e.g., trauma, illness, surgery, or stress) are implicated, describe appropriate strategies to respond to these and similar situations in the future so the patient can avoid developing life-threatening complications.
- Provide education about survival skills again to patients who may not be able to recall the instructions.
- If necessary, explore reasons a patient has omitted insulin or oral antidiabetic agents that have been prescribed and address issues to prevent future recurrence and readmissions for treatment of these complications.
- Educate (or remind) the patient about the need for maintaining blood glucose at a normal level and learning about diabetes management and survival skills.

DECREASING ANXIETY

Educate the patient about cognitive strategies that may be useful for relieving tension overcoming anxiety, decreasing fear, and achieving relaxation including imagery, distraction, optimistic self-recitation, or music.

MONITORING AND MANAGING POTENTIAL COMPLICATIONS

- Fluid overload: Monitor the patient closely during treatment by measuring vital signs and intake and output at frequent intervals; initiate central venous pressure monitoring and hemodynamic monitoring to provide additional measures of fluid status; focus physical examination on assessment of cardiac rate and rhythm, breath sounds, venous distention, skin turgor, and urine output; monitor fluid intake and keep careful records of IV and other fluid intake, along with urine output measurements.
- Hypokalemia: Ensure cautious replacement of potassium; however, prior to administration, it is important to ensure that a patient's kidneys are functioning; because of the adverse effects of hypokalemia on cardiac function; monitor cardiac rate, cardiac rhythm, ECG, and serum potassium levels.
- Cerebral edema: Assist with gradual reduction of the blood glucose level; use an hourly flow sheet to enable close monitoring of the blood glucose level, serum electrolyte levels, fluid intake, urine output, mental status, and neurologic signs. Take precautions to minimize activities that could increase intracranial pressure.

EDUCATING PATIENTS ABOUT SELF-CARE

- Educate patient about survival skills, including treatment modalities (diet, insulin administration, monitoring of blood glucose and, for type 1 diabetes, monitoring of urine ketones), recognition, treatment, and prevention of DKA.
- The educational plan should also address those factors leading to DKA.
- Arrange follow-up education with a home care nurse and dietitian or an outpatient diabetes education center.
- Reinforce the importance of self-monitoring and of monitoring and follow-up by primary health care providers; remind the patient about the importance of keeping follow-up appointments.

Evaluation

EXPECTED OUTCOMES

- Achieves fluid and electrolyte balance
- Demonstrates knowledge about DKA

- Exhibits decreased anxiety
- Has absence of complications

For more information, see Chapter 51 in Hinkle, J. L., & Cheever, K. H. (2014). *Brunner and Suddarth's textbook of medical-surgical nursing* (13th ed.). Philadelphia: Lippincott Williams & Wilkins.

D

Diarrhea

Diarrhea is a condition defined by an increased frequency of bowel movements (more than three per day), increased amount of stool (more than 200 g per day), and altered consistency (liquid stool). It is usually associated with urgency, perianal discomfort, incontinence, or a combination of these factors. Diarrhea can result from any condition that causes increased intestinal secretions, decreased mucosal absorption, or altered (increased) motility.

Pathophysiology

Types of diarrhea include secretory, osmotic, malabsorptive, infectious, and exudative. The disorder can be acute (self-limiting and often associated with infection) or chronic (persists for a long period and may return sporadically). It can be caused by certain medications, tube feeding formulas, metabolic and endocrine disorders, and viral (e.g., norovirus), parasitic (*Giardia*), and bacterial infections (e.g., *Shigella*, *Clostridium difficile*). Other causes are nutritional and malabsorptive disorders, anal sphincter deficit, Zollinger–Ellison syndrome, acquired immunodeficiency syndrome (AIDS), and laxative misuse.

Clinical Manifestations

- Increased frequency and fluid content of stool
- Abdominal cramps, distention, intestinal rumbling (borborygmus), anorexia, and thirst
- Painful spasmodic contractions of the anus and ineffectual straining (tenesmus) with each defecation

Other symptoms, depending on the cause and severity and related to dehydration and fluid and electrolyte imbalances, include the following:

- Watery stools, which may indicate small bowel disease
- Loose, semisolid stools, which are associated with disorders of the large bowel

D

- Voluminous greasy stools, which suggest intestinal malabsorption
- Blood, mucus, and pus in the stools, which denote inflammatory enteritis or colitis
- Oil droplets on the toilet water, which are diagnostic of pancreatic insufficiency
- Nocturnal diarrhea, which may be a manifestation of diabetic neuropathy
- C. *difficile* infection possible in all patients with unexplained diarrhea who are taking or have recently taken antibiotics

Complications

Complications of diarrhea include cardiac dysrhythmias due to fluid and electrolyte (potassium) imbalance, loss of bicarbonate (can lead to metabolic acidosis), urinary output less than 30 mL per hour, muscle weakness, paresthesia, hypotension, anorexia, drowsiness (report if potassium level is less than 3.5 mEq/L [3.5 mmol/L]), skin care issues related to irritant dermatitis, and death if imbalances become severe.

Assessment and Diagnostic Findings

When the cause is not obvious, obtain complete blood cell count; serum chemistries; urinalysis; routine stool examination; and stool examinations for infectious or parasitic organisms, bacterial toxins, blood, fat, electrolytes, and white blood cells. Endoscopy or barium enema may assist in identifying the cause.

🌿 Gerontologic Considerations

Older patients can become dehydrated quickly and develop low potassium levels (i.e., hypokalemia) as a result of diarrhea. The nurse observes for clinical manifestations of muscle weakness, dysrhythmias, or decreased peristaltic motility that may lead to paralytic ileus. The older patient taking digitalis (e.g., digoxin [Lanoxin]) must be made aware of how quickly dehydration and hypokalemia can occur with diarrhea. The nurse educates the patient to recognize the symptoms of hypokalemia because low levels of potassium potentiate the action of digitalis, leading to digitalis toxicity.

Medical Management

- Primary medical management is directed at controlling symptoms, preventing complications, and eliminating or treating the underlying disease.
- Effective infection control measures can limit transmission of infectious organisms (e.g., C. *difficile*–associated diarrhea).

- Certain medications (e.g., antibiotics, anti-inflammatory agents) and antidiarrheal agents (e.g., loperamide [Imodium], diphenoxylate atropine [Lomotil]) may reduce the severity of diarrhea and the disease. Antidiarrheals should not be used until *C. difficile* has been ruled out.
- Increase oral fluids; oral glucose and electrolyte solution may be prescribed.
- Antimicrobial agents are prescribed when the infectious agent has been identified or diarrhea is severe.
- IV therapy is used for rapid hydration in very young or older patients.
- Some research supports the use of probiotic medications (e.g., *Saccharomyces boulardii* or lactobacillus species) in some forms of diarrhea.

Nursing Management

- Elicit a complete health history to identify character and pattern of diarrhea and the following: any related signs and symptoms, current medication therapy, daily dietary patterns and intake, past related medical and surgical history, and recent exposure to an acute illness or travel to another geographic area.
- Perform a complete physical assessment, paying special attention to auscultation (characteristic bowel sounds), palpation for abdominal tenderness, and inspection of stool (obtain a sample for testing).
- Inspect mucous membranes and skin to determine hydration status, and assess perianal area for skin excoriation.
- Encourage bed rest, liquids, and foods low in bulk until acute period subsides.
- Recommend bland diet (semisolids to solids) when food intake is tolerated.
- Encourage patient to limit intake of caffeine and carbonated beverages and avoid very hot and cold foods because these increase intestinal motility.
- Advise patient to restrict intake of milk products, fat, whole grain products, fresh fruits, and vegetables for several days.
- Administer antidiarrheal drugs as prescribed.
- Monitor serum electrolyte levels closely.
- Report evidence of dysrhythmias or change in level of consciousness immediately.
- Encourage patient to follow a perianal skin care routine to decrease irritation and excoriation.

> ▶ *Quality and Safety Nursing Alert*
>
> Skin in older patients is sensitive to rapid perianal excoriation because of decreased turgor and reduced subcutaneous fat layers. Gentle cleansing with a perineal cleansing solution (i.e., wet wiping method) and use of a barrier cream or a liquid skin sealant will prevent and/or treat the excoriation.

For more information, see Chapter 48 in Hinkle, J. L., & Cheever, K. H. (2014). *Brunner and Suddarth's textbook of medical-surgical nursing* (13th ed.). Philadelphia: Lippincott Williams & Wilkins.

Disseminated Intravascular Coagulation

Disseminated intravascular coagulation (DIC) is a potentially life-threatening sign (not a disease itself) of a serious underlying disease mechanism. DIC may be triggered by sepsis, trauma, cancer, shock, abruptio placentae, toxins, allergic reactions, and other conditions. The severity of DIC is variable, but it is potentially life-threatening. Mortality rates can exceed 80% in severe DIC with ischemic thrombosis, frank hemorrhage, and multiple organ dysfunction syndrome (MODS).

Pathophysiology

In DIC, the normal hemostatic mechanisms are altered so that tiny clots form within the microcirculation of the body. These clots consume platelets and clotting factors, eventually causing coagulation to fail and bleeding to result. This bleeding disorder is characterized by low platelet and fibrinogen levels; prolonged prothrombin time (PT), partial thromboplastin time (PTT), and thrombin time; and by elevated fibrin degradation products (D-dimers). The primary prognostic factor is the ability to treat the underlying condition that precipitated DIC.

Clinical Manifestations

Clinical manifestations of DIC are primarily reflected in compromised organ function or failure, usually a result of excessive clot formation (with resultant ischemia to all or part of the organ) or, less often, bleeding.

- Patient may bleed from mucous membranes, venipuncture sites, and gastrointestinal and urinary tracts.

D

- Bleeding can range from minimal occult internal bleeding to profuse hemorrhage from all orifices.
- Patients typically develop MODS, and they may exhibit renal failure and pulmonary and multifocal central nervous system infarctions, as a result of microthrombosis, macrothrombosis, or hemorrhage.
- Initially, the only manifestation is a progressive decrease in the platelet count; then, progressively, the patient exhibits signs and symptoms of thrombosis in the organs involved. Eventually, bleeding occurs (at first subtle, advancing to frank hemorrhage). Signs and symptoms depend on the organs involved.

Assessment and Diagnostic Findings

- Clinically, the diagnosis of DIC is often established by laboratory tests that reflect consumption of platelets and clotting factors (i.e., a drop in platelet count, an elevation in fibrin degradation products including D-dimer, an increase in PT and PTT and low fibrinogen levels). D-dimer levels are more accurate than other fibrin degradation products.
- The International Society on Thrombosis and Haemostasis has developed a highly sensitive and specific scoring system using the platelet count, fibrin degradation products, PT, and fibrinogen level to diagnose DIC. This system is also useful in predicting the severity of the disease over time and subsequent mortality.

Medical Management

The most important issue in managing DIC is treating its underlying cause. A second goal is to correct the secondary effects of tissue ischemia by improving oxygenation, replacing fluids, correcting electrolyte imbalances, and administering vasopressor medications. If serious hemorrhage occurs, the depleted coagulation factors and platelets may be replaced based on the extent of the hemorrhage (i.e., cryoprecipitate to replace fibrinogen and factors V and VII; fresh-frozen plasma to replace other coagulation factors).

A heparin infusion, which is a controversial management method, may be used to interrupt the thrombosis process. In the absence of frank bleeding, prophylactic doses of unfractionated heparin or low-molecular-weight heparin (LMWH) are recommended to prevent venous thromboembolism (VTE).

Nursing Management

Maintaining Hemodynamic Status
- Lab values must be monitored frequently for trends over time, including rate of change and actual results.
- Avoid procedures and activities that can increase intracranial pressure, such as coughing and straining.
- Closely monitor vital signs, including neurologic checks, and assess for the amount of external bleeding.
- Avoid medications that interfere with platelet function, if possible (e.g., beta-lactam antibiotic agents, acetylsalicylic acid [aspirin], nonsteroidal anti-inflammatory drugs).
- Avoid rectal probes and rectal or intramuscular injection medications.
- Use low pressure with any suctioning.
- Administer oral hygiene carefully: Use sponge-tipped swabs and salt or soda mouth rinses; avoid lemon-glycerin swabs, hydrogen peroxide, and commercial mouthwashes.
- Avoid dislodging any clots, including those around IV sites, injection sites, and so forth.

Maintaining Skin Integrity
- Assess skin, with particular attention to bony prominences and skin folds.
- Reposition carefully; use pressure-reducing mattress and lamb's wool between digits and around ears and soft absorbent material in skin folds, as needed.
- Perform skin care every 2 hours; administer oral hygiene carefully.
- Use prolonged pressure (5 minutes minimum) after essential injections.

Monitoring for Imbalanced Fluid Volume
- Auscultate breath sounds every 2 to 4 hours.
- Monitor extent of edema.
- Monitor volume of IV medications and blood products; decrease volume of IV medications if possible.
- Administer diuretic agents as prescribed.

Assessing for Ineffective Tissue Perfusion
Related to Microthrombi
- Assess neurologic, pulmonary, and skin systems.
- Monitor response to heparin therapy via anticoagulation laboratory values.

- Assess extent of bleeding.
- Stop epsilon-aminocaproic acid if symptoms of thrombosis occur.

Reducing Fear and Anxiety

- Identify previous coping mechanisms, if possible; encourage patient to use them as appropriate.
- Explain all procedures and rationale in terms that the patient and family can understand.
- Assist family in supporting patient.
- Use services from behavioral medicine and clergy, if desired.

For more information, see Chapter 33 in Hinkle, J. L., & Cheever, K. H. (2014). *Brunner and Suddarth's textbook of medical-surgical nursing* (13th ed.). Philadelphia: Lippincott Williams & Wilkins.

Diverticular Disease

A diverticulum is a saclike herniation of the lining of the bowel that extends through a defect in the muscle layer. Diverticulosis exists when multiple diverticula are present without inflammation or symptoms. Diverticulitis is an inflammatory condition caused by food and bacteria retained in the diverticulum.

Pathophysiology

Diverticula may occur anywhere in the small intestine or colon but most commonly occur in the sigmoid colon. Diverticulosis exists when multiple diverticula are present without inflammation or symptoms; it is most common in people older than 80 years. A low intake of dietary fiber is considered a major predisposing factor. Diverticulitis results when food and bacteria retained in the diverticulum produce infection and inflammation, which can weaken the colonic wall. The inflammation of the weakened colonic wall can cause it to perforate, giving rise to irritability and spasticity of the colon. In addition, abscesses may develop and eventually perforate, leading to peritonitis. Diverticulitis may occur in acute attacks or persist as a chronic, smoldering infection. A congenital predisposition is likely when the disorder is present in those younger than 40 years. Symptoms of diverticulitis generally manifest from its complications, which include abscess, fistula (abnormal tract) formation, obstruction, perforation, peritonitis, and hemorrhage.

Clinical Manifestations

Diverticulosis
- Frequently, no problematic symptoms; often, chronic constipation preceding development by many years
- Bowel irregularity with intervals of diarrhea, nausea, and anorexia, and bloating or abdominal distention
- Cramps, narrow stools, and increased constipation or, at times, intestinal obstruction
- Weakness, fatigue, and anorexia

Diverticulitis
- Acute onset of mild to severe pain in the left lower quadrant
- Nausea, vomiting, fever, chills, and leukocytosis
- If untreated, peritonitis and septicemia

Assessment and Diagnostic Findings
- Colonoscopy and possibly barium enema studies; however, colonoscopy contraindicated in acute diverticulitis and barium enema contraindicated with symptoms of peritoneal irritation
- CT scan with contrast agent
- Abdominal x-ray
- Laboratory tests: complete blood cell count, revealing an elevated white blood cell count, and elevated erythrocyte sedimentation rate (ESR)

🍂 Gerontologic Considerations
The incidence of diverticular disease increases with age because of degeneration and structural changes in the circular muscle layers of the colon and cellular hypertrophy. Symptoms are less pronounced among older adult patients, who may not experience abdominal pain until infection occurs. They may delay reporting symptoms because they fear surgery or cancer. Blood in stool may frequently be overlooked because of failure to examine the stool or inability to see changes because of impaired vision.

Medical Management

Dietary and Pharmacologic Management
- Diverticulitis can usually be treated on an outpatient basis with diet and medication; symptoms are treated with rest, analgesic agents, and antispasmodic medications.
- The patient is instructed to ingest clear liquids until inflammation subsides, then a high-fiber, low-fat diet. Antibiotic agents are prescribed for 7 to 10 days, and a bulk-forming laxative is also prescribed.

- Patients with significant symptoms and often older adults and those who are immunocompromised or taking corticosteroids are hospitalized. The bowel is rested by withholding oral intake, administering IV fluids, and instituting nasogastric suctioning.
- Broad-spectrum antibiotic agents and analgesic drugs are prescribed, and an opioid is prescribed for pain relief. Oral intake is increased as symptoms subside. A low-fiber diet may be necessary until signs of infection decrease.
- Antispasmodic agents such as propantheline bromide (Probanthine) and oxyphencyclimine (Daricon) may be prescribed.
- Normal stools can be achieved by administering bulk preparations (psyllium), stool softeners (docusate), warm oil enemas, and evacuant suppositories (bisacodyl).
- Probiotic agents have been suggested as a way to prevent relapse by creating a better balance of microbes in the gut and augmenting immune competencies.

Surgical Management

Surgery (resection) is usually necessary only if complications (e.g., perforation, peritonitis, hemorrhage, obstruction) occur. The type of surgery performed varies according to the extent of complications (one-stage resections or multistaged procedures). In some cases, fecal diversion (colostomy) may be performed. Laparascopic lavage has been suggested to avoid bowel resection and creation of a stoma in selected younger patients without comorbidities.

NURSING PROCESS

The Patient With Diverticulitis

Assessment

- Assess health history, including onset and duration of pain, dietary habits (fiber intake), and past and present elimination patterns (straining at stool, constipation with diarrhea, tenesmus [spasm of the anal sphincter with pain and persistent urge to defecate], abdominal bloating, and distention).
- Auscultate for presence and character of bowel sounds; palpate for tenderness, pain, or firm mass over left lower quadrant.
- Inspect stool for pus, mucus, or blood.
- Monitor blood pressure, temperature, and pulse for abnormal variations.

Diagnosis

Nursing Diagnoses
- Constipation related to narrowing of the colon secondary to thickened muscular segments and strictures
- Acute pain related to inflammation and infection

Collaborative Problems/Potential Complications
- Peritonitis
- Abscess formation
- Bleeding

Planning and Goals

The major goals of the patient may include attainment and maintenance of normal elimination patterns, pain relief, and absence of complications.

Nursing Interventions

Maintaining Normal Elimination Patterns
- Increase fluid intake to 2 L per day within limits of patient's cardiac and renal reserve.
- Promote foods that are soft but have increased fiber content.
- Encourage individualized exercise program to improve abdominal muscle tone.
- Review patient's routine to establish a set time for meals and defecation.
- Encourage daily intake of bulk laxatives (e.g., psyllium [Metamucil]); encourage the use of stool softeners, osmotic laxatives (e.g., polyethylene glycol 3350 [MiraLAX]), or oil-retention enemas as needed or as prescribed.
- Urge patients to try to identify food triggers (e.g., nuts and popcorn) that may bring on an attack of diverticulitis and to avoid them.

Relieving Pain
- Administer analgesic agents (usually opioid analgesic agents) for pain and antispasmodic medications.
- Record and monitor intensity, duration, and location of pain and pain relief.

Monitoring and Managing Potential Complications
- Identify patients at risk and manage their symptoms as needed.
- Assess for indicators of perforation: increased abdominal pain and tenderness accompanied by abdominal rigidity, elevated white blood cell count, elevated ESR, increased temperature, tachycardia, and hypotension.

- Perforation is a surgical emergency: Monitor vital signs and urine output and administer IV fluids as prescribed.

Evaluation

EXPECTED PATIENT OUTCOMES

- Attains a normal pattern of elimination
- Reports decreased pain
- Recovers without complications

For more information, see Chapter 48 in Hinkle, J. L., & Cheever, K. H. (2014). *Brunner and Suddarth's textbook of medical-surgical nursing* (13th ed.). Philadelphia: Lippincott Williams & Wilkins.

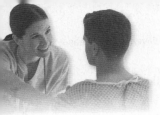

Empyema

Empyema is an accumulation of thick, purulent fluid within the pleural space. At first, the pleural fluid is thin, with a low leukocyte count, but it frequently progresses to a fibropurulent stage and then to a stage where it encloses the lung within a thick exudative membrane (loculated empyema).

Clinical Manifestations

- The patient is acutely ill with signs and symptoms similar to those of an acute respiratory infection or pneumonia (e.g., fever, night sweats, pleural pain, cough, dyspnea, anorexia, weight loss).
- Symptoms may be vague if the patient is immuno-compromised.
- Symptoms may be less obvious if the patient has received antimicrobial therapy.

Assessment and Diagnostic Findings

- Chest auscultation demonstrates decreased or absent breath sounds over the affected area, dullness on chest percussion, or decreased fremitus.
- Conduct chest computed tomography (CT) and thoracentesis (under ultrasound guidance).

Medical Management

The objectives of treatment are to drain the pleural cavity and to achieve complete expansion of the lung. The fluid is drained, and appropriate antibiotics (usually IV) for 4 to 6 weeks, in large doses, are prescribed on the basis of the causative organism. Drainage of the pleural fluid depends on the stage of the disease and is accomplished by one of the following methods:

- Needle aspiration (thoracentesis) if volume is small and fluid is not too thick
- Tube thoracostomy with fibrinolytic agents instilled through chest tube when indicated

- Open-chest drainage via thoracotomy to remove thickened pleura, pus, and debris and to remove the underlying diseased pulmonary tissue
- Decortication (surgical removal) of exudate if inflammation has been long-standing
- Drainage tube possibly remaining for weeks to months
- Monitoring of drainage and serial chest x-rays

Nursing Management
- Provide care specific to method of pleural fluid drainage.
- Help patient cope with condition; instruct in lung-expanding breathing exercises to restore normal respiratory function.
- Instruct patient and family about care of drainage system and drain site; measure and observe drainage.
- Educate patient and family in signs and symptoms of infection and how and when to contact the health care provider.

For more information, see Chapter 23 in Hinkle, J. L., & Cheever, K. H. (2014). *Brunner and Suddarth's textbook of medical-surgical nursing* (13th ed.). Philadelphia: Lippincott Williams & Wilkins..

Endocarditis, Infective

Infective endocarditis is a microbial infection of the endothelial surface of the heart. Development of infective endocarditis occurs in the following patient populations:

- Patients with prosthetic heart valves, cardiac devices (pacemaker or implantable cardioverter–defibrillator), or structural cardiac defects (e.g., valve disorders, hypertrophic cardiomyopathy)
- Older patients, who are more likely to have degenerative or calcified valve lesions, reduced immunologic response to infection, and the metabolic alterations associated with aging
- IV drug abusers, who have a higher risk of developing staphylococcal endocarditis in the right side of the heart
- Patients with debilitating disease or indwelling catheters and those receiving hemodialysis or prolonged IV fluid or antibiotic therapy, in whom hospital-acquired endocarditis occurs most often
- Patients taking immunosuppressive medications or corticosteroids, who are more susceptible to fungal endocarditis
- Patients receiving invasive procedures, particularly those involving mucosal surfaces (e.g., manipulation of gingival

tissue or periapical regions of teeth), and patients with body piercings (especially oral, nasal, and nipple), branding, and tattooing

Pathophysiology

A deformity or injury of the endocardium leads to accumulation on the endocardium of fibrin and platelets (clot formation). Infectious organisms, usually staphylococci, streptococci, enterococci, or pneumococci, invade the clot and endocardial lesion. Other causative microorganisms include fungi (e.g., *Candida*, *Aspergillus*) and Rickettsiae. Vegetations may embolize to other tissues throughout the body. As the clot on the endocardium continues to expand, the infecting organism is covered by new clot and concealed from the body's normal defenses. Infection may erode through the endocardium into underlying structures, causing tears or other deformities of valve leaflets, dehiscence of prosthetic valves, deformity of chordae tendineae, or mural abscesses.

Infective endocarditis signs and symptoms develop from toxic effects of the infection, destruction of heart valves, and embolization of fragments of vegetative growths on the endocardium. Systemic emboli occur with infective endocarditis of the left side of the heart; pulmonary emboli occur with infective endocarditis of the heart's right side.

Clinical Manifestations

- Primary presenting symptoms are fever and a heart murmur. Fever may be intermittent or absent, especially in patients receiving antibiotics or corticosteroids, or those who are older and those who have heart failure or renal failure. Murmurs worsen over time.
- Vague complaints of malaise, anorexia, weight loss, cough, and back and joint pain may occur.
- Small, painful nodules (Osler nodes) may be present in the pads of fingers or toes.
- Irregular, red or purple, painless, flat macules (Janeway lesions) may be present on the palms, fingers, hands, soles, and toes.
- Hemorrhages with pale centers (Roth spots) caused by emboli may be observed in the fundi of the eyes. Splinter hemorrhages (i.e., reddish brown lines and streaks) may be seen under the fingernails and toenails.
- Petechiae may appear in the conjunctiva and mucous membranes.
- Cardiomegaly, heart failure, tachycardia, or splenomegaly may occur.

- Central nervous system manifestations include headache, temporary or transient cerebral ischemia, and strokes.
- Embolization may be a presenting symptom, and it may occur at any time and may involve other organ systems; embolic phenomena may occur.
- Valvular stenosis or regurgitation, myocardial damage and mycotic (fungal) aneurysms, and first-degree, second-degree, and third-degree atrioventricuar blocks are potential cardiac complications.
- Emboli, immunologic responses, abscess of the spleen, mycotic aneurysms, cerebritis, and hemodynamic deterioration may cause complications in other organs.

Assessment and Diagnostic Findings

A definitive diagnosis is made when a microorganism is found in two separate blood cultures or in a vegetation or abscess.

- Elevated white blood cell (WBC) counts, anemia, positive rheumatoid factor, elevated erythrocyte sedimentation rate (ESR) or C-reactive protein and microscopic hematuria
- Transesophageal echocardiography

Prevention

A key strategy is primary prevention in high-risk patients with antibiotic prophylaxis immediately before and sometimes after the following procedures:

- Dental procedures that manipulate gingival tissue or periapical area of teeth or perforation of oral mucosa
- Tonsillectomy or adenoidectomy
- Surgical procedures that involve respiratory mucosa
- Bronchoscopy with biopsy or incision of respiratory tract mucosa
- Cystoscopy or urinary tract manipulation with enterococcal urinary tract infections or colonization
- Surgery involving infected skin or musculoskeletal tissue

The type of antibiotic prophylaxis varies with the type of procedure and degree of risk. Patients are instructed to take 2 g of amoxicillin (Amoxil) orally 1 hour before the procedure. If patients are allergic to penicillin, clindamycin (Cleocin), cephalexin (Keflex), cefazolin (Ancef, Kefzol), ceftriaxone (Rocephin), azithromycin (Zithromax), or clarithromycin (Biaxin) may be used.

Regular professional oral care combined with good personal oral care may reduce the risk of bacteremia. Personal oral care includes using a soft toothbrush and toothpaste to brush teeth, gums, tongue and oral mucosa at least twice daily, as well as rinsing the mouth with an antiseptic mouthwash for 30 seconds intermittently between tooth brushing. Patients are advised to:

- Avoid using toothpicks or other sharp objects in the oral cavity.
- Avoid nail biting.
- Avoid body piercing, branding, tattooing.
- Minimize outbreaks of acne, psoriasis.
- Avoid use of intrauterine devices (IUDs) for female patients.
- Report any fever of more than 7 days' duration to a primary care provider.

To assist in prevention, increased vigilance with IV catheters during invasive procedures is recommended. Remove all catheters, tubes, drains, and other devices as soon as they are no longer needed or no longer function.

Medical Management

Objectives of treatment are to eradicate the invading organism through adequate doses of an appropriate antimicrobial agent (continuous IV infusion for 2 to 6 weeks every 4 hours or continuously by IV infusion or once daily by intramuscular injection at home). Treatment measures include the following:

- Monitoring serum levels of the antibiotic and blood cultures to gauge effectiveness of therapy
- Monitoring patient's temperature at regular intervals for effectiveness of the treatment

Surgical Management

Surgical intervention may be required if the infection does not respond to medications or the patient has prosthetic heart valve endocarditis or a vegetation larger than 1 cm or develops complications such as a septal perforation. Surgical interventions include aortic or mitral valve debridement or excision, débridement of vegetations, débridement and closure of an abscess, and closure of a fistula in patients who:

- Develop congestive heart failure despite adequate medical treatment.
- Have more than one serious systemic embolic episode.
- Develop a valve obstruction.

- Develop a periannular (heart valve), myocardial, or aortic abscess.
- Have uncontrolled infection, persistent or recurrent infection, or fungal endocarditis.

Nursing Management

- Monitor patient's temperature; a fever may be present for weeks. Encourage fluids to keep urine light yellow, use fan or tepid water baths or compresses with light layers.
- Administer prescribed antibiotics, antifungals, or antivirals and nonsteroidal anti-inflammatory agents.
- Assess heart sounds for new or worsening murmur.
- Monitor for signs and symptoms of systemic embolization or, for patients with right heart endocarditis, signs and symptoms of pulmonary infarction and infiltrates.
- Assess for signs and symptoms of organ damage such as stroke, meningitis, heart failure, myocardial infarction, glomerulonephritis, and splenomegaly.
- Instruct patient and family about spacing activities and planned rest periods, medications, and signs and symptoms of infection.
- Provide psychosocial support while patient is confined to hospital or home with restrictive IV therapy.
- Reinforce that antibiotic prophylaxis is recommended for patients who have had infective endocarditis and who are undergoing invasive procedures.
- If patient received surgical treatment, provide postsurgical care and instruction.
- Refer to home care nurse who can supervise and monitor IV antibiotic therapy in the home.

For additional nursing interventions, please see Perioperative Nursing Management in Section P.

For more information, see Chapter 28 in Hinkle, J. L., & Cheever, K. H. (2014). *Brunner and Suddarth's textbook of medical-surgical nursing* (13th ed.). Philadelphia: Lippincott Williams & Wilkins.

Endocarditis, Rheumatic

Acute rheumatic fever, which occurs most often in school-age children, may develop after an episode of group A beta-hemolytic streptococcal pharyngitis (or "strep" throat). Patients with rheumatic fever may develop rheumatic heart disease as evidenced by a new heart murmur, cardiomegaly, pericarditis, and heart failure.

The *Streptococcus* is spread by direct contact with oral or respiratory secretions. Although the bacteria are the causative agents, malnutrition, overcrowding, poor hygiene, and lower socioeconomic status may predispose individuals to rheumatic fever. Incidence of rheumatic fever in the United States and other developed countries has generally decreased, but the exact incidence is difficult to determine because the infection may go unrecognized, and people may not seek treatment. Clinical diagnostic criteria are not standardized, and autopsies are not performed routinely.

Prevention of acute rheumatic fever is dependent on effective antibiotic treatment of streptococcal pharyngitis (see Pharyngitis, Acute in Section P). Antibiotic prophylaxis for recurrent rheumatic fever with rheumatic carditis may require 10 or more years of antibiotic coverage (e.g., penicillin G intramuscularly every 4 weeks, penicillin V orally twice daily, sulfadiazine orally daily, or erythromycin orally twice daily). Further information about rheumatic fever and rheumatic endocarditis can be found in pediatric nursing books.

For more information, see Chapter 28 in Hinkle, J. L., & Cheever, K. H. (2014). *Brunner and Suddarth's textbook of medical-surgical nursing* (13th ed.). Philadelphia: Lippincott Williams & Wilkins.

Endometriosis

Endometriosis is a chronic disease characterized by benign lesions with cells similar to those lining the uterus, growing aberrantly in the pelvic cavity outside the uterus. There is a high incidence among patients who bear children later and have fewer children. It is usually found in nulliparous women between 25 and 35 years of age and in adolescents, particularly those with dysmenorrhea that does not respond to nonsteroidal anti-inflammatory drugs (NSAIDs) or oral contraceptives. There appears to be a familial predisposition to endometriosis. It is a major cause of chronic pelvic pain and infertility.

Pathophysiology

Misplaced endometrial tissue responds to and depends on ovarian hormonal stimulation. During menstruation, this ectopic endometrial tissue is sloughed off, mostly into areas having no outlet, which causes pain and adhesions. Endometrial tissue can also be spread by lymphatic or venous channels. Extensive endometriosis causes few symptoms, whereas an isolated lesion may produce severe symptoms.

Clinical Manifestations
- Symptoms vary but include dysmenorrhea, dyspareunia, and pelvic discomfort or pain (some patients have no pain).
- Dyschezia (pain with bowel movements) and radiation of pain to the back or leg may occur.
- Depression, inability to work due to pain, and difficulties in personal relationships may result.
- Infertility may occur.

Assessment and Diagnostic Findings
A health history, including an account of the menstrual pattern, is necessary to elicit specific symptoms. On bimanual pelvic examination, fixed tender nodules are sometimes palpated, and uterine mobility may be limited, indicating adhesions. Laparoscopic examination confirms the diagnosis and enables clinicians to determine the disease's stage.

Medical Management
Treatment depends on symptoms, desire for pregnancy, and extent of the disease. In asymptomatic cases, routine examination may be all that is required. Other therapy for varying degrees of symptoms may be NSAIDs, oral contraceptives, gonadotropin-releasing hormone (GnRH) agonists, or surgery. Pregnancy often alleviates symptoms because neither ovulation nor menstruation occurs.

Pharmacologic Therapy
- Palliative measures (e.g., use of medications, such as analgesic agents and prostaglandin inhibitors) for pain may be initiated.
- Oral contraceptives are used.
- Synthetic androgen, danazol (Danocrine), causes atrophy of the endometrium and subsequent amenorrhea. (Danazol is expensive and may cause troublesome side effects such as fatigue, depression, weight gain, oily skin, decreased breast size, mild acne, hot flashes, and vaginal atrophy.)
- GnRH agonists decrease estrogen production and cause subsequent amenorrhea. Side effects are related to low estrogen levels (e.g., hot flashes and vaginal dryness).

Surgical Management

- Laparoscopy to fulgurate endometrial implants and to release adhesions
- Laser surgery to vaporize or coagulate endometrial implants, thereby destroying the tissue
- Other surgical procedures, including endocoagulation and electrocoagulation, laparotomy, abdominal hysterectomy, oophorectomy, bilateral salpingo-oophorectomy, and appendectomy; hysterectomy a possible option for some women

Nursing Management

- Obtain health history and physical examination, concentrating on identifying when and how long specific symptoms have been bothersome, the effect of prescribed medications, and the woman's reproductive plans.
- Explain various diagnostic procedures to alleviate anxiety.
- Provide emotional support to the woman and her partner who wish to have children.
- Respect and address the psychosocial impact of the realization that pregnancy is not easily possible. Discuss alternatives, such as in vitro fertilization (IVF) or adoption.
- Encourage patient to seek care of dysmenorrhea or abnormal bleeding patterns.
- Direct patient to the Endometriosis Association for more information and support.

For more information, see Chapter 57 in Hinkle, J. L., & Cheever, K. H. (2014). *Brunner and Suddarth's textbook of medical-surgical nursing* (13th ed.). Philadelphia: Lippincott Williams & Wilkins.

Epididymitis

Epididymitis is an infection of the epididymis, which usually spreads from an infected urethra, bladder, or prostate. The incidence is less than 1 in 1,000 males per year; prevalence is greatest in men 19 to 35 years of age. Risk factors include recent surgery or instrumentation of the urinary tract, high-risk sexual activities, personal history of sexually transmitted infections (STIs), past prostate infections or urinary tract infections (UTIs), lack of circumcision, history of an enlarged prostate, and the presence of a chronic indwelling urinary catheter.

Pathophysiology

In prepubertal males, older men, and homosexual men, the predominant causal organism is *Escherichia coli,* although in older men the condition may also be a result of urinary obstruction. In sexually active men ages 35 years and younger, the pathogens are usually related to bacteria associated with STIs (e.g., *Chlamydia trachomatis, Neisseria gonorrhoeae*). The infection moves in an upward direction, through the urethra and the ejaculatory duct, and then along the vas deferens to the epididymis.

E

Clinical Manifestations

- Often slowly develops over 1 to 2 days, beginning with a low-grade fever, chills, and heaviness in the affected testicle
- Unilateral pain and soreness in the inguinal canal along the course of the vas deferens.
- Pain and swelling in the scrotum and groin
- Possible discharge from the urethra, blood in the semen, pus (pyuria) and bacteria (bacteriuria) in the urine, and pain during intercourse and ejaculation
- Urinary frequency, urgency, or dysuria, and testicular pain aggravated by bowel movement

Assessment and Diagnostic Findings

- Urinalysis, Gram stain of urethral drainage, urethral culture or DNA probe
- Complete blood count
- Referral for STI testing in sexually active patients (syphilis, chlamydia, gonorrhea, and HIV)

Medical Management

If epididymitis is associated with an STI, the patient's partner should also receive antimicrobial therapy; selection of antibiotic depends on culture results. Patient's spermatic cord may be infiltrated with a local anesthetic agent for analgesia if patient is seen within the first 24 hours after onset of pain. Urethral instrumentation is avoided. Chronic epididymitis requires a 4 to 6 week course of antibiotics; infertility may result from inability of sperm to pass through the obstructed epididymis. Epididymectomy (excision of the epididymis from the testes) may be performed for patients who have recurrent, refractory, incapacitating episodes of this infection.

E

Nursing Management

- Place patient on bed rest with scrotum elevated with a scrotal bridge or folded towel to prevent traction on spermatic cord, to improve venous drainage, and to relieve pain.
- Give antimicrobial medications as prescribed.
- Provide intermittent cold compresses to scrotum to help ease pain; later, local heat or sitz baths may hasten resolution of inflammatory process.
- Give analgesic agents as prescribed for pain relief.
- Instruct patient to avoid straining, lifting, and sexual stimulation until infection is under control.
- Instruct patient to continue with analgesic and antibiotic medications as prescribed and to use ice packs as necessary for discomfort.
- Explain that it may take 4 weeks or longer for the epididymis to return to normal.

For more information, see Chapter 59 in Hinkle, J. L., & Cheever, K. H. (2014). *Brunner and Suddarth's textbook of medical-surgical nursing* (13th ed.). Philadelphia: Lippincott Williams & Wilkins.

Epilepsies

The epilepsies are a symptom complex of several disorders characterized by unprovoked paroxysmal and transient disturbances of brain function. There may be associated loss of consciousness, excess movement, or loss of muscle tone or movement and disturbances of behavior, mood, sensation, and perception. Epilepsy can be primary (idiopathic) or secondary (when the cause is known and the epilepsy is a symptom of another underlying condition, such as a brain tumor).

Pathophysiology

The basic problem in epilepsies is an electrical disturbance (dysrhythmia) in the nerve cells in one section of the brain, causing them to emit abnormal, recurring, uncontrolled electrical discharges. The characteristic epileptic seizure is a manifestation of this excessive neuronal discharge. In most cases, the cause is unknown (idiopathic). Susceptibility to some types may be inherited. Epilepsies often follow many medical disorders, traumas, and drug or alcohol intoxication. They are also associated with brain tumors, abscesses, and congenital malformations. Epilepsy affects an estimated 3% of people during their lifetime, and most forms of epilepsy occur in childhood. Epilepsy is not synonymous with mental retardation or illness; it is not associated with intellectual level.

Clinical Manifestations

Seizures range from simple staring episodes to prolonged convulsive movements with loss of consciousness. Seizures are classified as partial, generalized, and unclassified according to the area of brain involved; the initial pattern of the seizures often indicates the region of the brain in which the seizure originates. Aura, a premonitory or warning sensation, may occur before a seizure (e.g., seeing a flashing light, hearing a sound).

Simple Partial Seizures
- Only a finger or hand may shake; the mouth may jerk uncontrollably.
- Patient may talk unintelligibly, may be dizzy, or may experience unusual or unpleasant sights, sounds, odors, or taste—all without loss of consciousness.

Complex Partial Seizures
- Patient remains motionless or moves automatically but inappropriately for time and place.
- Patient may experience excessive emotions of fear, anger, elation, or irritability.
- Patient does not remember episode when it is over.

Generalized Seizures (Grand Mal Seizures)
Generalized seizures involve both hemispheres of the brain.

- Intense rigidity of the entire body, followed by alternations of muscle relaxation and contraction (generalized tonic–clonic contraction)
- Simultaneous contractions of diaphragm and chest muscles, producing characteristic epileptic cry
- Tongue chewing; patient incontinent of urine and stool
- Convulsive movements lasting 1 or 2 minutes
- Relaxation followed by deep coma and noisy breathing; respirations chiefly abdominal

Postictal State
- After the seizure, patients are often confused and difficult to arouse.
- Patient may sleep for hours.
- Many complain of headache, sore muscles, fatigue, and depression.

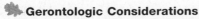Gerontologic Considerations

Older adults have a high incidence of new-onset epilepsy; increased incidence is also associated with head injury, dementia, infection, alcoholism, and aging. Cerebrovascular disease is the leading cause of seizures in the older adult; treatment depends on the underlying cause. Because many older adults have chronic health problems, they may be taking other medications that can interact with medications prescribed for seizure control. In addition, the absorption, distribution, metabolism, and excretion of medications are altered in the older adult as a result of age-related changes in renal and liver function. Therefore, older adult patients must be monitored closely for adverse and toxic effects of antiseizure medications and for osteoporosis. The cost of antiseizure medications can lead to poor adherence to the prescribed regimen in older adult patients on fixed incomes.

Assessment and Diagnostic Findings

- Developmental history (including pregnancy and childbirth) are obtained to identify any preexisting injury or head trauma, and physical and neurologic examinations are done to determine the type, frequency, and severity of seizures. Biochemical, hematologic, and serologic studies are included.
- MRI is performed to detect structural lesions such as focal abnormalities, cerebrovascular abnormalities, and cerebral degenerative changes.
- Electroencephalograms (EEGs) aid in classifying the type of seizure.
- Single photon emission CT (SPECT) may be used to identify the epileptogenic zone.

Medical Management

The management of epilepsy is individualized to meet the needs of the patient, not merely to manage and prevent seizures. Management differs from patient to patient, because some forms of epilepsy arise from brain damage and others result from altered brain chemistry.

Pharmacologic Therapy

Medications are used to achieve seizure control; the objective is to do so with minimal site effects. The usual treatment begins with single-drug therapy.

Surgical Management

- Surgery is indicated when epilepsy results from intracranial tumors, abscesses, cysts, or vascular anomalies.

- Surgical removal of the epileptogenic focus is performed for seizures that originate in a well-circumscribed area of the brain that can be excised without producing significant neurologic defects.
- For seizures that are refractory to medication in adolescents and adults with focal seizures, a pulse generator with a lead attached to the vagus nerve may be implanted to deliver electrical signals to the brain via the vagus nerve to control and reduce seizure activity.

E

NURSING PROCESS

The Patient With Epilepsy

Assessment

- Obtain a complete seizure history. Ask about factors or events that precipitate the seizures; document alcohol intake.
- Determine whether the patient has an aura before an epileptic seizure, which may indicate the origin of the seizure. (For example, seeing a flashing light may indicate that the seizure originated in the occipital lobe.)
- Observe and assess neurologic condition during and after a seizure. Assess vital and neurologic signs continuously. Patient may die from cardiac involvement or respiratory depression.
- Assess effects of epilepsy on lifestyle.

Diagnosis

NURSING DIAGNOSES
- Risk for injury related to seizure activity
- Fear related to possibility of having seizures
- Ineffective coping related to stresses imposed by epilepsy
- Deficient knowledge about epilepsy and its control

COLLABORATIVE PROBLEMS/POTENTIAL COMPLICATIONS
Status epilepticus (see the *Status Epilepticus* box) and toxicity related to medications are potential complications.

Planning and Goals

Major goals include prevention of injury, control of seizures, achievement of a satisfactory psychosocial adjustment, acquisition of knowledge and understanding about the condition, and absence of complications.

Status Epilepticus

Status epilepticus (acute, prolonged seizure activity) is a series of generalized seizures that occur without full recovery of consciousness between attacks. The condition is a medical emergency that is characterized by continuous clinical or electrical seizures lasting at least 30 minutes. Repeated episodes of cerebral anoxia and edema may lead to irreversible and fatal brain damage. Common factors that precipitate status epilepticus include withdrawal of antiseizure medication, fever, and concurrent infection.

Nursing Interventions

PREVENTING INJURY RELATED TO SEIZURE ACTIVITY

- Provide privacy and protect patient from curious onlookers.
- Ease the patient to the floor, if possible.
- Protect the head with a pad to prevent striking a hard surface.
- Loosen constrictive clothing.
- Push aside any furniture that may injure the patient during a seizure.
- If the patient is in bed, remove pillows and raise side rails.
- Do not attempt to pry open jaws that are clenched in a spasm or try to insert anything; do not attempt to restrain patient during seizure.
- Turn patient to side-lying position with head flexed forward to assist in draining pharyngeal secretions.
- Have suction equipment available if necessary to clear secretions.

REDUCING FEAR OF SEIZURES

- Reduce fear that a seizure may occur unexpectedly by encouraging compliance with prescribed treatment.
- Emphasize that prescribed antiepileptic medication must be taken on a continuing basis and is not habit forming; periodic monitoring is necessary to assess adequacy of treatment.
- Assess lifestyle and environment to determine factors that precipitate seizures, such as emotional disturbances, environmental stressors, onset of menstruation, or fever. Encourage patient to avoid such stimuli.

- Encourage patient to follow a regular and moderate routine in lifestyle, diet (avoiding excessive stimulants), exercise, and rest (regular sleep patterns).
- Advise patient to avoid photic stimulation (e.g., bright flickering lights, television viewing); dark glasses or covering one eye may help.
- Encourage patient to attend classes on stress management.

IMPROVING COPING MECHANISMS
- Understand that epilepsy imposes feelings of stigmatization, alienation, depression, and uncertainty.
- Provide counseling to patient and family to help them understand the condition and limitations imposed.
- Encourage patient to participate in social and recreational activities.
- Educate patient and family about symptoms and their management.
- Refer for counseling if indicated.

PROMOTING HOME- AND COMMUNITY-BASED CARE
Educating Patients About Self-Care
- Prevent or control gingival hyperplasia, a side effect of phenytoin (Dilantin) therapy, by educating patient to perform thorough oral hygiene and gum massage and to seek regular dental care.
- Instruct patient to notify physician if unable to take medications owing to illness.
- Instruct patient and family about medication side effects and toxicity.
- Provide specific guidelines to assess and report signs and symptoms of medication overdose.
- Encourage patient to keep a drug and seizure chart, noting when medications are taken and any seizure activity.
- Instruct patient to take showers rather than tub baths to avoid drowning and to never swim alone.
- Encourage realistic attitude toward the disease; provide facts concerning epilepsy.
- Instruct patient to carry an emergency medical identification card or wear an identification bracelet.
- Advise patient to seek preconception and genetic counseling if desired. (Inherited transmission of epilepsy has not been proved.)

Continuing Care
- Financial considerations: Epilepsy Foundation of America offers a mail-order program for medications at minimum cost and access to life insurance as well as information on vocational rehabilitation and coping with epilepsy.
- Vocational rehabilitation: The state vocational rehabilitation agency, Epilepsy Foundation of America, and federal and state agencies may be of assistance in cases of job discrimination.

Evaluation

EXPECTED PATIENT OUTCOMES
- Sustains no injuries from seizure activity
- Indicates a decrease in fear
- Displays effective individual coping
- Exhibits knowledge and understanding of epilepsy
- Experiences no complications of seizures (injury) or complications of status epilepticus

For more information, see Chapter 66 in Hinkle, J. L., & Cheever, K. H. (2014). *Brunner and Suddarth's textbook of medical-surgical nursing* (13th ed.). Philadelphia: Lippincott Williams & Wilkins.

Epistaxis (Nosebleed)

Epistaxis, a hemorrhage from the nose, is caused by the rupture of tiny, distended vessels in the mucous membrane of any area of the nose. The anterior septum is the most common site, where three major blood vessels enter the nasal cavity: (1) the anterior ethmoidal artery, (2) the sphenopalatine artery, and (3) the internal maxillary branches.

Risk factors include infections, low humidity, nasal inhalation of illicit drugs, trauma (including vigorous nose blowing and nose picking), arteriosclerosis, hypertension, nasal tumors, thrombocytopenia, aspirin use, liver disease, and hemorrhagic syndromes.

Medical Management

A nasal speculum, penlight, or headlight may be used to identify the site of bleeding in the nasal cavity. Initial treatment may include pinching the soft outer portion of the nose against the midline septum with continuous direct pressure for 5 or

10 minutes as the patient sits upright with the head tilted forward to prevent swallowing and aspiration of blood. Application of anesthetic agents and nasal decongestants (phenylephrine, one or two sprays) to act as vasoconstrictors may be necessary. Visible bleeding sites may be cauterized with silver nitrate or electrocautery (high-frequency electrical current). A supplemental patch of Surgicel or Gelfoam may be used.

Alternatively, a cotton tampon may be used to try to stop the bleeding. Suction may be used to remove excess blood and clots from the field of inspection. If the origin of the bleeding cannot be identified, the nose may be packed with gauze impregnated with petrolatum jelly or antibiotic ointment; a topical anesthetic spray and decongestant agent may be used before the gauze packing is inserted, or a balloon-inflated catheter may be used. Alternatively, a compressed nasal sponge may be used. Once the sponge becomes saturated with blood or is moistened with a small amount of saline, it will expand and produce tamponade to halt the bleeding. The packing may remain in place for 3 to 4 days if necessary to control bleeding. Antibiotics may be prescribed because of the risk of iatrogenic rhinosinusitis and toxic shock syndrome.

Nursing Management

- Monitor vital signs, airway, and breathing and assist in control of bleeding.
- Provide tissues and an emesis basin for expectoration of blood.
- Reassure patient in a calm, efficient manner that bleeding can be controlled.
- Provide IV normal saline infusion with cardiac and pulse oximetry monitoring for patient with significant hemorrhage.

Educating Patients About Self-Care

- Instruct patient to avoid vigorous exercise for several days and to avoid hot or spicy foods and tobacco once bleeding is controlled.
- Educate patient about ways to prevent epistaxis: avoid forceful nose blowing, straining, high altitudes, and nasal trauma (including nose picking).
- Educate patient about adequate humidification to prevent drying of nasal passages.
- Instruct patient in ways to apply direct pressure to nose with thumb and index finger for 15 minutes for recurrent nosebleeds.

- Instruct patient to seek medical attention if recurrent bleeding cannot be stopped.

For more information, see Chapter 22 in Hinkle, J. L., & Cheever, K. H. (2014). *Brunner and Suddarth's textbook of medical-surgical nursing* (13th ed.). Philadelphia: Lippincott Williams & Wilkins.

Esophageal Varices, Bleeding

Bleeding or hemorrhage from esophageal varices is one of the major causes of death in patients with cirrhosis. Esophageal varices are dilated tortuous veins usually found in the submucosa of the lower esophagus; they may develop higher in the esophagus or extend into the stomach. The condition is nearly always caused by portal hypertension. Risk factors for hemorrhage include muscular strain from lifting heavy objects; straining at stool; sneezing, coughing, or vomiting; esophagitis; irritation of vessels (poorly chewed food or irritating fluids); reflux of stomach contents (especially alcohol); and salicylates or any medication that erodes the esophageal mucosa.

Clinical Manifestations
- Hematemesis, melena, or general deterioration in mental or physical status are usual; often a history of alcohol abuse is reported.
- Signs and symptoms of shock (cool clammy skin, hypotension, tachycardia) may be present.

Assessment and Diagnostic Findings
- Endoscopy, ultrasonography, CT, angiography, and endoscopic videocapsule
- Neurologic and portal hypertension assessment (dilated abdominal veins and hemorrhoids)
- Liver function tests (serum aminotransferases, bilirubin, alkaline phosphatase, and serum proteins)
- Splenoportography, hepatoportography, and celiac angiography

Medical Management
- Transfer to ICU for aggressive medical care including evaluation of extent of bleeding and continuous monitoring of vital signs if hematemesis and melena are present.
- Signs of potential hypovolemia are noted; blood volume is monitored with a central venous catheter or pulmonary artery catheter.

- Oxygen is administered to prevent hypoxia and to maintain adequate blood oxygenation; IV fluids, electrolytes, and volume expanders are provided to restore fluid volume and replace electrolytes.
- Transfusion of blood components may also be required.
- Nonsurgical treatment is preferable because of the high mortality associated with emergency surgery to control bleeding from esophageal varices and because of the poor physical condition of most patients with severe liver dysfunction. Nonsurgical measures include the following:
  - Pharmacologic therapy: preferred treatment—octreotide (Sandostatin); other treatments—somatostatin, vasopressin (Pitressin) with nitroglycerin, beta-blocking agents, and nitrates
  - Balloon tamponade, saline lavage, and endoscopic injection sclerotherapy
  - Esophageal banding therapy and variceal banding (endoscopic variceal ligation)
  - Transjugular intrahepatic portosystemic shunting (TIPS)

Surgical Management

If necessary, surgery may involve the following:

- Direct surgical ligation of varices
- Portal-systemic shunt: splenorenal, mesocaval, and portacaval venous shunts
- Devascularization and transection

Additional possible therapies:

- Endoscopically placed tissue adhesives and fibrin glue
- Coated expandable stents (placed via endoscope)

Nursing Management

Provide postoperative care similar to that for any thoracic or abdominal operation. See Perioperative Nursing Management in Section P for additional information.

 Quality and Safety Nursing Alert

The risk for postsurgical complications (hypovolemic or hemorrhagic shock, hepatic encephalopathy, electrolyte imbalance, metabolic and respiratory alkalosis, alcohol withdrawal syndrome, and seizures) is high. Bleeding may recur as new collateral vessels develop as liver disease progresses.

- Monitor patient's physical condition and evaluate emotional responses and cognitive status.
- Monitor and record vital signs, especially blood pressure.
- Perform a neurologic assessment, monitoring for signs of hepatic encephalopathy (findings may range from drowsiness to encephalopathy and coma).
- Assess nutritional status; initiate parenteral nutrition (PN), if complete rest of the esophagus is indicated because of bleeding.
- After the surgical or endoscopic procedure, observe for bleeding, perforation of the esophagus, aspiration pneumonia, and esophageal stricture; administer antacids, histamine-2 antagonists such as cimetidine (Tagamet), or proton pump inhibitors such as pantoprazole (Protonix) as prescribed.
- Assist patient to avoid straining and vomiting. Maintain gastric suction to keep the stomach as empty as possible.
- Provide frequent oral hygiene and moist sponges to the lips to relieve thirst.
- Administer vitamin K therapy and multiple blood transfusions as ordered for blood loss.
- Provide a quiet environment and calm reassurance to reduce anxiety and agitation.
- Provide support and careful explanations during and after procedure regarding medical and nursing interventions.
- Monitor closely to detect and manage complications, including hypovolemic or hemorrhagic shock, hepatic encephalopathy, electrolyte imbalance, metabolic and respiratory alkalosis, alcohol withdrawal syndrome, and seizures.

For more information, see Chapter 49 in Hinkle, J. L., & Cheever, K. H. (2014). *Brunner and Suddarth's textbook of medical-surgical nursing* (13th ed.). Philadelphia: Lippincott Williams & Wilkins.

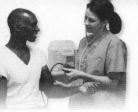

Fractures

A fracture is a complete or incomplete disruption in the continuity of bone structure and is defined according to its type and extent.

Pathophysiology

Fractures occur when the bone is subjected to stress greater than it can absorb. Fractures can be caused by a direct blow, crushing force, sudden twisting motion, or even extreme muscle contractions. When the bone is broken, adjacent structures are also affected, resulting in soft tissue edema, hemorrhage into the muscles and joints, joint dislocations, ruptured tendons, severed nerves, and damaged blood vessels. Body organs may be injured by the force that caused the fracture or by the fracture fragments.

Types of Fractures

- Complete fracture: a break across the entire cross section of the bone, which is frequently displaced from its normal position
- Incomplete fracture, also called *greenstick fracture*: a break occurring only through part of the cross section of the bone
- Comminuted fractures: a break with several bone fragments
- Closed fracture, or simple fracture: does not produce a break in the skin
- Open fracture, or compound or complex fracture: a break in which the skin or mucous membrane wound extends to the fractured bone; graded as follows:
  - Grade I: a clean wound less than 1 cm long
  - Grade II: a larger wound without extensive soft tissue damage
  - Grade III: a highly contaminated wound that has extensive soft tissue damage (most severe type)
- Fractures also described according to anatomic placement of fragments, particularly if displaced or nondisplaced
- Intra-articular fracture: extends into joint surface of a bone

Clinical Manifestations

Not all of these manifestations are present in every fracture; symptoms may be specific for the area of injury:

- Acute pain and loss of function
- Deformity, shortening of the extremity
- Crepitus
- Localized edema and ecchymosis

F

> **Quality and Safety Nursing Alert**
>
> Avoid testing for crepitus because testing can cause further tissue damage. Subtle personality changes, restlessness, irritability, or confusion in a patient who has sustained a fracture are indications for immediate blood gas studies.

Assessment and Diagnostic Findings

The diagnosis of a fracture depends on the symptoms, the physical signs, and radiographic examination. Usually, the patient reports an injury to the area. MRI and arthroscopy may be used to identify the fracture and confirm the diagnosis.

Medical Management

Emergency Management

- The affected body part should be immobilized immediately after the injury and before the patient is moved.
- The injured area should be splinted, including joints proximal and distal to the fracture, to prevent movement of fracture fragments.
- Immobilization of the long bones of the lower extremities is typically accomplished by bandaging the legs together, with the unaffected extremity serving as a splint for the injured one.
- In an upper extremity injury, the arm may be bandaged to the chest, or an injured forearm may be placed in a sling.
- Neurovascular status distal to the injury is assessed both before and after splinting to determine adequacy of peripheral tissue perfusion and nerve function.
- The wound of an open fracture is covered with a sterile dressing to prevent contamination of deeper tissues.

Reduction of Fractures

The fracture is reduced as soon as possible after the injury; reduction becomes more difficult as the injury heals.

Closed Reduction
- Bone fragments are brought into anatomic alignment through manipulation and manual traction; extremity is held in aligned place while cast, splint, or other immobilizing device is applied.
- Immobilizing device maintains reduction and stabilizes bone for healing.
- Traction may be used to maintain reduction prior to surgical fixation.

F

Open Reduction
- Fracture fragments are aligned via a surgical approach.
- Internal fixation devices (metallic pins, wires, screws, plates, nails, or rods) may be used to hold fragments in place.
- Devices may be attached to the side of the bone or inserted through bony fragments or directly into the medullary cavity of bone.

Immobilization
After reduction, immobilization holds the bone in correct position and alignment until union occurs. Immobilization is accomplished by external fixation (bandages, casts, splints, continuous traction, and external fixators) or internal fixation.

Maintaining and Restoring Function
- Function is maintained and restored by controlling swelling by elevating the injured extremity and applying ice as prescribed.
- Neurovascular status (circulation, motion, and sensation) is monitored frequently distal to the injury; compromise may occur due to edema and swelling.
- Restlessness, anxiety, and discomfort are controlled using a variety of approaches (e.g., reassurance, position changes, and pain relief strategies, including use of analgesics).
- Isometric and muscle-setting exercises are encouraged to minimize atrophy and to promote circulation. With internal fixation, the surgeon determines the amount of movement and weight-bearing stress the extremity can withstand and prescribes the level of activity.

Clinical Manifestations of Complications
Early complications of fractures include shock, fat embolism syndrome (FES), compartment syndrome, disseminated intravascular coagulation (DIC), and venous thromboemboli (deep vein thrombosis [DVT], pulmonary embolism [PE]). Delayed

complications include delayed union, malunion, nonunion, avascular necrosis (AVN) of bone, reaction to internal fixation devices, complex regional pain syndrome (CRPS, formerly called *reflex sympathetic dystrophy* [RSD]), and heterotopic ossification.

Hypovolemic Shock

Hypovolemic shock resulting from hemorrhage is more frequently noted in trauma patients with pelvic fractures and in patients with a displaced or open femoral fracture in which the femoral artery is torn by bone fragments. Early symptoms of hypovolemic shock are anxiety, rapid respiration, increasing pulse, decreasing systolic pressure, and decrease or narrowing of pulse pressure. See Shock, Hypovolemic in Section S for additional information.

Fat Embolism Syndrome

If FES occurs, with blockage of the small blood vessels that supply the brain, lungs, kidneys, and other organs (sudden onset, usually occurring within 12 to 48 hours but may occur up to 10 days after injury), the following may be noted: hypoxia, tachypnea, tachycardia, and pyrexia; dyspnea, crackles, wheezes, precordial chest pain, cough, large amounts of thick white sputum; blood gas values with PaO_2 below 60 mm Hg, with an early respiratory alkalosis and later respiratory acidosis; mental status changes varying from headache and mild agitation to delirium and coma. The chest radiograph exhibits a typical "snowstorm" infiltrate. Eventually, acute pulmonary edema, acute respiratory distress syndrome (ARDS), and heart failure may develop.

With systemic embolization, the patient appears pale. Petechiae appear in the buccal membranes and conjunctival sacs, on the hard palate, and over the chest and anterior axillary folds. Fever (temperature above 39.5°C [103°F]) develops. Free fat may be found in the urine when emboli reach the kidneys. Acute tubular necrosis and renal failure may develop.

Compartment Syndrome

Compartment syndrome is a sudden and severe decrease in blood flow to the tissues distal to the injury. Acute compartment syndrome may produce deep, throbbing, unrelenting pain not controlled by opioid medications (can be due to a tight cast or constrictive dressing or an increase in muscle compartment contents because of edema or hemorrhage). Cyanotic (blue-tinged) nail beds and pale or dusky and cold fingers or toes are present; nail bed capillary refill times are prolonged (greater than 3 seconds); pulse may be diminished (Doppler) or absent; and motor weakness, paralysis, and paresthesia may occur.

Disseminated Intravascular Coagulation

Manifestations of DIC include unexpected bleeding after surgery and bleeding from the mucous membranes, venipuncture sites, and gastrointestinal and urinary tracts. See Disseminated Intravascular Coagulation in Section D for additional information.

F

Other Complications

- Symptoms of infection may include tenderness, pain, redness, swelling, local warmth, elevated temperature, and purulent drainage.
- Delayed union manifests when healing does not occur within the expected time frame for the location and type of fracture, but the fracture does eventually heal.
- Nonunion is manifested by persistent discomfort and abnormal movement at the fracture site. Some risk factors include infection at the fracture site, interposition of tissue between the bone ends, inadequate immobilization or manipulation that disrupts callus formation, excessive space between bone fragments, limited bone contact, and impaired blood supply resulting in AVN.
- *Malunion* is healing of the fractures bones in a maligned position.
- AVN of the bone occurs when the bone loses its blood supply and dies.
- CRPS manifests as an infrequent, painful, sympathetic nervous system problem characterized by severe burning pain, local edema, hyperesthesia, stiffness, discoloration, vasomotor skin changes (i.e., fluctuating warm, red, dry, and cold, sweaty, cyanotic), and trophic changes that may include glossy, shiny skin and increased hair and nail growth.
- Manifestations of other complications may be noted (DVT, thromboembolism, PE). See specific disorders for additional information.

Management of Complications

Early Complications

- Treatment of hypovolemic shock consists of stabilizing the fracture to prevent further hemorrhage, restoring blood volume and circulation, relieving the patient's pain, providing proper immobilization, and protecting the patient from further injury and other complications. See "Nursing Management" under Shock, Hypovolemic in Section S for additional information.

- Prevention and management of FES involve immediate immobilization of fractures, including early surgical fixation, minimal fracture manipulation, adequate support for fractured bones during turning and positioning, and maintenance of fluid and electrolyte balance. Prompt initiation of respiratory support with prevention of respiratory and metabolic acidosis and correction of homeostatic disturbances is essential. Corticosteroids as well as vasopressor medications may be given.

> ### Quality and Safety Nursing Alert
>
> Subtle personality changes, restlessness, irritability, or confusion in a patient who has sustained a fracture are indications for immediate arterial blood gas studies.

- Compartment syndrome is managed by maintaining the extremity at the heart level (*not above heart level*), and opening and bivalving the cast or opening the splint, if one or the other are present.
- A fasciotomy (surgical decompression with excision of the fascia) may be needed to relieve the constrictive muscle fascia. The wound remains open and covered with moist sterile saline dressings for 3 to 5 days. The limb is splinted and elevated to the level of the heart. Prescribed passive range of motion (ROM) exercises may be performed every 4 to 6 hours.
- Other complications are treated as indicated (see specific disorders for additional information).

Delayed Complications

- Nonunion (failure of the ends of a fractured bone to unite) is treated with internal fixation, bone grafting (osteogenesis, osteoconduction, osteoinduction), electrical bone stimulation, or a combination of these.
- Management of CRPS involves elevating the extremity; relieving pain; performing ROM exercises; and helping patients with chronic pain, disuse atrophy, and osteoporosis. Blood pressure readings or venipuncture should be avoided in the affected extremity.

- Other complications are treated as indicated (see specific disorders for additional information).

Nursing Management

Managing Closed Fractures

- Instruct the patient regarding the proper methods to control edema and pain (e.g., elevate extremity to heart level, take analgesic agents as prescribed).
- Educate patient regarding exercises to maintain the health of unaffected muscles and to strengthen muscles needed for transferring and for using assistive devices (e.g., crutches, walker).
- Instruct patients regarding how to use assistive devices safely.
- Arrange to help patients modify their home environment as needed and to secure personal assistance if necessary.
- Provide patient education, including self-care, medication information, monitoring for potential complications, and the need for continuing health care supervision.

Managing Open Fractures

- The objectives of management are to prevent infection of the wound, soft tissue, and bone and to promote healing of bone and soft tissue. In an open fracture, there is the risk of osteomyelitis, tetanus, and gas gangrene.
- Administer IV antibiotics immediately on the patient's arrival in the hospital, along with tetanus toxoid if needed; obtain wound culture if indicated.
- Wound irrigation and debridement is initiated in the operating room as soon as possible.
- Elevate the extremity to minimize edema.
- Assess neurovascular status frequently.
- Take the patient's temperature at regular intervals and monitor for signs of infection.

Managing Fractures at Specific Sites

Fractures may require weeks to months to heal; maximum functional recovery is the goal of management. Ongoing neurovascular assessment of the extremity distal to the fracture to evaluate the extent of injury and possible involvement of the nerves and blood vessels is essential.

Clavicle

- Fracture of the clavicle (collar bone) is a common injury that results from a fall or a direct blow to the shoulder.
- Monitor the circulation and nerve function of the affected arm and compare with the unaffected arm to determine

variations, which may indicate disturbances in neurovascular status.

- Immobilization of the shoulder is accomplished by placing the arm on the affected side in a sling.
- Caution the patient not to elevate the arm above shoulder level until the fracture has healed (about 6 weeks).
- Encourage the patient to exercise the elbow, wrist, and fingers as soon as possible and, when prescribed, to perform shoulder exercises; vigorous activity is limited for 3 months.

Humeral Neck

- Impacted fractures of the humeral neck are seen most frequently in older women after a fall on an outstretched arm.
- Active middle-aged patients who are injured in a fall may suffer severely displaced humeral neck fractures with associated rotator cuff damage.
- Symptoms include affected arm hanging limp at the side or supported by the uninjured hand.
- Educate the patient to support the arm and immobilize it by a sling and swathe that secure the supported arm to the trunk; fractures require approximately 4 to 10 weeks to heal.
- Begin pendulum exercises as soon as tolerated by the patient. Educate the patient to avoid vigorous activity for an additional 4 weeks after the bone has healed.
- Inform the patient that residual stiffness, aching, and some limitation of ROM may persist for 6 or more months. When a humeral neck fracture is displaced with required fixation, exercises are started only after a prescribed period of immobilization.
- Use well-padded splints to immobilize the upper arm initially and to support the arm in 90 degrees of flexion at the elbow, use a sling or collar and cuff to support the forearm, and use external fixators to treat open fractures of the humeral shaft. Functional bracing may also be used for these fractures.
- Encourage patient to perform isometric exercises as prescribed.

Elbow

- Elbow fractures (distal humerus) may result in injury to the median, radial, or ulnar nerves as a result of motor vehicle accidents, falls on the elbow, or direct blows.
- Monitor neurovascular status closely and assess for signs of Volkmann contracture (an acute compartment syndrome) as well as for hemarthrosis (blood in the joint).

- Reinforce information regarding reduction and fixation of the fracture and planned active motion when swelling has subsided and healing has begun.
- Explain care if the arm is immobilized in a cast or posterior splint and sling.
- Encourage active finger exercises; provide demonstrations of and encourage patient to do gentle ROM exercise of the injured joint about 1 week after internal fixation.

Radial Head

- Radial head fractures are common and usually produced by a fall on the outstretched hand with the elbow extended.
- If the fracture is not displaced, instruct patient in use of a splint for immobilization; educate patient not to lift with the affected arm for approximately 4 weeks.
- If the fracture is displaced, surgery is typically required. Reinforce the need for postoperative immobilization of the arm in a posterior plaster splint and sling.
- Encourage the patient to carry out a program of active motion of the elbow and forearm when prescribed.

Radial and Ulnar Shafts

- Radial and ulnar shaft fractures occur more frequently in children than adults; displacement occurs when both bones are fractured.
- If fragments are not displaced, fracture is treated with closed reduction and a long arm cast; neurovascular assessment is essential after the cast is applied.
- Advise the patient to elevate the arm and perform frequent finger flexion to reduce edema; active ROM of the involved shoulder is essential.
- Fracture is immobilized about 12 weeks; in the last 6 weeks, arm may be placed in a functional forearm brace that allows exercise of the wrist. Advise patent to avoid lifting and twisting.
- Displaced fractures are managed surgically with open-reduction internal fixation (ORIF) and are immobilized postoperatively with plaster splint or cast. Arm is elevated to control swelling; regular neurovascular assessments are essential.

Wrist

- Wrist fractures (distal radius [Colles' fracture]) usually result from a fall on an open, dorsiflexed hand; they are frequently seen in older women with osteoporotic bones and weak soft tissues that do not dissipate the energy of a fall.

- Treatment usually consists of closed reduction and immobilization; reinforce care of the cast or, with more severe fractures requiring ORIF with wire insertion, educate about incision care.
- Instruct patient to keep the wrist and forearm elevated for 48 hours after reduction.
- Begin active ROM of the fingers and shoulder to reduce swelling and prevent stiffness with the hand held at the level of the heart.
- Encourage use of the hand in functional activities.
- Actively exercise the shoulder and elbow, including complete ROM exercises of both joints.
- Assess the sensory function of the median nerve by pricking the distal aspect of the index finger, and assess the motor function by testing patient's ability to touch the thumb to the little finger. If diminished circulation and nerve function are noted, treat promptly.

Hand and Fingers

- The most common type of metacarpal fracture in adults is a "boxer's fracture," which occurs when a closed fist bangs against a hard surface, fracturing the neck of the fifth finger; falls and occupational injuries (e.g., machinery injuries, crushes) are the most common cause of phalangeal injury in adults.
- The objective of treatment is always to regain maximum function of the hand and minimize cosmetic deformities.
- With a nondisplaced fracture, the finger is splinted for 3 to 4 weeks to relieve pain and protect the fingertip from further trauma; splinting may consist of "buddy tapping" the fractured finger to an adjacent nonfractured finger.
- Displaced fractures and open fractures may require ORIF.
- Evaluate the neurovascular status of the injured hand. Educate the patient to control swelling by elevating the hand. Encourage functional use of the uninvolved portions of the hand.

Pelvis

- Pelvic fractures may be caused by falls, motor vehicle crashes, or crush injuries and are more commonly seen in younger and middle-aged adults.
- Pelvic fractures are categorized as stable or unstable; treatment is determined by type of pelvic fracture.
- Monitor for symptoms, including ecchymosis; tenderness over the symphysis pubis, anterior iliac spines, iliac crest, sacrum, or coccyx; local edema; numbness or tingling of the

pubis, genitals, and proximal thighs; and inability to bear weight without discomfort.

- Complete a neurovascular assessment of the lower extremities to detect injury to pelvic blood vessels and nerves.
- Monitor for hemorrhage and shock, two of the most serious consequences that may occur. Palpate both lower extremities for absence of peripheral pulses, which may indicate a torn iliac artery or one of its branches.
- Assess for injuries to the bladder, rectum, intestines, other abdominal organs, and pelvic vessels and nerves. Examine urine for blood to assess for urinary tract injury. In male patients, do not insert a catheter until the status of the urethra is known.
- Monitor for diffuse and intense abdominal pain, hyperactive or absent bowel sounds, and abdominal rigidity and resonance (free air) or dullness to percussion (blood), which suggest injury to the intestines or abdominal bleeding.
- If patient has a stable pelvic fracture, maintain patient on bed rest for a few days and provide symptom management until the pain and discomfort are controlled. Treatment of unstable fractures generally involves external fixation or ORIF after the patient is hemodynamically stable.
- Provide fluids, dietary fiber, ankle and leg exercises, antiembolism stockings to aid venous return, logrolling, deep breathing, and skin care to reduce the risk of complications and to increase comfort.
- Monitor bowel sounds. If patient has a fracture of the coccyx and experiences pain on sitting and with defecation, assist with sitz baths as prescribed to relieve pain and administer stool softeners to prevent the need to strain on defecation.
- As pain resolves, instruct patient to resume activity gradually, using assistive mobility devices for protected weight bearing.
- Promote hemodynamic stability and comfort and encourage early mobilization.

Acetabulum

- A type of intra-articular fracture, the typical mechanism of injury is from an external force that drives the femoral shaft into the hip joint, fracturing the acetabulum.
- Treatment is dependent upon the pattern of fracture.
- Stable, nondisplaced fractures may be managed with traction and protective weight bearing; displaced and unstable fractures are treated with ORIF, joint débridement, or arthroplasty.

Hip

- Two major types of hip fractures occur: intracapsular (fractures of the neck of the femur) and extracapsular (fractures of the trochanteric and subtrochanteric regions).
- With fractures of the femoral neck, the leg is shortened, adducted, and externally rotated. The patient reports pain in the hip and groin or in the medial side of the knee.
- Fractures are treated with Buck's extension traction, a type of temporary skin traction. Surgical treatment consists of ORIF or closed reduction of the fracture, replacement of the femoral head with a prosthesis (hemiarthroplasty), or closed reduction with percutaneous stabilization for an intracapsular fracture.
- Displaced femoral neck fracture is an emergency and must be repaired within 24 hours.
- Goals of treatment include pain management, prevention of secondary medical problems, and early mobilization of the patient so that independent functioning can be restored.
- Potential early complications include neurovascular complications, venous thromboembolism, pulmonary complications (e.g., atelectasis, pneumonia), skin breakdown, and loss of bladder control (incontinence or retention). Late complications include infection, nonunion, and AVN.

Gerontologic Considerations

Older adults (particularly women) who have low bone density from osteoporosis and who tend to fall frequently have a high incidence of hip fracture. Stress and immobility related to the trauma predispose the older adult to atelectasis, pneumonia, sepsis, venous thromboemboli, pressure ulcers, and reduced ability to cope with other health problems. Many older adults hospitalized with hip fractures exhibit delirium as a result of the stress of the trauma, unfamiliar surroundings, sleep deprivation, and medications. In addition, delirium that develops in some older adult patients may be caused by mild cerebral ischemia or mild hypoxemia. Other factors associated with delirium include responses to medications and anesthesia, malnutrition, dehydration, infectious processes, mood disturbances, and blood loss. The same factors that may cause delirium may exacerbate the manifestations of dementia in the older adult with a fractured hip.

Femoral Shaft

- Femoral shaft fractures are most often seen in young adults involved in a motor vehicle crash or a fall from a high place.

Frequently, these patients have associated multiple trauma and develop shock, because a loss of 1,000 mL of blood is common with these fractures.

- Symptoms include an edematous, deformed, painful thigh and patient's inability to move the hip or the knee; fractures may be transverse, oblique, spiral, or comminuted.
- Assess neurovascular status of the extremity, especially circulatory perfusion of the lower leg and foot (popliteal, posterior tibial, and pedal pulses and toe capillary refill time, as well as Doppler ultrasound monitoring).
- Note signs of dislocation of the hip and knee, as well as knee effusion, which may suggest ligament damage and possible instability of the knee joint.
- Apply and maintain skeletal traction or splint to immobilize the fracture fragments and achieve muscle relaxation and alignment of the fracture fragments before ORIF procedures and, later, a cast brace. Internal fixation permits early mobilization, which is associated with improved outcomes and recovery.
- Assist patient in prescribed partial weight bearing when indicated and progress to full weight bearing as tolerated.
- Instruct in and encourage patient to perform ROM exercises of lower leg, foot, and toes on a regular basis. Assist patient in performing active and passive knee exercises as soon as possible, depending on the management approach and the stability of the fracture and knee ligaments.
- Long-term complications may include malrotation, malunion, delayed union, and nonunion.

Tibia and Fibula

- Tibia and fibula fractures (most common fractures below the knee) tend to result from a direct blow, falls with the foot in a flexed position, or a violent twisting motion. Symptoms include pain, deformity, obvious hematoma, and considerable edema.
- Closed nondisplaced fractures that do not involve the ankle joint are treated with closed reduction and immobilization and usually heal within 4 to 6 weeks. Displaced, open, or articular fractures are treated with traction, ORIF, or external fixation and typically heal within 6 to 10 weeks.
- Instruct patient in care of skeletal traction, if applicable. Encourage patient to perform hip, foot, and knee exercises within the limits of the immobilizing device.

- Instruct patient to begin weight bearing when prescribed (usually in about 4 to 8 weeks).
- Instruct patient to elevate extremity to control edema.
- Perform continuous neurovascular evaluation and assess for acute compartment syndrome.

Rib

- Rib fractures occur frequently in adults and usually result in no impairment of function but produce painful respirations.
- Assist patient to cough and take deep breaths by splinting the chest with hands or pillow during cough.
- Reassure patient that pain associated with rib fracture diminishes significantly in 3 or 4 days, and the fracture heals within 6 weeks; nonsteroidal anti-inflammatory medications may be prescribed for analgesic relief.
- Monitor for complications, which may include atelectasis, pneumonia, a flail chest, pneumothorax, and hemothorax. (See specific disorders for nursing management.)

Thoracolumbar Spine

- Fractures of the thoracolumbar spine may involve the vertebral body, the laminae and articulating processes, and the spinous processes or transverse processes; the T12 to L2 are the most vulnerable to fracture. Osteoporosis contributes to vertebral collapse.
- Fractures can be stable (disruption of either anterior or posterior structural columns) or unstable (disruptions of both anterior and posterior structural columns).
- Symptoms include acute tenderness (worse with moving, coughing, or weight bearing), swelling, paravertebral muscle spasm, and change in the normal curves or in the gap between spinous processes.
- Immobilization is essential prior to diagnosis. Stable spinal fractures are treated with bed rest and analgesic agents; bracing may be applied for support during ambulation, and activities are restricted for 6 months. Unstable fractures are treated initially with bed rest followed by ORIF within 24 hours of injury.
- Monitor neurologic status closely during the preoperative and postoperative periods.

For more information, see Chapter 43 in Hinkle, J. L., & Cheever, K. H. (2014). *Brunner and Suddarth's textbook of medical-surgical nursing* (13th ed.). Philadelphia: Lippincott Williams & Wilkins.

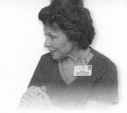

Gastritis

Gastritis is inflammation of the stomach mucosa and is a common gastrointestinal (GI) problem. It affects women and men equally and is more common in older adults. Gastritis may be acute or chronic and is further classified as erosive or nonerosive based on the pathological signs in the stomach wall. Acute gastritis lasts several hours to a few days and is often caused by dietary indiscretion (eating irritating food that is highly seasoned or food that is infected). Acute gastritis can also develop in acute illnesses (e.g., major traumatic injuries; burns; severe infection; hepatic, renal, or respiratory failure; or major surgery). Other causes include excessive use of aspirin and other nonsteroidal anti-inflammatory drugs (NSAIDs), excessive alcohol intake, bile reflux, and radiation therapy. A more severe form of acute gastritis is caused by ingestion of strong acids or alkali, which may cause the mucosa to become gangrenous or to perforate. Gastritis may also be the first sign of acute systemic infection.

Chronic gastritis is a prolonged inflammation of the stomach that may be caused either by benign or malignant ulcers of the stomach or by bacteria such as *Helicobacter pylori* (*H. pylori*). Chronic gastritis caused by *H. pylori* infection is implicated in the development of peptic ulcers, gastric cancer, and mucosa-associated lymphoid tissue (MALT) lymphoma. Chronic gastritis may be associated with autoimmune diseases such as pernicious anemia.

Nonerosive gastritis (acute and chronic) is most often caused by *H. pylori* infection. Erosive gastritis is most often caused by long-term use of NSAIDs; alcohol abuse and recent exposure to radiation are also implicated.

Pathophysiology

In gastritis, the gastric mucous membrane becomes edematous and hyperemic (congested with fluid and blood) and undergoes superficial erosion. It secretes a scanty amount of gastric juice, containing very little acid but much mucus. Superficial ulceration may occur as a result of erosive disease and may lead to hemorrhage.

Clinical Manifestations

Acute Gastritis
- May have rapid onset of symptoms
- Complaints of abdominal discomfort, headache, lassitude, nausea, anorexia, vomiting, and hiccuping lasting from a few hours to a few days
- Erosive gastritis possibly causing bleeding manifested as black tarry stools (melena) or bright red bloody stool (hematochezia)

Chronic Gastritis
- May be asymptomatic
- Complaints of anorexia, heartburn after eating, belching, a sour taste in the mouth, or nausea and vomiting
- May have mild epigastric discomfort, intolerance to spicy or fatty foods, or pain relieved by eating
- May not be able to absorb vitamin B_{12} and usually having evidence of malabsorption of vitamin B_{12}; may lead to pernicious anemia

Assessment and Diagnostic Findings
- Gastritis is sometimes associated with achlorhydria or hypochlorhydria (absence or low levels of hydrochloric acid) or with high acid levels.
- Upper gastrointestinal (UGI) x-ray series and upper endoscopy are useful.
- Biopsy with histologic examination are performed.
- Serologic testing for antibodies to the *H. pylori* antigen and a breath test may be performed.

Medical Management

Acute Gastritis
The gastric mucosa is capable of repairing itself after an episode of gastritis. As a rule, the patient recovers in about 1 day, although the appetite may be diminished for an additional 2 or 3 days. The patient should refrain from alcohol and eating until symptoms subside. Then the patient can progress to a nonirritating diet. If symptoms persist, intravenous fluids may be necessary. If bleeding is present, management is similar to that of upper GI tract hemorrhage. Supportive therapy may include antacids and histamine-2 receptor antagonist (H_2 blockers; e.g., famotidine [Pepcid], ranitidine [Zantac], proton pump inhibitors, such as lansoprazole [Prevacid]); nasogastric (NG) intubation and IV fluids may be required.

If gastritis is due to ingestion of strong acids or alkali, dilute and neutralize the acid with common antacids (e.g., aluminum hydroxide); neutralize alkali with diluted lemon juice or diluted vinegar. If corrosion is extensive or severe, avoid emetics and lavage because of danger of perforation.

Fiberoptic endoscopy may be necessary; emergency surgery may be required to remove gangrenous or perforated tissue; gastric resection (gastrojejunostomy) may be necessary to treat pyloric obstruction.

G

Chronic Gastritis

Diet modification, rest, stress reduction, avoidance of alcohol and NSAIDs, and supportive pharmacotherapy including antacids, H_2 blockers, or proton pump inhibitors are key treatment measures. Gastritis related to *H. pylori* infection is treated with selected drug combinations that may include multiple antibiotics and a proton pump inhibitor.

Nursing Management

Reducing Anxiety

- Carry out emergency measures for ingestion of strong acids or alkalies.
- Offer supportive therapy to patient and family during treatment and after the ingested acid or alkali has been neutralized or diluted.
- Assess mood to determine whether ingestion may have been intentional.
- Prepare patient for additional diagnostic studies (endoscopy) or surgery.
- Calmly listen to and answer questions as completely as possible; explain all procedures and treatments.

Promoting Optimal Nutrition

- Provide physical and emotional support for patients with acute gastritis.
- Help patient manage symptoms (e.g., nausea, vomiting, heartburn, and fatigue).
- Avoid foods and fluids by mouth for hours or days until acute symptoms subside.
- Offer ice chips and clear liquids when symptoms subside.
- Encourage patient to report any symptoms suggesting a repeat episode of gastritis as food is introduced.
- Discourage caffeinated beverages (caffeine increases gastric activity and pepsin secretion), alcohol, and cigarette

smoking (nicotine inhibits neutralization of gastric acid in the duodenum).
- Refer patient for alcohol counseling and smoking cessation when appropriate.

Promoting Fluid Balance
- Monitor daily intake and output for dehydration (minimal intake of 1.5 L per day and urine output of 0.5 mL/kg per hour). Infuse intravenous fluids if prescribed.
- Assess electrolyte values every 24 hours for fluid imbalance.
- Be alert for indicators of hemorrhagic gastritis (hematemesis, tachycardia, hypotension) and notify physician.
- Assess all stools for presence of frank or occult bleeding.

Relieving Pain
- Instruct patient to avoid foods and beverages that may irritate the gastric mucosa.
- Instruct patient in the correct use of medications to relieve chronic gastritis.
- Assess pain and attainment of comfort through use of medications and avoidance of irritating substances.

Promoting Home- and Community-Based Care

Educating Patients About Self-Care
- Assess knowledge about gastritis and develop an individualized education plan that incorporates patient's pattern of eating, daily caloric needs, and food preferences.
- Provide a list of substances to avoid (e.g., caffeine, nicotine, spicy foods, irritating or highly seasoned foods, alcohol); consult with nutritionist if indicated.
- Educate about antibiotic agents, antacids, H_2 blockers, proton pump inhibitors, bismuth salts, sedative medications, or anticholinergic agents that may be prescribed.
- When necessary, reinforce the importance of completing the medication regimen as prescribed to eradicate *H. pylori* infection.

Continuing Care
- Reinforce previous instructions and conduct ongoing assessment of patient's symptoms and progress.
- If malabsorption of B_{12} is an issue, educate patient and family in proper injection technique for B_{12} therapy or provide appropriate referrals for home care.

For more information, see Chapter 47 in Hinkle, J. L., & Cheever, K. H. (2014). *Brunner and Suddarth's textbook of medical-surgical nursing* (13th ed.). Philadelphia: Lippincott Williams & Wilkins.

Glaucoma

The term *glaucoma* is used to refer to a group of ocular conditions characterized by optic nerve damage. Most cases are asymptomatic until extensive and irreversible damage has occurred. Glaucoma affects people of all ages but is more prevalent with increasing age (older than 40 years). Others at risk are patients with diabetes, African Americans, those individuals with a family history of glaucoma, and people with previous eye trauma or surgery or those who have had long-term steroid treatment. There is no cure for glaucoma, but the disease can be controlled. Glaucoma is the second leading cause of blindness among adults in the United States.

Pathophysiology

Aqueous humor flows between the iris and the lens, nourishing the cornea and lens. Intraocular pressure (IOP) is determined by the rate of aqueous production, the resistance encountered by the aqueous humor as it flows out of the passages, and the venous pressure of the episcleral veins that drain into the anterior ciliary vein. When aqueous fluid is inhibited from flowing out, pressure builds up within the eye. Increased IOP damages the optic nerve and nerve fiber layer, but the degree of harm is highly variable. The degree of damage to the optic nerve is related to the elevations in IOP caused by the congestion of aqueous humor in the eye.

Classification of Glaucomas

There are several types of glaucoma. Current clinical forms of glaucoma are identified as open-angle glaucoma, angle-closure glaucoma (also called *pupillary block*), congenital glaucoma, and glaucoma associated with other conditions. Glaucoma can be primary or secondary, depending on whether associated factors contribute to the rise in IOP. The two common clinical forms of glaucoma encountered in adults are primary open-angle glaucoma (POAG) and angle-closure glaucoma, which are differentiated by the mechanisms that cause impaired aqueous outflow.

Clinical Manifestations

- Most patients are unaware that they have the disease until they have experienced visual changes and vision loss.
- Symptoms may include blurred vision or "halos" around lights, difficulty focusing, difficulty adjusting eyes in low

lighting, loss of peripheral vision, aching or discomfort around the eyes, and headache.
- Pallor and cupping of the optic nerve disc are seen; as the optic nerve damage increases, visual perception in the area is lost.

Assessment and Diagnostic Findings
- Ocular and medical history (to investigate predisposing factors)
- Diagnostic tests: tonometry (measures IOP), ophthalmoscopy (to inspect the optic nerve), gonioscopy (to examine the filtration angle of the anterior chamber), and perimetry (visual fields assessment)

Medical Management
The aim of all glaucoma treatment is prevention of optic nerve damage. Lifelong therapy is almost always necessary because glaucoma cannot be cured. Treatment focuses on pharmacologic therapy, laser procedures, surgery, or a combination of these approaches, all of which have potential complications and side effects. The objective is to achieve the greatest benefit at the least risk, cost, and inconvenience to the patient. Although treatment cannot reverse optic nerve damage, further damage can be controlled. The goal is to maintain an IOP within a range unlikely to cause further damage. Periodic follow-up examinations are essential to monitor IOP, the appearance of the optic nerve, the visual fields, and side effects of medications. Therapy takes into account the patient's health and stage of glaucoma.

Pharmacologic Therapy
Medical management of glaucoma relies on systemic and topical ocular medications that lower IOP.

- Patient is usually started on the lowest dose of topical medication and then advanced to increased concentrations until the desired IOP level is reached and maintained.
- One eye is treated first, with the other eye used as a control in determining the efficacy of the medication. If the IOP is elevated in both eyes, both are treated.
- Several types of ocular medications are used to treat glaucoma, including miotic agents (medications that cause pupillary constriction), adrenergic agonists (i.e., sympathomimetic agents), beta-blockers (preferred initial topical medications), alpha$_2$-agonists (i.e., adrenergic agents), carbonic anhydrase

inhibitors (decreases aqueous humor production), and prostaglandins (increases aqueous humor outflow).

Surgical Management

- Laser trabeculoplasty or iridotomy is indicated when IOP is inadequately controlled by medications.
- Filtering procedures create an opening or a fistula in the trabecular meshwork; trabeculectomy is standard technique.
- Drainage implant or shunt surgery may be performed.
- Trabectome surgery is reserved for patients in whom pharmacologic treatment and/or laser trabeculoplasty do not control the IOP sufficiently.

G

Nursing Management

Promoting Home- and Community-Based Care

Educating Patients About Self-Care
- Educate patient regarding the nature of the disease and the importance of strict adherence to the medication regimen to help ensure compliance.
- Review the patient's medication program including administration techniques for eye drops, particularly the interactions of glaucoma control medications with other medications.
- Explain effects of glaucoma control medications on vision (e.g., miotic drugs and sympathomimetic agents result in altered focus; therefore, patients need to be cautious in navigating their surroundings).

Continuing Care
- Refer patient to services that assist in performing activities of daily living, if needed.
- Refer patients with impaired mobility for low vision and rehabilitation services; patients who meet the criteria for legal blindness should be offered referrals to agencies that can assist them in obtaining federal assistance.
- Provide reassurance and emotional support.
- Integrate patient's family into the plan of care and, because the disease has a familial tendency, encourage family members to undergo examinations at least once every 2 years to detect glaucoma early.

For more information, see Chapter 63 in Hinkle, J. L., & Cheever, K. H. (2014). *Brunner and Suddarth's textbook of medical-surgical nursing* (13th ed.). Philadelphia: Lippincott Williams & Wilkins.

Glomerulonephritis, Acute

Acute nephritic syndrome is the clinical manifestation of glomerular inflammation. Glomerulonephritis is an inflammation of the glomerular capillaries that can occur in acute and chronic forms. Primary glomerular diseases include postinfectious glomerulonephritis, rapidly progressive glomerulonephritis, membrane proliferative glomerulonephritis, and membranous glomerulonephritis. Postinfectious causes are group A beta-hemolytic streptococcal infection of the throat, impetigo (infection of the skin), and acute viral infections (upper respiratory tract infections, mumps, varicella zoster virus, Epstein-Barr virus, hepatitis B, and HIV infection). Antigens outside the body such as medications or foreign serum may initiate the process in some patients. In other patients, the kidney tissue itself serves as the inciting antigen.

Clinical Manifestations

Primary presenting features of an acute glomerular inflammation include the following:

- Hematuria, edema, azotemia, an abnormal concentration of nitrogenous wastes in the blood, and proteinuria or excess protein in the urine; cola-colored because of red blood cells (RBCs) and protein plugs or casts
- Possible increase in blood urea nitrogen (BUN) and serum creatinine levels as urine output decreases
- Anemia
- Headache, malaise, and flank pain
- In older patients, possible circulatory overload with dyspnea, engorged neck veins, cardiomegaly, and pulmonary edema

Assessment and Diagnostic Findings

- Kidneys become large, edematous, and congested. All renal tissues including the glomeruli, tubules, and blood vessels are affected to varying degrees.
- Blood studies related to renal failure progression include hyperkalemia, metabolic acidosis, anemia, hypoalbuminemia, decreased serum calcium and increased serum phosphorus, and hypermagnesemia.
- Electron microscopy and immunofluorescent analysis help identify the nature of the lesion; however, a kidney biopsy may be needed for definitive diagnosis.

Medical Management

- Symptoms are treated with an attempt to preserve kidney function, and any complications must be treated promptly.

- If treatment is effective, diuresis will begin, resulting in decreased edema and blood pressure.
- Corticosteroid agents are prescribed to help manage hypertension and control proteinuria.
- If residual streptococcal infection is suspected, penicillin is the agent of choice; however, other antibiotic agents may be prescribed.
- Dietary protein is restricted when renal insufficiency and nitrogen retention (elevated BUN) develop. Sodium is restricted when the patient has hypertension, edema, and heart failure.

Nursing Management

- Measure and record intake and output (I&O) and weigh the patient daily; provide fluids based on the patient's fluid losses and daily body weight. Insensible fluid loss through the lungs (300 mL) and skin (600 mL) is considered when estimating fluid loss.
- Monitor for proteinuria and microscopic hematuria, which may persist for many months.
- Educate patient about the disease process, managing symptoms, and monitoring for complications.
- Explain laboratory and other diagnostic tests, and prepare the patient for safe and effective self-care at home.
- Educate patient on managing symptoms and monitoring for complications.
- Review fluid and diet restrictions with the patient to avoid worsening of edema and hypertension.
- Instruct patient verbally and in writing to notify the primary provider if symptoms of renal failure occur (e.g., fatigue, nausea, vomiting, diminishing urine output) or at the first sign of any infection.
- Refer to community health or home care nurse for assessment of patient progress and continued education about problems to report to a health care provider.
- Remind patient and family of the importance of participation in health promotion activities, including health screening.
- Instruct patient to inform all health care providers about the diagnosis of glomerulonephritis.

For more information, see Chapter 54 in Hinkle, J. L., & Cheever, K. H. (2014). *Brunner and Suddarth's textbook of medical-surgical nursing* (13th ed.). Philadelphia: Lippincott Williams & Wilkins.

Glomerulonephritis, Chronic

Chronic glomerulonephritis may be due to repeated episodes of acute nephritic syndrome, hypertensive nephrosclerosis, hyperlipidemia, chronic tubulointerstitial injury, or hemodynamically mediated glomerular sclerosis. Secondary glomerular diseases that can have systemic effects include lupus erythematosus, Goodpasture syndrome (caused by antibodies to the glomerular basement membrane), diabetic glomerulosclerosis, and amyloidosis. The kidneys are reduced to as little as one-fifth of their normal size and consist largely of fibrous tissue. The cortex layer shrinks to 1 to 2 mm in thickness or less, scarring occurs, and the branches of the renal artery are thickened. The resulting severe glomerular damage can progress to stage 5 of chronic kidney disease (CKD) and require renal replacement therapies.

Clinical Manifestations

Symptoms are variable. Some patients with severe disease have no symptoms for many years.

- Hypertension or elevated blood urea nitrogen (BUN) and serum creatinine levels
- General symptoms: loss of weight and strength, increasing irritability, and an increased need to urinate at night (nocturia); headaches, dizziness, and digestive disturbances also common

Renal Insufficiency and Chronic Renal Failure

- Patient appears poorly nourished with a yellow-gray pigmentation of the skin, periorbital and peripheral edema, and pale mucous membranes.
- Blood pressure is normal or severely elevated.
- Retinal findings include hemorrhage, exudate, narrowed tortuous arterioles, and papilledema.
- Anemia causes pale membranes.
- Cardiomegaly, gallop rhythm, distended neck veins, and other signs of heart failure may be present.
- Crackles are audible in lungs.
- Possibly, peripheral neuropathy with diminished deep tendon reflexes are evident.
- Neurosensory changes occur late in the illness, resulting in confusion and limited attention span. Other late signs include pericarditis with pericardial friction rub and pulsus paradoxus.

Assessment and Diagnostic Findings

On laboratory analysis, the following abnormalities may be found:

- Urinalysis: fixed specific gravity of 1.010, variable protein-uria, and urinary casts
- Blood studies related to renal failure progression: hyperkalemia, metabolic acidosis, anemia, hypoalbuminemia, decreased serum calcium and increased serum phosphorus, and hypermagnesemia
- Impaired nerve conduction; mental status changes
- Cardiac enlargement and pulmonary edema on chest x-rays
- Electrocardiogram (ECG): normal or may reflect left ventricular hypertrophy
- On CT and MRI scans, a decrease in the size of the renal cortex

Medical Management

The treatment of ambulatory patients is guided by symptoms.

- If hypertension is present, the blood pressure is lowered with sodium and water restriction, antihypertensive agents, or both.
- Weight is monitored daily, and diuretic medications are prescribed to treat fluid overload.
- Proteins of high biologic value are provided to support good nutritional status (dairy products, eggs, meats).
- Urinary tract infections are treated promptly.
- Dialysis is initiated early in the course of disease to keep patient in optimal physical condition, prevent fluid and electrolyte imbalances, and minimize the risk of complications of renal failure.

Nursing Management

- Observe for common fluid and electrolyte disturbances in renal disease; report changes in fluid and electrolyte status and in cardiac and neurologic status.
- Provide emotional support throughout the disease and treatment course by providing opportunities for patient and family to verbalize concerns. Answer questions and discuss options.
- Educate patient and family about prescribed treatment plan and the risk of noncompliance. Explain about need for follow-up evaluations of blood pressure, urinalysis for protein and casts, blood for BUN, and creatinine.
- If long-term dialysis is needed, educate the patient and family about the procedure, how to care for the access site,

dietary restrictions, and other necessary lifestyle modifications.

- Educate patient about recommended diet and fluid modifications and medications (purpose, desired effects, adverse effects, dosage, and administration schedule).
- Refer to community health or home care nurse for assessment of patient progress and continued education about problems to report to health care provider.
- Remind patient and family of the importance of participation in health promotion activities, including health screening.
- Instruct patient to inform all health care providers about the diagnosis of glomerulonephritis.

For more information, see Chapter 54 in Hinkle, J. L., & Cheever, K. H. (2014). *Brunner and Suddarth's textbook of medical-surgical nursing* (13th ed.). Philadelphia: Lippincott Williams & Wilkins.

Gout

Gout is a heterogeneous group of inflammatory arthritis in which crystals called *monosodium urate* are deposited within the joints and tissues. Gout results from hyperuricemia.

Pathophysiology

In gout, there is an increased serum uric acid, especially greater than 6.8 mg/dL. Uric acid is a by-product of purine metabolism; purines are basic chemical compounds found in high concentrations in meat products. Urate levels are affected by diet, medications, overproduction in the body, and inadequate excretion by the kidneys. Gout attacks occur when macrophages in the joint space phagocytize urate crystals. Through a series of immunologic steps, interleukin-1 beta (IL-1β) is secreted, increasing the inflammation, and is exacerbated by the presence of free fatty acids. Both alcohol and consumption of a large meal, especially with red meat, can lead to increases in free fatty acid concentrations, which are both triggers to acute gout attacks. More common in men, risk for gout increases with age, body mass index, alcohol and fructose-rich beverage consumption, hypertension, and diuretic use.

Primary hyperuricemia may be due to severe dieting or starvation, excessive intake of foods high in purines (shellfish, organ meats), or heredity. In secondary hyperuricemia, the gout is a clinical feature secondary to any of a number of genetic or acquired processes, including conditions with an increase in cell turnover (leukemias, multiple myeloma, psoriasis, some anemias) and an increase in cell breakdown.

Clinical Manifestations

Gout is characterized by deposits of uric acid in various joints. Four stages of gout can be identified: asymptomatic hyperuricemia, acute gouty arthritis, intercritical gout, and chronic tophaceous gout.

- Acute arthritis of gout is the most common early sign.
- The metatarsophalangeal joint of the big toe is most commonly affected; the tarsal area, ankle, or knee may also be affected.
- The acute attack may be triggered by trauma, alcohol ingestion, dieting, medication, surgical stress, or illness.
- Abrupt onset occurs at night, causing severe pain, redness, swelling, and warmth over the affected joint.
- Early attacks tend to subside spontaneously over 3 to 10 days without treatment.
- The next attack may not come for months or years; in time, attacks tend to occur more frequently, involve more joints, and last longer.
- Tophi are generally associated with frequent and severe inflammatory episodes.
- Higher serum concentrations of uric acid are associated with tophus formation.
- Tophi occur in the synovium, olecranon bursa, subchondral bone, infrapatellar and Achilles' tendons, subcutaneous tissue, and overlying joints.
- Tophi have also been found in aortic walls, heart valves, nasal and ear cartilage, eyelids, cornea, and sclerae.
- Joint enlargement may cause loss of joint motion.
- Uric acid deposits may cause renal stones and kidney damage.

Assessment and Diagnostic Findings

A definitive diagnosis of gouty arthritis is established by polarized light microscopy of the synovial fluid of the involved joint. Uric acid crystals are seen within the polymorphonuclear leukocytes in the fluid.

Medical Management

- Colchicine (oral or parenteral), a nonsteroidal anti-inflammatory drug (NSAID) such as indomethacin, or a corticosteroid is prescribed to relieve an acute attack of gout.

- Hyperuricemia, tophi, joint destruction, and renal problems are treated after the acute inflammatory process has subsided.
- Uricosuric agents, such as probenecid, may be used to correct hyperuricemia by increasing excretion of uric acid.
- Allopurinol is effective when renal insufficiency or renal calculi are a risk.
- Corticosteroids may be used in patients who have no response to other therapy.
- Patients with gout should avoid purine-rich foods, consider weight loss, decrease alcohol consumption, and avoid certain medications.
- Anakinra, an IL-1 receptor antagonist, is also suggested in the management of acute gout.
- Prophylactic treatment is considered if patient experiences several acute episodes or there is evidence of tophi formation.
- For refractory chronic gout not controlled with the preceding regimens, pegloticase, a urate lowering agent, may be used.

Nursing Management

- Encourage dietary restriction of foods high in purines, especially organ meats, and limiting alcohol intake.
- Encourage patient to maintain normal body weight. In an acute episode of gouty arthritis, pain management is essential.
- Review medications with patient and family stressing importance of continuing medications to maintain effectiveness to avoid acute episodes. See "Nursing Management" under Arthritis, Rheumatoid in Section A for additional information.
- Review factors that increase pain and inflammation, such as trauma, stress, and alcohol.

For more information, see Chapter 39 in Hinkle, J. L., & Cheever, K. H. (2014). *Brunner and Suddarth's textbook of medical-surgical nursing* (13th ed.). Philadelphia: Lippincott Williams & Wilkins.

Guillain-Barré Syndrome
(Polyradiculoneuritis)

Guillain-Barré syndrome (GBS) is an autoimmune (cell-mediated and humoral) inflammatory demyelination on the peripheral nerves. An antecedent event (most often a viral infection occurring 1 to 3 weeks prior to onset of symptoms) usually precipitates clinical presentation in the majority of cases. It is more frequent in males between 16 and 25 years of age and those older than 55 years of age. Results of studies on recovery rates differ, but most indicate that 60% to 75% of patients recover completely.

Pathophysiology

Guillain-Barré syndrome results in the acute, rapid segmental demyelination of peripheral nerves and some cranial nerves, producing ascending weakness with dyskinesia (inability to execute voluntary movements), hyporeflexia, and paresthesias (numbness). With the autoimmune attack, there is an influx of macrophages and other immune-mediated agents that attack myelin and cause inflammation and destruction, inter-ruption of nerve conduction, and axonal loss. The Schwann cell (which produces myelin in the peripheral nervous system) is spared in GBS, allowing for remyelination in the recovery phase of the disease.

Clinical Manifestations

- Classic clinical features of GBS include areflexia and ascend-ing weakness; variations in presentation occur. GBS does not affect cognitive function or level of consciousness.
- Initial symptoms include muscle weakness and diminished reflexes of the lower extremities; hyporeflexia and weakness may progress to tetraplegia; demyelination of the nerves that innervate the diaphragm and intercostal muscles results in neuromuscular respiratory failure.
- Sensory symptoms include paresthesias of the hands and feet and pain related to the demyelination of sensory fibers.
- Optic nerve demyelination may result in blindness.
- Bulbar muscle weakness related to demyelination of the glos-sopharyngeal and vagus nerves results in the inability to swal-low or clear secretions.
- Vagus nerve demyelination results in autonomic dysfunc-tion, manifested by instability of the cardiovascular system (tachycardia, bradycardia, hypertension, or orthostatic hypo-tension).

Assessment and Diagnostic Findings

- Clinical presentation (symmetric weakness, diminished reflexes, and upward progression of motor weakness); a history of recent viral infection suggests the diagnosis.
- Changes in vital capacity and negative inspiratory force are assessed to identify impending neuromuscular respiratory failure.

- Elevated protein levels are detected in cerebrospinal fluid (CSF) evaluation, without an increase in other cells.
- Evoked potential studies demonstrate a progressive loss of nerve conduction velocity.

Medical Management

GBS is considered a medical emergency; the patient is managed in an ICU. Respiratory problems may require respiratory therapy or mechanical ventilation. Elective intubation may be implemented before the onset of extreme respiratory muscle fatigue; emergent intubation may result in autonomic dysfunction, and mechanical ventilation may be required for an extended period. Anticoagulant agents and antiembolism stockings or sequential compression boots may be used to prevent venous thromboembolism and pulmonary emboli. The cardiovascular risks posed by autonomic dysfunction require continuous electrocardiographic (ECG) monitoring.

Pharmacologic Therapy

- Intravenous immunoglobulin (IVIG) is the drug of choice and may be used to directly affect the peripheral nerve myelin antibody level; plasmapheresis (plasma exchange) is also effective for treatment.
- Tachycardia and hypertension (due to autonomic dysfunction) are treated with short-acting medications such as alpha-adrenergic blocking agents. Hypotension is managed by increasing the amount of intravenous fluid administered.
- Anticoagulant agents and sequential compression boots are prescribed to prevent thrombosis and pulmonary emboli.

NURSING PROCESS

The Patient With GBS

Assessment (Ongoing and Critical)

Continually monitor the patient for life-threatening complications (e.g., respiratory failure, cardiac dysrhythmias, venous thromboembolism [VTE] including deep vein thrombosis [DVT] or pulmonary embolism [PE]) so that appropriate interventions can be initiated. Assess the patient's and family's ability to cope and their use of coping strategies.

Diagnosis

NURSING DIAGNOSES
- Ineffective breathing pattern and impaired gas exchange related to rapidly progressive weakness and impending respiratory failure
- Impaired physical mobility related to paralysis
- Imbalanced nutrition, less than body requirements, related to inability to swallow
- Impaired verbal communication related to cranial nerve dysfunction
- Fear and anxiety related to loss of control and paralysis

COLLABORATIVE PROBLEMS/POTENTIAL COMPLICATIONS
- Respiratory failure
- Autonomic dysfunction

Planning and Goals

Major goals include improved respiratory function, increased mobility, improved nutritional status, effective communication, decreased fear and anxiety, and absence of complications.

Nursing Interventions

MAINTAINING RESPIRATORY FUNCTION
- Encourage use of incentive spirometry and provide chest physiotherapy.
- Monitor for changes in vital capacity and negative inspiratory force; if vital capacity falls, mechanical ventilation will be necessary (discuss the potential need for mechanical ventilation with the patient and family on admission, to provide time for psychological preparation and decision making).
- Suction to maintain a clear airway.
- Assess blood pressure and heart rate frequently to identify autonomic dysfunction.

ENHANCING PHYSICAL MOBILITY
- Provide passive range-of-motion exercises at least twice daily; support the paralyzed extremities in functional positions. Change patient's position at least every 2 hours.
- Administer prescribed anticoagulant regimen to prevent VTE (DVT and PE); assist with physical therapy and position changes; use antiembolism stockings or sequential compression boots and provide adequate hydration.

- Place padding over bony prominences such as elbows and heels to reduce the risk of pressure ulcers.

PROVIDING ADEQUATE NUTRITION

- Collaborate with physician and dietitian to meet patient's nutritional and hydration needs. Provide adequate nutrition to prevent muscle wasting.
- Evaluate laboratory test results that may indicate malnutrition or dehydration (both of which conditions increase the risk for pressure ulcers).
- If patient has paralytic ileus, provide intravenous fluids and parenteral nutrition as prescribed and monitor for return of bowel sounds.
- Provide gastrostomy tube feedings if patient cannot swallow.
- Assess the return of the gag reflex and bowel sounds before resuming oral nutrition.

IMPROVING COMMUNICATION

- Establish communication through lip reading, use of picture cards, or eye blinking.
- Collaborate with speech therapist, as indicated.

DECREASING FEAR AND ANXIETY

- Refer patient and family to a support group.
- Allow and encourage family members to participate in physical care of patient after providing instruction and support.
- Provide patient with information about condition, emphasizing a positive appraisal of coping resources.
- Provide instruction for and encourage use of relaxation exercises and distraction techniques.
- Create a positive attitude and atmosphere.
- Encourage diversional activities to decrease loneliness and isolation. Encouraging visitors, engaging visitors or volunteers to read to the patient, listening to music or books on tape, and watching television are ways to alleviate the patient's sense of isolation.

MONITORING AND MANAGING POTENTIAL COMPLICATIONS

- Assess respiratory function at regular and frequent intervals; monitor respiratory rate, the quality of respirations, and vital capacity.
- Watch for breathlessness while talking, shallow and irregular breathing, use of accessory muscles, tachycardia, weak cough, and changes in respiratory pattern.

- Monitor for and report cardiac dysrhythmias (through electrocardiographic monitoring), transient hypertension, orthostatic hypotension, DVT, PE, and urinary retention.

PROMOTING HOME- AND COMMUNITY-BASED CARE

Educating Patients About Self-Care

- Provide education to patient and family about the disorder and its generally favorable prognosis.
- During the acute phase, instruct patient and family about strategies they can implement to minimize the effects of immobility and other complications.
- Explain care of patient and roles of patient and family in rehabilitation process.
- Use an interdisciplinary effort for family or caregiver education (nurse, physician, occupational and physical therapists, speech therapist, and respiratory therapist).

Continuing Care

- Provide care in a comprehensive inpatient program or an outpatient program, if patient can travel by car, or encourage a home program of physical and occupational therapy.
- Support patient and family through long recovery phase and promote involvement for return of former abilities.
- Remind or instruct patients and family members of the need for continuing health promotion and screening practices.

Evaluation

EXPECTED PATIENT OUTCOMES

- Maintains effective respirations and airway clearance
- Shows increasing mobility
- Receives adequate nutrition and hydration
- Demonstrates recovery of speech
- Shows lessening fear and anxiety
- Remains free of complications

For more information, see Chapter 69 in Hinkle, J. L., & Cheever, K. H. (2014). *Brunner and Suddarth's textbook of medical-surgical nursing* (13th ed.). Philadelphia: Lippincott Williams & Wilkins.

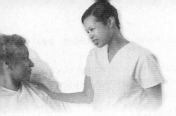

Head Injury (Brain Injury)

Injuries to the head involve trauma to the scalp, skull, and brain. A head injury may lead to conditions ranging from mild concussion to coma and death; the most serious form is known as a traumatic brain injury (TBI). The most common causes of TBIs are falls (35.2%), motor vehicle crashes (17.3%), being struck by objects (16.5%), and assaults (10%). Groups at highest risk for TBI are persons 15 to 19 years of age, with greater incidence in males in every age group. Adults ages 65 years or older have the highest TBI-related hospitalization and death rates. There are two forms of damage to the brain from traumatic injury. **Primary injury** is the initial damage to the brain that results from the traumatic event. Primary injuries include contusions, lacerations, and torn blood vessels due to impact, acceleration–deceleration, or foreign object penetration. **Secondary injury** evolves over the ensuing hours and days after the initial injury and results from inadequate delivery of nutrients and oxygen to the cells. Secondary injuries include intracranial hemorrhage, cerebral edema, increased intracranial pressure, hypoxic brain damage, and infection.

Clinical Manifestations

Symptoms, other than local, depend on the severity and the anatomic location of the underlying brain injury.

- Persistent, localized pain usually suggests fracture.
- Fractures of the cranial vault may or may not produce swelling in that region.
- Fractures of the base of the skull frequently produce hemorrhage from the nose, pharynx, or ears, and blood may appear under the conjunctiva.
- Ecchymosis may be seen over the mastoid (Battle's sign).
- Drainage of cerebrospinal fluid (CSF) from the ears (otorrhea) and the nose (rhinorrhea) suggests basal skull fracture.
- Drainage of CSF may cause serious infection (e.g., meningitis) through a tear in the dura mater.

- Bloody spinal fluid suggests brain laceration or contusion.
- Brain injury may have various signs, including altered level of consciousness (LOC), pupillary abnormalities, altered or absent gag reflex or corneal reflex, neurologic deficits, change in vital signs (e.g., respiration pattern, hypertension, bradycardia), hyperthermia or hypothermia, and sensory, vision, or hearing impairment.
- Signs of a postconcussion syndrome may include headache, dizziness, anxiety, irritability, and lethargy.
- In acute or subacute subdural hematoma, changes in LOC, pupillary signs, hemiparesis, coma, hypertension, bradycardia, and slowing respiratory rate are signs of expanding mass.
- Chronic subdural hematoma may result in severe headache, alternating focal neurologic signs, personality changes, mental deterioration, and focal seizures.

Assessment and Diagnostic Findings
- Physical examination and evaluation of neurologic status
- Radiographic studies: x-rays, CT, MRI
- Cerebral angiography

Scalp and Skull Injuries
- Scalp trauma may result in an abrasion (brush wound), contusion, laceration, or hematoma. The scalp bleeds profusely when injured. Scalp wounds are a portal of entry for intracranial infections.
- Fracture of the skull is a break in the continuity of the skull caused by forceful trauma. Fractures may occur with or without damage to the brain. They are classified as simple, comminuted, depressed, or basilar and may be open (dura is torn) or closed (dura is not torn).

Medical Management
- Nondepressed skull fractures generally do not require surgical treatment but require close observation of patient.
- Depressed skull fractures usually require surgery with elevation of the skull and debridement, usually within 24 hours of injury.

Concussion (Brain Injury)
A concussion after a head injury is a temporary loss of neurologic function with no apparent structural damage. A concussion (also referred to as a *mild TBI*) may or may not produce a brief loss of consciousness. The mechanism of injury is usually blunt trauma from an acceleration–deceleration force, a direct

blow, or a blast injury. If brain tissue in the frontal lobe is affected, the patient may exhibit bizarre irrational behavior, whereas involvement of the temporal lobe can produce temporary amnesia or disorientation. There are three grades of concussion as defined by the American Academy of Neurology.

- Grade 1: transient confusion, no loss of consciousness, and resolution of mental status abnormalities on examination in less than 15 minutes.
- Grade 2: transient confusion, no loss of consciousness, and concussion symptoms or mental status abnormalities on examination that last more than 15 minutes
- Grade 3: any loss of consciousness lasting from seconds to minutes

Nursing Management
- Provide information, explanations, and encouragement to reduce postconcussion syndrome.
- Educate family to look for the following signs and notify physician or clinic: difficulty in awakening or speaking; confusion; severe headache; vomiting; and weakness of one side of the body.

Contusion

In cerebral contusion, a moderate to severe head injury, the brain is bruised and damaged in a specific area because of severe acceleration–deceleration force or blunt trauma. The impact of the brain against the skull leads to a contusion. Contusions are characterized by loss of consciousness associated with stupor and confusion. Other characteristics can include tissue alteration and neurologic deficit without hematoma formation, alteration in consciousness without localizing signs, or hemorrhage into the tissue that varies in size and is surrounded by edema. The effects of injury (hemorrhage and edema) peak after about 18 to 36 hours. Patient outcome depends on the area and severity of the injury. Temporal lobe contusions carry a greater risk of swelling, rapid deterioration, and brain herniation. Deep contusions are more often associated with hemorrhage and destruction of the reticular activating fibers altering arousal.

Diffuse Axonal Injury

Diffuse axonal injury (DAI) results from widespread shearing and rotational forces that produce damage throughout the brain—to axons in the cerebral hemispheres, corpus callosum, and brain stem. The injured area may be diffuse, with no identifiable focal lesion. The patient has no lucid intervals and experiences immediate coma, decorticate and decerebrate posturing, and global cerebral edema. Diagnosis is made by clinical signs and a CT or MRI scan. Recovery depends on the severity of the axonal injury.

Intracranial Hemorrhage

Hematomas are collections of blood in the brain that may be epidural (above the dura), subdural (below the dura), or intracerebral (within the brain). Major symptoms are frequently delayed until the hematoma is large enough to cause distortion of the brain and increased intracranial pressure (ICP).

Epidural Hematoma

After a head injury, blood may collect in the epidural (extradural) space between the skull and the dura mater, resulting from a skull fracture that causes a rupture or laceration of the middle meningeal artery (the artery that runs between the dura and the skull inferior to a thin portion of temporal bone). Symptoms are caused by the pressure of the expanding hematoma: usually a momentary loss of consciousness at time of injury followed by an interval of apparent recovery while compensation for the increased volume occurs. When compensation is no longer possible, sudden signs of herniation may appear, including deterioration of consciousness and signs of focal neurologic deficits (dilation and fixation of a pupil or paralysis of an extremity); the patient's condition deteriorates rapidly. The most common type of herniation syndrome associated with an epidural hematoma is uncal herniation.

Medical Management

Epidural hematoma is an extreme emergency because marked neurologic deficit or respiratory arrest may occur within minutes. Burr holes are made to remove the clots and, to control bleeding (craniotomy, drain insertion).

Subdural Hematoma

Blood collects between the dura and the underlying brain and is more frequently venous in origin. The most common cause is trauma, but it can also occur as a result of coagulopathies or rupture of an aneurysm. Subdural hematoma may be acute (major head injury), subacute (sequelae of less severe contusions), or chronic (minor head injuries in older adults may be a cause; signs and symptoms fluctuate and may be mistaken for neurosis, psychosis, or stroke).

Intracerebral Hemorrhage and Hematoma

Bleeding occurs into the parenchyma of the brain. Hematoma is commonly seen when forces are exerted to the head over a small area (missile injuries or bullet wounds; stab injury). It may also result from systemic hypertension causing degeneration and rupture of a vessel; rupture of a saccular aneurysm; vascular anomalies; intracranial tumors; bleeding disorders such as leukemia, hemophilia, aplastic anemia, and thrombocytopenia; and complications of anticoagulant therapy. Its onset may be insidious, with neurologic deficits followed by headache.

Medical Management

Presume that a person with a head injury has a cervical spine injury until proven otherwise. Assessment and diagnosis of the extent of injury are accomplished by the initial physical and neurologic examinations. Diagnostic tools include CT, MRI, and positron emission tomography (PET). From the scene of the injury, the patient is transported on a board, with head and neck maintained in alignment with the axis of the body. Apply a cervical collar and maintain it until cervical spine x-rays have been obtained and the absence of cervical spinal cord injury documented. All therapy is directed toward preserving brain homeostasis and preventing secondary brain injury.

- Management involves control of ICP, supportive care (e.g., ventilatory support, seizure prevention, fluid and electrolyte maintenance, nutritional support, and management of pain and anxiety), or craniotomy.
- Increased ICP is managed by adequate oxygenation, mannitol administration, ventilatory support, hyperventilation, elevation of the head of the bed, maintenance of fluid and electrolyte balance, nutritional support, pain and anxiety management, or neurosurgery.

See "Medical Management" and "Nursing Process" under Increased Intracranial Pressure in Section I for additional information.

NURSING PROCESS

The Patient With a TBI

Assessment

Obtain health history, including time of injury, cause of injury, direction and force of the blow, loss of consciousness, and condition after injury. Detailed neurologic information (LOC, ability to respond to verbal commands if patient is conscious), response to tactile stimuli (if patient is unconscious), pupillary response to light, corneal and gag reflexes, motor function, and system assessments provide baseline data. The Glasgow Coma Scale (GCS) serves as a guide for assessing LOCs based on three criteria: (1) eye opening, (2) verbal responses, and (3) motor responses to a verbal command or painful stimulus.

MONITORING VITAL SIGNS
- Monitor patient at frequent intervals to assess intracranial status.
- Assess for increasing ICP, including slowing of pulse, increasing systolic pressure, and widening pulse pressure. As brain compression increases, vital signs are reversed, pulse and respirations become rapid, and blood pressure may decrease.
- Monitor for rapid rise in body temperature; keep temperature below 38°C (100.4°F) to avoid increased metabolic demands on the brain.
- Keep in mind that tachycardia and hypotension may indicate bleeding elsewhere in the body.

ASSESSING MOTOR FUNCTION
- Observe spontaneous movements; ask patient to raise and lower extremities; compare strength and equality of the upper and lower extremities at periodic intervals.
- Note presence or absence of spontaneous movement of each extremity.
- Determine patient's ability to speak; note quality of speech.
- Assess responses to painful stimuli in absence of spontaneous movement; abnormal response carries a poorer prognosis.

OTHER NEUROLOGIC SIGNS
- Evaluate spontaneous eye opening.
- Evaluate size of pupils and reaction to light (unilaterally dilated and poorly responding pupils may indicate

developing hematoma). If both pupils are fixed and dilated, it usually indicates overwhelming injury and poor prognosis.

- The patient with a head injury may develop deficits such as anosmia (lack of sense of smell), eye movement abnormalities, aphasia, memory deficits, and posttraumatic seizures or epilepsy.
- Patients may be left with residual psychosocial deficits and may lack insight into their emotional responses.

Diagnosis

NURSING DIAGNOSES

- Ineffective airway clearance and impaired gas exchange related to brain injury
- Risk for ineffective cerebral tissue perfusion related to increased ICP, decreased cerebral perfusion pressure (CPP), and possible seizures
- Deficient fluid volume related to decreased LOC and hormonal dysfunction
- Imbalanced nutrition (less than body requirements) related to increased metabolic demands, fluid restriction, and inadequate intake
- Risk for injury (self-directed and directed at others) related to seizures, disorientation, restlessness, or brain damage
- Risk for imbalanced body temperature related to damaged temperature-regulating mechanisms in the brain
- Risk for impaired skin integrity related to bed rest, hemiparesis, hemiplegia, immobility, or restlessness
- Ineffective coping related to brain injury
- Disturbed sleep pattern related to brain injury and frequent neurologic checks
- Interrupted family processes related to unresponsiveness of patient, unpredictability of outcome, prolonged recovery period, and the patient's residual physical disability and emotional deficit
- Deficient knowledge about brain injury, recovery, and the rehabilitation process

COLLABORATIVE PROBLEMS/POTENTIAL COMPLICATIONS

- Decreased cerebral perfusion
- Cerebral edema and herniation
- Impaired oxygenation and ventilation
- Impaired fluid, electrolyte, and nutritional balance
- Risk for posttraumatic seizures

Planning and Goals

Goals may include maintenance of a patent airway, adequate CPP, fluid and electrolyte balance, adequate nutritional status, prevention of secondary injury, maintenance of normal body temperature, maintenance of skin integrity, improvement of coping, prevention of sleep deprivation, effective family coping, increased knowledge about the rehabilitation process, and absence of complications.

Nursing Interventions

MONITORING NEUROLOGIC FUNCTION

- Monitor LOC using the GCS at regular intervals. A score of 3 is least responsive, and a score of 15 is most responsive. A GCS reading between 3 and 8 is generally accepted as indicating a severe head injury.
- Monitor vital signs at frequent intervals to assess the intracranial status.
- Monitor for signs of increasing ICP include slowing of the heart rate (bradycardia), increasing systolic blood pressure, and widening pulse pressure (Cushing's reflex).
- Maintain temperature less than 38°C (100.4°F). Tachycardia and arterial hypotension may indicate that bleeding is occurring elsewhere in the body.

> **Quality and Safety Nursing Alert**
>
> In a patient with a head injury, a rapid increase in body temperature is unfavorable because hyperthermia increases the metabolic demands of the brain and may indicate brain stem damage.

MAINTAINING THE AIRWAY

- Position the unconscious patient to facilitate drainage of secretions; elevate the head of the bed 30 degrees to decrease intracranial venous pressure.
- Establish effective suctioning procedures.
- Guard against aspiration and respiratory insufficiency.
- Monitor arterial blood gases (ABGs) to assess adequacy of ventilation.
- Monitor patient on mechanical ventilation for pulmonary complications (acute respiratory distress syndrome [ARDS] and pneumonia).

MAINTAINING FLUID AND ELECTROLYTE BALANCE

Fluid and electrolyte balance is particularly important in patients receiving osmotic diuretic drugs, those with the syndrome of inappropriate antidiuretic hormone (SIADH) secretion, and those with posttraumatic diabetes insipidus.

- Monitor serum and urine electrolyte levels (including blood glucose and urine acetone), osmolality, and intake and output to evaluate endocrine function.
- Record daily weights (which may indicate fluid loss from diabetes insipidus).

PROMOTING ADEQUATE NUTRITION

- Parenteral nutrition (PN) via a central line or enteral feedings administered via a nasogastric or nasojejunal feeding tube may be used.
- Monitor laboratory values closely in patients receiving PN.
- Elevate the head of the bed and aspirate the enteral tube for evidence of residual feeding before administering additional feedings. This will help prevent distention, regurgitation, and aspiration; a continuous-drip infusion or pump may be used to regulate the feeding.
- Continue enteral or parenteral feedings until the swallowing reflex returns and the patient can meet caloric requirements orally.

PREVENTING INJURY

- Observe for restlessness, which may be due to hypoxia, fever, pain, or a full bladder. Restlessness may also be a sign that the unconscious patient is regaining consciousness.
- Avoid restraints when possible because straining can increase ICP.
- Avoid bladder distention.
- Protect patient from self-injury and dislodging tubes (padded side rails, hands wrapped in mitts).
- Avoid using opioid drugs for restlessness because they depress respiration, constrict pupils, and alter LOC.
- Reduce environmental stimuli by keeping the room quiet, limiting visitors, speaking calmly, and providing frequent orientation information.
- Provide adequate lighting to prevent visual hallucinations.
- Minimize disruption of patient's sleep and wake cycles.
- Lubricate the patient's skin with oil or emollient lotion to prevent irritation due to rubbing against the sheet.

- Use an external sheath catheter for a male patient with incontinence to prevent infection from an indwelling catheter.

Maintaining Body Temperature
- Monitor temperature every 2 to 4 hours.
- If temperature rises, try to identify the cause and administer acetaminophen and cooling blankets to maintain normothermia.
- Monitor for infection related to fever.

Maintaining Skin Integrity
- Assess all body surfaces and document skin integrity every 8 hours.
- Turn and reposition patient every 2 hours.
- Provide skin care every 4 hours.
- Assist patient in getting out of bed three times a day as appropriate.

Improving Cognitive Functioning
- Develop patient's ability to devise problem-solving strategies through cognitive rehabilitation over time; use a multidisciplinary approach.
- Be aware that there are fluctuations in orientation and memory and that these patients are easily distracted.
- Do not push to a level greater than patient's impaired cortical functioning allows because fatigue, anger, and stress (headache, dizziness) may occur; the Rancho Los Amigos Levels of Cognitive Function scale is frequently used to assess cognitive function and evaluate ongoing recovery from head injury.

Preventing Sleep Pattern Disturbance
- Group nursing activities so that patient is disturbed less frequently.
- Decrease environmental noise and dim room lights.
- Provide strategies (e.g., back rubs) to increase comfort.

Supporting Family Coping
- Provide family with accurate and honest information.
- Encourage family to continue to set well-defined, mutual, short-term goals.
- Encourage family counseling to deal with feelings of loss and helplessness and provide guidance in the management of inappropriate behaviors.

- Refer family to support groups that provide a forum for networking, sharing problems, and gaining assistance in maintaining realistic expectations and hope. The Brain Injury Association provides information and other resources.
- Assist patient and family in making decisions to end life support and permit donation of organs.

MONITORING AND MANAGING POTENTIAL COMPLICATIONS
- Take measures to control CPP (e.g., elevate the head of the bed and increase IV fluids).
- Take measures to control ICP (see section on "Increased Intracranial Pressure" in Section I).
- Monitor for a patent airway, altered breathing pattern, and hypoxemia and pneumonia. Assist with intubation and mechanical ventilation.
- Provide enteral feedings, IV fluids and electrolytes, or insulin as prescribed.
- Initiate PN as ordered if patient is unable to eat.
- Assess carefully for development of posttraumatic seizures.

PROMOTING HOME- AND COMMUNITY-BASED CARE
Educating Patients About Self-Care
- Reinforce information provided to the family about patient's condition and prognosis early in the course of head injury.
- As patient's status changes over time, focus educational plans on interpretation and explanation of changes in patient's responses.
- Instruct patient and family about limitations that can be expected and complications that may occur if patient is to be discharged.
- Explain to the patient and family, verbally and in writing, how to monitor for complications that merit contacting the neurosurgeon.
- Educate about self-care management strategies, if patient's status indicates.
- Educate about side effects of medications and importance of taking medications as prescribed.

Continuing Care
- Encourage patient to continue rehabilitation program after discharge. Improvement may take 3 or more years after injury, during which time the family and their coping skills need frequent assessment.
- Encourage patient to return to normal activities gradually.

- Remind the patient and family of the need for continuing health promotion and screening practices after the initial phase of care.

Evaluation

EXPECTED PATIENT OUTCOMES

- Attains or maintains effective airway clearance, ventilation, and brain oxygenation
- Achieves satisfactory fluid and electrolyte balance
- Attains adequate nutritional status
- Avoids injury
- Maintains normal body temperature
- Demonstrates intact skin integrity
- Shows improvement in cognitive function and improved memory
- Demonstrates normal sleep/wake cycle
- Demonstrates absence of complications
- Experiences no post-traumatic seizures
- Adaptive coping processes demonstrated by family
- Participates with family in rehabilitation process as indicated

For more information, see Chapter 68 in Hinkle, J. L., & Cheever, K. H. (2014). *Brunner and Suddarth's textbook of medical-surgical nursing* (13th ed.). Philadelphia: Lippincott Williams & Wilkins.

Headache

Headache (cephalgia) is one of the most common of all human physical complaints. Headache is actually a symptom rather than a disease entity and may indicate organic disease (neurologic), a stress response, vasodilation (migraine), skeletal muscle tension (tension headache), or a combination of these factors. A primary headache is one for which no organic cause can be identified. These types of headache include migraine, tension-type, and cluster. A secondary headache is a symptom associated with organic causes, such as a brain tumor or aneurysm, subarachnoid hemorrhage, stroke, severe hypertension, meningitis, and head injury.

Pathophysiology

A migraine headache is a complex of symptoms characterized by periodic and recurrent attacks of severe headache. The cerebral signs and symptoms of migraine result from a hyperexcitable brain that is susceptible to a phenomenon known as *cortical spreading depression* (CSD). CSD can be described as a wave of depolarization over the cerebral cortex, cerebellum, and hippocampus; vascular changes, inflammation, and a continuation of pain signal stimulation occur. The cause of migraine has not been clearly demonstrated, but it is primarily a vascular disturbance that occurs more commonly in women and has strong familial tendencies. Onset typically occurs in puberty, and the incidence is 18% in women and 6% in men. Migraines are often hereditary and associated with low brain magnesium levels. Attacks can be triggered by hormonal changes associated with menstrual cycles, bright lights, stress, depression, sleep deprivation, fatigue, and certain foods (e.g., those containing tyramine, monosodium glutamate, nitrites, milk products, or aged cheeses) or odors. Use of oral contraceptives may be associated with increased frequency and severity of migraine attacks in some women.

Emotional or physical stress may cause contraction of the muscles in the neck and scalp, resulting in tension headache. The pathophysiology of cluster headache is not fully understood; one theory is that it is caused by dilation of orbital and nearby extracranial arteries. Cranial arteritis is thought to represent an immune vasculitis, in which immune complexes are deposited within the walls of affected blood vessels, producing vascular injury and inflammation.

Clinical Manifestations

Migraines
The classic migraine attack with aura can be divided into four phases: prodrome, aura, headache, and recovery.

Prodrome Phase
- Prodrome phase is present in 60% of patients with migraine headache.
- Symptoms may occur consistently hours to days before onset of migraine.
- Depression, irritability, feeling cold, food cravings, anorexia, change in activity level, increased urination, diarrhea, or constipation may be noted with each migraine.
- Prodrome is usually the same for each patient with each migraine headache.

Aura Phase
- Occurs in a minority of patients and lasts less than 1 hour

- Focal neurologic symptoms (predominantly visual disturbances such as light flashes and bright spots); may be hemi-
  anopic (loss of vision occurring in half of the visual field)
- Numbness and tingling of lips, face, or hands; mild confusion; slight weakness of an extremity; or drowsiness and dizziness possible

Headache Phase

- Headache itself involves throbbing, is unilateral in 60% of
  patients, and intensifies over several hours.
- Pain is severe and incapacitating, often associated with photophobia, nausea, and vomiting.
- Duration varies from about 4 to 72 hours.

Recovery Phase (Termination and Postdrome)

- Pain gradually subsides.
- Muscle contraction in the neck and scalp are common
  and associated with muscle ache and localized tenderness,
  exhaustion, and mood changes.
- Any physical exertion exacerbates the headache pain.
- Patient may sleep for an extended period.

Other Headache Types

Tension-Type Headaches

Tension-type headache is characterized by a steady, constant feeling of pressure that usually begins in the forehead,
temple, or back of the neck. It is often described as bandlike or
"a weight on top of my head."

Cluster Headaches

- Severe form of vascular headache, seen mostly in men
- Unilateral and come in clusters of one to eight daily
- Excruciating pain localized to the eye and orbit and radiating
  to the facial and temporal regions; also involves watering of
  the eye and nasal congestion
- Duration of 15 minutes to 3 hours and may have a crescendo–
  decrescendo pattern; described as penetrating

Cranial Arteritis

- Inflammation of the cranial arteries is characterized by a
  severe headache localized in the temporal artery region;
  inflammation may be generalized or focal.
- Older adults, particularly those over age 70, are affected.
- Onset often is marked by general manifestations, such as
  fatigue, malaise, weight loss, and fever.

- Clinical manifestations associated with inflammation (heat, redness, swelling, tenderness, or pain over the involved artery) usually are present.
- A tender, swollen, or nodular temporal artery is visible.
- Vision problems are caused by ischemia of the involved structures.

Assessment and Diagnostic Findings

- Detailed health and headache assessment and history; medication history (including over-the-counter preparations and supplements); family history
- Assessment of any psychosocial factors or occupational exposure hazards that may precipitate headaches
- Physical assessment of head and neck
- Neurologic examination
- Cerebral angiography, CT or MRI if abnormalities are present on neurologic examination
- Electromyography (EMG) and laboratory tests (complete blood cell [CBC] count, electrolytes, glucose, creatinine, erythrocyte sedimentation rate, electrolytes, glucose, and thyroid hormone levels)

Medical Management

Therapy is divided into preventive and abortive (symptomatic) approaches. A preventive approach is used for those who have frequent attacks at regular or predictable intervals and may have medical conditions that preclude abortive therapies. Abortive approach is used for frequent attacks and is aimed at relieving or limiting a headache at the onset or while in progress.

Prevention

Prevention begins by helping the patient identify triggers known to initiate headaches and discussing strategies to avoid exposure to such triggers (e.g., alcohol, nitrites, vasodilators, and histamines). Elimination of these triggers helps prevent the headaches. For some, preventive medical management of migraine involves the daily use of one or more agents that are thought to block the physiologic events leading to an attack.

Pharmacologic Therapy

- Daily use of medications is thought to block the headache attack.

- Medications used to prevent migraine include antiepileptics (divalproex sodium, valproate [Depakote], topiramate [Topamax]), beta-blockers (metoprolol [Lopressor], propranolol [Inderal], timolol [Blocadren]), and triptans (frovatriptan [Frova]).
- Other medications that are prescribed for migraine prevention include antidepressive agents (amitriptyline [Elavil], venlafaxine [Effexor]) and additional beta-blockers (atenolol [Tenormin], nadolol [Corgard]) and triptans (naratriptan [Amerge], zolmitriptan [Zomig]).

Management of Acute Attack

Treatment varies greatly; close monitoring is indicated.

- Triptans (considered first-line therapy for moderate to severe migraine pain): sumatriptan (Imitrex), naratriptan (Amerge), rizatriptan (Maxalt), zolmitriptan (Zomig), and almotriptan (Axert). Triptan nasal sprays are useful for patients experiencing nausea and vomiting.
- Ergotamine preparations may be effective if taken early. Ergotamine preparations may be taken by mouth (*per os* [PO]), by subcutaneous (SC) or intramuscular (IM) injections, sublingually, or rectally, or they may be inhaled. Cafergot is a combination of ergotamine and caffeine.

> ▶ *Quality and Safety Nursing Alert*
>
> None of the triptan medications should be taken concurrently with medications containing ergotamine, because of the potential for a prolonged vasoactive reaction.

- For some patients, giving 100% oxygen by facemask for 15 minutes is effective.
- Symptomatic therapy includes analgesic, sedative, antianxiety, and antiemetic agents.

Nursing Management

Enhancing Pain Relief

- Individualized treatment depends on the type of headache.
- Attempt to abort migraine headache early.
- Provide comfort measures (e.g., a quiet, dark environment and elevating the head of bed 30 degrees) and symptomatic treatment (e.g., administration of antiemetic medication).

- Symptomatic pain relief for tension headache may be obtained by application of local heat or massage, analgesic agents, antidepressant medications, and muscle relaxants.
- Administer medications if nonpharmacologic measures are ineffective.

Promoting Home- and Community-Based Care

Educating Patients About Self-Care

- Educate patient about the type of headache and its mechanism (if known).
- Educational plans should include identifying and avoiding precipitating factors, implementing possible lifestyle or habit changes that may be helpful, and pharmacologic measures.
- Inform patient that regular sleep, meals, exercise, relaxation, and avoiding dietary triggers may be helpful in preventing headaches.
- Instruct and reassure the patient with tension headaches that the headache is not the result of a brain tumor (common unspoken fear).
- Stress reduction techniques, such as biofeedback, exercise programs, and meditation, may prove helpful.
- Remind patient about the importance of following the prescribed treatment regimen, keeping follow-up appointments, and participating in health promotion activities and recommended health screenings.

Continuing Care

The National Headache Foundation provides a list of clinics in the United States and the names of physicians who are members of the American Association for the Study of Headaches.

For more information, see Chapter 66 in Hinkle, J. L., & Cheever, K. H. (2014). *Brunner and Suddarth's textbook of medical-surgical nursing* (13th ed.). Philadelphia: Lippincott Williams & Wilkins.

Heart Failure

Heart failure (HF), sometimes referred to as *congestive HF*, results from structural or functional cardiac disorders that impair the ability of the ventricles to fill or eject blood. HF is a clinical syndrome characterized by signs and symptoms of fluid overload or inadequate tissue perfusion. The underlying mechanism of HF involves impaired contractile properties of the heart (systolic dysfunction) or filling of the heart (diastolic dysfunction), which leads to a lower than normal cardiac output. The low cardiac output can lead to compensatory mechanisms that cause increased workload on the heart and eventual resistance to the filling of the heart.

HF is a progressive, lifelong condition that is managed with lifestyle changes and medications, designed to prevent episodes of acute decompensated HF. These episodes are characterized by an increase in symptoms, decreased cardiac output (CO), and low perfusion. HF results from a variety of cardiovascular conditions, including chronic hypertension, coronary artery disease, and valvular disease. These conditions can result in systolic failure, diastolic failure, or both. Several systemic conditions (e.g., progressive renal failure and uncontrolled hypertension) can contribute to the development and severity of cardiac failure.

Clinical Manifestations
The signs and symptoms of HF can be related to the ventricle that is affected. *Left-sided HF* (left ventricular failure) causes different manifestations than *right-sided HF* (right ventricular failure). In chronic HF, patients may have signs and symptoms of both left and right ventricular failure.

Left-Sided HF
- Most often precedes right-sided cardiac failure
- Pulmonary congestion: dyspnea, cough, pulmonary crackles, and low oxygen saturation levels; an extra heart sound, the S_3, or "ventricular gallop," possibly detected on auscultation
- Dyspnea on exertion (DOE), orthopnea, paroxysmal nocturnal dyspnea (PND)
- Cough, initially dry and nonproductive; may become moist over time
- Large quantities of frothy sputum, which is sometimes pink (blood-tinged)
- Bibasilar crackles advancing to crackles in all lung fields
- Inadequate tissue perfusion
- Oliguria and nocturia
- With progression of HF: altered digestion; dizziness, lightheadedness, confusion, restlessness, and anxiety; skin that is pale or ashen and cool and clammy
- Tachycardia; weak, thready pulse; fatigue

Right-Sided HF

- Congestion of the viscera and peripheral tissues
- Edema of the lower extremities (dependent edema), hepatomegaly (enlargement of the liver), ascites (accumulation of fluid in the peritoneal cavity), anorexia and nausea, and weakness and weight gain due to fluid retention

Assessment and Diagnostic Findings

- Signs and symptoms of pulmonary and peripheral edema
- Assessment of ventricular function
- Echocardiogram, chest x-ray, electrocardiogram (ECG)
- Laboratory studies: serum electrolytes, blood urea nitrogen (BUN), creatinine, thyroid-stimulating hormone (TSH), complete blood cell count (CBC), brain natriuretic peptide (BNP), and routine urinalysis
- Cardiac stress testing, cardiac catheterization

Medical Management

The overall goals of management of HF are to relieve patient symptoms, to improve functional status and quality of life, and to extend survival. Treatment options vary according to the severity of the patient's condition and may include oral and IV medications, major lifestyle changes, supplemental oxygen, implantation of assistive devices, and surgical approaches (including cardiac transplantation). Lifestyle recommendations include restriction of dietary sodium; avoidance of excessive fluid intake, alcohol, and smoking; weight reduction when indicated; and regular exercise.

Pharmacologic Therapy

- Alone or in combination: vasodilator therapy (angiotensin-converting enzyme [ACE] inhibitors), angiotensin II receptor blockers (ARBs), select beta-blockers, calcium channel blockers, diuretic therapy, cardiac glycosides (digitalis), and others
- IV infusions: nesiritide, milrinone, dobutamine
- Medications for diastolic dysfunction
- Possibly anticoagulants, medications that manage hyperlipidemia (statins)

Surgical Management

HF may be managed with coronary bypass surgery, percutaneous transluminal coronary angioplasty (PTCA), or other innovative therapies as indicated (e.g., mechanical assistance devices, transplantation).

NURSING PROCESS

The Patient With HF

Assessment

The nursing assessment for the patient with HF focuses on observing for effectiveness of therapy and for the patient's ability to understand and implement self-management strategies. Signs and symptoms of pulmonary and systemic fluid overload are recorded and reported immediately.

- Note sleep disturbances due to shortness of breath, and number of pillows used for sleep.
- Ask patient about edema, abdominal symptoms, altered mental status, activities of daily living, and the activities that cause fatigue.
- Respiratory: Auscultate lungs to detect crackles and wheezes. Note rate and depth of respirations.
- Cardiac: Auscultate for S_3 heart sound (sign of heart beginning to fail); document heart rate and rhythm.
- Assess sensorium and level of consciousness (LOC).
- Periphery: Assess dependent parts of body for perfusion and edema; assess the liver for hepatojugular reflux; assess jugular venous distention.
- Measure intake and output to detect oliguria or anuria; weigh patient daily.

Diagnosis

NURSING DIAGNOSES

- Activity intolerance and fatigue related to decreased CO
- Excess fluid volume related to the HF syndrome
- Anxiety related to breathlessness from inadequate oxygenation
- Powerlessness related to chronic illness and hospitalizations
- Ineffective therapeutic regimen management related to lack of knowledge

COLLABORATIVE PROBLEMS/POTENTIAL COMPLICATIONS

- Hypotension, poor perfusion, and cardiogenic shock
- Dysrhythmias
- Thromboembolism
- Pericardial effusion and cardiac tamponade

Planning and Goals

Major goals for the patient may include promoting activity and reducing fatigue; relieving fluid overload symptoms; decreasing anxiety or increasing the patient's ability to manage anxiety; encouraging the patient to verbalize his or her ability to make decisions and influence outcomes; and educating the patient about the self-care program.

Nursing Interventions

PROMOTING ACTIVITY TOLERANCE

- Monitor patient's response to activities. Instruct patient to avoid prolonged bed rest; patient should rest if symptoms are severe but otherwise should assume regular activity.
- Encourage patient to perform an activity more slowly than usual, for a shorter duration, or with assistance initially.
- Identify barriers that could limit patient's ability to perform an activity, and discuss methods of pacing an activity (e.g., chop or peel vegetables while sitting at the kitchen table rather than standing at the kitchen counter).
- Take vital signs, especially pulse, before, during, and immediately after an activity to identify whether these are within the predetermined range; heart rate should return to baseline within 3 minutes. If patient tolerates the activity, develop short-term and long-term goals to gradually increase the intensity, duration, or frequency of activity.
- Refer to a cardiac rehabilitation program as needed, especially for patients with a recent myocardial infarction, recent open heart surgery, or increased anxiety.

REDUCING FATIGUE

- Collaborate with patient to develop a schedule that promotes pacing and prioritization of activities. Encourage patient to alternate activities with periods of rest and avoid having two significant energy-consuming activities occur on the same day or in immediate succession.
- Explain that small, frequent meals tend to decrease the amount of energy needed for digestion while still providing adequate nutrition.
- Help patient develop a positive outlook focused on strengths, abilities, and interests.

MANAGING FLUID VOLUME

- Administer diuretics early in the morning so that diuresis does not disturb nighttime rest.

- Monitor fluid status closely: Auscultate lungs, compare daily body weights, and monitor intake and output.
- Educate patient to adhere to a low-sodium diet by reading food labels and avoiding commercially prepared convenience foods.
- Assist patient to adhere to any fluid restriction by planning the fluid distribution throughout the day, while maintaining dietary preferences.
- Monitor IV fluids closely; contact physician or pharmacist about the possibility of double-concentrating any medications.
- Place patient in a position that facilitates breathing (increase number of pillows, elevate the head of bed), or educate patient on how to assume such position; alternatively, patient may prefer to sit in a comfortable armchair to sleep.
- Assess for skin breakdown, and institute preventive measures (frequent changes of position, positioning to avoid pressure, leg exercises).

CONTROLLING ANXIETY
- Decrease anxiety so that patient's cardiac work is also decreased.
- Administer oxygen during the acute stage to diminish the work of breathing and to increase comfort.
- When patient exhibits anxiety, promote physical comfort and psychological support; a family member's presence may provide reassurance; pet visitation or animal-assisted therapy can also be beneficial.
- When patient is comfortable, teach ways to control anxiety and avoid anxiety-provoking situations (relaxation techniques).
- Assist in identifying factors that contribute to anxiety.
- Screen for depression, which often accompanies or results from anxiety.

> *Quality and Safety Nursing Alert*

In cases of confusion and anxious reactions that affect the patient's safety, the use of restraints should be avoided. Restraints are likely to be resisted, and resistance inevitably increases the cardiac workload.

MINIMIZING POWERLESSNESS

- Assess for factors contributing to a sense of powerlessness and intervene accordingly.
- Listen actively to patient; encourage patient to express concerns and questions.
- Provide patient with decision-making opportunities with increasing frequency and significance; provide encouragement and praise while identifying patient's progress; assist patient to differentiate between factors that can be controlled and those that cannot.

MONITORING AND MANAGING POTENTIAL COMPLICATIONS

Many potential problems associated with HF therapy relate to the use of diuretics:

- Monitor for hypokalemia caused by diuresis (potassium depletion). Signs are ventricular dysrhythmias, hypotension, muscle weakness, and generalized weakness.
- Monitor for hyperkalemia, especially with the use of ACE inhibitors, ARBs, or spironolactone.
- Hyponatremia (deficiency of sodium in the blood) can occur, which results in disorientation, apprehension, weakness, fatigue, malaise, and muscle cramps.
- Volume depletion from excessive fluid loss may lead to dehydration and hypotension (ACE inhibitors and beta-blockers may contribute to the hypotension).
- Other problems associated with diuretics include increased serum creatinine and hyperuricemia (excessive uric acid in the blood), which leads to gout.

PROMOTING HOME- AND COMMUNITY-BASED CARE

Educating Patients About Self-Care

- Provide patient education and involve patient in implementing the therapeutic regimen to promote understanding and compliance.
- Support patient and family and encourage them to ask questions so that information can be clarified.
- Adapt teaching plan according to cultural factors.
- Educate patients and family on how progression of the disease is influenced by compliance with the treatment plan.

Continuing Care

- Refer patient for home care if indicated (elderly patients or patients who have long-standing heart disease and whose physical stamina is compromised). The home care nurse assesses the physical environment of the home and the patient's support system, and then suggests adaptations in the home to meet patient's activity limitations.

- Reinforce and clarify information about dietary changes and fluid restrictions, the need to monitor symptoms and daily body weights, and the importance of obtaining follow-up health care.
- Encourage patient to increase self-care and responsibility for accomplishing the daily requirements of the therapeutic regimen.
- Refer patient to an HF clinic if necessary.

Evaluation

EXPECTED PATIENT OUTCOMES

- Demonstrates tolerance for desired activity
- Maintains fluid balance
- Experiences decrease in anxiety
- Makes sound decisions regarding care and treatment
- Adheres to self-care regimen

For more information, see Chapter 29 in Hinkle, J. L., & Cheever, K. H. (2014). *Brunner and Suddarth's textbook of medical-surgical nursing* (13th ed.). Philadelphia: Lippincott Williams & Wilkins.

Hemophilia

Hemophilia is a relatively rare disease. Two inherited bleeding disorders—hemophilia A and hemophilia B—are clinically indistinguishable but can be separated by laboratory tests:. Hemophilia A is due to a genetic defect that results in deficient or defective factor VIII. Hemophilia B (also called *Christmas disease*) stems from a genetic defect that causes deficient or defective factor IX. Hemophilia A is more common; it occurs about four times more often than hemophilia B. Both types are inherited as X-linked traits, so almost all affected people are males; females can be carriers but are almost always asymptomatic. All ethnic groups are affected. The disease is usually recognized in early childhood, usually in toddlers. Mild hemophilia may not be diagnosed until trauma or surgery.

Clinical Manifestations

The frequency and severity of bleeding depend on the degree of factor deficiency and the intensity of trauma.

- Hemorrhage occurs into various body parts (large, spreading bruises and bleeding into muscles, joints, and soft tissues) after even minimal trauma.
- Most bleeding occurs in joints (most often in knees, elbows, ankles, shoulders, wrists, and hips); pain in joints may occur before swelling and limitation of motion are apparent.
- Chronic pain, ankylosis (fixation), or arthropathy of the joint may occur with recurrent hemorrhage; many patients are crippled by joint damage before adulthood.
- Spontaneous hematuria and gastrointestinal bleeding can occur. Hematomas within the muscle can cause peripheral nerve compression with decreased sensation, weakness, and atrophy of the area.
- Bleeding may also occur in the muscles, mucous membranes, and soft tissue.
- The most dangerous site of hemorrhage is in the head (intracranial or extracranial); any head trauma requires prompt evaluation and treatment.
- Surgical procedures typically result in excessive bleeding at the surgical site; bleeding is most commonly associated with dental extraction. Wound healing is also impaired.

Assessment and Diagnostic Findings

Laboratory tests include clotting factor measurement and complete blood cell (CBC) count.

Medical Management

- Recombinant forms of factors VIII and IX concentrates are available and decrease the need for using factor concentrates. These are given when active bleeding occurs or as a preventive measure before traumatic procedures (e.g., lumbar puncture, dental extraction, surgery).
- Plasmapheresis or concurrent immunosuppressive therapy may be required for patients who develop antibodies (inhibitors) to factor concentrates.
- Aminocaproic acid inhibits fibrinolysis and may slow the dissolution of blood clots; desmopressin acetate (DDAVP) induces transient increase in factor VIII.

- Desmopressin is useful for patients with mild forms of hemophilia A; however, it is not effective in severe factor VIII deficiency.

Nursing Management

- Assist family and patient in coping with the condition because it is chronic, places restrictions on their lives, and is an inherited disorder that can be passed to future generations.
- From childhood, help patients to cope with the disease and to identify the positive aspects of their lives.
- Encourage patients to be self-sufficient and to maintain independence by preventing unnecessary trauma.
- Patients with mild factor deficiency that were not diagnosed until adulthood need extensive education about activity restrictions and self-care measures to diminish the chance of hemorrhage and complications of bleeding; emphasize safety at home and in the workplace.
- Instruct patients to avoid any agents that interfere with platelet aggregation, such as aspirin, nonsteroidal anti-inflammatory drugs (NSAIDs), some herbal and nutritional supplements (e.g., chamomile, nettle, alfalfa), and alcohol. (Also applies to over-the-counter medications such as cold remedies.)
- Instruct patients and family members in ways to administer factor concentrates at home at the first sign of bleeding; prophylactic use can be effective in reducing morbidity associated with repeat bleeding.
- Promote good dental hygiene as a preventive measure because dental extractions are hazardous.
- Instruct patient that applying pressure to a minor wound may be sufficient to control bleeding if the factor deficiency is not severe; avoid nasal packing.
- Splints and other orthopedic devices may be useful in patients with joint or muscle hemorrhages.
- Avoid all injections; minimize invasive procedures (e.g., endoscopy, lumbar puncture) or perform after administration of appropriate factor replacement.
- Carefully assess bleeding during hemorrhagic episodes; patients at risk for significant compromise (e.g., bleeding into the respiratory tract or brain) warrant close observation and systematic assessment for emergent complications (e.g., respiratory distress, altered level of consciousness).

- If patient has had recent surgery, frequently and carefully assess the surgical site for bleeding; frequent monitoring of vital signs is needed until the nurse is certain that there is no excessive postoperative bleeding.
- Administer analgesics as required; allow warm baths but avoid during bleeding episodes.
- Patients who have been exposed to infections (e.g., HIV infection, hepatitis) through previous transfusions may need assistance in coping with the diagnosis and consequences.
- Recommend genetic testing and counseling to female carriers so that they can make informed decisions regarding having children and managing pregnancy.
- Encourage patients to carry or wear medical identification (e.g., MedicAlert bracelets). Patients and their families should have a written emergency plan including what to do in specific situations as well as important contact information in case of an emergency.

Gerontologic Considerations

The older adult patient with hemophilia was likely managed with blood component transfusion, at least early in life. Thus, hepatitis B and C infection are very common in this population, particularly hepatitis C; HIV is also common. Patients with HIV or hepatitis C are at increased risk for liver disease, which can be fatal. Intracranial hemorrhage is the third most common cause of death after HIV and hepatitis and may not result from trauma. The major cause of morbidity in these patients is joint disease; arthropathy is often common in four or more joints. Pain management can be challenging as the use of NSAIDs is contraindicated due to the increased risk of bleeding. The likelihood of acquiring inhibitors, especially hemophilia A inhibitors, increases with increasing age. Therefore, these patients are at increased risk not only of bleeding but also of thrombosis. Though patients with hemophilia less commonly have concomitant cardiovascular disease, it is difficult to manage when it is present because both medical and surgical treatments for cardiovascular disease increase risk of bleeding; coordination of care with a hematologist can improve outcomes.

For more information, see Chapter 33 in Hinkle, J. L., & Cheever, K. H. (2014). *Brunner and Suddarth's textbook of medical-surgical nursing* (13th ed.). Philadelphia: Lippincott Williams & Wilkins.

Hepatic Encephalopathy and Hepatic Coma

Hepatic encephalopathy, or portosystemic encephalopathy (PSE), is a life-threatening complication of liver disease that occurs with profound liver failure. Ammonia is considered the major etiologic factor in the development of encephalopathy. Patients have no overt signs but do have abnormalities on neuropsychologic testing. Hepatic encephalopathy is the neuropsychiatric manifestation of hepatic failure associated with portal hypertension and the shunting of blood from the portal venous system into the systemic circulation. Circumstances that increase serum ammonia levels precipitate or aggravate hepatic encephalopathy, such as digestion of dietary and blood proteins and ingestion of ammonium salts. Other factors that may cause hepatic encephalopathy include excessive diuresis, dehydration, infections, fever, surgery, some medications and, additionally, elevated levels of serum manganese and changes in the types of circulating amino acids, mercaptans, and levels of dopamine and gamma-aminobutyric acid (GABA) neurotransmitters in the central nervous system.

Clinical Manifestations

- Earliest symptoms of hepatic encephalopathy include minor mental changes and motor disturbances. Slight confusion and alterations in mood occur; the patient becomes unkempt, experiences disturbed sleep patterns, and tends to sleep during the day and to experience restlessness and insomnia at night.
- With progression, patient may be difficult to awaken and be completely disoriented with respect to time and place; with further progression, the patient lapses into frank coma and may have seizures.
- Asterixis (flapping tremor of the hands) may be seen in stage II encephalopathy. Simple tasks, such as handwriting, become difficult. Inability to reproduce a simple figure is referred to as *constructional apraxia*.
- In early stages, patient's deep reflexes are hyperactive; with worsening encephalopathy, reflexes disappear, and extremities become flaccid.
- Occasionally fetor hepaticus, a characteristic breath odor like freshly mowed grass, acetone, or old wine, may be noticed.

Assessment and Diagnostic Findings
- Electroencephalogram (EEG) shows generalized slowing, an increase in the amplitude of brain waves, and characteristic triphasic waves.
- Serum ammonia measurements are evaluated.
- Daily handwriting or drawing samples can be assessed if hepatic encephalopathy is suspected; constructional apraxia reveals progression.

Medical Management
- Lactulose (Cephulac) is administered to reduce serum ammonia level. Patient should be observed for watery diarrheal stools, which indicate lactulose overdose, and monitored for hypokalemia and dehydration.
- IV glucose is administered to minimize protein breakdown, and vitamins are administered to correct deficiencies and electrolyte imbalances (especially potassium).
- Antibiotic agents are administered if needed—such as Neomycin, metronidazole (Flagyl), and rifaximin (Xifaxan)—to reduce levels of ammonia-forming bacteria in the colon; no benefit has been shown for long-term treatment with these antibiotic drugs.
- Patients who are comatose or who have encephalopathy that is refractory to lactulose and antibiotic therapy should have their protein intake moderately restricted; enteral feeding is provided for patients whose encephalopathic state persists.
- Medications that may precipitate encephalopathy (e.g., sedative medications, tranquilizers, analgesic agents) should be discontinued.
- Benzodiazepine antagonists (flumazenil) can be administered.

Nursing Management
- Maintain a safe environment to prevent bleeding, injury, and infection.
- Administer the prescribed treatments and monitor the patient for the numerous potential complications.
- Assess neurologic and mental status.
- Record fluid input and output (I&O) and body weight daily and vital signs every 4 hours.
- Assess potential sites of infection (peritoneum, lungs); report abnormal findings promptly.
- Monitor serum ammonia level daily.

- Encourage deep breathing and position changes to prevent the development of atelectasis, pneumonia, and other respiratory complications.
- Communicate with the patient's family to inform them about the patient's status and support them by explaining the procedures and treatments that are part of the patient's care.
- Ask the family to observe patient for subtle signs of recurrent encephalopathy. Explain that rehabilitation after recovery is likely to be prolonged.
- Advise on caloric intake and protein intake: 35 to 40 kcal/kg body weight per day and 1.0 to 1.5 g/kg body weight per day.
- Educate patient about ways to administer lactulose and monitor for side effects.
- Refer patient for home care nurse visits to assess home environment to identify risk of falls and other injuries.
- Reinforce previous education and remind the patient and family about the importance of dietary restrictions, close monitoring, and follow-up.
- Assess patient's physical and mental status and compliance with prescribed therapeutic regimen.
- Refer to psychologists, psychiatric liaison nurses, case managers, social workers, spiritual advisor, or therapists to assist family members with coping. Provide support and education if alcohol played a role in the liver disease and refer to Alcoholics Anonymous or Al-Anon.

For more information, see Chapter 49 in Hinkle, J. L., & Cheever, K. H. (2014). *Brunner and Suddarth's textbook of medical-surgical nursing* (13th ed.). Philadelphia: Lippincott Williams & Wilkins.

Hepatic Failure, Fulminant

Fulminant hepatic failure is the clinical syndrome of sudden and severely impaired liver function in a previously healthy person. Fulminant hepatic failure develops within 8 weeks after the first symptoms of jaundice with patterns of the progression to encephalopathy of time-based classifications. Three categories are frequently cited: hyperacute (0 to 7 days), acute (8 to 28 days), and subacute (28 to 72 days). The hepatic lesion is potentially reversible, and survival rates are approximately 20% to 50%, depending greatly on the cause of liver failure. Those who do not survive die of massive hepatocellular injury and necrosis. Viral hepatitis is a common cause; other causes include toxic medications and chemicals, metabolic disturbances, and structural changes.

Clinical Manifestations
- Jaundice and profound anorexia
- Often accompanied by coagulation defects, renal failure and electrolyte disturbances, cardiovascular abnormalities, infection, hypoglycemia, encephalopathy, and cerebral edema

Medical Management
- Liver transplantation is the treatment of choice.
- Liver support systems, such as hepatocytes within synthetic fiber columns, extracorporeal liver assist devices, and bio-artificial liver, may be used until transplantation is possible.
- The use of antidotes for certain conditions may be indicated—such as N-acetylcysteine for acetaminophen toxicity and penicillin for mushroom poisoning.
- Blood or plasma exchanges (plasmapheresis) and prostaglandin therapy may be indicated.

Nursing Management
- Monitor intracranial pressure, fluid balance, and hemodynamic assessments; provide a quiet environment.
- Administer mannitol (Osmitrol), an osmotic diuretic agent, as directed; a barbiturate anesthesia or pharmacologic paralysis and sedation may be required.
- Monitor for and treat hypoglycemia, coagulopathies, and infection.

For more information, see Chapter 49 in Hinkle, J. L., & Cheever, K. H. (2014). *Brunner and Suddarth's textbook of medical-surgical nursing* (13th ed.). Philadelphia: Lippincott Williams & Wilkins.

Hepatitis, Viral: Types A, B, C, D, E, and G

Hepatitis A Virus
Hepatitis A (HAV) is caused by an RNA virus of the enterovirus family. This form of hepatitis is transmitted primarily through the fecal–oral route, by the ingestion of food or liquids infected by the virus. The virus is found in the stool of infected patients before the onset of symptoms and during the first few

days of illness. The incubation period is estimated to be 2 to 6 weeks, with a mean of approximately 4 weeks. The course of illness may last 4 to 8 weeks. The virus is present only briefly in the serum; by the time jaundice appears, the patient is likely to be noninfectious. A person who is immune to hepatitis A may contract other forms of hepatitis. Recovery from hepatitis A is usual; it rarely progresses to acute liver necrosis and fulminant hepatitis. No carrier state exists, and no chronic hepatitis is associated with hepatitis A.

Clinical Manifestations
- Many patients are anicteric (without jaundice) and symptomless.
- When symptoms appear, they are those of a mild, flulike, upper respiratory infection with low-grade fever.
- Anorexia is an early symptom and is often severe.
- Later, jaundice and dark urine may be apparent.
- Indigestion is present in varying degrees, marked by vague epigastric distress, nausea, heartburn, and flatulence.
- Liver and spleen are often moderately enlarged for a few days after onset.
- Patient may have a strong aversion to cigarette smoke and strong odors; symptoms tend to clear when jaundice reaches its peak.
- Symptoms may be mild in children; in adults, they may be more severe and the course of the disease prolonged.

Assessment and Diagnostic Findings
- Stool analysis for hepatitis A antigen
- Serum hepatitis A virus antibodies; immunoglobulin

Prevention
- Scrupulous hand washing, safe water supply, proper control of sewage disposal
- Hepatitis vaccine
- Administration of immune globulin, if not previously vaccinated, to prevent hepatitis A (if given within 2 weeks of exposure)
- Immune globulin vaccination recommended for household members and for those in sexual contact with people with hepatitis A
- Pre-exposure prophylaxis recommended for those traveling to developing countries, for travelers to settings with poor or uncertain sanitation conditions, or for those with insufficient

time to acquire protection by administration of hepatitis A vaccine

Nursing Management
- Encourage a nutritious diet, as well as bed rest during the acute stage.
- Provide small, frequent feedings supplemented by IV glucose if necessary during period of anorexia.
- Promote gradual but progressive ambulation to hasten recovery. Patient is usually managed at home unless symptoms are severe.
- Assist patient and family to cope with temporary disability and fatigue, both common problems associated with hepatitis.
- Educate patient and family about seeking additional health care if the symptoms persist or worsen.
- Instruct patient and family regarding diet, rest, follow-up blood work, avoidance of alcohol, and sanitation and hygiene measures (hand washing) to prevent spread of disease.
- Educate patient and family about reducing risk for contracting hepatitis A: good personal hygiene with careful hand washing; environmental sanitation with safe food and water supply and sewage disposal.

Hepatitis B Virus
Hepatitis B virus (HBV) is a DNA virus transmitted primarily through blood (percutaneous and permucosal routes), semen, and vaginal secretions. It can be transmitted through mucous membranes and breaks in the skin. Hepatitis B has a long incubation period (1 to 6 months). It replicates in the liver and remains in the serum for long periods, allowing transmission of the virus. Those at risk include all health care workers, patients in hemodialysis and oncology units, sexually active homosexual and bisexual men, and IV drug users. About 10% of patients progress to a carrier state or develop chronic hepatitis. Hepatitis B remains a major worldwide cause of cirrhosis and hepatocellular carcinoma.

Gerontologic Considerations
The immune system is altered in older adults, which may be responsible for the increased incidence and severity of hepatitis B among this demographic and the increased incidence of liver abscesses secondary to decreased phagocytosis by the Kupffer cells. The older patient with hepatitis B has a serious risk of severe liver cell necrosis or fulminant hepatic failure, particularly if other illnesses are present.

Clinical Manifestations

- Symptoms may be insidious and variable; subclinical episodes frequently occur, but fever and respiratory symptoms are rare; some patients have arthralgias and rashes.
- Loss of appetite, dyspepsia, abdominal pain, general aching, malaise, and weakness may occur.
- Jaundice may or may not be evident. With jaundice, there are light-colored stools and dark urine.
- Liver may be tender and enlarged; spleen is enlarged and palpable in a few patients. Posterior cervical lymph nodes may also be enlarged.

Assessment and Diagnostic Findings

HBV is a DNA virus composed of the following antigenic particles:

- HBcAg—hepatitis B core antigen (antigenic material in an inner core)
- HBsAg—hepatitis B surface antigen (antigenic material on the viral surface, a marker of active replication and infection)
- HBeAg—an independent protein circulating in the blood
- HBxAg—gene product of X gene of HBV DNA

Each antigen elicits its specific antibody and is a marker for different stages of the disease process:

- anti-HBc—antibody to core antigen of HBV; persists during the acute phase of illness; may indicate continuing HBV in the liver
- anti-HBs—antibody to surface determinants on HBV; detected during late convalescence; usually indicates recovery and development of immunity
- anti-HBe—antibody to hepatitis B e-antigen; usually signifies reduced infectivity
- anti-HBxAg—antibody to the hepatitis B x-antigen; may indicate ongoing replication of HBV

HepBsAg appears in the blood of up to 80% to 90% of patients. Additional antigens help to confirm the diagnosis.

Prevention

- Screening of blood donors
- Use of disposable syringes, needles, and lancets; introduction of needleless IV administration systems

- Glove wearing when handling all blood and body fluids
- Good personal hygiene
- Education
- Hepatitis B vaccine

Medical Management
- Alpha-interferon has shown promising results.
- Lamivudine (Epivir) and adefovir (Hepsera) are useful agents.
- Bed rest and restriction of activities are advisable until hepatic enlargement, elevation of serum bilirubin, and elevation of liver enzymes have disappeared.
- Adequate nutrition should be maintained; restrict proteins when the ability of the liver to metabolize protein byproducts is impaired.
- Administer antacid and antiemetic agents for dyspepsia and general malaise; avoid all medications if patient is vomiting.
- Provide hospitalization and fluid therapy if vomiting persists.

Nursing Management
- Convalescence may be prolonged and recovery may take 3 to 4 months; encourage gradual activity after jaundice is completely clear.
- Identify psychosocial issues and concerns, particularly the effects of separation from family and friends if the patient is hospitalized; if not hospitalized, the patient will be unable to work and must avoid sexual contact.
- Include family in planning, to help reduce their fears and anxieties about the spread of the disease.
- Educate patient and family in home care and convalescence.
- Instruct patient and family that adequate rest and nutrition are essential.
- Inform family and intimate friends about risks of contracting hepatitis B.
- Arrange for family and intimate friends to receive hepatitis B vaccine or hepatitis B immune globulin as prescribed.
- Caution patient to avoid drinking alcohol and eating raw shellfish.
- Educate family that follow-up visits by home care nurses are indicated to assess progress and understanding, reinforce teaching, and answer questions.
- Encourage patient to use strategies to prevent exchange of body fluids, such as abstinence or using condoms.

- Emphasize importance of keeping follow-up appointments and participating in other health promotion activities and recommended health screenings.

Hepatitis C Virus

Blood transfusions and sexual contact once accounted for most cases of hepatitis C in the United States, but today the disease is primarily contracted by parenteral means (sharing contaminated needles, needlesticks or injuries to health care workers). The incubation period is variable and may range from 15 to 160 days. The clinical course of hepatitis C is similar to that of hepatitis B; symptoms are usually mild. A chronic carrier state occurs frequently. There is an increased risk for cirrhosis and liver cancer after contracting hepatitis C. The protease inhibitors telaprevir (Incivek) and boceprevir (Victrelis) are used for the treatment of hepatitis C genotype 1 in combination with peginterferon alpha 2-b (Peg-Intron) and ribavirin. Neither protease inhibitor may be used as monotherapy for the disease. This triple therapy of protease inhibitor, pegintrferon, and ribavirin is recommended as standard treatment for hepatitis C by the American Association for the Study of Liver Diseases.

Hepatitis D Virus

Hepatitis D (delta agent) occurs in some cases of hepatitis B. Because the virus requires hepatitis B surface antigen for its replication, only patients with hepatitis B are at risk. Hepatitis D is common among IV drug users, hemodialysis patients, and recipients of multiple blood transfusions. Sexual contact is an important mode of transmission of hepatitis B and D. Incubation varies between 30 and 150 days. The symptoms are similar to those of hepatitis B, except that patients are more likely to have fulminant hepatitis and progress to chronic active hepatitis and cirrhosis. Treatment is similar to that for other forms of hepatitis. Currently, interferon-alpha is the only licensed drug for the treatment of hepatitis D viral infection. The rate of recurrence is high and the efficacy of interferon is related to the dose and duration of treatment. High-dose, long-duration therapy for at least 1 year is recommended.

Hepatitis E Virus

The hepatitis E virus (HEV) is transmitted by the fecal–oral route, principally through contaminated water and poor sanitation. Incubation is variable and is estimated to range between

15 and 65 days. In general, hepatitis E resembles hepatitis A. It has a self-limited course with an abrupt onset. Jaundice is almost always present. Chronic forms do not develop. The major method of prevention is avoiding contact with the virus through hygiene (hand washing). The effectiveness of immune globulin in protecting against hepatitis E virus is uncertain.

Hepatitis G Virus and GB Virus-C

Hepatitis G virus (HGV) and GB virus-C (GBV-C) are post-transfusion hepatitis viruses with an incubation period of 14 to 145 days. Autoantibodies are absent. The risk factors are similar to those for hepatitis C. There is no clear relationship between HGV/GBV-C infection and progressive liver disease. Persistent infection does occur but does not affect the clinical course.

For more information, see Chapter 49 in Hinkle, J. L., & Cheever, K. H. (2014). *Brunner and Suddarth's textbook of medical-surgical nursing* (13th ed.). Philadelphia: Lippincott Williams & Wilkins.

Hiatal Hernia

In a hiatal (hiatus) hernia, the opening in the diaphragm through which the esophagus passes becomes enlarged, and part of the upper stomach tends to move up into the lower portion of the thorax. There are two types of hernias: sliding and paraesophageal. Sliding, or type I, hiatal hernia occurs when the upper stomach and the gastroesophageal junction are displaced upward and slide in and out of the thorax; this occurs in about 90% of patients with esophageal hiatal hernias. The less frequent paraesophageal hernias are classified by extent of herniation (type II, III, or IV) and occur when all or part of the stomach pushes through the diaphragm beside the esophagus. Hiatal hernia occurs more often in women than men.

Clinical Manifestations

Sliding Hernia
- Heartburn, regurgitation, and dysphagia; at least 50% of patients asymptomatic
- Often implicated in reflux

Paraesophageal Hernia
- Sense of fullness or chest pain occurs after eating or may be asymptomatic.

- Reflux does not usually occur.
- Complications of hemorrhage, obstruction, and strangulation are possible.

Assessment and Diagnostic Findings

Diagnosis is confirmed by x-ray studies, barium swallow, and CT scan.

Medical Management

- Provide frequent, small feedings that easily pass through the esophagus.
- Advise patient not to recline for 1 hour after eating (prevents reflux or hernia movement).
- Elevate the head of bed on 4- to 8-in blocks to prevent hernia from sliding upward.
- Surgery is indicated in about 15% of patients; paraesophageal hernias may require emergency surgery.
- Medical and surgical management of paraesophageal hernias is similar to that for gastroesophageal reflux: antacids, histamine blockers, proton pump inhibitors, or prokinetic agents (metoclopramide [Reglan]).

NURSING PROCESS

The Patient With an Esophageal Condition and Reflux

Assessment

- Complete a comprehensive health history, including pain assessment and nutrition assessment.
- Determine whether patient appears emaciated.
- Auscultate chest to determine presence of pulmonary complications.

Diagnosis

NURSING DIAGNOSES

- Imbalanced nutrition: less than body requirements related to difficulty swallowing
- Risk for aspiration due to difficulty in swallowing or tube feeding
- Acute pain related to difficulty in swallowing, ingestion of abrasive agent, a tumor, or reflux
- Deficient knowledge about the esophageal disorder, diagnostic studies, treatments, and rehabilitation

Planning and Goals

Major goals may include adequate nutritional intake, avoidance of respiratory compromise from aspiration, relief of pain, and increased knowledge level.

Nursing Interventions

ENCOURAGING ADEQUATE NUTRITIONAL INTAKE

- Encourage patient to eat slowly and chew all food thoroughly.
- Recommend small, frequent feedings of nonirritating foods; sometimes drinking liquids with food helps passage.
- Prepare food in an appealing manner to help stimulate appetite; avoid irritants (tobacco, alcohol).
- Obtain a baseline weight, and record daily weights; assess nutrient intake.

DECREASING RISK OF ASPIRATION

- If patient has difficulty in swallowing or handling secretions, keep him or her upright in at least a semi-Fowler's position.
- Instruct patient in the use of oral suction to decrease risk of aspiration.

RELIEVING PAIN

- Educate patient to eat small meals frequently (six to eight daily).
- Advise patient to avoid any activities that increase pain and to remain upright for 1 to 4 hours after each meal to prevent reflux.
- Elevate the head of bed on 4- to 8-in blocks; discourage eating before bed.
- Advise patient not to use over-the-counter antacids because of possible rebound acidity.
- Instruct in use of prescribed antacids, PPIs, or histamine antagonists.

PROMOTING HOME- AND COMMUNITY-BASED CARE

Educating Patients About Self-Care

- Help patient plan for needed physical and psychological adjustments and follow-up care if condition is chronic.
- Educate patient and family to use special equipment (enteral or parenteral feeding devices, suction).
- Help in planning meals, using medications as prescribed, and resuming activity.
- Educate about nutritional requirements and ways to measure the adequacy of nutrition (particularly in the older adult and debilitated patients). See "Nursing Process: The Hospitalized

Postoperative Patient" in Perioperative Nursing Management in Section P for additional information.

Continuing Care
- Arrange for home health care nursing support and assessment when indicated.
- Educate patient to prepare soft food (e.g., with a blender) if indicated.
- Assist patient to adjust medication schedule to daily activities when possible.
- Arrange for nutritionist, social worker, or hospice care when indicated.

Evaluation

EXPECTED PATIENT OUTCOMES
- Achieves an adequate nutritional intake
- Does not aspirate or develop pneumonia
- Is free of pain or able to control pain within a tolerable level
- Increases knowledge level of esophageal condition, treatment, and prognosis

For more information, see Chapter 46 in Hinkle, J. L., & Cheever, K. H. (2014). *Brunner and Suddarth's textbook of medical-surgical nursing* (13th ed.). Philadelphia: Lippincott Williams & Wilkins.

Hodgkin Lymphoma

Hodgkin lymphoma (Hodgkin's disease) is a rare cancer of unknown cause that spreads along the lymphatic system. Disease occurrence has a familial pattern; it is somewhat more common in men and tends to peak in the early 20s and after the 50s. It is seen more commonly in patients receiving chronic immunosuppressive therapy (e.g., for renal transplantation), in veterans of the military who were exposed to the herbicide Agent Orange, and in patients with IgA or certain types of IgG deficiency. The 5-year survival rate is 88%; survival is more than 92% for those younger than 45 years of age.

Pathophysiology

Unlike other lymphomas, Hodgkin lymphoma is unicentric in origin in that it initiates in a single node. The disease spreads by contiguous extension along the lymphatic system. The Reed–Sternberg cell, a gigantic morphologically unique tumor cell that is thought to be of immature lymphoid origin, is the pathologic hallmark and essential diagnostic criterion for Hodgkin lymphoma. The cause of Hodgkin lymphoma is unknown, but a viral etiology is suspected. Although fragments of the Epstein-Barr virus have been found in some Reed-Sternberg cells, the precise role of this virus in the development of Hodgkin lymphoma remains unknown. Hodgkin lymphoma is customarily classified into five subgroups, based on pathologic analyses that reflect the natural history of the malignancy and suggest the prognosis. Most patients with Hodgkin lymphoma have the types currently designated *nodular sclerosis* or *mixed cellularity*. The nodular sclerosis type tends to occur more often in young women (and at an earlier stage) but has a worse prognosis than the mixed cellularity subgroup, which occurs more commonly in men and causes more constitutional symptoms.

Clinical Manifestations

- Painless enlargement of the lymph nodes occurs on one side of the neck. Individual nodes are firm; common sites are the cervical, supraclavicular, and mediastinal nodes.
- Mediastinal lymph nodes may be visible on x-ray films and are large enough to compress the trachea and cause dyspnea.
- Pruritus is common and can be distressing; the cause is unknown. Herpes zoster infection (shingles) is common.
- Some patients experience brief but severe pain after drinking alcohol, usually at the site of the tumor.
- Symptoms may result from the tumor compressing other organs, causing cough and pulmonary effusion (from pulmonary infiltrates), jaundice (from hepatic involvement or bile duct obstruction), abdominal pain (from splenomegaly or retroperitoneal adenopathy), or bone pain (from skeletal involvement).
- Constitutional symptoms, for prognostic purposes referred to as *B symptoms*, are found in 40% of patients and are more common in advanced disease; these include fever (without chills), drenching sweats (particularly at night), and unintentional weight loss of more than 10% of body weight.
- Mild anemia develops; leukocyte count may be elevated or decreased; platelet count is typically normal, unless the tumor has invaded the bone marrow, suppressing hematopoiesis.
- Impaired cellular immunity (evidenced by an absence of, or decreased response to, skin sensitivity tests such as candidal infection, mumps) may be noted.

- Erythrocyte sedimentation rates (ESR) and serum copper level evaluations are sometimes used to assess disease activity.

Assessment and Diagnostic Findings

- Because many manifestations are similar to those occurring with infection, diagnostic studies are performed to rule out an infectious origin for the disease.
- Excisional lymph node biopsy and the finding of the Reed-Sternberg cell confirm the diagnosis.
- Assess for any B symptoms; perform physical examination to evaluate the lymph node chains as well as the size of the spleen and liver.
- Chest x-ray and a CT scan of the chest, abdomen, and pelvis are used; positron emission tomography (PET) scan may identify residual disease.
- Laboratory tests include complete blood cell count, platelet count, ESR, and liver and renal function studies.
- Bone marrow biopsy and sometimes bilateral biopsies can be used.
- Bone scans may be performed.

Medical Management

The goal in the treatment of Hodgkin lymphoma is cure. Treatment is determined by the stage of the disease instead of the histologic type. Treatment of limited-stage Hodgkin lymphoma commonly involves a short course (2 to 4 months) of chemotherapy followed by radiation therapy to the specific involved area. Combination chemotherapy with doxorubicin (Adriamycin), bleomycin (Blenoxane), vinblastine (Velban), and dacarbazine (DTIC) is referred to as *ABVD* and is considered the standard treatment for more advanced disease (stages III and IV and all stages with B symptoms). Other combinations of chemotherapy may afford higher response rates but result in more toxicity. Chemotherapy is often successful in obtaining remission even when relapse occurs. Transplantation is used for advanced or refractory disease. The development of complications from treatment may not occur for years, so long-term surveillance is crucial. In large, population-based studies of Hodgkin lymphoma survivors, the estimated risk of developing a second cancer was between 18% and 26%. Hematologic malignancies are the most common; solid tumors can also occur. Cardiovascular toxicity is the second leading cause of death after malignancy.

Nursing Management

See "Nursing Management" under "Cancer" for additional information about nursing interventions for patients undergoing chemotherapy and radiation treatments.

- Address the potential development of a second malignancy with the patient when treatment decisions are made; it is also important to tell patients that Hodgkin lymphoma is often curable.
- Encourage patients to reduce other factors that increase the risk of developing second cancers, such as use of tobacco and alcohol, and exposure to environmental carcinogens and excessive sunlight.
- Screen for late effects of treatment (e.g., immune dysfunction, herpes infections [zoster and varicella]; pneumococcal sepsis).
- Provide education about relevant self-care strategies and disease management.

For more information, see Chapter 34 in Hinkle, J. L., & Cheever, K. H. (2014). *Brunner and Suddarth's textbook of medical-surgical nursing* (13th ed.). Philadelphia: Lippincott Williams & Wilkins.

Huntington Disease

Huntington disease (HD) is a chronic, progressive hereditary disease of the nervous system that results in progressive involuntary choreiform (jerky) movements and dementia. Neuronal dysfunction and eventually cell death result from a genetic disease mutation in certain brain areas. HD affects men and women of all races. It is transmitted as an autosomal dominant genetic disorder; therefore, each child of a parent with HD has a 50% risk of inheriting the illness. Onset of physical symptoms usually occurs between 35 and 45 years of age.

Clinical Manifestations

- The most prominent clinical features are abnormal involuntary movements (chorea), cognitive decline and, often, emotional disturbance.
- Constant writhing, twisting, and uncontrollable movements of the entire body occur as the disease progresses.
- Facial movements produce tics and grimaces; speech becomes slurred, hesitant, often explosive, and then eventually unintelligible.

- Chewing and swallowing are difficult, and aspiration and choking are dangers.
- Gait becomes disorganized, and ambulation is eventually impossible; patient is eventually confined to a wheelchair.
- Bowel and bladder control is lost.
- Progressive cognitive impairment occurs with eventual dementia.
- Personality changes may result in nervous, irritable, or impatient behaviors. The early stages of illness exhibit uncontrollable fits of anger; profound, often suicidal depression; apathy; anxiety; psychosis; or euphoria.
- Hallucinations, delusions, and paranoid thinking may precede appearance of disjointed movements.
- Patient dies in 10 to 20 years from heart failure (HF), pneumonia, or infection or as a result of a fall or choking.

Assessment and Diagnostic Findings

- Diagnosis is made based on the clinical presentation of characteristic symptoms, a positive family history, a positive genetic test, and exclusion of other causes.
- HD arises from a genetic mutation in the gene for a cellular protein called *huntingtin*. Mutant huntingtin disrupts neuronal function and eventually leads to cell death in certain brain areas. A genetic test clearly defines who will or will not get the disease, but it offers no hope of cure or even specific determination of onset.

Medical Management

No treatment stops or reverses the process; palliative care is given.

- Tetrabenazine (Xenazine) is the only approved drug for the treatment of the chorea, although haloperidol, which predominantly block dopamine receptors, has been used in the past. Benzodiazepines (clonazepam [Klonopin]) and neuroleptic drugs (valproic acid [Depakote]) have also been reported to control chorea.
- Motor signs are continually assessed and evaluated. Akathisia (motor restlessness) in the overmedicated patient can be overlooked and should be watched for.
- Psychotherapy aimed at allaying anxiety and reducing stress may be beneficial; selective serotonin-reuptake inhibitors and tricyclic antidepressants are given for depression or suicidal ideation; psychotic symptoms usually respond to antipsychotic medications.
- Patient's needs and capabilities are the focus of treatment.

Nursing Management

- Educate patient and family about medications, including signs indicating need for change in dosage or medication.
- Address strategies to manage symptoms (chorea, swallowing problems, ambulation problems, or altered bowel or bladder function).
- Arrange for consultation with a speech therapist, if needed.
- Provide supportive care, as HD exacts enormous emotional, physical, social, and financial tolls on every member of the patient's family.
- Emphasize the need for regular follow-up.
- Refer for home care nursing assistance, respite care, day care centers, and eventually skilled long-term care to assist patient and family to cope.
- Provide information about the Huntington's Disease Society of America, which gives information, referrals, education, and support for research.

For more information, see Chapter 70 in Hinkle, J. L., & Cheever, K. H. (2014). *Brunner and Suddarth's textbook of medical-surgical nursing* (13th ed.). Philadelphia: Lippincott Williams & Wilkins.

Hyperglycemic Hyperosmolar Syndrome

Hyperglycemic hyperosmolar syndrome (HHS) is a metabolic disorder resulting from a relative insulin deficiency initiated by an illness or physiologic stressor (e.g., infection, surgery, cerebrovascular injury [CVA] or myocardial infarction [MI]) that raises demand for insulin. This condition occurs most frequently in older people (50 to 70 years of age) who have no known history of diabetes or who have type 2 diabetes. The acute development of the condition can be traced to some precipitating event, such as an acute illness (e.g., pneumonia, CVA), medications (e.g., thiazides) that exacerbate hyperglycemia, or treatments such as dialysis.

Pathophysiology

HHS is a serious condition in which hyperglycemia and hyperosmolarity predominate with alterations of consciousness (sense of awareness). Ketosis is minimal or absent. The basic biochemical defect is lack of effective insulin (insulin resistance). Persistent hyperglycemia causes osmotic diuresis, resulting in water and electrolyte losses. Although there is not enough insulin to prevent hyperglycemia, the small amount of insulin present is enough to prevent fat breakdown.

Clinical Manifestations
- History of days to weeks of polyuria with adequate fluid intake
- Hypotension, tachycardia
- Profound dehydration (dry mucous membranes, poor skin turgor)
- Variable neurologic signs (alterations of consciousness, seizures, hemiparesis)

Assessment and Diagnostic Findings
- Laboratory tests, including blood glucose, electrolytes, blood urea nitrogen (BUN), complete blood cell (CBC) count, serum osmolality, and arterial blood gasses (ABGs)
- Clinical picture of severe dehydration

Medical Management
The overall treatment of HHS is similar to that of diabetic ketoacidosis (DKA): fluids, electrolytes, and insulin. Because patients with HHS are typically older, close monitoring of volume and electrolyte status is important for prevention of fluid overload, heart failure, and cardiac dysrhythmias. Fluid treatment is started with 0.9% sodium chloride or NaCl (normal saline) or 0.45% sodium chloride (half-strength normal saline), depending on the patient's sodium level and the severity of volume depletion. Central venous or hemodynamic pressure monitoring guides fluid replacement. Potassium is added to IV fluids when urinary output is adequate and is guided by continuous electrocardiography (ECG) monitoring and frequent laboratory determinations of potassium. Insulin is usually given at a continuous low rate to treat hyperglycemia, and dextrose is added to replacement fluids when the glucose level decreases to 250 to 300 mg/dL. Other therapeutic modalities are determined by the underlying illness and results of continuing clinical and laboratory evaluation, and treatment is continued until metabolic abnormalities are corrected; it may take 3 to 5 days for neurologic symptoms to resolve.

Nursing Management
See "Nursing Management" under Diabetes in Section D and "Nursing Process: The Patient With DKA" under Diabetic Ketoacidosis in Section D additional information.

- Assess vital signs, fluid status, and laboratory values. Fluid status and urine output are closely monitored because of the high risk of renal failure secondary to severe dehydration.
- Blood glucose should be checked hourly.
- Because HHS tends to occur in older patients, the physiologic changes that occur with aging should be considered.
- Careful assessment of cardiovascular, pulmonary, and renal function throughout the acute and recovery phases of HHS is important.

For more information, see Chapter 51 in Hinkle, J. L., & Cheever, K. H. (2014). *Brunner and Suddarth's textbook of medical-surgical nursing* (13th ed.). Philadelphia: Lippincott Williams & Wilkins.

H

Hypertension (and Hypertensive Crisis)

Hypertension is defined as a systolic blood pressure greater than 140 mm Hg and a diastolic pressure greater than 90 mm Hg, based on two or more measurements. Primary (also referred to as *essential*) hypertension (most common) refers to hypertension in which there is no identifiable cause; *secondary hypertension* is used to describe hypertension in which the cause is identified (e.g., renal parenchymal disease, pheochromocytoma, certain medications, pregnancy). Hypertension can be classified as follows:

- Normal: systolic less than 120 mm Hg; diastolic less than 80 mm Hg
- Prehypertension: systolic 120 to 139 mm Hg; diastolic 80 to 89 mm Hg
- Stage 1: systolic 140 to 159 mm Hg; diastolic 90 to 99 mm Hg
- Stage 2: systolic ≥160 mm Hg; diastolic ≥100 mm Hg

Hypertension is a major risk factor for atherosclerotic cardiovascular disease, heart failure (HF), stroke, and kidney failure. Hypertension carries the risk for premature morbidity or mortality, which increases as systolic and diastolic pressures rise. Prolonged blood pressure elevation damages blood vessels in target organs (heart, kidneys, brain, and eyes). **Hypertensive emergency** and **hypertensive urgency** are conditions that require immediate intervention (see the *Emergency! Hypertensive Crisis* box).

Emergency! Hypertensive Crisis

Hypertensive emergency and **hypertensive urgency** (pressures above 180 mm Hg systolic or above 120 mm Hg diastolic) require immediate intervention and may occur in patients whose hypertension has been poorly controlled or undiagnosed or in those who have abruptly discontinued their medications. A **hypertensive emergency** is an acute, life-threatening situation in which blood pressures are extremely elevated and must be lowered immediately (not necessarily to less than 140/90 mm Hg) to halt or prevent damage to the target organs; these patients require intravenous vasodilators in the intensive care setting. A **hypertensive urgency** describes a situation in which blood pressure is very elevated but there is no evidence of impending or progressive target organ damage. Elevated blood pressures associated with severe headaches, nosebleeds, or anxiety are classified as urgencies. In these situations, oral agents can be administered with the goal of normalizing blood pressure within 24 to 48 hours. Extremely close hemodynamic monitoring of the patient's blood pressure and cardiovascular status is required during treatment of hypertensive emergencies and urgencies. The exact frequency of monitoring is a matter of clinical judgment and varies with the patient's condition.

Pathophysiology

Blood pressure is the product of cardiac output (CO) multiplied by peripheral resistance. Hypertension can result from increases in CO, increases in peripheral resistance (constriction of the blood vessels), or both. Increases in CO are often related to an expansion in vascular volume. Although no precise cause can be identified for most cases of hypertension, it is understood that hypertension is a multifactorial condition. Because hypertension can be a sign, it is most likely to have many causes. For hypertension to occur, there must be a change in one or more factors affecting peripheral resistance or CO. The tendency to develop hypertension is inherited; however, genetic profiles alone cannot predict who will or will not develop hypertension. Suggested causes include increased sympathetic tone related to dysfunction of the autonomic nervous system; increased renal absorption of sodium, chloride, and water due to genetic variations; increased activity of the renal–angiotensin–aldosterone system: decreased vasodilatation of the arterioles related to dysfunction of the vascular endothelium; resistance to insulin action; and activation of an immune response that may contribute to renal inflammation and dysfunction.

Gerontologic Considerations

Structural and functional changes in the heart, blood vessels, and kidneys contribute to increases in blood pressure that occur with aging. These changes include accumulation of atherosclerotic plaque, fragmentation of arterial elastins, increased collagen deposits, impaired vasodilation, and renal dysfunction. The result of these changes is decreased elasticity of the major blood vessels and volume expansion. Consequently, the aorta and large arteries are less able to accommodate the volume of blood pumped out by the heart (stroke volume), and the energy that would have stretched the vessels instead elevates the systolic blood pressure. This results in an elevated systolic pressure without a change in diastolic pressure. This condition, known as *isolated systolic hypertension,* is more common in older adults and is associated with significant cardiovascular and cerebrovascular morbidity and mortality.

Clinical Manifestations

- Physical examination may reveal no abnormality other than high blood pressure.
- Changes in the retinas with hemorrhages, exudates, narrowed arterioles, cotton–wool spots (small infarctions), and papilledema may be seen in severe hypertension.
- Symptoms usually indicate vascular damage related to organ systems served by involved vessels.
- Coronary artery disease with angina or myocardial infarction are common consequences.
- Left ventricular hypertrophy may occur; HF may ensue.
- Pathologic changes may occur in the kidney (nocturia and increased blood urea nitrogen [BUN] and creatinine levels).
- Cerebrovascular involvement may lead to cerebrovascular accident (CVA, stroke, or brain attack), transient ischemic attack (TIA) with symptoms of alterations in vision or speech, dizziness, weakness, a sudden fall, or transient or permanent hemiplegia.

Assessment and Diagnostic Findings

- History and physical examination, including retinal examination

- Laboratory studies to assess organ damage, including urinalysis, blood chemistry (sodium, potassium, creatinine, fasting glucose, total and high-density lipoprotein cholesterol)
- Electrocardiogram and echocardiography to assess left ventricular hypertrophy
- Additional studies, such as creatinine clearance, renin level, urine tests, and 24-hour urine protein
- Risk factor assessment as advocated by the Seventh Report of the Joint National Committee on Prevention, Detection, Evaluation, and Treatment of High Blood Pressure (JNC 7)

Medical Management

The goal of any treatment program is to prevent complications and death by achieving and maintaining, whenever possible, an arterial blood pressure at or below 140/90 mm Hg (130/80 mm Hg for people with diabetes or chronic kidney disease). Nonpharmacologic approaches include lifestyle modifications such as weight reduction, reduced alcohol and sodium intake, and regular physical exercise. A DASH (Dietary Approaches to Stop Hypertension) diet high in fruits, vegetables, and low-fat dairy products has been shown to lower elevated pressures.

Pharmacologic Therapy

The medications used for treating hypertension decrease peripheral resistance, blood volume, or the strength and rate of myocardial contraction.

- First-line medications include diuretic agents, beta blockers, or both, beginning with low doses; doses are gradually increased until hypertension is controlled. Additional medications may be added.
- If blood pressure is less than 140/90 mm Hg for at least 1 year, reductions in dosing may be considered.
- Promote compliance by avoiding complicated drug schedules; single or multiple agents may be combined into a single pill.

Gerontologic Considerations

Hypertension, particularly elevated systolic blood pressure, increases the risk of death, stroke, and HF in people older than age 50 years, and treatment reduces this risk. Like younger patients, older patients should begin treatment with lifestyle modifications. If medications are needed to achieve the blood pressure goal of less than 140/90 mm Hg, the starting dose should be the lowest available and then gradually increased with a second medication from a different class (added if control is difficult to achieve). It is recommended that a diuretic be included as either the first or second treatment choice. As older adults often have other co-morbid conditions, awareness of possible drug interactions is critical. In addition, older adults are at increased risk for the side effects of hyperkalemia and orthostatic hypotension, putting them at increased risk for falls and fractures.

H

NURSING PROCESS

The Patient With Hypertension

Assessment

- Assess blood pressure at frequent intervals to determine treatment; know baseline level. Note changes in pressure that would require a change in medication.
- Use appropriate-sized cuff and standard techniques for measuring blood pressure.
- Assess for signs and symptoms that indicate target organ damage (e.g., angina; shortness of breath; alterations in speech, vision, or balance; nosebleeds; headaches; dizziness; or nocturia).
- Inquire about any obstructive sleep apnea with patient's partner.
- Note the apical and peripheral pulse rate, rhythm, and character.
- Assess the extent to which hypertension has affected patient personally, socially, or financially.

Diagnosis

NURSING DIAGNOSES
- Deficient knowledge regarding the relationship between the treatment regimen and control of the disease process
- Noncompliance with therapeutic regimen related to side effects of prescribed therapy

COLLABORATIVE PROBLEMS/POTENTIAL COMPLICATIONS
- Left ventricular hypertrophy
- Myocardial infarction

- HF
- TIA
- CVA
- Renal insufficiency and failure
- Retinal hemorrhage

Planning and Goals

The major goals for the patient include understanding of the disease process and its treatment, participation in a self-care program, and absence of complications.

Nursing Interventions

H

INCREASING KNOWLEDGE
- Emphasize the concept of controlling hypertension (with lifestyle changes and medications) rather than curing it.
- Arrange a consultation with a dietitian to help develop a plan for improving nutrient intake or for weight loss.
- Advise patient to limit alcohol intake and avoid use of tobacco.

PROMOTING ADHERENCE TO THE THERAPEUTIC REGIMEN
- Adherence to the therapeutic regimen increases when patients actively participate in self-care (including self-monitoring of blood pressure and diet), possibly because patients receive immediate feedback and have a greater sense of control.
- Continued education and encouragement are usually needed to enable patients to formulate an acceptable plan.
- Support patients in making small changes with each visit that move them toward their goals; assess progress at each visit.
- Recommend support groups for weight control, smoking cessation, and stress reduction.
- Assist the patient to develop and adhere to an appropriate exercise regimen.

PROMOTING HOME- AND COMMUNITY-BASED CARE
Educating Patients About Self-Care
- Help the patient achieve blood pressure control through education about managing blood pressure, setting goal blood pressures, and providing assistance with social support;

encourage family members to support the patient's efforts to control hypertension.

- Provide written information about the expected effects and side effects of medications; ensure patient understands importance of reporting side effects to the appropriate health care provider when they occur.
- Inform patient that rebound hypertension can occur if antihypertensive medications are suddenly stopped; advise patient to have an adequate supply of medication. Discuss packing medication for travel in carry-on luggage.
- Inform patients that some medications, such as beta-blockers, may cause sexual dysfunction and that other medications are available if problems occur.
- Provide education and encourage patients to correctly measure their blood pressure at home; inform patients that blood pressure varies continuously and that the their blood pressure range should be monitored.

Gerontologic Considerations

Adherence to the therapeutic program may be more difficult for older adults. The medication regimen can be difficult to remember, and the expense can be a problem. Monotherapy (treatment with a single agent), if appropriate, may simplify the medication regimen and make it less expensive. Ensure that the older adult patient understands the regimen and can see and read instructions, open the medication container, and get the prescription refilled. Include family members or caregivers in the teaching program so that they (1) understand the patient's needs, (2) can encourage adherence to the treatment plan, and (3) know when and whom to call if problems arise or information is needed.

Continuing Care

- Reinforce importance of regular follow-up care.
- Update patient history and perform physical examination at each clinic visit.
- Assess for medication-related problems (orthostatic hypotension).
- Provide continued education and encouragement to enable patients to formulate an acceptable plan that helps them live with their hypertension and adhere to the treatment plan.

◢ *Quality and Safety Nursing Alert*

The patient and caregivers should be cautioned that anti-hypertensive medications might cause hypotension. Low blood pressure or postural hypotension should be reported immediately. Older adults have impaired cardiovascular reflexes and thus are more sensitive to the extracellular volume depletion caused by diuretic drugs and to the sympathetic inhibition caused by adrenergic antagonists. The nurse educates patients to change positions slowly when moving from a lying or sitting position to a standing position. The nurse also counsels older adult patients to use supportive devices such as handrails and walkers to prevent falls that could result from dizziness.

MONITORING AND MANAGING POTENTIAL COMPLICATIONS
- Assess all body systems when patient returns for follow-up care to detect any evidence of target organ or vascular damage.
- Question patient about blurred vision, spots, or diminished visual acuity.
- Report any significant findings promptly to determine whether additional studies or changes in medications are required.

Evaluation

EXPECTED PATIENT OUTCOMES
- Reports knowledge of disease management sufficient to maintain adequate tissue perfusion
- Adheres to self-care program
- Experiences no complications

For more information, see Chapter 34 in Hinkle, J. L., & Cheever, K. H. (2014). *Brunner and Suddarth's textbook of medical-surgical nursing* (13th ed.). Philadelphia: Lippincott Williams & Wilkins.

Hyperthyroidism (Graves' Disease)

Hyperthyroidism, a common endocrine disorder, is a form of thyrotoxicosis resulting in excessive synthesis and secretion of endogenous or exogenous thyroid hormones by the thyroid. The most common cause is Graves' disease, an autoimmune disorder that results from an excessive output of thyroid hormones due to abnormal stimulation of the thyroid gland by circulating immunoglobulins. The disorder affects women eight times more frequently than men and peaks between the second and fourth decades of life. It may appear after an emotional shock, stress, or infection, but the exact significance of these relationships is not understood. Other common causes include thyroiditis and excessive ingestion of thyroid hormone (e.g., from the treatment of hypothyroidism).

Clinical Manifestations
Hyperthyroidism presents a characteristic group of signs and symptoms (thyrotoxicosis).

- Nervousness (emotionally hyperexcitable), irritability, apprehensiveness; inability to sit quietly; palpitations; rapid pulse on rest and exertion
- Poor tolerance of heat; excessive perspiration; skin that is flushed, with a characteristic salmon color, and likely to be warm, soft, and moist
- Dry skin and diffuse pruritus
- Fine tremor of the hands
- Exophthalmos (bulging eyes) in some patients
- Increased appetite and dietary intake, progressive loss of weight, abnormal muscle fatigability, weakness, amenorrhea, and changes in bowel function (constipation or diarrhea)
- Osteoporosis and fracture
- Cardiac effects: atrial fibrillation, sinus tachycardia or dysrhythmias, increased pulse pressure, and palpitations; myocardial hypertrophy and heart failure (HF) (especially in older adult patients, which may occur if the hyperthyroidism is severe and untreated)
- Possible remissions and exacerbations, terminating with spontaneous recovery in a few months or years
- May progress relentlessly, causing emaciation, intense nervousness, delirium, disorientation, and eventually HF

Assessment and Diagnostic Findings
- Thyroid gland is enlarged; it is soft and may pulsate; a thrill may be felt and a bruit heard over thyroid arteries.

- Laboratory tests show a decrease in serum thyroid-stimulating hormone (TSH), increased free T_4, and an increase in radioactive iodine uptake.

Medical Management

Treatment is directed toward reducing thyroid hyperactivity to relieve symptoms and prevent complications. Four forms of primary treatment are available:

- Radioactive iodine therapy for destructive effects on the thyroid gland
- Antithyroid medications
- Surgical removal of most of the thyroid gland
- Beta-adrenergic blocking agents (e.g., propranolol [Inderal], atenolol [Tenormin], metoprolol [Lopressor]) as adjunctive therapy for symptomatic relief, particularly in transient thyroiditis

Radioactive Iodine (^{131}I)

- ^{131}I is given to destroy the overactive thyroid cells (most common treatment in older adults).
- ^{131}I is contraindicated in pregnancy and for nursing mothers because radioiodine crosses the placenta and is secreted in breast milk.

Antithyroid Medications

- The objective of pharmacotherapy is to inhibit hormone synthesis or release and reduce the amount of thyroid tissue.
- Use of an ablative dose of radioactive iodine initially causes an acute release of thyroid hormone from the thyroid gland and may cause increased symptoms. The patient is observed for signs of thyroid storm (a life-threatening condition manifested by cardiac dysrhythmias, fever, and neurologic impairment). See Thyroid Storm in Section T for more information.
- The most commonly used medications are propylthiouracil (PropylThyracil, PTU) and methimazole (Tapazole) until patient is euthyroid.
- Maintenance dose is established, followed by gradual withdrawal of the medication over the next several months.
- Antithyroid drugs are contraindicated in late pregnancy because of a risk for goiter and cretinism in the fetus.
- Thyroid hormone may be administered to put the thyroid to rest.

Adjunctive Therapy
- Potassium iodide (KI), Lugol's solution, and saturated solution of potassium iodide (SSKI) may be added.
- Beta-adrenergic agents may be used to control the sympathetic nervous system effects that occur in hyperthyroidism; for example, propranolol (Inderal) is used for nervousness, tachycardia, tremor, anxiety, and heat intolerance.

Surgical Intervention
- Surgical intervention (reserved for special circumstances) removes about five-sixths of the thyroid tissue.
- Surgery to treat hyperthyroidism is performed after thyroid function has returned to normal (4 to 6 weeks).
- Before surgery, patient is given propylthiouracil until signs of hyperthyroidism have disappeared.
- Iodine is prescribed to reduce blood loss and thyroid size and vascularity. Patient is monitored carefully for evidence of iodine toxicity (swelling buccal mucosa, excessive salivation, skin eruptions).
- Risk for relapse and complications necessitates long-term follow-up of patient undergoing treatment of hyperthyroidism.

Gerontologic Considerations

Older patients commonly present with atypical vague and non-specific signs and symptoms. The only presenting manifestations may be anorexia and weight loss, absence of ocular signs, or isolated atrial fibrillation. (New or worsening HF or angina is more likely to occur in older than in younger patients.) These signs and symptoms may mask the underlying thyroid disease. Spontaneous remission of hyperthyroidism is rare in older adults. Measurement of TSH uptake is indicated in older adult patients with unexplained physical or mental deterioration. Use of radioactive iodine is generally recommended for treatment of thyrotoxicosis rather than surgery, unless an enlarged thyroid gland is pressing on the airway. Thyrotoxicosis must be controlled by medications before radioactive iodine is used because radiation may precipitate thyroid storm, which has a mortality rate of 10% in older adults. Beta-adrenergic blocking agents may be indicated. Use these agents with extreme caution and monitor closely for granulocytopenia. Modify dosages of other medications because of the altered rate of metabolism in hyperthyroidism.

NURSING PROCESS

The Patient With Hyperthyroidism

Assessment

- Obtain a health history and examination, including family history of hyperthyroidism, and note reports of irritability or increased emotional reaction; note the impact of these changes on patient's interaction with family, friends, and coworkers.
- Assess stressors and patient's ability to cope with stress.
- Evaluate nutritional status and presence of symptoms; note excessive nervousness, changes in vision, and appearance of eyes.
- Assess and monitor cardiac status periodically (heart rate, blood pressure, heart sounds, and peripheral pulses).
- Assess emotional state and psychological status.

Diagnosis

NURSING DIAGNOSES

- Imbalanced nutrition: less than body requirements related to exaggerated metabolic rate, excessive appetite, and increased gastrointestinal activity
- Ineffective coping related to irritability, hyperexcitability, apprehension, and emotional instability
- Situational low self-esteem related to changes in appearance, excessive appetite, and weight loss
- Risk for imbalanced body temperature

COLLABORATIVE PROBLEMS/POTENTIAL COMPLICATIONS

- Thyrotoxicosis or thyroid storm
- Hypothyroidism

Planning and Goals

Goals of the patient may be improved nutritional status, improved coping ability, improved self-esteem, maintenance of normal body temperature, and absence of complications.

Nursing Interventions

IMPROVING NUTRITIONAL STATUS

- Provide several small, well-balanced meals (up to six meals a day) to satisfy patient's increased appetite.

- Replace food and fluids lost through diarrhea and diaphoresis and control diarrhea that results from increased peristalsis.
- Reduce diarrhea by avoiding highly seasoned foods and stimulants such as coffee, tea, cola, and alcohol; encourage high-calorie, high-protein foods.
- Provide quiet atmosphere during mealtime to aid digestion.
- Record weight and dietary intake daily.

ENHANCING COPING MEASURES

- Reassure the patient that the emotional reactions being experienced are a result of the disorder and that, with effective treatment, those symptoms will be controlled.
- Reassure family and friends that symptoms are expected to disappear with treatment.
- Maintain a calm, unhurried approach and minimize stressful experiences.
- Keep the environment quiet and uncluttered.
- Provide information regarding thyroidectomy and preparatory pharmacotherapy to alleviate anxiety.
- Assist patient to take medications as prescribed and encourage adherence to the therapeutic regimen.
- Repeat information often and provide written instructions as indicated due to short attention span.

IMPROVING SELF-ESTEEM

- Convey to patient an understanding of concerns regarding problems with appearance, appetite, and weight and assist in developing coping strategies.
- Provide eye protection if patient experiences eye changes secondary to hyperthyroidism; instruct patient with correct installation of eye drops or ointment to soothe the eyes and protect the exposed cornea. Discourage smoking.
- Arrange for patient to eat alone, if desired, and if embarrassed by the large meals consumed due to increased metabolic rate. Avoid commenting on intake.

MAINTAINING NORMAL BODY TEMPERATURE

- Provide a cool, comfortable environment and fresh bedding and gown as needed.
- Give cool baths and provide cool fluids; monitor body temperature.

MONITORING AND MANAGING POTENTIAL COMPLICATIONS
- Monitor closely for signs and symptoms indicative of thyroid storm.
- Assess cardiac and respiratory function: vital signs, cardiac output, electrocardiographic (ECG) monitoring, arterial blood gases (ABGs), pulse oximetry.
- Administer oxygen to prevent hypoxia, to improve tissue oxygenation, and to meet the high metabolic demands.
- Give IV fluids to maintain blood glucose levels and replace lost fluids.
- Administer antithyroid medications to reduce thyroid hormone levels.
- Administer propranolol and digitalis to treat cardiac symptoms.
- Implement strategies to treat shock if needed.
- Monitor for hypothyroidism; encourage continued therapy.
- Educate patient and family about the importance of continuing therapy after discharge and about the consequences of failing to take medication.

PROMOTING HOME- AND COMMUNITY-BASED CARE
Educating Patients About Self-Care
- Instruct patient about how and when to take prescribed medications.
- Educate patient on ways the medication regimen fits in with the broader therapeutic plan.
- Provide an individualized written plan of care for use at home.
- Educate patient and family about the desired effects and side effects of medications.
- Instruct patient and family about which adverse effects should be reported to the health care provider.
- Educate patient about what to expect from a thyroidectomy if this is to be performed.
- Educate patient to avoid situations that have the potential of stimulating thyroid storm.

Continuing Care
- Refer to home care for assessment of the home and family environment.
- Stress long-term follow-up care because of the possibility of hypothyroidism after thyroidectomy or treatment with antithyroid drugs or radioactive iodine.

- Assess for changes indicating return to normal thyroid function; assess for physical signs of hyperthyroidism and hypothyroidism.
- Remind the patient and family about the importance of health promotion activities and recommended health screening.

Evaluation

EXPECTED PATIENT OUTCOMES

- Improves nutritional status
- Demonstrates effective coping methods in dealing with family, friends, and coworkers
- Achieves increased self-esteem
- Maintains normal body temperature
- Displays absence of complications

For more information, see Chapter 52 in Hinkle, J. L., & Cheever, K. H. (2014). *Brunner and Suddarth's textbook of medical-surgical nursing* (13th ed.). Philadelphia: Lippincott Williams & Wilkins.

Hypoglycemia (Insulin Reaction)

Hypoglycemia is defined as low blood glucose levels of less than 70 mg/dL; severe hypoglycemia is defined as blood glucose levels of less than 40 mg/dL.

Pathophysiology

Hypoglycemia can be caused by too much insulin or oral hypoglycemic agents, too little food, or excessive physical activity and may occur at any time. It often occurs before meals, especially if meals are delayed or if snacks are omitted. Midmorning hypoglycemia may occur when the morning regular insulin is peaking, whereas hypoglycemia that occurs in the late afternoon coincides with the peak of the morning NPH or Lente insulin. Middle-of-the-night hypoglycemia may occur because of peaking evening NPH or Lente insulins, especially in patients who have not eaten a bedtime snack.

Gerontologic Considerations

Older adults frequently live alone and may not recognize the symptoms of hypoglycemia. With decreasing renal function, it takes longer for oral hypoglycemic agents to be excreted by the kidneys. Educate older patients to avoid skipping meals because of decreased appetite or financial limitations. Decreased visual acuity may lead to errors in insulin administration.

Clinical Manifestations

The symptoms of hypoglycemia may be grouped into two categories: adrenergic symptoms and central nervous system (CNS) symptoms; these may occur suddenly and unexpectedly and vary from person to person.

Mild Hypoglycemia

The sympathetic nervous system is stimulated, producing adrenergic symptoms including sweating, tremor, tachycardia, palpitations, nervousness, and hunger.

Moderate Hypoglycemia

Moderate hypoglycemia produces impaired function of the CNS, including inability to concentrate, headache, light-headedness, confusion, memory lapses, numbness of the lips and tongue, slurred speech, impaired coordination, emotional changes, irrational or combative behavior, double vision, and drowsiness, or any combination of these symptoms.

Severe Hypoglycemia

In severe hypoglycemia, CNS function is further impaired. The patient needs the assistance of another for treatment. Symptoms may include disoriented behavior, seizures, difficulty arousing from sleep, or loss of consciousness.

Assessment and Diagnostic Findings

Measurement of serum glucose levels; decreased hormonal (adrenergic) response to hypoglycemia may contribute to lack of symptoms of hypoglycemia despite low blood glucose.

Medical Management

Management of Hypoglycemia in the Conscious Patient

Immediate treatment must be given when hypoglycemia occurs. The usual recommendation is for initial treatment with 15 g of a fast-acting concentrated source of carbohydrate orally (e.g., two or three commercially prepared glucose tablets; 1 tube of glucose gel, 4 to 6 oz of fruit juice) followed by a snack including a starch and protein (e.g., cheese and crackers, milk and crackers, half sandwich). Patient should avoid adding table sugar to juice, even "unsweetened" juice, which may cause a sharp increase in glucose, resulting in hyperglycemia hours later. Close monitoring for 24 hours after a hypoglycemic episode is indicated because the patient is at increased risk of another episode.

Management of Hypoglycemia in the Unconscious Patient

- Glucagon, 1 mg subcutaneously or intramuscularly for patients who cannot swallow or who refuse treatment; patient may take up to 20 minutes to regain consciousness. Provide a concentrated source of carbohydrate followed by a snack when awake.
- From 25 to 50 mL of 50% dextrose in water is administered IV to patients who are unconscious or unable to swallow (in a hospital setting).

Nursing Management

- Educate patient to prevent hypoglycemia by following a consistent, regular pattern for eating, administering insulin, and exercising. Advise patient to consume between-meal and bedtime snacks to counteract the maximum insulin effect.
- Reinforce that routine blood glucose tests are performed so that changing insulin requirements may be anticipated and the dosage adjusted.
- Encourage patients taking insulin to wear an identification bracelet or tag indicating they have diabetes.
- Instruct patient to notify physician after severe hypoglycemia has occurred.
- Instruct patients and family about symptoms of hypoglycemia and use of glucagon; encourage patients to share information about recognizing symptoms of hypoglycemia with coworkers.
- Educate family that hypoglycemia can cause irrational and unintentional behavior.
- Reinforce with the patient the importance of performing self-monitoring of blood glucose on a frequent and regular basis.
- Educate patients who have diabetes and take oral sulfonylurea agents that symptoms of hypoglycemia may also develop.
- Patients with diabetes should carry a form of simple sugar with them at all times.
- Patients are discouraged from eating high-calorie, high-fat dessert foods to treat hypoglycemia, because high-fat snacks may slow absorption of the glucose.

For more information, see Chapter 51 in Hinkle, J. L., & Cheever, K. H. (2014). *Brunner and Suddarth's textbook of medical-surgical nursing* (13th ed.). Philadelphia: Lippincott Williams & Wilkins.

Hypoparathyroidism

The most common causes of hypoparathyroidism are inadequate secretion of parathyroid hormone after interruption of the blood supply, or surgical removal of parathyroid gland tissue during thyroidectomy, parathyroidectomy, or radical neck dissection. Atrophy of the parathyroid glands of unknown etiology is a less common cause. Symptoms are due to deficiency of parathormone, which results in an elevation of blood phosphate (hyperphosphatemia) and a decrease in blood calcium levels (hypocalcemia).

Clinical Manifestations

- Tetany is the chief symptom.
- Latent tetany is characterized by numbness, tingling, and cramps in the extremities; stiffness in the hands and feet.
- Overt tetany is marked by bronchospasm, laryngeal spasm, carpopedal spasm, dysphagia, photophobia, cardiac dysrhythmias, and seizures.
- Other symptoms include anxiety, irritability, depression, and delirium. Electrocardiogram (ECG) changes and hypotension may also occur.

Assessment and Diagnostic Findings

- Latent tetany is suggested by a positive Trousseau's sign (in which carpopedal spasm is induced by occluding the blood flow to the arm for 3 minutes with a blood pressure cuff) or a positive Chvostek's sign (in which sharp tapping over the facial nerve just in front of the parotid gland and anterior to the ear causes spasm or twitching of the mouth, nose, and eye);
- Diagnosis is difficult because of vague symptoms such as aches and pains; laboratory studies show increased serum phosphate, with serum calcium of 5 to 6 mg/dL (1.2 to 1.5 mmol/L) or lower; x-rays of bone show increased density and calcification of the subcutaneous or paraspinal basal ganglia of the brain.

Medical Management

- Raise serum calcium level to 9 to 10 mg/dL (2.2 to 2.5 mmol/L).
- When hypocalcemia and tetany occur after thyroidectomy, IV calcium gluconate is given immediately. Sedative agents (pentobarbital) may be administered. Parenteral parathormone may be given, but watch for an allergic reaction and changes in serum calcium levels.

- Neuromuscular irritability is reduced by providing an environment that is free of noise, drafts, bright lights, or sudden movement.
- Tracheostomy, or mechanical ventilation and bronchodilating medications, may become necessary if the patient develops respiratory distress.
- Chronic hypoparathyroidism is treated with a diet high in calcium and low in phosphorus. Patient should avoid milk, milk products, egg yolk, and spinach.
- Provide combinations of calcitriol, calcium, magnesium, and vitamin D_2 (ergocalciferol) or vitamin D_3 (cholecalciferol), the latter being preferred. Administer a thiazide diuretic (e.g., hydrochlorothiazide) to help decrease urinary calcium excretion. Oral calcium tablets and vitamin D preparations, as well as aluminum hydroxide gel or aluminum carbonate, may be given after meals.

Nursing Management

- Detect early signs of hypocalcemia and anticipate signs of tetany, seizures, and respiratory difficulties.
- Keep calcium gluconate at the bedside; if patient has a cardiac disorder, is subject to dysrhythmias, or is receiving digitalis, the calcium gluconate is administered slowly and cautiously.
- Provide continuous cardiac monitoring and careful assessment; calcium and digitalis increase systolic contraction and also potentiate each other; this can produce potentially fatal dysrhythmias.
- Educate patient about medications and diet therapy, the reason for high calcium and low phosphate intake, and the symptoms of hypocalcemia and hypercalcemia.
- Direct patient to contact physician if symptoms occur.

For more information, see Chapter 52 in Hinkle, J. L., & Cheever, K. H. (2014). *Brunner and Suddarth's textbook of medical-surgical nursing* (13th ed.). Philadelphia: Lippincott Williams & Wilkins.

Hypopituitarism

Abnormalities of pituitary function are caused by oversecretion or undersecretion of any of the hormones produced or released by the gland. Abnormalities of the anterior and posterior portions of the gland may occur independently. Hypopituitarism, a hypofunction of the pituitary gland, or hypophysis, can result from disease of the pituitary gland itself or disease of the hypothalamus; the result is essentially the same. Hypopituitarism also may result from destruction of the anterior lobe of the pituitary gland and from radiation therapy to the head and neck area. The total destruction of the pituitary gland by trauma, tumor, or vascular lesion removes all stimuli that are normally received by the thyroid, the gonads, and the adrenal glands. The result is extreme weight loss, emaciation, atrophy of all endocrine glands and organs, hair loss, impotence, amenorrhea, hypometabolism, and hypoglycemia. Coma and death occur if the missing hormones are not replaced.

For more information, see Chapter 52 in Hinkle, J. L., & Cheever, K. H. (2014). *Brunner and Suddarth's textbook of medical-surgical nursing* (13th ed.). Philadelphia: Lippincott Williams & Wilkins.

Hypothyroidism and Myxedema

Hypothyroidism results from suboptimal levels of thyroid hormone. Types of hypothyroidism include **primary**, which refers to dysfunction of the thyroid gland (more than 95% of cases); **central**, due to failure of the pituitary gland, hypothalamus, or both; **secondary** (or pituitary), which is due entirely to a pituitary disorder; and **hypothalamic** (or tertiary), due to a disorder of the hypothalamus resulting in inadequate secretion of thyroid-stimulating hormone (TSH) from decreased stimulation by thyroid-releasing hormone (TRH). Hypothyroidism occurs most often in older women. Its causes include autoimmune thyroiditis (Hashimoto's thyroiditis, most common type in adults); therapy for hyperthyroidism (radioiodine, surgery, or antithyroid drugs); radiation therapy for head and neck cancer; infiltrative diseases of the thyroid (amyloidosis and scleroderma); iodine deficiency; and iodine excess. When thyroid deficiency is present at birth, the condition is known as *cretinism*. The term *myxedema* refers to the accumulation of mucopolysaccharides in subcutaneous and other interstitial tissue and is used only to describe the extreme symptoms of severe hypothyroidism.

Clinical Manifestations

- Extreme fatigue
- Hair loss, brittle nails, dry skin, and numbness and tingling of fingers
- Husky voice and hoarseness
- Menstrual disturbances (e.g., menorrhagia or amenorrhea); loss of libido
- Severe hypothyroidism: subnormal temperature and pulse rate; weight gain without corresponding increase in food intake; cachexia; elevated serum cholesterol level; atherosclerosis; coronary artery disease; poor left ventricle function
- Thickened skin, thinning hair or alopecia; expressionless and masklike facial features
- Sensation of being cold in a warm environment
- Subdued emotional responses as the condition progresses; dulled mental processes and apathy
- Slow speech; enlarged tongue, hands, and feet; constipation; possibly deafness
- Advanced hypothyroidism: personality and cognitive changes, pleural effusion, pericardial effusion, and respiratory muscle weakness
- Hypothermia: abnormal sensitivity to sedatives, opiate drugs, and anesthetic agents (administer with extreme caution)
- Myxedema coma (rare): initial signs of depression, diminished cognitive status, lethargy, and somnolence; progression resulting in respiratory depression, hyponatremia, hypoglycemia, hypoventilation, hypotension, bradycardia, and hypothermia

Gerontologic Considerations

The higher prevalence of hypothyroidism in older adults may be related to alterations in immune function with age. Depression, apathy, or decreased mobility or activity may be the major initial symptom. In all patients with hypothyroidism, the effects of analgesic agents, sedatives, and anesthetic agents are prolonged; special caution is necessary in administering these agents to older adult patients because of concurrent changes in liver and renal function. Thyroid hormone replacement must be started with low doses and gradually increased to prevent serious cardiovascular and neurologic side effects, such as angina. Regular testing of serum TSH is recommended for people older than 60 years. Myxedema and myxedema coma generally occur in patients older than 50 years.

> ◄ *Quality and Safety Nursing Alert*
>
> Monitor patients for signs and symptoms of acute coronary syndrome (ACS), which can occur in response to therapy in patients with severe, longstanding hypothyroidism or myxedema coma, especially during the early phase of treatment. ACS must be aggressively treated at once to avoid morbid complications (e.g., myocardial infarction [MI]).

Medical Management

The primary objective is to restore a normal metabolic state by replacing thyroid hormone. Additional treatment in severe hypothyroidism consists of maintaining vital functions, monitoring arterial blood gas (ABG) values, and administering fluids cautiously because of the danger of water intoxication.

Pharmacologic Therapy

- Synthetic levothyroxine (Synthroid or Levothroid) is the common treatment for hypothyroidism and for suppressing nontoxic goiters.
- High-dose glucocorticoids (hydrocortisone) every 8 to 12 hours for 24 hours followed by low-dose therapy is recommended until coexisting adrenal insufficiency is ruled out.
- Concentrated glucose may be given if hypoglycemia is evident.
- If myxedema coma is present, thyroid hormone is given intravenously until consciousness is restored.

Prevention of Medication Interactions

- Thyroid hormone absorption decreases when taking magnesium-containing antacids.
- Thyroid hormones increase blood glucose levels, which may necessitate adjustment in doses of insulin or oral hypoglycemic agents.
- Thyroid hormone may increase the pharmacologic effect of digitalis glycosides, anticoagulant medications, and indomethacin, requiring careful observation and assessment for side effects of these drugs.
- The effects of thyroid hormone may be increased by phenytoin and tricyclic antidepressants.

> ◄ *Quality and Safety Nursing Alert*
>
> Medications are administered to the patient with hypothyroidism with extreme caution because of the potential for altered metabolism and excretion and depressed metabolic rate and respiratory status.

Nursing Management

Promoting Home- and Community-Based Care

Educating Patients About Self-Care
Oral and written instructions should be provided regarding the following:

- Desired actions and side effects of medications
- Correct medication administration
- Importance of continuing to take the medications as prescribed even after symptoms improve
- Time to seek a health care provider
- Importance of nutrition and diet to promote weight loss and normal bowel patterns
- Importance of periodic follow-up testing

The patient and family should be informed that many of the symptoms observed during the course of the disorder will disappear with effective treatment.

Continuing Care
- Before hospital discharge, monitor the patient's recovery and ability to cope with the recent changes, along with the patient's physical and cognitive status. Be sure the family understands the instructions provided.
- Document and report to the patient's primary health care provider subtle signs and symptoms that may indicate either inadequate or excessive thyroid hormone.

For more information, see Chapter 52 in Hinkle, J. L., & Cheever, K. H. (2014). *Brunner and Suddarth's textbook of medical-surgical nursing* (13th ed.). Philadelphia: Lippincott Williams & Wilkins.

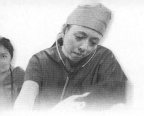

Immune Thrombocytopenic Purpura

Immune thrombocytopenic purpura (ITP) is an autoimmune disorder characterized by a destruction of normal platelets by an unknown stimulus. The disease affects all ages but is more common in children and young women. Other names for the disorder are *idiopathic thrombocytopenic purpura* or *immune thrombocytopenia*. Primary ITP is defined as a platelet count of less than $100 \times 10^9/L$ with an inexplicable absence of a cause for thrombocytopenia and occurs in isolation; secondary ITP often results from an autoimmune disease (e.g., antiphospholipid antibody syndrome, viral infections, HIV infections, and various drugs). Although the precise cause remains unknown, viral infection sometimes precedes the disease in children. Other conditions (e.g., systemic lupus erythematosus, pregnancy) or medications (e.g., sulfa drugs) can also produce ITP.

Pathophysiology

In patients with ITP, antiplatelet autoantibodies develop in the blood and then bind to the patient's platelets. These antibody-bound platelets are ingested and destroyed by the reticuloendothelial system (RES) or tissue macrophage system. The body attempts to compensate for this destruction by increasing platelet production within the marrow. There are two forms of ITP: acute (primarily in children) and chronic.

Clinical Manifestations

- Many patients asymptomatic
- Petechiae and easy bruising (dry purpura)
- Heavy menses and mucosal bleeding (wet purpura; high risk of intracranial bleeding)
- Platelet count generally below 20,000/mm^3
- Acute form self-limiting, possibly with spontaneous remissions

Assessment and Diagnostic Findings

A careful history and physical assessment must be made to exclude causes of thrombocytopenia and to identify evidence of bleeding. Usually, the diagnosis is based on the decreased platelet count, survival time, and increased bleeding time after ruling out other causes of thrombocytopenia. Key diagnostic procedures include platelet count, complete blood cell count, and bone marrow aspiration, which shows an increase in megakaryocytes (platelet precursors). Patients should be tested for hepatitis C and HIV. Many patients are infected with *Helicobacter pylori*. To date, effectiveness of *H. pylori* treatment in relation to management of ITP is unknown.

Medical Management

The primary goal of treatment is a safe platelet count (e.g., counts exceeding 30,000/mm^3). If the patient is taking a medication known to be associated with ITP (e.g., quinine, sulfa-containing medications), the medication should be stopped. Splenectomy is sometimes performed (thrombocytopenia may return months or years later).

Pharmacologic Therapy

Immunosuppressive medications, such as corticosteroids, are the treatment of choice. The bone mineral density of patients receiving chronic corticosteroid therapy needs to be monitored. These patients may benefit from calcium and vitamin D supplementation or bisphosphonate therapy to prevent significant bone disease.

- Intravenous gamma globulin (very expensive) and the chemotherapy agent vincristine are also effective.
- Certain monoclonal antibodies (e.g., rituximab) may increase platelet count.
- Another approach involves using anti-D (WinRho) for patients who are Rh(D) positive.
- Thrombopoietin receptor agonists (romiplostin [Nplate] and eltromopag [Promacta]) have been approved in steroid-refractory ITP.
- Epsilon aminocaproic acid (EACA; Amicar) may be useful for patients with significant mucosal bleeding who are refractory to other treatment modalities.
- Platelet infusions are avoided except to stop catastrophic bleeding.

Nursing Management

- Assess patient's lifestyle to determine the risk of bleeding from activity.

- Obtain history of medication use, including over-the-counter medications, herbs, and nutritional supplements; recent viral illness; or complaints of headache or visual disturbances (intracranial bleed). Be alert for sulfa-containing medications and medications that alter platelet function (e.g., aspirin or other nonsteroidal anti-inflammatory drugs [NSAIDs]). Physical assessment should include a thorough search for signs of bleeding, neurologic assessment, and vital sign measurement.
- Educate patient to recognize exacerbations of disease (petechiae, ecchymoses); how to contact health care personnel; and the names of medications that induce ITP.
- Educate patient regarding the prevalence of fatigue in patients with ITP, explore the extent to which the patient experiences fatigue, and offer strategies to ameliorate fatigue.
- Provide information about medications (tapering schedule, if relevant), frequency of platelet count monitoring, and medications to avoid.
- To minimize bleeding, instruct patient to avoid all agents that interfere with platelet function, including herbal therapies and over-the-counter products. Avoid administering medications by injection or rectal route; rectal temperature measurements should not be performed.
- Instruct patient to avoid constipation, the Valsalva maneuver (e.g., straining at stool), and vigorous tooth flossing.
- Encourage patient to use electric razor for shaving and soft-bristled toothbrushes instead of stiff-bristled brushes.
- Advise patient to refrain from vigorous sexual intercourse when platelet count is less than 10,000/mm³.
- Monitor for complications of long-term corticosteroid use, including osteoporosis, proximal muscle wasting, cataract formation, and dental caries.

For more information, see Chapter 33 in Hinkle, J. L., & Cheever, K. H. (2014). *Brunner and Suddarth's textbook of medical-surgical nursing* (13th ed.). Philadelphia: Lippincott Williams & Wilkins.

Impetigo

Impetigo is a superficial infection of the skin caused by staphylococci, streptococci, or multiple bacteria. Exposed areas of the body, face, hands, neck, and extremities are most frequently involved. Impetigo is contagious and may spread to other parts of the skin; it can also be spread to other family members who touch the patient or who use towels or combs that are soiled with the exudate of the lesion. Impetigo is seen in people of all races and ages. It is particularly common among children living in poor hygienic conditions. Chronic health problems, poor hygiene, and malnutrition may predispose adults to impetigo; it is more prevalent in warm, humid climates (i.e., more common in southeastern United States than in northern climates).

Pathophysiology

Disruptions in the integrity of the skin allow bacteria to colonize below the skin surface. The resulting symptoms are manifestations of the bacterial infection. Bacteria can be spread into the skin by autoinoculation (scratching oneself and spreading the bacteria from the original lesion to a different area). Risk factors include immunosuppression (from medication or systemic disease), trauma, insect bites, or any circumstance that disrupts the skin integrity.

Clinical Manifestations

- Lesions begin as small, red macules that become discrete, thin-walled vesicles. These vesicles rupture and become covered with a honey-yellow crust.
- These crusts, when removed, reveal smooth, red, moist surfaces on which new crusts develop.
- Bullous impetigo, a deep-seated infection of the skin caused by *Staphylococcus aureus*, is characterized by the formation of bullae from original vesicles. The bullae rupture, leaving a raw, red area.

Medical Management

Pharmacologic Therapy

- Topical antibacterial therapy (e.g., mupirocin [Bactroban]), retapamulin [Altabax]) is the usual treatment for impetigo that is limited to a small area. The topical preparation is applied to lesions several times daily for 1 week. Lesions are soaked or washed with antibacterial soap solution to remove the central site of bacterial growth and to give the topical antibiotic an opportunity to reach the infected site.
- Systemic antibiotic agents amoxicillin-clavulanate (Augmentin), cloxacillin (Cloxapen), or dicloxacillin (Dynapen) may be prescribed to treat infections that are widespread or in cases where there are systemic manifestations (e.g., a fever is present). These antibiotic drugs are effective in reducing

contagious spread and as well as treating deep infections and preventing acute glomerulonephritis (kidney infection), which may occur as a consequence of streptococcal skin diseases.

- In cases where methicillin-resistant *Staphylococcus aureus* (MRSA) is present, antibiotic agents may include clindamycin (Cleocin), trimethoprim-sulfamethoxazole (Bactrim), or vancomycin (Vancocin).

Nursing Management

- Wear gloves when caring for patients with impetigo.
- Use antiseptic solutions (chlorhexidine [Hibiclens]) to cleanse the skin at least once daily to reduce bacterial content and prevent spread.
- Educate patient and family members to practice meticulous hand hygiene when touching a lesion, until the lesions are completely healed, to prevent spread of lesion from one skin area to another and from one person to another. Each family member should have a separate towel and washcloth.

For more information, see Chapter 61 in Hinkle, J. L., & Cheever, K. H. (2014). *Brunner and Suddarth's textbook of medical-surgical nursing* (13th ed.). Philadelphia: Lippincott Williams & Wilkins.

Increased Intracranial Pressure

Increased intracranial pressure (ICP) is an excess of the amount of brain tissue, blood, or cerebrospinal fluid (CSF) within the skull at any one time.

Pathophysiology

The volume and pressure of these three components are usually in a state of equilibrium and collectively comprise ICP. Because there is limited space for brain tissue expansion within the skull, an increase in any of these components causes a change in the volume of the others. Compensation is typically accomplished by displacing or shifting CSF, increasing the absorption or diminishing the production of CSF, or decreasing cerebral blood volume. Without such compensatory changes, ICP rises. Although elevated ICP is most commonly associated with head injury, an elevated pressure may be seen secondary to brain tumors, subarachnoid hemorrhage, and toxic and viral encephalopathies. Increased ICP from any cause decreases cerebral perfusion, stimulates further swelling, and may shift brain tissue. The result is herniation, a dire and frequently fatal event.

Clinical Manifestations

When ICP increases to the point where the brain's ability to compensate has reached its limits, neural function is impaired. Increased ICP is manifested by changes in level of consciousness and abnormal respiratory and vasomotor responses.

- Lethargy is the earliest sign of increasing ICP. Agitation, slowing of speech, and delay in response to verbal suggestions are early indicators.
- Sudden change in condition, such as restlessness (without apparent cause), confusion, or increasing drowsiness, has neurologic significance.
- Decreased cerebral perfusion pressure (CPP) can result in a Cushing's response (increase in systolic blood pressure, widening of the pulse pressure, and reflex slowing of the heart rate) and Cushing's triad (bradycardia, bradypnea, and hypertension); widening pulse pressure is an ominous sign.
- As pressure increases, patient becomes stuporous and may react only to loud auditory or painful stimuli. This indicates serious impairment of brain circulation, and immediate surgical intervention may be required. With further deterioration, coma and abnormal motor responses in the form of decortication (abnormal flexion of the upper extremities and extension of the lower extremities), decerebration (extreme extension of the upper and lower extremities), or flaccidity may occur.
- When coma is profound, pupils are dilated and fixed, respirations are impaired, and death is usually inevitable.

Assessment and Diagnostic Findings

- Assess vital signs.
- CT and MRI are the most common diagnostic tests.
- Cerebral angiography, positron emission tomography (PET), and single photon emission tomography (SPECT) imaging are used.
- ICP monitoring provides useful information (ventriculostomy, subarachnoid bolt or screw, epidural monitor, fiberoptic monitor).
- Use transcranial Doppler to assess cerebral blood flow; *evoked potential* monitoring measures the electrical potentials produced by nerve tissue in response to external stimulation (auditory, visual, or sensory).
- Avoid lumbar puncture; sudden release in increased ICP can cause brain to herniate.

Complications

- Brain stem herniation (causes cessation of blood flow to the brain, leading to irreversible brain anoxia and brain death)
- Diabetes insipidus (decreased secretion of antidiuretic hormone [ADH])
- Syndrome of inappropriate antidiuretic hormone (SIADH), an increased secretion of ADH

Medical Management

Increased ICP is a true emergency and must be treated promptly. Immediate management involves invasive monitoring of ICP, decreasing cerebral edema, lowering the volume of CSF, or decreasing cerebral blood volume while maintaining cerebral perfusion. These goals are accomplished by administering osmotic diuretic drugs, restricting fluids, draining CSF, controlling fever, maintaining systemic blood pressure and oxygenation, and reducing cellular metabolic demands.

Pharmacologic Therapy

- Osmotic diuretic agents (e.g., mannitol) and possibly corticosteroids (if due to the mass effect of a tumor) are administered.
- Fluid is restricted to decrease cerebral edema.
- CSF is cautiously drained; excessive drainage may result in collapse of the ventricles and herniation.
- Fever is controlled (using antipyretic medications, hypothermia blanket, and chlorpromazine [Thorazine] to control shivering).
- If patient does not respond to conventional treatment, cellular metabolic demands may be reduced by administering high doses of barbiturates or administering pharmacologic paralyzing agents, such as pancuronium (Pavulon).
- Patient requires care in a critical care unit.

NURSING PROCESS

The Patient With ICP

Assessment

- Obtain patient history with subjective data, including events leading to present illness and pertinent medical history; may require input from family or friends.
- Complete a neurologic examination as patient's condition allows. Evaluate mental status, level of consciousness (LOC),

cranial nerve function, cerebellar function (balance and coordination), reflexes, and motor and sensitivity function.
- Ongoing assessment is more focused, including pupil checks, assessment of selected cranial nerves, frequent measurements of vital signs and ICP, and use of the Glasgow Coma Scale.
- Assess the unconscious patient's level of responsiveness, pattern of respiration, eye movements, corneal reflex, facial symmetry, presence of spontaneous swallowing or drooling, neck movements, response of extremity to noxious stimuli, reflexes, and abnormal posturing.

Diagnosis

NURSING DIAGNOSES
- Ineffective airway clearance related to diminished protective reflexes (cough, gag)
- Ineffective breathing patterns related to neurologic dysfunction (brain stem compression, structural displacement)
- Ineffective cerebral tissue perfusion related to the effects of increased ICP
- Deficient fluid volume related to fluid restriction
- Risk for infection related to ICP monitoring system (fiberoptic or intraventricular catheter)

COLLABORATIVE PROBLEMS/POTENTIAL COMPLICATIONS
- Brain stem herniation
- Diabetes insipidus
- SIADH

Planning and Goals

The major goals of the patient may include maintenance of a patent airway, normalization of respiration, adequate cerebral tissue perfusion through reduction in ICP, restoration of fluid balance, absence of infection, and absence of complications.

Nursing Interventions

MAINTAINING A PATENT AIRWAY
- Maintain patency of the airway; oxygenate patient before and after suctioning.
- Discourage coughing and straining.
- Auscultate lung fields for adventitious sounds or congestion every 8 hours.
- Elevate the head of bed to help clear secretions and improve venous drainage of the brain.

ACHIEVING AN ADEQUATE BREATHING PATTERN
- Monitor constantly for respiratory irregularities.
- Collaborate with respiratory therapist in monitoring arterial carbon dioxide pressure ($PaCO_2$), which is usually maintained below 30 mm Hg when hyperventilation therapy is used.
- Maintain continuous neurologic observation record with repeated assessments.

OPTIMIZING CEREBRAL TISSUE PERFUSION
- Keep patient's head in a neutral (midline) position, maintained with the use of a cervical collar if necessary, to promote venous drainage. Elevation of the head is maintained at 30 to 45 degrees unless contraindicated.
- Avoid extreme rotation and flexion of the neck, because compression or distortion of the jugular veins increases ICP.
- Avoid extreme hip flexion; this position causes an increase in intra-abdominal and intrathoracic pressures, which produce a rise in ICP.
- Rotating beds, turning sheets, and holding the patient's head during turning may minimize the stimuli that increase ICP.
- Instruct patient to avoid the Valsalva maneuver; instruct patient to exhale while moving or turning in bed.
- Provide stool softeners and a high-fiber diet if patient can eat; note any abdominal distention; avoid enemas and cathartic agents.
- Avoid suctioning longer than 15 seconds; pre-oxygenate and hyperventilate on ventilator with 100% oxygen before suctioning.
- Space interventions to prevent transient increases in ICP. During nursing care, ICP should not rise above 25 mm Hg and should return to baseline within 5 minutes.
- Maintain a calm atmosphere and reduce environmental stimuli; avoid emotional stress and frequent arousal from sleep.

MAINTAINING NEGATIVE FLUID BALANCE
- Administer corticosteroids and diuretic drugs as ordered.
- Assess skin turgor, mucous membranes, urine output, and serum and urine osmolality for signs of dehydration.
- Administer IV fluids by pump at a slow to moderate rate; monitor patients receiving mannitol for congestive heart failure and pulmonary edema.

- Monitor vital signs to assess fluid volume status.
- Insert indwelling catheter to assess renal and fluid status.
- Monitor urine output every hour in the acute phase.
- Ensure careful and frequent oral hygiene for mouth dryness.

PREVENTING INFECTION
- Strictly adhere to the facility's written protocols for managing ICP monitoring systems.
- Use aseptic technique at all times when managing the ventricular drainage system and changing drainage bag.
- Check carefully for any loose connections that cause leaking and contamination of the ventricular system and contamination of CSF; check for inaccurate ICP readings.
- Check character of CSF drainage for signs of infection (cloudiness or blood). Report changes.
- Monitor for signs and symptoms of meningitis: fever, chills, nuchal (neck) rigidity, and increasing or persistent headache.

MONITORING AND MANAGING POTENTIAL COMPLICATIONS
Detecting Early Indications of Increasing ICP
Assess for, and immediately report, any of the following early signs or symptoms of increasing ICP: disorientation, restlessness, increased respiratory effort, purposeless movements, or mental confusion; pupillary changes and impaired extra-ocular movements; weakness in one extremity or on one side of the body; headache that is constant, increasing in intensity, and aggravated by movement or straining.

Detecting Later Indications of Increasing ICP
- Assess for and immediately report any of the following later signs and symptoms: LOC that continues to deteriorate until patient is comatose; decreased or erratic pulse rate and respiratory rate, increased blood pressure and temperature, widened pulse pressure, rapidly fluctuating pulse; altered respiratory patterns (Cheyne–Stokes breathing and ataxic breathing); projectile vomiting; hemiplegia; decorticate or decerebrate posturing; loss of brain stem reflexes.
- ICP elevation: Monitor ICP closely for continuous elevation or significant increase over baseline; assess vital signs at time of ICP increase. Assess for, and immediately report, manifestations of increasing ICP.

- Impending brain herniation: Monitor for increase in blood pressure, decrease in pulse, and change in pupillary response.

Monitoring for Secondary Complications

- Diabetes insipidus requires fluid and electrolyte replacement and administration of vasopressin; monitor serum electrolytes for replacement.
- SIADH requires fluid restriction and serum electrolyte monitoring.

Evaluation

EXPECTED PATIENT OUTCOMES

- Maintains patent airway
- Attains optimal breathing pattern
- Demonstrates optimal cerebral tissue perfusion
- Attains desired fluid balance
- Has no signs or symptoms of infection
- Remains free of complications

For more information, see Chapter 66 in Hinkle, J. L., & Cheever, K. H. (2014). *Brunner and Suddarth's textbook of medical-surgical nursing* (13th ed.). Philadelphia: Lippincott Williams & Wilkins.

Influenza

Influenza is an acute viral disease that causes worldwide epidemics every 2 to 3 years and exhibits a highly variable degree of severity. The term *upper respiratory infection* (URI) is used when the causative virus is influenza (the flu). The virus is easily spread from host to host through droplet exposure by coughing, sneezing, or nasal secretions. The virus is shed for about 2 days before the symptoms appear and during the first part of the symptomatic phase. Previous infection with influenza does not guarantee protection from future exposure. Mortality is probably attributable to accompanying pneumonia (viral or superimposed bacterial pneumonia) and exacerbations of chronic obstructive pulmonary disease (COPD) and reduced pulmonary function.

Prevention

Annual influenza vaccinations are recommended for all people 6 months of age and older, especially those at high risk for complications of influenza. These include people age 65 or older, children 6 to 59 months of age, pregnant women, residents of nursing homes or other chronic-care facilities, and those with chronic medical diseases or disabilities. In addition, health care providers and household contacts of those at high risk should also receive the vaccine.

Management

Goals of medical and nursing management include relieving symptoms, treating complications, and preventing transmission. See the "Medical Management" and "Nursing Management" sections under Pharyngitis and Pneumonia for additional information.

For more information, see Chapters 22 and 23 in Hinkle, J. L., & Cheever, K. H. (2014). *Brunner and Suddarth's textbook of medical-surgical nursing* (13th ed.). Philadelphia: Lippincott Williams & Wilkins.

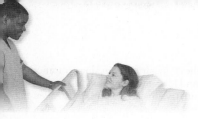

Kaposi's Sarcoma

Kaposi's sarcoma (KS) is the most common HIV-related malignancy and involves the endothelial layer of blood and lymphatic vessels. In people with AIDS, epidemic KS is most often seen among male homosexuals and bisexuals. AIDS-related KS exhibits a variable and aggressive course, ranging from localized cutaneous lesions to disseminated disease involving multiple organ systems.

Clinical Manifestations
- Cutaneous lesions can occur anywhere on the body and are usually brownish pink to deep purple. They characteristically present as lower-extremity skin lesions.
- Lesions may be flat or raised and surrounded by ecchymosis and edema; they develop rapidly and cause extensive disfigurement.
- The location and size of the lesions can lead to venous stasis, lymphedema, and pain. Common sites of visceral involvement include the lymph nodes, gastrointestinal tract, and lungs.
- Involvement of internal organs may eventually lead to organ failure, hemorrhage, infection, and death.

Assessment and Diagnostic Findings
- Diagnosis is confirmed by biopsy of suspected lesions.
- Prognosis depends on extent of tumor, presence of other symptoms of HIV infection, and the CD4+ cell count.
- Pathologic findings indicate that death occurs from tumor progression but more often from other complications of HIV infection.

Medical Management
Treatment goals are to reduce symptoms by decreasing the size of the skin lesions, to reduce discomfort associated with edema and ulcerations, and to control symptoms associated with mucosal or visceral involvement. No one treatment has been shown to improve survival rates. Radiation therapy is effective

as a palliative measure to relieve localized pain due to tumor mass (especially in the legs) and for KS lesions that are in sites such as the oral mucosa, conjunctiva, face, and soles of the feet.

Pharmacologic Therapy

- Patients with cutaneous KS treated with interferon alpha (IFN-α) have experienced tumor regression and improved immune system function.
- IFN-α is administered by the IV, intramuscular, or subcutaneous route. Patients may self-administer interferon at home or receive interferon in an outpatient setting.
- Nonsteroidal anti-inflammatory drugs (NSAIDs) and opioids can be used.

Nursing Management

- Provide thorough and meticulous skin care involving regular turning, cleansing, and application of medicated ointments and dressings.
- Provide analgesic agents at regular intervals around the clock.
- Educate patient about relaxation and guided imagery, which may be helpful in reducing pain and anxiety.
- Educate patient to self-administer IFN-α at home or arrange for patient to receive it in an outpatient setting.
- Support patient in coping with disfigurement from the condition; stress that lesions are temporary, when applicable (after immunotherapy is discontinued).
- Provide supportive care and treatment as ordered to minimize pain and edema, address complications, and promote healing.

For more information, see Chapter 37 in Hinkle, J. L., & Cheever, K. H. (2014). *Brunner and Suddarth's textbook of medical-surgical nursing* (13th ed.). Philadelphia: Lippincott Williams & Wilkins.

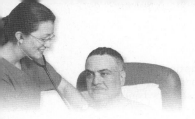

Leukemia

Leukemia is a neoplastic proliferation of one particular cell type (granulocytes, monocytes, lymphocytes [type of white blood cell involved in immune functions], or, infrequently, erythrocytes or megakaryocytes). The leukemias are commonly classified according to the stem cell line involved, either lymphoid (referring to stem cells that produce lymphocytes) or myeloid (referring to stem cells that produce nonlymphoid blood cells). Leukemia is also classified as acute (abrupt onset) or chronic (evolves over months to years). Its cause is unknown. There is some evidence that genetic influence and viral pathogenesis may be involved.

Pathophysiology
Hematopoiesis is characterized by a rapid, continuous turnover of blood cells. Normally, production of specific blood cells from their stem cell precursors is carefully regulated according to the body's needs. If the mechanisms that control the production of these cells are disrupted, the cells can proliferate excessively, as seen in the development of hematologic neoplasms. The common feature of the leukemias is an unregulated proliferation of leukocytes in the bone marrow, leaving little room for normal cell production. Also seen are a proliferation of leukocytes in the liver and spleen and invasion of other organs, such as the meninges, lymph nodes, gums, and skin. There is some evidence that genetic influence and viral pathogenesis may be involved. Bone marrow damage from radiation exposure or chemicals such as benzene and alkylating agents can also cause leukemia.

Clinical Manifestations
Cardinal signs and symptoms may vary based on the particular leukemia and may include weakness, pallor, fatigue, bleeding tendencies, petechiae and ecchymoses, pain, headache, vomiting, fever, infection, lymphadenopathy or splenomegaly, and bone pain.

Assessment and Diagnostic Findings

Blood and bone marrow studies confirm proliferation of white blood cells (WBCs, leukocytes) in the bone marrow.

The Patient With Leukemia

Assessment

- Identify range and duration of signs and symptoms reported by patient in nursing history and physical examination.
- Assess results of blood studies and report alterations of WBCs, absolute neutrophil count (ANC), hematocrit, platelet, creatinine and electrolyte levels, hepatic function tests, and culture results.

Diagnosis

NURSING DIAGNOSES

- Risk for infection and bleeding
- Risk for impaired skin integrity related to toxic effects of chemotherapy, alteration in nutrition, and impaired mobility
- Impaired gas exchange
- Impaired tissue integrity related to damaged mucous membranes from changes in epithelial lining of the gastrointestinal (GI) tract, resulting from chemotherapy or antimicrobial medications
- Imbalanced nutrition: less than body requirements related to hypermetabolic state, anorexia, mucositis, pain, and nausea
- Acute pain and discomfort related to mucositis, leukocytic infiltration of systemic tissues, fever, and infection
- Hyperthermia related to tumor lysis and infection
- Fatigue and activity intolerance related to anemia, infection, and deconditioning
- Impaired physical mobility due to anemia, malaise, discomfort, and protective isolation
- Risk for excess fluid volume related to renal dysfunction, hypoproteinemia, need for multiple IV medications and blood products
- Diarrhea due to altered GI flora, mucosal denudation, prolonged use of broad-spectrum antibiotic medications
- Risk for deficient fluid volume related to potential for diarrhea, bleeding, infection, and increased metabolic rate

- Self-care deficits related to fatigue, malaise, and protective isolation or prolonged hospitalization
- Anxiety due to knowledge deficit and uncertain future
- Disturbed body image related to change in appearance, function, and roles
- Grieving related to anticipatory loss and altered role functioning
- Risk for spiritual distress
- Deficient knowledge of disease process, treatment, complication management, and self-care measures

COLLABORATIVE PROBLEMS/POTENTIAL COMPLICATIONS
- Infection
- Bleeding/disseminated intravascular coagulation (DIC)
- Renal dysfunction
- Tumor lysis syndrome
- Nutritional depletion
- Mucositis
- Depression and anxiety

Planning and Goals

The major goals of the patient may include absence of complications and pain; attainment and maintenance of adequate nutrition; activity tolerance; ability to provide self-care and to cope with the diagnosis and prognosis; positive body image; and an understanding of the disease process and its treatment.

Nursing Interventions

PREVENTING OR MANAGING BLEEDING
- Assess for thrombocytopenia, granulocytopenia, and anemia.
- Report any increase in petechiae, melena, hematuria, or nosebleeds.
- Avoid trauma and injections; use small-gauge needles when analgesic agents are administered parenterally, and apply pressure after injections to avoid bleeding.
- Use acetaminophen instead of aspirin for analgesia.
- Provide prescribed hormone therapy to prevent menses.
- Manage hemorrhage with bed rest and transfuse red blood cells and platelets as ordered.

PREVENTING INFECTION
- Assess vital signs for temperature elevation, flushed appearance, chills, tachycardia, and appearance of white patches in the mouth; monitor WBC.

- Observe for redness, swelling, heat, or pain in eyes, ears, throat, skin, joints, abdomen, and rectal and perineal areas.
- Assess for cough and for changes in character or color of sputum.
- Provide frequent oral hygiene.
- Wear sterile gloves to start infusions.
- Provide daily IV site care; inspect all port-of-entry sites for signs of infection; change all catheter dressings and intravenous infusion sets per institutional frequency protocols.
- Obtain cultures prior to initiation of antimicrobial treatment.
- Ensure normal elimination; use stool softeners to avoid constipation; avoid rectal thermometers, enemas, and rectal trauma; avoid vaginal tampons.
- Avoid catheterization unless essential. Practice scrupulous asepsis if catheterization is necessary.
- Educate patient and family regarding food hygiene and safe food-handling.

> **Quality and Safety Nursing Alert**
>
> The usual manifestations of infection are altered in patients with leukemia. Corticosteroid therapy may blunt the normal febrile and inflammatory responses to infection.

MANAGING MUCOSITIS
- Assess the oral mucosa thoroughly and daily, using same assessment scale; identify and describe lesions; note color and moisture (remove dentures first).
- Encourage patient to report any oral symptoms, including decreased tolerance for food.
- Assist patient with oral hygiene by using a soft-bristle toothbrush.
- Avoid drying agents, such as lemon–glycerin swabs and commercial mouthwashes (use saline or saline–baking soda).
- Emphasize the importance of oral rinse medications to prevent yeast infections.
- Use water-based moisturizers to protect lips.
- Instruct patient to cleanse the perirectal area after each bowel movement; monitor frequency of stools and stop stool softener on presence of loose stool.

Improving Nutritional Intake
- Provide frequent oral hygiene (before and after meals) to promote appetite; with oral anesthetic drugs, caution patient to prevent self-injury and to chew carefully.
- Consider a dietician consultation to coordinate home and institutional intake.
- Maintain nutrition with palatable, small, frequent feedings of soft nonirritating foods; provide nutritional supplements as prescribed; promote relaxation during meals.
- Avoid foods that are spicy, hard to chew, or extreme in temperature.
- Assess for dehydration in severe cases; consult provider to implement oral or topical anesthetic agents if intake is impaired.
- Administer prescribed antiemetic drugs, sedatives, and corticosteroids before chemotherapy and afterward as needed.
- Assess and address other factors contributing to nausea and vomiting.
- Record daily body weight and intake and output to monitor fluid status.
- Perform calorie counts and other more formal nutritional assessments.
- Provide parenteral nutrition, if required.
- Encourage activity levels as tolerated to promote appetite.

Easing Pain and Discomfort
- Administer acetaminophen rather than aspirin for fever reduction and analgesia.
- Sponge patient with cool water for fever; avoid cold water or ice packs; frequently change bedclothes; provide gentle back and shoulder massage.
- Provide oral hygiene (for mucositis), and assist the patient with use of patient-controlled analgesia (PCA) for pain.
- Use creative strategies to permit uninterrupted sleep (a few hours). Assist the patient when awake to balance rest with activity to prevent deconditioning.
- Listen actively to patients enduring pain.

Decreasing Fatigue and Deconditioning
- Help patient avoid fatigue by providing assistance in choosing activities; help patient balance activity and rest; suggest a stationary bicycle and sitting up in chair.
- Assist patient in using a high-efficiency particulate air (HEPA) filter mask to ambulate outside room.

- Encourage patient to sit up in a chair while awake (versus lying in bed).
- Arrange for physical therapy when indicated.

MAINTAINING FLUID AND ELECTROLYTE BALANCE
- Measure intake and output accurately; weigh the patient daily.
- Assess for signs of fluid overload or dehydration.
- Monitor laboratory tests (electrolytes, blood urea nitrogen [BUN], creatinine, and hematocrit), and replace blood, fluids, and electrolyte components as ordered and indicated.
- Treatment with amphotericin increases risk for dehydration.

IMPROVING SELF-CARE
- Encourage the patient to do as much as possible; however, nurse must perform hygiene measures if patient is unable.
- Listen empathetically to the patient.
- Encourage and assist patient to resume more self-care during recovery from treatment.
- Coordinate appropriate home care services as needed.

MANAGING ANXIETY AND GRIEF
- Provide emotional support, and discuss the impact of uncertain future.
- Assess how much information patient wants to have regarding the illness, its treatment, and potential complications; reassess information needs at regular intervals.
- Assist patient to identify the source of grief, and encourage patient to allow time to adjust to the major life changes rendered by the illness.
- Arrange to have communication with nurses across care settings to reassure patient that he or she has not been abandoned.

ENCOURAGING SPIRITUAL WELL-BEING
- Assess the patient's spiritual and religious practices and offer relevant services.
- Assist the patient to maintain realistic hope over the course of the illness (initially, for a cure; in latter stages, for a quiet, dignified death).

PROMOTING HOME- AND COMMUNITY-BASED CARE
Educating Patients About Self-Care
- Ensure that patients and their families have a clear understanding of the disease and complications (risk for infection and bleeding).

- Educate family members about home care while patient is still in the hospital, particularly vascular-access device management if applicable.

Continuing Care
- Maintain communication between the patient and nurses across care settings.
- Provide specific instructions regarding when and how to seek care from the physician.
- Identify which provider to call for which problem.

Terminal Care
- Respect the patient's choices about treatment, including measures to prolong life and other end-of-life measures. Advance directives, including living wills, provide patients with some measure of control during terminal illness.
- Support families and coordinate home care services to alleviate anxiety about managing the patient's care in the home.
- Provide respite for the caregivers and patient with hospice volunteers.
- Provide the patient and caregivers assistance to cope with changes in their roles and responsibilities (i.e., anticipatory grieving).
- Provide information on hospital-based hospice programs for patients to receive palliative care in the hospital when care at home is no longer possible.

Evaluation

EXPECTED PATIENT OUTCOMES
- Shows no evidence of infection
- Experiences no bleeding
- Exhibits intact oral mucous membranes
- Attains optimal level of nutrition
- Reports satisfaction with pain and discomfort levels
- Experiences less fatigue and increases activity
- Maintains fluid and electrolyte balance
- Participates in self-care
- Copes with anxiety and grief
- Experiences absence of complications

For more information, see Chapter 34 in Hinkle, J. L., & Cheever, K. H. (2014). *Brunner and Suddarth's textbook of medical-surgical nursing* (13th ed.). Philadelphia: Lippincott Williams & Wilkins.

Leukemia, Lymphocytic, Acute

Acute lymphocytic leukemia (ALL) results from an uncontrolled proliferation of immature cells (lymphoblasts) from the lymphoid stem cell. It is most common in young children; boys are affected more frequently than girls, with a peak incidence at 4 years of age. Increasing age is associated with diminished survival. After age 15 years, ALL is uncommon until age 50 years, when the incidence rises again. ALL is very responsive to treatment; therapy for this childhood leukemia has improved to the extent that about 80% of children survive at least 5 years; however, survival rates for adults with ALL are much lower.

Pathophysiology

In ALL, the cell of origin is the precursor to the B lymphocyte in approximately 75% of cases; T lymphocytes occur in the remaining 25% of cases. Immature lymphocytes proliferate in the marrow and impede the development of normal myeloid cells. As a result, normal hematopoiesis is inhibited, resulting in reduced numbers of granulocytes, erythrocytes, and platelets.

Clinical Manifestations

- Leukocyte counts are low or high but always include immature cells (lymphoblasts).
- Fevers (high and low), fatigue, petechiae, and pallor occur.
- Manifestations of leukemic cell infiltration into other organs are more common with ALL than with other forms of leukemia and include pain from an enlarged liver or spleen and bone pain.
- The central nervous system is frequently a site for leukemic cells; thus, patients may exhibit headache and vomiting because of meningeal involvement.
- Other extranodal sites include the testes and breasts.

Assessment and Diagnostic Findings

- Complete blood cell count, platelet count, metabolic panel (including uric acid), electrolytes, phosphorus, and serum lactate dehydrogenase (LDH)
- Immunophenotyping to determine lineage (B cell versus T cell)
- Bone marrow aspirate and lumbar puncture
- Baseline electrocardiogram and echocardiogram (if use of anthracycline agents is anticipated)
- Testicular ultrasonography (to assess enlarged testes)

Medical Management

Because ALL frequently invades the central nervous system, preventive intrathecal chemotherapy (e.g., methotrexate) is also a key part of the treatment plan. Initial induction chemotherapy includes corticosteroids (dexamethasone) and vinca alkaloids as an integral part of the initial induction therapy. Typically, an anthracycline is included, sometimes with asparaginase (Elspar). Once the patient is in remission, special testing to assess minimal residual disease (MRD) is performed as a useful prognostic indicator, enabling decisions to be made for consolidation therapy. Once the patient is in remission, consolidation chemotherapy ensues. In the adult with ALL, allogeneic transplant may be used for intensification therapy. When transplant is not an option (or is reserved for relapse), a prolonged maintenance phase ensues, when lower doses of medications are given for up to 3 years. Medical management also includes management of adverse effects related to treatment, including increased susceptibility to infection due to immunosuppression and hepatic toxicity.

Nursing Management

See "Nursing Process" under "Leukemia" for additional information.

For more information, see Chapter 34 in Hinkle, J. L., & Cheever, K. H. (2014). *Brunner and Suddarth's textbook of medical-surgical nursing* (13th ed.). Philadelphia: Lippincott Williams & Wilkins.

Leukemia, Lymphocytic, Chronic

Chronic lymphocytic leukemia (CLL) is a common cancer of older adults characterized by an excess of lymphocytes; in the early stage, an elevated lymphocyte can exceed 100,000/mm^3, The average age at diagnosis is 72 years. CLL is the most common form of leukemia in the United States and Europe; it is infrequently seen in persons of Asian descent and rarely seen in Native Americans. A family history of CLL may be the most important risk factor for developing the disease. The disease is classified into three or four stages; two classification systems are in use. The disease is usually diagnosed during physical examination or treatment for another disease. On average, most patients with CLL survive over 20 years, although some patients may survive for shorter time periods (e.g., 2 to 4 years).

Pathophysiology

CLL is derived from a malignant clone of B lymphocytes. One possible mechanism that explains this oncogenesis is that these cells can escape apoptosis (programmed cell death), resulting in an excessive accumulation of the cells in the marrow and circulation. Most of the leukemia cells in CLL are fully mature, so it tends to be a mild disorder as compared with the acute form. Prognostic markers such as beta$_2$-microglobulin, immunophenotyping, and other special cytogenetic analyses (e.g., fluorescence in situ hybridization [FISH]) are used to guide prognosis and therapy. Autoimmune complications can occur at any stage, as either autoimmune hemolytic anemia or idiopathic thrombocytopenic purpura. Patients with CLL also have a greater risk for developing other cancers, typically bone, lung, and skin. A small minority of patients may experience a gradual transformation in which the disease becomes refractory to chemotherapy; others may experience a sudden transformation to a very aggressive lymphoma (Richter's lymphoma).

Clinical Manifestations

- Many cases are asymptomatic.
- Lymphocytosis is always present.
- Erythrocyte and platelet counts may be normal or decreased in later stages.
- Lymphadenopathy (enlargement of lymph nodes) is common and sometimes severe and painful, and splenomegaly (enlargement of spleen) may be noted.
- CLL patients can develop "B symptoms": fevers, sweats (especially night sweats), and unintentional weight loss. Infections are common.

Medical Management

A major paradigm shift has occurred in CLL therapy. For years, there appeared to be no survival advantage in treating CLL in its early stages. However, with the advent of more sensitive means of assessing therapeutic response, it has been demonstrated that achieving a complete remission—and eradicating even minimal residual disease—results in improved survival. As a result, treatment may be initiated sooner in the illness trajectory; clinical trials are ongoing to assess for an advantage in survival with this approach.

Pharmacologic Therapy

- The chemotherapy agents fludarabine (Fludara) and cyclo-phosphamide (Cytoxan) are often given in combination with the monoclonal antibody rituximab (Rituxan).
- Another alkylating agent, bendamustine (Treanda), is also effective, particularly when combined with rituximab.
- The monoclonal antibody alemtuzumab (Campath) is often used in combination with other chemotherapeutic agents when (1) the disease is refractory to fludarabine, (2) the patient has very poor prognostic markers, or (3) it is necessary to eradicate residual disease after initial treatment.
- Prophylactic use of antiviral agents and antibiotics (e.g., trimethoprim/sulfamethoxazole [Bactrim, Septra]) is recommended for patients receiving alemtuzumab who are at increased risk of infection due to alemtuzumab.
- IV immunoglobulin may prevent recurrent bacterial infections in selected patients.

Nursing Management

See "Nursing Process" under "Leukemia" for additional information.

For more information, see Chapter 34 in Hinkle, J. L., & Cheever, K. H. (2014). *Brunner and Suddarth's textbook of medical-surgical nursing* (13th ed.). Philadelphia: Lippincott Williams & Wilkins.

Leukemia, Myeloid, Acute

Acute myeloid leukemia (AML) is the most common non-lymphocytic leukemia. AML can be further classified into seven different subgroups based on cytogenetics, histology, and morphology (appearance) of the blasts. All age groups are affected; incidence rises with age and peaks at 67 years. Prognosis is highly variable; patient age is a significant factor, in that younger patients have greater 5-year survival rates. The development of AML in people with preexisting myelodysplastic syndrome (MDS) or myeloproliferative disorders, or in those who previously received alkylating agents for cancer, is associated with a more dire prognosis. Secondary AML tends to be more resistant to treatment, resulting in a much shorter duration of remission. Death usually occurs secondary to infection or hemorrhage.

Pathophysiology

AML results from a defect in the hematopoietic stem cell that differentiates into all myeloid cells: monocytes, granulocytes (e.g., neutrophils, basophils, eosinophils), erythrocytes, and platelets. The hematopoietic stem cells become arrested in an early stage of development and do not mature; these resulting cells are called *blasts*. The presence of blasts limits the ability of the bone marrow to produce the normal blood cell population (e.g., erythrocytes, platelets, leukocytes).

Clinical Manifestations

- AML develops without warning, with symptoms typically occurring over a period of weeks.
- Most signs and symptoms evolve from insufficient production of normal blood cells: fever and infection (neutropenia); weakness, dyspnea on exertion, pallor, and fatigue (anemia); petechiae, ecchymoses, and bleeding tendencies (thrombocytopenia).
- Proliferation of leukemic cells within organs leads to a variety of additional symptoms: pain from an enlarged liver or spleen, hyperplasia of the gums, and bone pain from expansion of marrow.
- Leukemic cells can also infiltrate the gingiva or synovial spaces of joints.

Assessment and Diagnostic Findings

- Complete blood cell count (CBC; decreased platelet count and erythrocyte count)
- Leukocyte count low, normal, or high; percentage of normal cells usually vastly decreased
- Bone marrow specimen (excess of immature blast cells)
- Cytogenetic, histologic, and morphologic studies to classify types of blasts

Medical Management

The objective is to achieve complete remission, typically with chemotherapy (induction therapy), which in some instances results in remissions lasting a year or longer.

Pharmacologic Therapy

Chemotherapy consists of induction and consolidation treatment phases.

Induction

- Cytarabine (Cytosar, Ara-C) and daunorubicin (Cerubidine)
- Mitoxantrone (Novantrone) or idarubicin (Idamycin)

- Sometimes etoposide (VP-16, VePesid) added
- In older patients, standard therapy often not well tolerated; lower-intensity therapy (e.g., low doses of cytarabine) possibly required
- Eradicates both leukemic and normal cells; can result in severe neutropenia

Consolidation
- Postremission therapy consists of multiple treatment cycles with chemotherapeutic agents; induction treatments may be repeated but at lower dosages.
- Some form of cytarabine is usually included.

Supportive Care
- Administration of blood products (packed red blood cells [PRBCs] and platelets)
- Prompt treatment of infections
- Granulocyte colony-stimulating factor (G-CSF) (filgrastim [Neupogen]) or granulocyte-macrophage colony-stimulating factor (GM-CSF) (sargramostim [Leukine]) to decrease neutropenia
- Antimicrobial therapy and transfusions as needed
- Occasionally, hydroxyurea (Hydrea) or low-dose cytarabine used briefly to control the increase of blast cells

Hematopoietic Stem Cell Transplantation (Bone Marrow Transplantation)
Hematopoietic stem cell transplantation (HSCT) is used when a tissue match can be obtained. The hematopoietic function of the patient's bone marrow is destroyed with aggressive chemotherapy and, possibly, radiation. It is then "rescued" with an infusion of stem cells from a matched donor to reconstitute normal hematopoietic function. Patients who undergo HSCT have a significant risk for infection, graft-versus-host disease (GVHD, in which the donor's lymphocytes [graft] recognize the patient's body as foreign and set up reactions to attack the foreign host), and other complications. Patients with a poorer prognosis may benefit from early HSCT; those with a good prognosis may not need transplantation at all.

Nursing Management
See "Nursing Process" under "Leukemia" for additional information.

For more information, see Chapter 34 in Hinkle, J. L., & Cheever, K. H. (2014). *Brunner and Suddarth's textbook of medical-surgical nursing* (13th ed.). Philadelphia: Lippincott Williams & Wilkins.

Leukemia, Myeloid, Chronic

Chronic myeloid leukemia (CML) is a myeloproliferative disorder that is characterized by increased production of the granulocytic cell line without loss of the ability to differentiate. CML is uncommon before 20 years of age, but the incidence increases with age (mean age is 65 years). CML has three stages: (1) chronic, (2) transformation, and (3) accelerated or blast crisis.

Pathophysiology

CML arises from a mutation in the myeloid stem cells. Normal myeloid cells continue to be produced, but there is a pathologic increase in the production of forms of blast cells. Marrow expands into cavities of the long bones, and cells are formed in the liver and spleen, with resultant painful enlargement problems. A cytogenetic abnormality termed the *Philadelphia chromosome* is found in 90% to 95% of patients. Patients diagnosed with CML in the chronic phase have few symptoms and complications, with an overall median life expectancy well exceeding 5 years. The transformation phase can be insidious or rapid; it marks the process of evolution (or transformation) to the acute form of leukemia (blast crisis). If the disease transforms to the acute phase (blast crisis), the disease becomes more difficult to treat. Infection and bleeding are rare until the disease transforms to the acute phase.

Clinical Manifestations

- Many patients are asymptomatic, and leukocytosis is detected by a complete blood cell count (CBC) performed for some other reason.
- Leukocyte count commonly exceeds $100,000/mm^3$.
- Patients with extremely high leukocyte counts may be somewhat short of breath or slightly confused because of leukostasis.
- Splenomegaly with tenderness and hepatomegaly are common; lymphadenopathy is rare.
- Some patients have insidious symptoms, such as malaise, anorexia, and weight loss.

Medical Management

Pharmacologic Therapy

- An oral formulation of a tyrosine kinase inhibitor, imatinib mesylate (Gleevec), is prescribed; this is most useful in the chronic stages.

- Other tyrosine kinase inhibitors (dasatinib [Sprycel] or nilotinib [Tasigna]) are also approved for primary therapy; each has a slightly (but importantly) different toxicity profile.
- In those instances where imatinib (at conventional doses) does not elicit a molecular remission, or when that remission is not maintained, other treatment options may be considered.
- Hematopoietic stem cell transplantation (HSCT) is an additional treatment strategy for patients younger than 65 years.
- In the acute form of CML (blast crisis), treatment may resemble induction therapy for acute leukemia, using the same medications as for AML or ALL.
- Oral chemotherapeutic agents, typically hydroxyurea (Hydrea) or busulfan (Myleran), may be used, as may leukapheresis (for leukocyte count greater than 300,000/mm^3). An anthracycline chemotherapeutic agent (e.g., daunomycin [Cerubidine]) may be prescribed for purely palliative approach (rare).

Nursing Management

Nursing management is similar to that for CLL. See "Nursing Process" under "Leukemia" for additional information.

For more information, see Chapter 34 in Hinkle, J. L., & Cheever, K. H. (2014). *Brunner and Suddarth's textbook of medical-surgical nursing* (13th ed.). Philadelphia: Lippincott Williams & Wilkins.

L

Lung Abscess

A lung abscess is necrosis of the pulmonary parenchyma caused by microbial infection. A lung abscess is generally caused by aspiration of anaerobic bacteria and is defined by chest x-ray as a cavity of at least 2 cm. Patients at risk for foreign material aspiration with lung abscess development include those with impaired cough reflexes, loss of glottal closures, or swallowing difficulties. Other at-risk patients include those with central nervous system disorders (e.g., seizure, stroke), drug addiction, alcoholism, esophageal disease, or compromised immune function; patients without teeth and those receiving nasogastric tube feedings; and patients with an altered state of consciousness due to anesthesia.

Pathophysiology

Most lung abscesses are a complication of bacterial pneumonia or are caused by oral anaerobe aspiration into the lung. Abscesses also may occur secondary to mechanical or functional obstruction of the bronchi by a tumor, foreign body, or bronchial stenosis or from necrotizing pneumonias, tuberculosis, pulmonary embolism, or chest trauma.

The site of the lung abscess is related to gravity and is determined by position. For patients who are confined to bed, the posterior segment of an upper lobe and the superior segment of the lower lobe are the most common areas. Atypical presentations may occur, depending on the position of the patient when the aspiration occurred.

Initially, the lung cavity may or may not extend directly into a bronchus. Eventually, the abscess becomes encapsulated by a wall of fibrous tissue. The necrotic process may extend until it reaches the lumen of a bronchus or the pleural space and establishes communication with the respiratory tract, the pleural cavity, or both. Purulent contents are expectorated as sputum if the bronchus is involved. An empyema results if the pleura is involved. A connection between the bronchus and pleura is known as a *bronchopleural fistula*.

Organisms frequently associated with lung abscesses are *S. aureus, Klebsiella,* and other gram-negative species. However, anaerobic organisms may also be present. The organisms vary, depending on underlying predisposing factors.

Clinical Manifestations

- Clinical features vary from a mild productive cough to acute illness.
- Fever is accompanied by a productive cough of moderate to copious amounts of foul-smelling, sometimes bloody sputum.
- Leukocytosis may be present.
- Pleurisy, or dull chest pain, dyspnea, weakness, anorexia, and weight loss are common.

Assessment and Diagnostic Findings

Chest dullness on percussion and decreased or absent breath sounds are found, with an intermittent pleural friction rub and possibly crackles on auscultation. Chest x-ray, sputum culture and, in some cases, fiberoptic bronchoscopy are performed. A CT scan of the chest may be required for more detailed images.

Prevention

To reduce the risk for lung abscess, give appropriate antibiotic therapy before dental procedures and maintain adequate dental and oral hygiene. Give appropriate antimicrobial therapy for pneumonia.

Medical Management

Findings of the history, physical examination, chest x-ray, and sputum culture indicate type of organism and treatment.

- Chest physiotherapy (percussion/postural drainage) may be performed for adequate drainage.
- Percutaneous catheter may be placed for long-term drainage.
- Bronchoscopy for abscess drainage is uncommon.
- Patient is advised to eat a high-protein, high-calorie diet.
- Surgical intervention is rare. Pulmonary resection (lobectomy) is performed when there is massive hemoptysis or no response to medical management.
- IV antimicrobial therapy depends on sputum culture and sensitivity results. Clindamycin (Cleocin) is the standard medication for anaerobic lung infections. Large IV doses are required because the antibiotic must penetrate necrotic tissue and abscess fluid.
- Antibiotics are administered orally instead of intravenously after signs of improvement (normal temperature, decreased white blood cell count, and improvement on chest x-ray showing resolution of infiltrate, reduction in size of cavity, and absence of fluid). Oral antibiotic therapy may last 4 to 12 weeks.

Nursing Management

- Administer antibiotic and IV therapy as prescribed, and monitor for adverse effects.
- Initiate chest physiotherapy, as prescribed, to drain abscess.
- Assess patient for adequate cough; educate patient regarding deep-breathing and coughing exercises.
- Encourage a diet high in protein and calories.
- Provide emotional support as the abscess may take a long time to resolve.

Promoting Home- and Community-Based Care

Educating Patients About Self-Care

- Educate patient or caregivers regarding method of changing the dressings to prevent skin excoriation and odor; method of monitoring for signs and symptoms of infection; and way to care for and maintain the drain or tube.

- Remind patient to perform deep-breathing and coughing exercises every 2 hours during the day.
- Demonstrate chest percussion and postural drainage techniques to caregivers.

Continuing Care

A patient may need review for home care visits. During home visits, the nurse will perform as follows:

- Assess the patient's physical condition, nutritional status, and home environment and patient's and caregiver's ability to carry out the therapeutic regimen.
- Reinforce education by providing counseling for attaining and maintaining an optimal state of nutrition.
- Emphasize importance of completing antibiotic regimen, rest, and appropriate activity levels to prevent relapse.
- Arrange home care nurses to initiate IV antibiotic therapy and evaluate its administration by the patient or caregiver.
- Address health promotion strategies and health screening.

For more information, see Chapter 23 in Hinkle, J. L., & Cheever, K. H. (2014). *Brunner and Suddarth's textbook of medical-surgical nursing* (13th ed.). Philadelphia: Lippincott Williams & Wilkins.

Lymphedema and Elephantiasis

Lymphedema is classified as primary (congenital malformations) or secondary (acquired obstruction). The most common type is congenital lymphedema (lymphedema praecox), caused by hypoplasia of the lymphatic system of the lower extremity. It is usually seen in women and appears first between the ages of 15 and 25 years.

Pathophysiology

Tissues in the extremities swell because of an increased quantity of lymph that results from an obstruction of the lymphatic vessels. It is especially marked when the extremity is in a dependent position. Initially, the edema is soft and pitting. As the condition progresses, the edema becomes firm, nonpitting, and unresponsive to treatment. The obstruction may be in both the lymph nodes and the lymphatic vessels. At times, it is seen in the arm after a radical mastectomy and in the leg in association with varicose veins or a chronic thrombophlebitis (from lymphangitis). When chronic swelling is present, there may be frequent bouts of infection (high fever and chills) and increased residual edema after inflammation resolves. These lead to chronic fibrosis, thickening of the subcutaneous tissues, and hypertrophy of the skin. Lymphatic obstruction caused by a parasite (filaria) is seen frequently in the tropics; the infection causes extreme swelling in the lower extremities. The condition in which chronic swelling of the extremity recedes only slightly with elevation is referred to as elephantiasis.

Medical Management

- The goal of therapy: to reduce and control edema and prevent infection
- Active and passive exercise to assist in moving lymphatic fluid into the bloodstream; also manual lymphatic drainage (a massage technique)
- External compression devices; custom-fitted elastic stockings, when patient is ambulatory
- Strict bed rest with leg elevation to help mobilize fluids
- Manual lymphatic drainage in combination with multilayer compression bandages, exercises, skin care, pressure gradient sleeves, and pneumatic pumps (depending on the severity and stage of the lymphedema)

Pharmacologic Therapy

- Diuretic therapy, initially with furosemide (Lasix) to prevent fluid overload, and other diuretic therapy palliatively for lymphedema
- Antibiotic therapy in presence of lymphangitis or cellulitis

Surgical Management

- Excision of the affected subcutaneous tissue and fascia, with skin grafting to cover the defect
- Surgical relocation of superficial lymphatic vessels into the deep lymphatic system by means of a buried dermal flap to provide a conduit for lymphatic drainage

Nursing Management

- If the patient undergoes surgery, provide standard post-surgical care of skin grafts and flaps, elevate the affected extremity, and continuously observe for complications (e.g., flap necrosis, hematoma, or abscess under the flap, cellulitis).

- Instruct patient or caregiver to inspect the dressing daily; unusual drainage or any inflammation around the wound margin should be reported to the surgeon.
- Inform patient that there may be a loss of sensation in the skin graft area.
- Instruct patient to avoid the application of heating pads or exposure to sun to prevent burns or trauma to the area.

For more information, see Chapter 30 in Hinkle, J. L., & Cheever, K. H. (2014). *Brunner and Suddarth's textbook of medical-surgical nursing* (13th ed.). Philadelphia: Lippincott Williams & Wilkins.

Lymphomas, Non-Hodgkin

The non-Hodgkin lymphomas (NHLs) are a heterogeneous group of cancers that originate from the neoplastic growth of lymphoid tissue. NHL is the seventh most common type of cancer diagnosed in the United States; incidence rates have almost doubled in the last 35 years, with a median age at diagnosis of 65 years. The incidence of NHL has increased in the following groups: people with immunodeficiencies or autoimmune disorders; who have received prior treatment for cancer; who were prior organ transplant recipients; and who had viral infections (including Epstein-Barr virus and HIV). Prognosis varies by subtype: For example, the most common diffuse large B cell has 5-year survival rates of 26% to 30% and the less common follicular lymphoma has a 5-year survival rate of 70%. Other factors associated with a poorer prognosis include excessive alcohol intake, obesity, and smoking.

Pathophysiology

Most NHLs involve malignant B lymphocytes; only 5% involve T lymphocytes. In contrast to Hodgkin lymphoma, the lymphoid tissues involved in NHL are largely infiltrated with malignant cells. The spread of these malignant lymphoid cells occurs unpredictably, and true localized disease is uncommon. Lymph nodes from multiple sites may be infiltrated, as may sites outside the lymphoid system (extranodal tissue).

Clinical Manifestations

- Early symptoms may be absent or very minor; symptoms tend to appear in later stages.
- Lymphadenopathy is most common and may wax and wane.

- B symptoms (fever, drenching night sweats, and unintentional weight loss) may be seen in one-third of patients.
- Lymphomatous masses can compromise organ function (e.g., mediastinal mass may cause respiratory distress).
- Involvement of the central nervous system with lymphoma is becoming increasingly common.

Assessment and Diagnostic Findings

- Disease is classified based on histopathology, immunophenotyping, and cytogenetic analyses of the malignant cells. Classification has prognostic implications.
- NHL for a given patient is assigned one of four stages at diagnosis. Staging is done with CT and positron emission tomography (PET) scans, bone marrow biopsies and, occasionally, analysis of cerebrospinal fluid.
- Two prognostic classification systems have been developed that are particularly useful in the older patient population: the International Prognostic Index (IPI) and, for follicular lymphomas, the Follicular Lymphoma International Prognostic Index (FLIPI).

Medical Management

Treatment is determined by the classification of disease, the stage of disease, prior treatment (if any), and the patient's ability to tolerate therapy as dictated by the patient's renal, hepatic, and cardiac function; the presence of concurrent diseases; functional status; and age. There is no standard therapy for follicular lymphoma; "watchful waiting," where therapy is delayed until symptoms develop, has often been used in those with indolent disease. Radiation alone may be used for localized disease that is not an aggressive cell type; with aggressive types of NHL, aggressive combinations of chemotherapeutic agents are used. Cranial radiation or intrathecal chemotherapy is used, in addition to systemic chemotherapy for central nervous system involvement. Immunotherapy and conventional chemotherapy, along with radiopharmaceutical agents, are used for follicular lymphomas. Treatment after relapse is controversial; hematopoietic stem cell transplantation (HSCT) may be considered for patients younger than 60 years.

Pharmacologic Therapy

- With aggressive types of lymphomas, standard treatment for common lymphomas is the combination of the monoclonal antibody rituximab (Rituxan) with conventional chemotherapy protocols referred to as *R-CHOP* (includes cytoxan, doxorubicin, vincristine, and prednisone).

- In follicular lymphomas, immunotherapy (e.g., rituximab) is often used in combination with conventional chemotherapy.
- Radiopharmaceutical agents (e.g., ibritumomab tiuxetan [Zevalin] or tositumomab/iodine-131 [Bexxar]) are also used, although they cause technical difficulties with administration due to the radioactivity of the agent.
- More aggressive treatment (often R-CHOP or R-Bendamustine [Levact]) may provide a longer duration of remission during which additional treatment is not needed.

Nursing Management

See "Nursing Management" under Cancer in Section C for additional information about nursing interventions for patients undergoing chemotherapy and radiation treatments.

- When caring for patients with lymphoma, it is extremely important for the nurse to know the specific disease type, stage of disease, treatment history, and current treatment plan. Most care takes place in the outpatient setting.
- Additional complications depend on the location of the lymphoma. Therefore, the nurse must know the tumor location so that assessments can be targeted appropriately.
- Educate patients and families that while many lymphomas can be cured, survivors should be screened regularly for the development of second malignancies.

For more information, see Chapter 34 in Hinkle, J. L., & Cheever, K. H. (2014). *Brunner and Suddarth's textbook of medical-surgical nursing* (13th ed.). Philadelphia: Lippincott Williams & Wilkins.

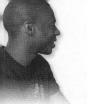
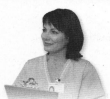

Mastoiditis and Mastoid Surgery

Mastoiditis is an inflammation of the mastoid resulting from an infection of the middle ear (otitis media). Since the discovery of antibiotic agents, acute mastoiditis has been rare. Chronic otitis media may cause chronic mastoiditis. Chronic mastoiditis can lead to the formation of cholesteatoma (a cystlike lesion in the middle ear) that may require surgical removal.

Clinical Manifestations
- Pain and tenderness behind the ear (postauricular)
- Foul-smelling discharge from the middle ear (otorrhea)
- Mastoid area that becomes erythematous and edematous

Medical Management
General symptoms are usually successfully treated with antibiotic agents; occasionally, myringotomy is required.

Surgical Management
If recurrent or persistent tenderness, fever, headache, and discharge from the ear are evident, mastoidectomy may be necessary to remove the cholesteatoma and gain access to diseased structures.

NURSING PROCESS

The Patient Undergoing Mastoid Surgery

Assessment

- During the health history, collect data about the ear problem, including infection, otalgia, otorrhea, hearing loss and vertigo, duration and intensity, causation, prior treatments, health problems, current medications, family history, and drug allergies.
- During the physical assessment, observe for erythema, edema, otorrhea, lesions, and odor and color of discharge.
- Review results of audiogram.

Diagnosis

NURSING DIAGNOSES

- Anxiety related to surgical procedure, potential loss of hearing, potential taste disturbance, and potential loss of facial movement
- Acute pain related to mastoid surgery
- Risk for infection related to mastoidectomy, placement of grafts, prostheses, or electrodes; surgical trauma to surrounding tissues and structures
- Disturbed auditory sensory perception related to ear disorder, surgery, or packing
- Risk for trauma related to impaired balance or vertigo during the immediate postoperative period, or from dislodgment of the graft or prosthesis
- Disturbed sensory perception related to potential damage to facial nerve (cranial nerve VII) and chorda tympani nerve
- Deficient knowledge about mastoid disease, surgical procedure, and postoperative care and expectations

Planning and Goals

Major goals for the patient undergoing mastoidectomy include reduction of anxiety; freedom from pain and discomfort; prevention of infection; stable or improved hearing and communication; absence of vertigo and related injury; absence of, or adjustment to, sensory or perceptual alterations; and increased knowledge regarding the disease, surgical procedure, and postoperative care.

Nursing Interventions

REDUCING ANXIETY

- Reinforce information that the otologic surgeon has discussed: anesthesia, the location of the incision (postauricular), and expected surgical results (hearing, balance, taste, and facial movement).
- Encourage patient to discuss any anxiety or concerns.

RELIEVING PAIN

- Administer prescribed analgesic agent for the first 24 hours postoperatively and then only as needed.
- If a tympanoplasty is also performed, inform patient that he or she may have packing or a wick in the external auditory canal and may experience sharp shooting pains in the ear for 2 to 3 weeks postoperatively.

- Inform patient that throbbing pain accompanied by fever may indicate infection and should be reported to the physician.

PREVENTING INFECTION
- Explain the prescribed prophylactic antibiotic regimen to the patient; ear packing may contain antibiotic.
- Instruct patient to keep water from entering the ear for 6 weeks and to keep postauricular incision dry for 2 days; a cotton ball or lamb's wool covered with a water-insoluble substance (e.g., petroleum jelly) and placed loosely in the ear canal usually prevents water contamination during exposure.
- Observe for and report signs of infection (fever, purulent drainage).
- Inform patient that some serosanguineous drainage is normal postoperatively.

IMPROVING HEARING AND COMMUNICATION
- Initiate measures to improve hearing and communication: Reduce environmental noise, face patient when speaking, and speak clearly and distinctly without shouting. Provide good lighting if patient must speech-read (also called lip-reading), and use nonverbal clues.
- Instruct family that patient will have temporarily reduced hearing from surgery as a result of edema, packing, and fluid in middle ear; instruct family in ways to improve communication with patient.

PREVENTING INJURY
- Administer antiemetic or antivertiginous medications (e.g., antihistamine agents) as prescribed if a balance disturbance or vertigo occurs.
- Assist patient with ambulation to prevent falls and injury.
- Instruct patient to avoid heavy lifting, straining, exertion, and nose blowing for two to three weeks after surgery; this will help to prevent dislodging of the tympanic membrane graft or ossicular prosthesis.

PREVENTING ALTERED SENSORY PERCEPTION
- Reinforce to patient that a taste disturbance and dry mouth may be experienced on the operated side for several months, until the nerve regenerates.
- Instruct patient to immediately report any evidence of facial nerve (cranial nerve VII) weakness, such as drooping of the mouth on the operated side.

PROMOTING HOME- AND COMMUNITY-BASED CARE
- Provide instructions about prescribed medications: analgesic medications, antivertiginous agents, and antihistamine drugs for balance disturbance.
- Inform patient about the expected effects and potential side effects of the medications.
- Instruct patient about any activity restrictions.
- Educate patient to monitor for possible complications, such as infection, facial nerve weakness, or taste disturbances, including specific signs and symptoms; report these immediately to the surgeon.
- Refer patients, particularly elderly patients, for home care nursing.
- Caution caregiver and patient that patient may experience some vertigo and will therefore require help with ambulation to avoid falling.
- Stress the importance of scheduling and keeping follow-up appointments.

Evaluation

EXPECTED PATIENT OUTCOMES
- Demonstrates reduced anxiety about surgical procedure
- Remains free of discomfort or pain
- Demonstrates no signs or symptoms of infection
- Exhibits signs that hearing has stabilized or improved
- Remains free of injury and trauma
- Adjusts to, or remains free of, altered sensory perception
- Verbalizes the reasons for, and methods of, care and treatment

For more information, see Chapter 64 in Hinkle, J. L., & Cheever, K. H. (2014). *Brunner and Suddarth's textbook of medical-surgical nursing* (13th ed.). Philadelphia: Lippincott Williams & Wilkins.

Ménière's Disease

Ménière's disease is an abnormal inner-ear fluid balance (too much endolymph fluid) caused by malabsorption in the endolymphatic sac or blockage in the duct. Endolymphatic hydrops, a dilation in the endolymphatic space, develops. Either increased pressure in the system or rupture of the inner ear membranes occurs, producing symptoms. Although it has been reported in children, Ménière's disease is more common in adults, with the average age of onset in the 40s. There is no cure. Two possible subsets of the disease exist: cochlear and vestibular.

Cochlear Disease
Cochlear disease is recognized as a fluctuating, progressive sensorineural hearing loss associated with tinnitus and aural pressure in the absence of vestibular symptoms or findings.

Vestibular Disease
Vestibular disease is characterized as the occurrence of episodic vertigo associated with aural pressure but without cochlear symptoms.

Clinical Manifestations
Symptoms of Ménière's disease include fluctuating, progressive sensorineural hearing loss; tinnitus or a roaring sound; a feeling of pressure or fullness in the ear; and episodic, incapacitating vertigo, often accompanied by nausea and vomiting. At the onset, only one or two symptoms may be manifested.

Assessment and Diagnostic Findings
- Disease is not diagnosed until the four major symptoms, as noted above, are present; careful history of vertigo, as well as episodes of nausea and vomiting, contribute to diagnosis.
- There is no absolute diagnostic test for this disease.
- Audiovestibular diagnostic procedures, including Weber's test and audiometry, are used to detect sensorineural hearing loss in the affected ear.
- Electronystagmogram may be normal or may show reduced vestibular response.
- Electrocochleography is used to assess inner ear pressures.

Medical Management
Goals of treatment include reduction of symptoms (e.g., vertigo) and prevention of additional episodes. This may be accomplished by recommending a salt-restricted diet, use of diuretics and steroids. The treatment is designed to eliminate vertigo or to stop the progression of, or stabilize, the disease. Psychological evaluation may be indicated if the patient is anxious, uncertain, fearful, or depressed.

Dietary Management
- Low sodium (1,000 to 1,500 mg per day or less)
- Avoidance of alcohol, monosodium glutamate (MSG), aspirin and aspirin-containing medications

Pharmacologic Therapy

- Antihistamine medications, such as meclizine (Antivert), to shorten the attack; tranquilizers such as diazepam (Valium) to help control vertigo; antiemetic agents such as promethazine (Phenergan) suppositories to control the nausea, vomiting, and vertigo
- Diuretics (hydrochlorothiazide alone [Aquazide] or with triamterene [Dyazide] or acetazolamine [Diamox]) to lower pressure in the endolymphatic system
- Intratympanic injection of gentamicin (Garamycin) to ablate vestibular hair cells, though risk of hearing loss is high

Surgical Management

Surgical procedures include endolymphatic sac procedures and vestibular nerve section. However, hearing loss, tinnitus, and aural fullness may continue, because the surgical treatment of Ménière's disease is aimed at eliminating the attacks of vertigo.

NURSING PROCESS

The Patient With Vertigo

Preventing Injury

- Assess for vertigo.
- Reinforce vestibular and balance therapy as prescribed.
- Administer and educate patient about antivertiginous medication and vestibular sedation; instruct in side effects.
- Encourage patient to sit down when dizzy.
- Recommend that patient keep eyes open and stare straight ahead when lying down and experiencing vertigo; place pillows on side of head to restrict movement.
- Assist patient in identifying aura that suggests an impending attack.

Adjusting to Disability

- Encourage patient to identify personal strengths and roles that can be fulfilled.
- Provide information about vertigo and what to expect.
- Include family and significant others in rehabilitative process.
- Encourage patient in making decisions and assuming more responsibility for care.

Maintaining Fluid Volume

- Assess intake and output; monitor laboratory values.
- Assess indicators of dehydration.
- Encourage oral fluids as tolerated; avoid caffeine (a vestibular stimulant).
- Educate patient about antiemetic and antidiarrheal medications.

Relieving Anxiety

- Assess level of anxiety; help identify successful coping skills.
- Provide information about vertigo and its treatment.
- Encourage patient to discuss anxieties and explore concerns about vertigo attacks.
- Educate patient about stress management; provide comfort measures.

Educating Patients About Self-Care

- Show patient how to administer antiemetic and other prescribed medications to relieve nausea and vomiting.
- Encourage patient to care for bodily needs when free of vertigo.
- Review diet with patient and caregivers; offer fluids as necessary.

For more information, see Chapter 64 in Hinkle, J. L., & Cheever, K. H. (2014). *Brunner and Suddarth's textbook of medical-surgical nursing* (13th ed.). Philadelphia: Lippincott Williams & Wilkins.

M

Meningitis

Meningitis is an inflammation of the meninges (lining around the brain and spinal cord) caused by bacteria, viruses, or fungi. Meningitis is classified as aseptic or septic. The aseptic form may be viral or secondary to an impaired immune system as with lymphoma, leukemia, or human immunodeficiency virus (HIV). The septic form is caused by bacteria such as *Streptococcus pneumoniae* and *Neisseria meningitidis*. Outbreaks of *N. meningitidis* infection are most likely to occur in dense community groups, such as college campuses and military installations; peak incidence in the winter and early spring. Increased risk of bacterial meningitis is associated with tobacco use, viral upper respiratory infection, otitis media, mastoiditis and immune system deficiencies.

Pathophysiology

Meningeal infections generally originate in one of two ways: either through the bloodstream from other infections (cellulitis) or by direct extension (after a traumatic injury to the facial bones). The causative organism enters the bloodstream, crosses the blood–brain barrier, and triggers an inflammatory reaction in the meninges. Independent of the causative agent, inflammation of the subarachnoid and pia mater occurs. Increased intracranial pressure (ICP) results. Bacterial or meningococcal meningitis also occurs as an opportunistic infection in patients with acquired immunodeficiency syndrome (AIDS) and as a complication of Lyme disease. Bacterial meningitis is the most significant form. The common bacterial pathogens are N. meningitidis (meningococcal meningitis) and S. pneumoniae, accounting for 80% of cases of meningitis in adults. Haemophilus influenzae was once a common cause of meningitis in children, but, because of vaccination, infection with this organism is now rare in developed countries.

Clinical Manifestations

- Headache and fever are frequently the initial symptoms; fever tends to remain high throughout the course of the illness; the headache is usually either steady or throbbing and very severe as a result of meningeal irritation.
- Meningeal irritation results in a number of other well-recognized signs common to all types of meningitis:
  - Nuchal rigidity (stiff neck) is an early sign.
  - Positive Kernig's sign: When lying with thigh flexed on abdomen, patient cannot completely extend leg.
  - Positive Brudzinski's sign (a more sensitive indicator of meningeal irritation than Kernig's sign): Flexing patient's neck produces flexion of the knees and hips; passive flexion of lower extremity of one side produces similar movement for opposite extremity.
  - Photophobia (extreme sensitivity to light) is common.
  - Rash (N. meningitidis): ranges from petechial rash with purpuric lesions to large areas of ecchymosis.
  - Disorientation and memory impairment; behavioral manifestations are also common. As the illness progresses, lethargy, unresponsiveness, and coma may develop.
- Seizures can occur and are the result of areas of irritability in the brain; ICP increases secondary to diffuse brain swelling or hydrocephalus; initial signs of increased ICP include decreased level of consciousness and focal motor deficits.

- An acute fulminant infection occurs in about 10% of patients with meningococcal meningitis, producing signs of overwhelming septicemia: an abrupt onset of high fever, extensive purpuric lesions (over the face and extremities), shock, and signs of disseminated intravascular coagulation (DIC); death may occur within a few hours after onset of the infection.

Assessment and Diagnostic Findings

- Computed tomography (CT) scan or magnetic resonance imaging (MRI) scan should be performed to detect a shift in brain contents (which may lead to herniation) prior to a lumbar puncture.
- Key diagnostic tests include a bacterial culture and Gram staining of cerebrospinal fluid (CSF) and blood.

Prevention

The Advisory Committee on Immunization Practices of the Centers for Disease Control and Prevention (CDC) (2008) recommends that the initial meningococcal conjugated vaccine be given to adolescents entering high school with a booster given to college freshmen living in dormitories. Vaccination should also be considered as an adjunct to antibiotic chemoprophylaxis for anyone living with a person who develops meningococcal infection. Vaccination against *H. influenzae* and *S. pneumoniae* should be encouraged for children and at-risk adults.

People in close contact with patients with meningococcal meningitis should be treated with antimicrobial chemoprophylaxis using rifampin (Rifadin), ciprofloxacin hydrochloride (Cipro), or ceftriaxone sodium (Rocephin). Therapy should be started within 24 hours after exposure because a delay in the initiation of therapy limits the effectiveness of the prophylaxis.

Medical Management

Early administration of antibiotics (optimally within 30 minutes of hospital arrival) that cross the blood–brain barrier halt the multiplication of bacteria. Dehydration and shock are treated with fluid volume expanders. Seizures, which may occur early in the course of the disease, are controlled with phenytoin (Dilantin). Increased ICP is treated as necessary.

Pharmacologic Therapy

Choice of antibiotic is based upon sensitivities; however, initial empiric treatment may be given prior to obtaining culture results including:

- Ampicillin (or vancomycin) in combination with one of the cephalosporins (e.g., ceftriaxone sodium, cefotaxime sodium) is administered by intravenous (IV) injection.
- Dexamethasone (Decadron) has been shown to be beneficial as adjunct therapy in the treatment of acute bacterial meningitis and in pneumococcal meningitis.
- Seizures, which may occur early in the course of the disease, are controlled with phenytoin (Dilantin).

Nursing Management

Prognosis depends largely on the supportive care provided. Related nursing interventions include the following:

- Institute infection control precautions until 24 hours after initiation of antibiotic therapy (oral and nasal discharge is considered infectious).
- Assess neurologic status and vital signs constantly. Determine oxygenation from arterial blood gas values and pulse oximetry.
- Insert cuffed endotracheal tube (or tracheostomy), and position patient on mechanical ventilation as prescribed.
- Assess blood pressure (usually monitored using an arterial line) for incipient shock, which precedes cardiac or respiratory failure.
- Rapid IV fluid replacement may be prescribed, but take care not to overhydrate patient because of risk of cerebral edema.
- Reduce high fever to decrease load on heart and brain from oxygen demands.
- Protect the patient from injury secondary to seizure activity or altered level of consciousness (LOC).
- Provide analgesia for pain management.
- Promote rest by providing a quiet, darkened room.
- Monitor daily body weight; serum electrolytes; and urine volume, specific gravity, and osmolality, especially if syndrome of inappropriate antidiuretic hormone (SIADH) is suspected.
- Prevent complications associated with immobility, such as pressure ulcers and pneumonia.
- Inform family about patient's condition and permit family to see patient at appropriate intervals.

For more information, see Chapter 69 in Hinkle, J. L., & Cheever, K. H. (2014). *Brunner and Suddarth's Textbook of Medical-Surgical Nursing* (13th ed.). Philadelphia: Lippincott Williams & Wilkins.

Mitral Regurgitation (Insufficiency)

Mitral regurgitation involves blood flowing back from the left ventricle into the left atrium during systole. Often, the edges of the mitral valve leaflets do not close during systole because leaflets and chordae tendineae have thickened and fibrosed, effecting the contraction. In developed countries, mitral valve degenerative changes and left ventricle ischemia are the most common causes, whereas in developing countries, rheumatic heart disease and its sequelae are the cause of mitral regurgitation. Myxomatous changes, infective endocarditis, collagen vascular diseases, cardiomyopathy, and ischemic heart disease are also conditions that lead to mitral regurgitation.

Pathophysiology

Mitral regurgitations may result from problems with one or more of the leaflets, the chordae tendineae, the annulus, or the papillary muscles. With each beat, the left ventricle forces some blood back into the left atrium, causing the atrium to dilate and hypertrophy. Backward flow of blood from the ventricle decreases blood flow from the lungs into the atrium and eventually causes the lungs to become congested, adding extra strain to the right ventricle, which dilates, resulting in systolic heart failure.

Clinical Manifestations

Chronic mitral regurgitation is often asymptomatic, but acute regurgitation (resulting from myocardial infarction [MI]) usually presents as severe congestive heart failure.

- Dyspnea, fatigue, and weakness are the most common symptoms.
- Palpitations, shortness of breath on exertion, and cough from pulmonary congestion also occur.

Assessment and Diagnostic Findings

A systolic murmur is a high-pitched, blowing sound at the apex. The pulse may be regular and of good volume, or it may be irregular as a result of extrasystolic beats or atrial fibrillation. Echocardiography is used to diagnose and monitor the progression of mitral regurgitation. Transesophageal echocardiography (TEE) provides the best images of the mitral valve.

Medical Management

Management is the same as for heart failure (see Heart Failure in Section H). Patients with mitral regurgitation and heart failure are treated with angiotensin-converting enzyme (ACE) inhibitors such as captopril (Capoten), enalapril (Vasotec), lisinopril (Prinivil, Zestril), ramipril (Altace), or with angiotensin receptor blockers (ARBs) such as losartan (Cozaar) or valsartan (Diovan); and with beta-blockers, such as carvedilol (Coreg), to help reduce afterload. Hydralazine (Apresoline) is used along with nitrates as a vasodilator to improve systolic function in select patients. Restriction of activity level will help to minimize symptoms.

Surgical Management
Surgical intervention consists of mitral valvuloplasty or mitral valve replacement.

For more information, see Chapter 28 in Hinkle, J. L., & Cheever, K. H. (2014). *Brunner and Suddarth's textbook of medical-surgical nursing* (13th ed.). Philadelphia: Lippincott Williams & Wilkins.

Mitral Stenosis

Mitral stenosis is an obstruction to blood flowing from the left atrium into the left ventricle. It most often is caused by rheumatic endocarditis, which progressively thickens mitral valve leaflets and chordae tendineae. Leaflets often fuse together. Eventually, the mitral valve orifice narrows and progressively obstructs blood flow into the ventricle.

Pathophysiology
A normal mitral valve orifice is about three fingers wide. In cases of severe stenosis, the orifice narrows to the width of a pencil. The left atrium has difficulty in moving blood into the ventricle because of increased resistance by the narrowed orifice. Poor left ventricular filling can cause decreased cardiac output. Increased blood volume in the left atrium causes it to dilate and hypertrophy. Because there is no valve to protect pulmonary veins from backward flow of blood from the left atrium, the pulmonary circulation becomes congested. As a result, the right ventricle must contract against abnormally high pulmonary arterial pressure and is subjected to excessive strain. The right ventricle hypertrophies and eventually dilates and fails. If heart rate increases, diastole is shortened, resulting in less time for forward flow of blood and in backflow of blood in the pulmonary veins. Therefore, as heart rate increases, cardiac output decreases, and pulmonary pressures increase.

Clinical Manifestations
- Dyspnea on exertion (due to pulmonary venous hypertension) is often the first symptom.

- Progressive fatigue and decreased exercise tolerance are results of low cardiac output.
- Dry cough or wheezing, hemoptysis, palpitations, orthopnea, paroxysmal nocturnal dyspnea (PND), and repeated respiratory infections are evident.
- Atrial dysrhythmias occur (owing to increased blood volume and pressure dilating the atrium).

Assessment and Diagnostic Findings
- Weak and often irregular pulse (because of atrial fibrillation) may also be noted.
- Low-pitched, rumbling diastolic murmur is heard at the apex.
- Echocardiography is used to diagnose and quantify mitral stenosis severity.
- Electrocardiography (ECG), exercise testing, and cardiac catheterization with angiography may be used to help determine the severity of the mitral stenosis.

Prevention
Prevention of mitral stenosis primarily is based on avoidance or treatment of bacterial infections. See Endocarditis, Rheumatic in Section E for more information on prevention.

Medical Management
Medical management measures include the following:

- Treat congestive heart failure as described in Heart Failure (see Section H).
- Administer anticoagulants to decrease the risk for developing atrial thrombus.
- Apply cardioversion if atrial fibrillation develops.
- Control ventricular rate with beta-blockers, digoxin, or calcium channel blockers.
- Educate patient to avoid strenuous exercise, competitive sports, and pregnancy.

Surgical Management
- Surgical intervention consists of valvuloplasty, usually a commissurotomy to open or rupture the fused commissures of the mitral valve.
- Percutaneous transluminal valvuloplasty or mitral valve replacement may be performed.

For more information, see Chapter 28 in Hinkle, J. L., & Cheever, K. H. (2014). *Brunner and Suddarth's textbook of medical-surgical nursing* (13th ed.). Philadelphia: Lippincott Williams & Wilkins.

Mitral Valve Prolapse

Mitral valve prolapse is a deformity of one or both mitral valve leaflets and usually produces no symptoms. It occurs more frequently in women. The cause may be an inherited connective tissue disorder but, in many cases, the cause is unknown.

Pathophysiology

In mitral valve prolapse, a portion of one or both mitral valve leaflets balloons back into the atrium during systole. Rarely, ballooning stretches the leaflet to the point that the valve does not remain closed during systole. Blood then regurgitates from the left ventricle back into the left atrium. About 15% of patients who develop murmurs eventually experience heart enlargement, atrial fibrillation, pulmonary hypertension, or heart failure.

Clinical Manifestations

The syndrome may produce no symptoms or, rarely, it progresses and can result in sudden death.

- Patients may experience shortness of breath (not correlated with activity), lightheadedness, dizziness, syncope, palpitations, chest pain, and anxiety.
- Fatigue may be present regardless of the person's activity level and amount of rest or sleep.

Assessment and Diagnostic Findings

- An extra heart sound, referred to as a *mitral* (systolic) *click*, is an early sign that a valve leaflet is ballooning into the left atrium.
- A mitral regurgitation murmur may be heard if the valve opens during systole and blood flows back into the left atrium.
- If mitral regurgitation exists, a patient may experience signs and symptoms of heart failure.
- Echocardiography is used to diagnose and monitor progression of mitral valve prolapse.

Medical Management

Medical management is directed at controlling symptoms.

- Advise dietary restrictions, the elimination of alcohol and caffeine, and cessation of tobacco products use.
- Antiarrhythmic medications may be prescribed.
- Prophylactic antibiotics are not recommended prior to dental or invasive procedures.

- Chest pain unresponsive to nitrates may respond to calcium channel blockers or beta-blockers.
- Heart failure from this cause is treated as it would be for any other case of heart failure.
- Patients with severe mitral regurgitation and symptomatic heart failure may require mitral valve repair or replacement.
- Women diagnosed with mitral valve prolapse without mitral regurgitation or other complications may complete pregnancies with vaginal deliveries.

Nursing Management

- Educate patient about the diagnosis and the possibility that the condition is hereditary.
- Instruct the patient regarding how to minimize risk for infective endocarditis, practicing good oral hygiene, obtaining routine dental care, avoiding body piercing and body branding, and not using toothpicks or other sharp objects in the oral cavity.
- Explain the need to inform the health care provider about any symptoms that may develop.
- Instruct patient to avoid alcohol and caffeine, and encourage patient to read over-the-counter product labels to avoid products with alcohol, caffeine, ephedrine, and epinephrine, which may stimulate dysrhythmias.
- Explore possible diet, activity, sleep, and other lifestyle factors that may correlate with symptoms.
- Discuss treatment of dysrhythmias, chest pain, heart failure, or other complications of mitral valve prolapse. (See Acute Coronary Syndrome and Myocardial Infarction in Section A, and Heart Failure in Section H).

For more information, see Chapter 28 in Hinkle, J. L., & Cheever, K. H. (2014). *Brunner and Suddarth's textbook of medical-surgical nursing* (13th ed.). Philadelphia: Lippincott Williams & Wilkins.

Multiple Myeloma

Multiple myeloma is a malignant disease of the most mature form of B lymphocyte and is the second most common hematologic cancer in the United States. The median 5-year survival rate for newly diagnosed patients is 39%. Currently, prognosis is based on two simple markers: serum albumin (presumed to be a negative acute-phase reactant) and serum beta-2 microglobulin (presumed to be an indirect measure of tumor burden, defined as an approximation of the number of cancer cells in the body).

Pathophysiology

Plasma cells secrete immunoglobulins, proteins necessary for antibody production to fight infection. The malignant plasma cells produce an increased amount of a specific immuno-globulin, referred to as M protein, that can be detected in the blood or urine and is nonfunctional. Functional types of immunoglobulin are still produced by nonmalignant plasma cells but in lower than normal quantity. Malignant plasma cells also secrete certain substances to stimulate the creation of new blood vessels (i.e., angiogenesis) to enhance the growth of these clusters of plasma cell. Occasionally, the plasma cells infiltrate other tissue, in which case they are referred to as *plasmacytomas*.

Clinical Manifestations

- The classic presenting symptom of multiple myeloma is bone pain, usually in the back or ribs; pain increases with move-ment and decreases with rest; patients may report that they have less pain on awakening but more during the day.
- Severe bone destruction results from substances secreted by the myeloma, causing vertebral collapse and fractures (including spinal fractures), which can impinge on the spinal cord and result in spinal cord compression.
- Hypercalcemia may develop from extensive bone destruc-tion; renal impairment and failure may also occur.

> **Quality and Safety Nursing Alert**
>
> Any older adult whose chief complaint is back pain and who has an elevated total protein level should be evaluated for possible myeloma.

- Anemia is a reduced number of leukocytes and platelets (late stage).
- Infection is a concern (most commonly occurring within the first 2 months of beginning therapy and usually with advanced, refractory disease) and is a frequent cause of death.
- Neurologic manifestations (e.g., spinal cord compression, peripheral neuropathy) may occur.

- Hyperviscosity (manifested by bleeding from the nose or mouth), headache, blurred vision, paresthesias, heart failure, and thromboembolic events are possible with high-dose corticosteroid use.

Assessment and Diagnostic Findings

- An elevated monoclonal protein spike in the serum (via serum protein electrophoresis), urine (via urine protein electrophoresis), or light chain (via serum-free light chain analysis) is considered to be a major criterion in the diagnosis of multiple myeloma.
- Evidence of end organ damage is necessary to establish diagnosis, manifested in four parts: elevations in calcium, renal insufficiency, anemia, and bone lesions (referred to by the acronym *CRAB*).
- The diagnosis of myeloma is confirmed by bone marrow biopsy.

🍁 Gerontologic Considerations

The incidence of multiple myeloma increases with age. The disease rarely occurs before age 40 years. Closely investigate any back pain, which is a common presenting complaint. Hematopoietic stem cell transplantation (HSCT) is usually not available to older adults; however, newer treatment options can be successfully used in the older patient but may require dose adjustments to diminish treatment-related toxicity.

Medical Management

There is no cure for multiple myeloma. Even autologous HSCT is considered to extend remission rather than provide a cure. However, for many patients, it is possible to control the illness and maintain their level of functioning quite well for several years or longer. For those who are not candidates for HSCT, chemotherapy is the primary treatment. Pharmacotherapeutic advances have resulted in significant improvement in response rates. Radiation therapy is very useful in strengthening the bone at a specific lesion, particularly one at risk for bone fracture or spinal cord compression; the radiation relieves bone pain and reduces the size of plasma cell tumors that occur outside the skeletal system. Vertebroplasty is often performed to manage vertebral compression fractures in conjunction with kyphoplasty. Plasmapheresis is used when patients have signs and symptoms of hyperviscosity.

Pharmacologic Therapy

- For those who are not candidates for transplantation, chemotherapy is the primary treatment.
- Corticosteroids, particularly dexamethasone (Decadron), are often combined with other agents (e.g., melphalan [Alkeran], thalidomide [Thalomid], lenalidomide [Revlimid], and bortezomib [Velcade]).
- Concomitant therapy with anticoagulant agents (e.g., low-dose aspirin to warfarin [Coumadin]) or low-molecular-weight heparins (e.g., enoxaparin [Lovenox]) to prevent deep vein thromboses is required with use of thalidomide and bortezomib.
- Some bisphosphonates, such as pamidronate (Aredia) and zoledronic acid (Zometa), have been shown to strengthen bone in multiple myeloma by diminishing survival of osteoclasts.
- Narcotic analgesics, thalidomide, and bortezomib may be used for refractory disease and severe pain.

Nursing Management

- Administer medications as recommended for pain relief (e.g., nonsteroidal anti-inflammatory drugs [NSAIDs] alone or in combination with opioid agents).
- Carefully monitor for renal function and assess for gastritis if NSAIDs are used.

Promoting Home- and Community-Based Care

Educating Patients About Self-Care

- Educate patient about activity restrictions (e.g., lifting no more than 10 lb, use of proper body mechanics); braces are occasionally needed to support the spinal column.
- Educate patient to recognize and report signs and symptoms of hypercalcemia.
- Encourage patient to maintain high urine output (3 L per day), which can be very useful in preventing or limiting renal failure.
- Observe for bacterial infections (pneumonia); instruct patient in appropriate infection prevention measures, including influenza and pneumococcal vaccinations.

Continuing Care

- Maintain mobility and use strategies that enhance venous return (e.g., antiembolism stockings, avoidance of crossing the legs).

- Educate patient and family to recognize symptoms related to peripheral neuropathy; home safety assessments should be made.

For more information, see Chapter 34 in Hinkle, J. L., & Cheever, K. H. (2014). *Brunner and Suddarth's textbook of medical-surgical nursing* (13th ed.). Philadelphia: Lippincott Williams & Wilkins.

Multiple Sclerosis

Multiple sclerosis (MS) is a chronic, degenerative, progressive disease of the central nervous system (CNS) characterized by small patches (plaques) of demyelination in the brain and spinal cord. Demyelination (destruction of myelin) results in impaired transmission of nerve impulses.

Pathophysiology

The cause of MS is not known, but a defective immune response probably plays a major role. In MS, sensitized T cells inhabit the CNS and facilitate the infiltration of other agents that damage the immune system. The immune system attack leads to inflammation that destroys myelin and oligodendroglial cells that produce myelin in the CNS. Plaques of sclerotic tissue appear on demyelinated axons, further interrupting the transmission of impulses.

MS may occur at any age but typically manifests in young adults between the ages of 20 and 40; it affects women more frequently than men. Geographic prevalence is highest in northern Europe, New Zealand, southern Australia, the northern United States, and southern Canada.

Disease Course

MS has various courses:

- Benign course: Symptoms are so mild that patients do not seek health care or treatment.
- Relapsing remitting (RR) course (80% to 85%): Patients experience complete recovery between relapses; 50% of these patients progress to a secondary progressive course, in which disease progression occurs with or without relapses.
- Primary progressive course (10%): Disabling symptoms steadily increase, with rare plateaus and temporary improvement; this course may result in quadriparesis, cognitive dysfunction, vision loss, and brain stem syndromes.

- Progressive relapsing course (least common, about 5%): This course is characterized by relapses with continuous disabling progression between exacerbations.

Clinical Manifestations
- Signs and symptoms varied and multiple and reflect location of the lesion (plaque) or combination of lesions
- Primary symptoms: fatigue, depression, weakness, numbness, difficulty in coordination, loss of balance, and pain
- Visual disturbances: blurring of vision, diplopia (double vision), patchy blindness (scotoma), and total blindness
- Spastic weakness of the extremities and loss of abdominal reflexes; ataxia and tremor
- Cognitive and psychosocial problems; depression, emotional lability, and euphoria
- Bladder, bowel, and sexual problems possible

Secondary Manifestations Related to Complications
- Urinary tract infections, constipation
- Pressure ulcers, contracture deformities, dependent pedal edema
- Pneumonia
- Reactive depression and osteoporosis
- Emotional, social, marital, economic, and vocational problems

Exacerbations and Remissions
Relapses may be associated with periods of emotional and physical stress.

Assessment and Diagnostic Findings
- MRI (primary diagnostic tool) to visualize plaques
- Electrophoresis study of the cerebrospinal fluid (CSF); abnormal immunoglobulin G antibody (oligoclonal banding)
- Evoked potential studies and urodynamic studies
- Neuropsychological testing as indicated to assess cognitive impairment
- Sexual history to identify changes in sexual function

Medical Management
Because no cure exists for MS, the goals of treatment are to delay the progression of the disease, manage chronic symptoms, and treat acute exacerbations. An individualized treatment program is indicated to relieve symptoms and provide support. Management strategies target the various motor and sensory symptoms and the effects of immobility that can occur.

Pharmacologic Therapy

Disease Modification

- Interferon beta-1a (Rebif) and interferon beta-1b (Betaseron) are administered subcutaneously. Another preparation of interferon beta-1a, Avonex, is administered intramuscularly once a week.
- Glatiramer acetate (Copaxone), to reduce the rate of relapse in the RR course of MS, is administered subcutaneously daily.
- IV methylprednisolone is administered to treat acute relapse in the RR course of MS.
- Mitoxantrone (Novantrone) is administered via IV infusion every 3 months for patients with secondary progressive or worsening RR MS.
- Fingolimod (Gilenya) can reduce relapse rate in RR MS by 50%; it is administered orally.

Symptom Management

- Baclofen (Lioresal) is the medication of choice for treating spasticity; benzodiazepines (Valium), tizanidine (Zanaflex), and dantrolene (Dantrium) may also be used to treat spasticity.
- Amantadine (Symmetrel), pemoline (Cylert), or dalfampridine (Ampyra) can be used to treat fatigue.
- Beta-adrenergic blockers (Inderal), antiseizure agents (Neurontin), and benzodiazepines (Klonopin) are given to treat ataxia.

Management of Related Bowel and Bladder Problems

Anticholinergic medications, alpha-adrenergic blockers, or antispasmodic agents may be used to treat problems related to elimination, and patients may be taught to perform intermittent self-catheterization as well. Additional measures include assessment of urinary tract infections; ascorbic acid treatment to acidify urine; and antibiotic use when appropriate.

NURSING PROCESS

The Patient With MS

Assessment

- Assess actual and potential problems associated with the disease: neurologic problems, secondary complications, and impact of disease on patient and family.
- Assess patient's function, particularly ambulation, when patient is well rested and when fatigued; look for weakness,

spasticity, visual impairment, incontinence, and disorders of swallowing and speech.
- Assess how MS has affected the patient's lifestyle, how the patient is coping, and what the patient would like to improve.

Diagnosis

NURSING DIAGNOSES

- Impaired physical mobility related to weakness, muscle paresis, spasticity
- Risk for injury related to sensory and visual impairment
- Impaired urinary and bowel elimination related to nervous system dysfunction
- Impaired verbal communication and risk for aspiration related to cranial nerve involvement
- Chronic confusion related to cerebral dysfunction
- Ineffective individual coping related to the uncertainty of the disease's progression
- Impaired home maintenance management related to physical, psychological, and social limits imposed by MS
- Potential for sexual dysfunction related to lesions or psychological reaction

Planning and Goals

The major goals of the patient may include promotion of physical mobility, avoidance of injury, achievement of bladder and bowel continence, promotion of speech and swallowing mechanisms, improvement of cognitive function, development of coping strengths, improved home maintenance management, and adaptation to sexual dysfunction.

Nursing Interventions

PROMOTING PHYSICAL MOBILITY

- Encourage relaxation and coordination exercises to promote muscle efficiency.
- Encourage progressive resistance exercises to strengthen weak muscles.
- Encourage walking exercises to improve gait.
- Apply warm packs to spastic muscles; avoid hot baths due to sensory loss.
- Encourage daily exercises for muscle stretching to minimize joint contractures.
- Encourage swimming, stationary bicycling, and progressive weight bearing to relieve spasticity in legs.

- Avoid hurrying patient in any activity, because hurrying increases spasticity.
- Encourage patient to work up to a point just short of fatigue.
- Advise patient to take frequent, short rest periods, preferably lying down, to prevent extreme fatigue.
- Prevent complications of immobility by assessment and maintenance of skin integrity and through coughing and deep-breathing exercises.

PREVENTING INJURY
- Teach patient to walk with feet wide apart to increase walking stability (if motor dysfunction causes lack of coordination).
- Teach patient to watch the feet while walking if there is a loss of position sense.
- Provide a wheelchair or motorized scooter if gait remains insufficient after gait training (walker, cane, braces, crutches, parallel bars, and physical therapy).
- Assess skin for pressure ulcers if patient is confined to wheelchair.

ENHANCING BLADDER AND BOWEL CONTROL
- Keep bedpan or urinal readily available, because the need to void must be heeded immediately.
- Set up a voiding schedule, with gradual lengthening of time intervals.
- Instruct patient to drink a measured amount of fluid every 2 hours and to attempt to void 30 minutes after drinking.
- Encourage patient to take prescribed medications for bladder spasticity.
- Teach intermittent self-catheterization, if necessary.
- Provide adequate fluids, dietary fiber, and a bowel training program for bowel problems, including constipation, fecal impaction, and incontinence.

MANAGING SPEECH AND SWALLOWING DIFFICULTIES
- Arrange for evaluation by a speech therapist. Reinforce this instruction and encourage patient and family to adhere to the plan.
- Reduce the risk for aspiration by careful feeding, proper positioning for eating, and having a suction apparatus available.

IMPROVING SENSORY AND COGNITIVE FUNCTION
- Provide an eye patch or eyeglass occluder to block visual impulses of one eye when diplopia (double vision) occurs.

- Advise patient about no-cost talking-book services.
- Refer patient and family to a speech-language pathologist when mechanisms of speech are involved.
- Provide compassion and emotional support to patient and family adapting to a new self-image and coping with a life disruption.
- Keep a structured environment; use lists and other memory aids to help patient maintain a daily routine.

STRENGTHENING COPING MECHANISMS
- Alleviate stress and make referrals for counseling and support to minimize adverse effects of dealing with chronic illness.
- Provide information on the illness to patient and family.
- Help patient define problems and develop alternatives for management.

IMPROVING HOME MANAGEMENT
- Suggest modifications that allow independence in self-care activities at home (raised toilet seat, bathing aids, telephone modifications, long-handled comb, tongs, modified clothing).
- Maintain moderate environmental temperature; heat increases fatigue and muscle weakness and extreme cold may increase spasticity.

PROMOTING SEXUAL FUNCTION
Suggest a sexual counselor to assist patient and partner with sexual dysfunction (e.g., erectile and ejaculatory disorders in men; orgasmic dysfunction and adductor spasms of the thigh muscles in women; bladder and bowel incontinence; urinary tract infections).

PROMOTING HOME- AND COMMUNITY-BASED CARE
Educating Patients About Self-Care
- Instruct patient and family in the use of assistive devices, self-catheterization, and administration of medications.
- Assist patient and family in dealing with new disabilities and changes as disease progresses.

Continuing Care
- Refer for home health care nursing assistance as indicated.
- Assess changes in patient's health status and coping strategies, provide physical care to the patient if required, coordinate outpatient services and resources, and encourage health promotion, appropriate health screenings, and adaptation.

- Encourage the patient to contact the primary care provider if changes in the disease or its course are noted.
- Encourage patient to contact the local chapter of the National Multiple Sclerosis Society for services, publications, and contact with others who have MS.

Evaluation

EXPECTED PATIENT OUTCOMES
- Reports improved physical mobility
- Remains free of injury
- Attains or maintains improved bladder and bowel control
- Participates in strategies to improve speech and swallowing
- Compensates for altered thought processes
- Demonstrates improved coping strategies
- Adheres to plan for home maintenance management
- Adapts to changes in sexual function

For more information, see Chapter 69 in Hinkle, J. L., & Cheever, K. H. (2014). *Brunner and Suddarth's textbook of medical-surgical nursing* (13th ed.). Philadelphia: Lippincott Williams & Wilkins.

M

Muscular Dystrophies

Muscular dystrophies are a group of incurable chronic muscle disorders characterized by a progressive weakening and wasting of the skeletal or voluntary muscles. Most are inherited. The pathologic features include degeneration and loss of muscle fibers, variation in muscle fiber size, phagocytosis and regeneration, and replacement of muscle tissue by connective tissue. Differences among these diseases center on the genetic pattern of inheritance, the muscles involved, the age at onset, and the rate of disease progression.

Clinical Manifestations
- Muscle wasting and weakness
- Gastrointestinal tract problems: gastric dilation, rectal prolapse, and fecal impaction
- Cardiomyopathy, a common complication in all forms of muscular dystrophy

Medical Management
Treatment focuses on supportive care and prevention of complications. Supportive management is intended to keep

patients active and functioning as normally as possible and to minimize functional deterioration. A therapeutic exercise program is individualized to prevent muscle tightness, contractures, and disuse atrophy. Night splints and stretching exercises are employed to delay joint contractures (especially ankles, knees, and hips). Braces may be used to compensate for muscle weakness. The patient may be fitted with an orthotic jacket to improve sitting stability, reduce trunk deformity, and support cardiovascular status. Spinal fusion may be performed to maintain spinal stability. All upper respiratory infections and fractures from falls are treated vigorously to minimize immobilization and to prevent joint contractures. Advise genetic counseling because of the genetic nature of this disease, and provide information about the Muscular Dystrophy Association. Also advise patient to consult with appropriate caregivers for dental and speech problems and gastrointestinal tract problems.

Nursing Management

The goals are to maintain function at optimal levels and enhance the quality of life.

- Attend to patient's physical requirements and emotional and developmental needs.
- Actively involve patient and family in decision making, including end-of-life decisions.
- During hospitalization for treatment of complications, assess knowledge and expertise of patient and family responsible for giving care in the home. Assist patient and family to maintain coping strategies used at home while in the hospital.
- Provide patient and family with information about the disorder, its anticipated course, and care and management strategies that will optimize patient's growth and development and physical and psychological status.
- Communicate recommendations to all members of the health care team so that they work toward common goals.
- Encourage patient to use self-help devices to achieve greater independence; assist adolescents to make transition to adulthood. Encourage education and job tracking as appropriate.
- When educating family to monitor patient for respiratory problems, give information regarding appropriate respiratory support, such as negative pressure devices and positive pressure ventilators.
- Encourage range-of-motion exercises to prevent disabling contractures.

- Assist family in adjusting home environment to maximize functional independence; patient may require manual or electric wheelchair, gait aids, seating systems, bathroom equipment, lifts, ramps, and additional activity of daily living aids.
- Assess for signs of depression, prolonged anger, bargaining, or denial, and help patient to cope and adapt to chronic disease. Arrange for referral to a psychiatric nurse clinician or other mental health professional, if indicated, to assist patient to cope and adapt to the disease.
- Provide a hopeful, supportive, and nurturing environment.

For more information, see Chapter 70 in Hinkle, J. L., & Cheever, K. H. (2014). *Brunner and Suddarth's textbook of medical-surgical nursing* (13th ed.). Philadelphia: Lippincott Williams & Wilkins.

Musculoskeletal Trauma
(Contusions, Strains, Sprains, and Joint Dislocations)

Injury to one part of the musculoskeletal system results in malfunction of adjacent muscles, joints, and tendons. The type and severity of injury affects the mobility of the injured area.

M

Pathophysiology

Contusions, Strains, and Sprains

A contusion is a soft tissue injury produced by blunt force (e.g., a blow, kick, or fall), causing small blood vessels to rupture and bleed into soft tissues (ecchymosis or bruising). A hematoma develops when the bleeding is sufficient to cause an appreciable collection of blood, leaving a characteristic "black and blue" appearance. Most contusions resolve in one to two weeks.

A strain is an injury to a muscle tendon from overuse, overstretching, or excessive stress. A **sprain** is an injury to the ligaments surrounding a joint, caused by a twisting motion or hyperextension (forcible) of a joint. A torn ligament causes a joint to become unstable. Blood vessels rupture, edema occurs, and the joint becomes painful. Strains and sprains are graded along a continuum based on postinjury symptoms and loss of function.

Joint Dislocations

A dislocation of a joint is a condition in which the articular surfaces of the bones forming the joint are no longer in anatomic alignment. In complete dislocation, the bones are literally "out of joint." A subluxation is a partial dislocation of the articulating surfaces. Traumatic dislocations are orthopedic emergencies because the associated joint structures, blood supply, and nerves are displaced and may be entrapped with extensive pressure on them. If a dislocation or subluxation is not treated promptly, avascular necrosis (AVN) may occur, which results in ischemia and subsequent tissue death (necrosis) due to anoxia and diminished blood supply.

Clinical Manifestations

- Contusion: local symptoms (pain, swelling, and discoloration)
- Strain: symptoms that vary by severity: edema, tenderness, muscle spasm, ecchymosis, soreness or sudden pain with local tenderness on muscle use, isometric contraction
- Sprain: edema, tenderness of the joint, painful movement; increased disability and pain in the first 2 to 3 hours after injury because of associated swelling and bleeding; abnormal joint motion
- Dislocation or subluxation: acute pain, change in positioning of the joint, shortening of the extremity, deformity, and decreased mobility

Assessment and Diagnostic Findings

Identifying the mechanism of the injury and physical examination are important for the diagnosis of strains and sprains. X-ray examinations of both the affected and unaffected joints are used to evaluate joint or bone injury.

Medical Management

Treatment of injury to the musculoskeletal system involves providing support for the injured part until healing is complete. Strains and sprains take weeks or months to heal. Splinting may be used to prevent re-injury. Severe sprains may require surgery or three to six weeks of immobilization before protected exercises are initiated.

With a dislocation, the affected joint needs to be immobilized while the patient is transported to the hospital. The dislocation is promptly reduced (i.e., displaced parts brought into normal position) to preserve joint function. Analgesia, muscle relaxing medications and, possibly, anesthesia are used to facilitate closed reduction. The joint is immobilized by bandages, splints, casts, or traction and is maintained in a stable position. After reduction, gentle, progressive, active, and passive movement three or four times a day is begun to preserve range of motion and restore strength. The joint is supported between exercise sessions.

Nursing Management

- Frequently assess and evaluate the injury and the distal extremity and complete full neurovascular assessment.
- Apply ice and a compression bandage and elevate the affected part (RICE: rest, ice, compression, elevation) at or above the level of the heart to reduce swelling for the first 72 hours. Avoid excessive cold because it could cause skin and tissue damage.
- An elastic compression bandage controls bleeding, reduces edema, and provides support for the injured tissues.
- Educate the patient and family regarding proper exercises and activities, as well as danger signs. Symptoms to look for include increasing pain (even with analgesic agents), numbness or tingling, and increased edema in the extremity.
- After the acute inflammatory stage (24 to 72 hours after injury), heat may be applied intermittently (for 15 to 30 minutes, four times daily) to relieve muscle spasm and to promote vasodilation, absorption, and repair.
- Depending on the severity of injury, progressive, passive, and active exercises may begin in two to five days.

For more information, see Chapter 43 in Hinkle, J. L., & Cheever, K. H. (2014). *Brunner and Suddarth's textbook of medical-surgical nursing* (13th ed.). Philadelphia: Lippincott Williams & Wilkins.

Myasthenia Gravis

Myasthenia gravis (MG) is an autoimmune disorder affecting the myoneural junction. Antibodies directed at the acetylcholine receptor sites impair transmission of impulses across the myoneural junction. Therefore, fewer receptors are available for stimulation, resulting in voluntary muscle weakness that escalates with continued activity. Women are affected more frequently than men, and they tend to develop the disease at an earlier age (20 to 40 years of age, versus 60 to 70 years for men).

Clinical Manifestations
MG is purely a motor disorder with no effect on sensation or coordination.

- Ocular muscles (e.g., diplopia and ptosis) involved in initial manifestation
- Weakness of the muscles of the face (resulting in a bland facial expression) and throat (bulbar symptoms), and generalized weakness
- Laryngeal involvement: dysphonia (voice impairment); increased risk of choking and aspiration
- Generalized weakness that affects all extremities and the intercostal muscles, resulting in decreasing vital capacity and respiratory failure

Assessment and Diagnostic Findings
- Injection of edrophonium (Tensilon) is used to confirm the diagnosis. (Have atropine available for side effects.) Improvement in muscle strength represents a positive test and usually confirms the diagnosis.
- MRI may demonstrate an enlarged thymus gland.
- Tests include (1) serum analysis for acetylcholine receptor antibodies and (2) electromyography (EMG) to measure electrical potential of muscle cells.

Complications
A myasthenic crisis is an exacerbation of the disease process characterized by severe generalized muscle weakness, and respiratory and bulbar weakness, that may result in respiratory failure. Crisis may result from disease exacerbation or a specific precipitating event. The most common precipitator is respiratory infection; others include medication change, surgery, pregnancy, and medications that exacerbate myasthenia. A cholinergic crisis caused by overmedication with cholinesterase inhibitors is rare; atropine sulfate should be on hand to treat bradycardia or respiratory distress. Neuromuscular respiratory failure is the critical complication in myasthenic and cholinergic crises.

Medical Management
Management of MG is directed at improving function and reducing and removing circulating antibodies. Therapeutic modalities include administration of anticholinesterase medications and immunosuppressive therapy, plasmapheresis, and

thymectomy. There is no cure for MG; treatments do not stop the production of the acetylcholine receptor antibodies.

Pharmacologic Therapy

Pyridostigmine bromide (Mestinon) is the first line of therapy. It provides symptomatic relief by inhibiting the breakdown of acetylcholine and increasing the relative concentration of available acetylcholine at the neuromuscular junction.

If pyridostigmine bromide does not improve muscle strength and control fatigue, the next agents used are the immunomodulating drugs. Immunosuppressive therapy aims to reduce the production of the antireceptor antibody or remove it directly by plasma exchange. Corticosteroids are given to suppress the immune response, decreasing the amount of blocking antibody. If response is inadequate, azathioprine (Imuran) can inhibit immune cell proliferation and reduce antibody levels. Leukopenia and hepatotoxicity are serious adverse effects, so monthly evaluation of liver enzymes and white blood cell count is necessary.

Intravenous immunoglobulin (IVIG) is also used to treat exacerbations. A number of medications are contraindicated for patients with myasthenia gravis because they exacerbate the symptoms. Procaine (Novocain) should be avoided.

Other Therapy

Plasma exchange (plasmapheresis) produces a temporary reduction in the titer of circulating antibodies. Thymectomy (surgical removal of the thymus) produces substantial remission, especially in patients with tumor or hyperplasia of the thymus gland.

Nursing Management

- Educate patient about self-care, including medication management, energy conservation, strategies to help with ocular manifestations, and prevention and management of complications.
- Ensure patient understands the actions of the medications and emphasize the importance of taking them on schedule and the consequences of delaying medication; stress the signs and symptoms of myasthenic and cholinergic crises.
- Encourage patient to determine the best times for daily dosing by keeping a diary to determine fluctuation of symptoms and to learn when the medication is wearing off.

> ▶ *Quality and Safety Nursing Alert*
>
> Maintenance of stable blood levels of anticholinesterase medications is imperative to stabilize muscle strength. Therefore, the anticholinesterase medications must be administered on time. Any delay in administration of medications may exacerbate muscle weakness and make it impossible for the patient to take medications orally.

- Instruct the patient in strategies to conserve energy. (For example, if the patient lives in a two-story home, suggest that frequently used items such as hygiene products, cleaning products, and snacks be kept on each floor to minimize travel between floors.)
- Help the patient identify the optimal times for rest throughout the day.
- Encourage the patient to apply for a handicapped license plate to minimize walking from parking spaces, and to schedule activities that coincide with peak energy and strength levels.
- Instruct patient to schedule mealtimes to coincide with the peak effects of anticholinesterase medication; encourage rest before meals to reduce muscle fatigue; advise the patient to sit upright during meals, with the neck slightly flexed to facilitate swallowing.
- Encourage meals of soft foods in gravy or sauces; if choking occurs frequently, suggest pureed food with a pudding-like consistency. Supplemental feedings may be necessary in some patients to ensure adequate nutrition.
- Ensure suction is available at home and that the patient and family are instructed in its use.
- Instruct the patient to tape the eyes closed for short intervals and to regularly instill artificial tears; patients who wear eyeglasses can have "crutches" attached to help lift the eyelids; patching of one eye can help with double vision.
- Remind the patient of the importance of maintaining health promotion practices and of following health care screening recommendations.
- Encourage patient to note and avoid these factors that exacerbate symptoms and potentially cause crisis: emotional stress, infections (particularly respiratory infections), vigorous physical activity, some medications, and high environmental temperature.

- Refer patient to the Myasthenia Gravis Foundation of America, which can provide support groups, services, and educational materials for patients and families.

For more information, see Chapter 69 in Hinkle, J. L., & Cheever, K. H. (2014). *Brunner and Suddarth's textbook of medical-surgical nursing* (13th ed.). Philadelphia: Lippincott Williams & Wilkins.

Myocarditis

Myocarditis is an inflammatory process involving the myocardium. When the muscle fibers of the heart are damaged, life is threatened. Myocarditis usually results from an infectious process (e.g., viral, bacterial, rickettsial, fungal, parasitic, metazoal, protozoal, or spirochetal); however, it may be immune-related and develop in patients receiving immunosuppressive therapy or those with infective endocarditis, Crohn's disease, or systemic lupus erythematosus. Myocarditis can cause heart dilation, thrombi on the heart wall (mural thrombi), infiltration of circulating blood cells around the coronary vessels and between the muscle fibers, and degeneration of the muscle fibers themselves.

Clinical Manifestations
- Symptoms may be moderate, mild, or absent.
- Symptoms depend on the type of infection, degree of myocardial damage, and capacity of the myocardium to recover.
- Fatigue and dyspnea, palpitations, and occasional discomfort in the chest and upper abdomen may be seen.
- Most common symptoms are flu-like.
- The patient may develop severe congestive heart failure or sustain sudden cardiac death.

Assessment and Diagnostic Findings
Cardiac enlargement, faint heart sounds (especially S_1), a gallop rhythm, or a systolic murmur may be found on clinical examination. Cardiac catheterization demonstrates normal coronary arteries. Cardiac MRI with contrast may be diagnostic and can guide clinicians to sites for endocardial biopsies. White blood cell (WBC) count and erythrocyte sedimentation rate (ESR) may be elevated.

Medical Management
- Patients are given specific treatment for the underlying cause if it is known (e.g., penicillin for hemolytic streptococci) and

are placed on bed rest to decrease cardiac workload, myocardial damage, and complications.

- In young patients, activities, especially athletics, should be limited for a 6-month period or at least until heart size and function have returned to normal; physical activity is increased slowly.
- If heart failure or dysrhythmia develops, management is essentially the same as for all causes of heart failure and dysrhythmias; beta-blockers are avoided.

> ### Quality and Safety Nursing Alert
>
> Nonsteroidal anti-inflammatory drugs (NSAIDS) should not be used for pain control as they not only have been shown to be ineffective in relieving the inflammatory process but have been linked to worsening inflammation of the myocardium. This also can contribute to an increased mortality from increased virulence of the pathogen.

Nursing Management

- Assess for resolution of tachycardia, fever, and any other clinical manifestations.
- Focus cardiovascular assessment on signs and symptoms of heart failure and dysrhythmias; patients with dysrhythmias should have continuous cardiac monitoring, with personnel and equipment readily available to treat life-threatening dysrhythmias.

> ### Quality and Safety Nursing Alert
>
> Patients with myocarditis are sensitive to digitalis. Nurses must closely monitor these patients for digitalis toxicity, which is evidenced by dysrhythmia, anorexia, nausea, vomiting, headache, and malaise.

Use graduated compression stockings and passive and active exercises, because embolization from venous thrombosis and mural thrombi can occur, especially in patients on bed rest.

For more information, see Chapter 28 in Hinkle, J. L., & Cheever, K. H. (2014). *Brunner and Suddarth's textbook of medical-surgical nursing* (13th ed.). Philadelphia: Lippincott Williams & Wilkins.

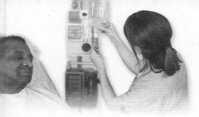

Nephritic Syndrome, Acute

Acute nephritic syndrome is the clinical manifestation of glomerular inflammation. Glomerulonephritis is an inflammation of the glomerular capillaries that can occur in acute and chronic forms.

Pathophysiology

Antigen–antibody complexes in the blood are trapped in the glomeruli, stimulating inflammation and producing injury to the kidney. Glomerulonephritis may also follow impetigo (infection of the skin) and acute viral infections (upper respiratory tract infections, mumps, varicella zoster virus, Epstein-Barr virus, hepatitis B, and HIV infections).

Clinical Manifestations

- Primary presenting features of an acute glomerular inflammation are hematuria, edema, azotemia, an abnormal concentration of nitrogenous wastes in the blood, and proteinuria or excess protein in the urine (urine may appear cola-colored).
- Some degree of edema and hypertension is present in most patients.
- Blood urea nitrogen (BUN) and serum creatinine levels may increase as urine output decreases; anemia may be present.
- In the more severe form of the disease, headache, malaise, and flank pain may occur.
- Older adults may have circulatory overload: dyspnea, engorged neck veins, cardiomegaly, and pulmonary edema.

Assessment and Diagnostic Findings

- Primary presenting feature is microscopic or gross (macroscopic) hematuria.
- Patients with an IgA nephropathy have an elevated serum IgA and low to normal complement levels.
- Electron microscopy and immunofluorescent analysis help identify the nature of the lesion; however, a kidney biopsy may be needed for definitive diagnosis.

Medical Management

Management consists primarily of treating symptoms, attempting to preserve kidney function, and treating complications promptly. Treatment may include using corticosteroid medications, managing hypertension, and controlling proteinuria. Pharmacologic therapy depends on the cause of acute glomerulonephritis. If residual streptococcal infection is suspected, penicillin is the agent of choice; however, other antibiotic agents may be prescribed. Dietary protein is restricted when renal insufficiency and nitrogen retention (elevated BUN) develop. Sodium is restricted when the patient has hypertension, edema, and heart failure.

Nursing Management

Although most patients with acute, uncomplicated glomerulonephritis are cared for as outpatients, nursing care is important in every setting.

Providing Care in the Hospital

- Give patient carbohydrates liberally to provide energy and reduce the catabolism of protein.
- Carefully measure and record intake and output; give fluids on the basis of the patient's fluid losses and daily body weight.
- Provide patient education about the disease process and explanations of laboratory and other diagnostic tests.
- Prepare the patient for safe and effective self-care at home.

Promoting Home- and Community-Based Care

Educating Patients About Self-Care
- Provide patient education for symptom management and monitoring for complications.
- Review fluid and diet restrictions with the patient to avoid worsening of edema and hypertension.
- Educate the patient verbally (and in writing) to notify the physician if symptoms of renal failure occur (e.g., fatigue, nausea, vomiting, diminishing urine output) or at the first sign of any infection.

Continuing Care
- Stress to the patient the importance of follow-up evaluations of blood pressure, urinalysis for protein, and BUN and serum creatinine levels to determine whether the disease has progressed.

- Refer for home care, if indicated, to assess the patient's progress and detect early signs and symptoms of renal insufficiency.
- Review with the patient the dosage, desired actions, and adverse effects of medications, and the precautions to be taken.

For more information, see Chapter 54 in Hinkle, J. L., & Cheever, K. H. (2014). *Brunner and Suddarth's textbook of medical-surgical nursing* (13th ed.). Philadelphia: Lippincott Williams & Wilkins.

Nephrotic Syndrome

Nephrotic syndrome is a primary glomerular disease characterized by proteinuria, hypoalbuminemia, diffuse edema, high serum cholesterol, and hyperlipidemia. It is seen in any condition that seriously damages the glomerular capillary membrane, causing increased glomerular permeability with loss of protein in the urine. It occurs with many intrinsic renal diseases and systemic diseases that cause glomerular damage. It is not a specific glomerular disease but rather a constellation of clinical findings that result from the glomerular damage.

Clinical Manifestations

- Major manifestation is edema. It is usually soft and pitting and commonly occurs around the eyes (periorbital), in dependent areas (sacrum, ankles, and hands), and in the abdomen (ascites).
- Malaise, headache, and irritability occur.
- Complications include infection (due to a deficient immune response), thromboembolism (especially of the renal vein), pulmonary emboli, acute kidney injury (due to hypovolemia), and accelerated atherosclerosis (due to hyperlipidemia).

Assessment and Diagnostic Findings

- Protein electrophoresis and immunoelectrophoresis are performed to determine type of proteinuria exceeding 3.5 g per day.
- Urine may contain increased white blood cells and granular and epithelial casts.
- Needle biopsy of the kidney is performed for histologic examination to confirm the diagnosis.

Medical Management

Treatment is focused on the underlying disease state causing proteinuria, slowing progression of chronic kidney disease

(CKD), and relieving symptoms. Typical treatment includes diuretics for edema, angiotensin-converting enzyme (ACE) inhibitors to reduce proteinuria, and lipid-lowering agents for hyperlipidemia.

Nursing Management

- In the early stages, nursing management is similar to that for acute glomerulonephritis.
- As the disease worsens, management is similar to that of end-stage renal disease.
- Provide adequate instruction about the importance of following all medication and dietary regimens so that the patient's condition can remain stable as long as possible.
- Convey to the patient the importance of communicating any health-related change to his or her health care provider as soon as possible, so that appropriate medication and dietary changes can be made before further changes occur within the glomeruli.

For more information, see Chapter 54 in Hinkle, J. L., & Cheever, K. H. (2014). *Brunner and Suddarth's textbook of medical-surgical nursing* (13th ed.). Philadelphia: Lippincott Williams & Wilkins.

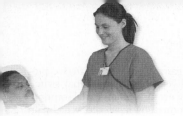

Obesity and Bariatric Surgery

Morbid obesity is the term applied to people who have a body mass index (BMI) that exceeds 40 kg/m² (BMI is the patient's weight in pounds divided by the patient's height in inches squared, multiplied by 703). Bariatric surgery, or surgery for obesity, is performed only after other nonsurgical attempts at weight control have failed. Most insurance companies will authorize bariatric surgery only after an obese patient tries 6 to 18 months of a medically supervised diet that fails to reach its weight loss goal. Patient selection is critical; therefore, patients need counseling before and after the surgery.

Pathophysiology
Bariatric surgical procedures work by (1) restricting a patient's ability to eat (restrictive procedure), (2) interfering with ingested nutrient absorption (malabsorptive procedures), or both.

Assessment and Diagnostic Findings
- Vital signs, including serial assessments of weight and BMI
- Documentation of diet and exercise history
- Assessment of life stressors that may drive dietary habits

Medical Management
Bariatric surgery involves a drastic change in the functioning of the digestive system. Different bariatric surgical procedures entail different lifestyle modifications, and patients must be well informed about the specific lifestyle changes, eating habits, and bowel habits that may result from a particular procedure. Roux-en-Y gastric bypass, gastric banding, vertical-banded gastroplasty, sleeve gastrectomy, and biliopancreatic diversion with duodenal switch are the current bariatric procedures of choice. The Roux-en-Y gastric bypass is a combined restrictive and malabsorptive procedure. The sleeve gastrectomy, gastric

banding, and vertical-banded gastroplasty are restrictive procedures, and biliopancreatic diversion with duodenal switch combines gastric restriction with intestinal malabsorption. These procedures may be performed by laparoscopy or by an open surgical technique.

NURSING PROCESS

The Patient Undergoing Bariatric Surgery

Assessment

- Assess for contraindications to major abdominal surgery.
- Encourage and support patient in making plans for lifestyle changes to reduce weight.
- Coordinate additional resources (e.g., dietitian or metal health providers) to assist patient in meeting lifestyle modification goals.
- Ensure the patient has been screened for mental and behavioral disorders that may interfere with postsurgical outcomes.
- General postoperative nursing care is similar to that for a patient recovering from a gastric resection but with great attention given to the risks of complications associated with morbid obesity.

Diagnosis

NURSING DIAGNOSES

- Deficient knowledge about dietary limitations during the immediate preoperative and postoperative phases
- Anxiety related to impending surgery
- Acute pain related to surgical procedure
- Risk for deficient fluid volume related to nausea, gastric irritation, and pain
- Risk for infection related to anastomotic leak
- Imbalanced nutrition, less than body requirement, related to dietary restrictions
- Disturbed body image, related to body changes from bariatric surgery
- Risk for constipation or diarrhea related to gastric irritation and surgical changes in anatomic structures from bariatric surgery

<small>COLLABORATIVE PROBLEMS/POTENTIAL COMPLICATIONS</small>
Potential complications that may develop include the following:

- Hemorrhage
- Bile reflux
- Dumping syndrome
- Dysphagia
- Bowel or gastric outlet obstruction

Planning and Goals

<small>PREOPERATIVE PLANNING AND GOALS</small>
- Increased knowledge about the preoperative and postoperative dietary routine and restrictions
- Decreased anxiety about bariatric surgery

<small>POSTOPERATIVE PLANNING AND GOALS</small>
- Relief of pain
- Maintenance of homeostatic fluid balance
- Absence of infection
- Adherence to prescribed dietary regimen with progression of food and fluid intake (according to plan)
- Increased knowledge about necessity of vitamin supplements and need for lifelong follow-up
- Maintenance of normal bowel habits

Nursing Interventions

<small>ENSURING DIETARY RESTRICTIONS</small>
- Counsel patient anticipating bariatric surgery to ingest nothing but clear liquids for specified time preoperatively (typically about 48 hours).
- Educate patient and family regarding dietary limitations postoperatively.

<small>REDUCING ANXIETY</small>
- Educate patient and family regarding expectations during and after surgery.
- Encourage patient to consider joining a bariatric surgery support group.

<small>RELIEVING PAIN</small>
- Administer analgesic drugs as prescribed; educate patient regarding use of patient-controlled analgesia and monitor effectiveness.

- Ensure adequate analgesia so that patient can perform pulmonary care activities (deep breathing and coughing) and leg exercises, turn from side to side, and ambulate.
- Positioning the patient in low Fowler's position promotes comfort and promotes emptying of the stomach after any type of gastric surgery, which includes bariatric procedures.

ENSURING FLUID AND VOLUME BALANCE
- Postoperatively, slowly introduce oral feedings beginning with small volumes (30 mL) of sugar-free oral fluids every 15 minutes.
- Encourage patients to stop ingesting fluids, however, if they feel nauseated or feel full.
- Antiemetic medications may be prescribed to relieve nausea and prevent vomiting, which may likewise cause strain on the surgical site.

> ### Quality and Safety Nursing Alert
>
> Insertion of nasogastric tubes is contraindicated in the patient after bariatric surgery. This procedure may disrupt the surgical suture line and cause anastomotic leak or hemorrhage.

PREVENTING INFECTION AND ANASTOMOTIC LEAK
- Disruption at the site of anastomosis (i.e., surgically resected site) may cause leakage of gastric contents into the peritoneal cavity, causing infection and possible sepsis; older male patients with greater body mass are at risk.
- Signs and symptoms of anastomotic leak are typically nonspecific—fever, abdominal pain, tachycardia, and leukocytosis—and may progress to sepsis.
- If anastomotic leak is suspected, patient may have an upper gastrointestinal series and a follow-up CT with contrast dye.

ENSURING ADEQUATE NUTRITIONAL STATUS
- After bowel sounds have returned and oral intake is resumed, six small feedings consisting of a total of 600 to 800 calories per day are provided; consumption of fluids between meals is encouraged to prevent dehydration.
- Educate the patient to eat slowly and to stop when feeling full to minimize vomiting or painful esophageal distention.
- Common dietary deficiencies include malabsorption of organic iron (which may require supplementation with oral or parenteral iron) and a low serum level of vitamin B_{12}; the

patient may be prescribed monthly vitamin B_{12} intramuscular injections to prevent pernicious anemia.

SUPPORTING BODY IMAGE CHANGES

- Educate the patient that the majority of weight loss will be in the first 6 months; however, some patients report lingering dissatisfaction with body image (e.g., loose skin folds).
- Support the patient who reports dissatisfaction with body image by acknowledging patient's feelings as real, sharing that these perceptions are not unusual, and providing links to supports groups or counselors.

ENSURING MAINTENANCE OF BOWEL HABITS

- Diarrhea is a more common occurrence after bariatric surgery than is constipation, particularly after malabsorptive procedures; however, some patients report constipation.
- Encourage consumption of a nutritious diet high in fiber, especially if constipation is a problem.
- Steatorrhea also may occur as a result of rapid gastric emptying, which prevents adequate mixing with pancreatic and biliary secretions.
- Persistent diarrhea or steatorrhea may warrant further diagnostic testing, such as an upper endoscopy or colonoscopy with biopsies to rule out the presence of additional pathology.

MONITORING AND MANAGING POTENTIAL COMPLICATIONS

Assess the patient for complications from the bariatric surgery, such as hemorrhage, bile reflux, dumping syndrome, dysphagia, and bowel or gastric outlet obstruction.

PROMOTING HOME- AND COMMUNITY-BASED CARE

The patient is usually discharged from the hospital in 4 days (this may be within 24 to 72 hours for patients who have had laparoscopic procedures) with detailed dietary instructions.

Educating Patients About Self-Care

- Provide information about nutrition, nutritional supplements, pain management, the importance of physical activity, and the symptoms of dumping syndrome; provide measures to prevent or minimize these symptoms.
- Emphasize the importance of routine follow-up outpatient appointments to ensure medical management of any side effects, which may include: increased risk of gallstones, nutritional and vitamin deficiencies, and potential to regain weight.

- For patients who undergo laparoscopic or open Roux-en-Y procedures and have one or more Jackson Pratt drains, educate the patient and family on how to empty, measure, and record the amount of drainage.

Continuing Care
- Emphasize importance of lifelong monitoring of weight loss, comorbidities, metabolic and nutritional status, and dietary and activity behaviors; patient is at risk for developing malnutrition or gaining weight.
- Women of childbearing age who have bariatric surgery are advised to use contraceptives for at least 18 months after surgery; patients are urged to avoid pregnancy until weight stabilizes.
- After weight loss, the patient may elect additional surgical interventions for body contouring.

Evaluation

EXPECTED PATIENT OUTCOMES
- Relief of pain
- Maintenance of fluid balance
- Maintenance of asepsis
- Achievement of nutritional balance
- Promotion of positive body image
- Maintenance of normal bowel habits

For more information, see Chapter 47 in Hinkle, J. L., & Cheever, K. H. (2014). *Brunner and Suddarth's textbook of medical-surgical nursing* (13th ed.). Philadelphia: Lippincott Williams & Wilkins.

Obesity, Morbid

Obesity is not merely a condition; rather, it is a metabolic disease that is characterized by fat that accumulates to the extent that health is impaired. Patients identified as overweight have body mass indices (BMI) of 25 to 29.9 kg/m², and those considered obese have BMIs that exceed 30 kg/m². *Morbid obesity* is the term applied to people who have a BMI that exceeds 40 kg/m². BMI is the patient's weight in pounds divided by the patient's height in inches squared, multiplied by 703.

Obesity-related mortality rates are 30% greater for every gain of 5 kg/m² of body mass beyond a BMI of 25 kg/m²; furthermore, the average lifespan for persons with BMIs in excess of

30 kg/m^2 is 3 years less than for persons with BMIs of 25 kg/m^2 or less. Patients with morbid obesity are at higher risk for such health complications as diabetes, heart disease, stroke, hypertension, gallbladder disease, osteoarthritis (OA), sleep apnea and other breathing problems, and some forms of cancer (uterine, breast, colorectal, kidney, and gallbladder). These patients frequently suffer from low self-esteem, impaired body image, and depression.

Pathophysiology

Though behaviors that are related to obesity include poor eating habits, and sedentary lifestyles may cause weight gain, various environmental, genetic, metabolic, cultural, and socioeconomic factors are all believed to interconnect in a complex—and still poorly understood—relationship that leads to obesity.

Assessment and Diagnostic Findings

- Vital signs including serial assessments of weight and BMI
- Diet and exercise history
- Assessment of life stressors that may drive dietary habits (e.g., low self-esteem, impaired body image, depression, and diminished quality of life)
- Assessment for presence of comorbidities (e.g., diabetes, hypertension, sleep apnea, and dyslipidemia)

Medical Management

There are three general approaches to treating obesity: lifestyle modifications, pharmacotherapy, and bariatric surgery.

Lifestyle Modifications

- Weight loss, in conjunction with behavioral modification and diet, is one approach
- Diet therapy includes dietitians in meal planning.
- Acupuncture, in combination with diet restrictions, has been found to be effective in enhancing weight loss and improving dyslipidemia
- Hypnosis, in combination with diet therapy for stress reduction and energy intake reduction, also has been shown to assist with weight loss.

Pharmacologic Management

- Sibutramine HCl (Meridia) decreases appetite by inhibiting the reuptake of serotonin and norepinephrine. Check drug precautions.

- Orlistat (Xenical) reduces caloric intake by inhibiting digestion of triglycerides. Review side effects; a multivitamin is usually recommended.
- Lorcaserin (Belviq), a new antiobesity drug, acts by stimulating serotonin receptors in the satiety and appetite centers of the hypothalamus in the brain, thus curbing appetite.
- Depression may contribute to weight gain, and treatment of the depression with an antidepressant agent may be helpful.

Surgical Management
- Bariatric surgery (surgery for morbid obesity) is considered only after medical management has failed.
- Gastric restriction procedures include gastric bypass and vertical banded gastroplasty (performed laparoscopically or by open surgical technique).
- Body contouring after weight loss involves lipoplasty to remove fat deposits or a panniculectomy to remove excess abdominal skinfolds.

Nursing Management
- Encourage and support patient in making plans for lifestyle changes to reduce weight.
- Coordinate additional resources (e.g., dietitian or mental health providers) to assist patient in meeting lifestyle modification goals.
- If the patient requires bariatric surgery, general postoperative nursing care is similar to that for a patient recovering from a gastric resection but with great attention given to the risks of complications associated with morbid obesity. See Nursing Process under Obesity and Bariatric Surgery.

For more information, see Chapter 47 in Hinkle, J. L., & Cheever, K. H. (2014). *Brunner and Suddarth's textbook of medical-surgical nursing* (13th ed.). Philadelphia: Lippincott Williams & Wilkins.

Osteoarthritis (Degenerative Joint Disease)

Osteoarthritis (OA), also known as *degenerative joint disease* or *osteoarthrosis*, is the most common and most frequently disabling joint disorder. It is characterized by a progressive loss of joint cartilage. Besides age, risk factors for OA include congenital and developmental disorders of the hip, obesity, previous joint damage, repetitive use (occupational or recreational), anatomic deformity, and genetic susceptibility. OA has been classified as primary (idiopathic) and secondary (resulting from previous joint injury or inflammatory disease). In addition to being a risk factor for OA, obesity, increases symptoms of the disease. OA peaks between the fifth and sixth decades of life.

Clinical Manifestations
- Primary manifestations are pain, stiffness, and functional impairment.
- Stiffness is most common in the morning after awakening. It usually lasts less than 30 minutes and decreases with movement.
- Functional impairment is due to pain on movement and limited joint motion when structural changes develop.
- OA occurs most often in weight-bearing joints (hips, knees, cervical and lumbar spine); finger joints are also involved.
- Bony nodes may be present (painless unless inflamed).

Assessment and Diagnostic Findings
- X-ray study shows narrowing of joint space and osteophytes (spurs) at the joint margins and on the subchondral bone. These two findings together are sensitive and specific.
- There is a weak correlation between joint pain and synovitis.
- Blood tests are not useful in the diagnosis of this disorder.

Prevention
- Weight reduction
- Prevention of injuries
- Perinatal screening for congenital hip disease
- Ergonomic modifications

Medical Management
Management focuses on slowing and treating symptoms, because there is no treatment available that stops the degenerative joint disease process.

Conservative Measures
- Heat, weight reduction, joint rest, and minimal use of the affected joint
- Orthotic devices to support inflamed joints (splints, braces)
- Isometric and postural exercises and aerobic exercise
- Occupational and physical therapy

Pharmacologic Therapy

- Acetaminophen; nonsteroidal anti-inflammatory drugs (NSAIDs)
- Cyclo-oxygenase 2 (COX-2) enzyme blockers (for patients with increased risk for gastrointestinal bleeding)
- Opioid medications and intra-articular corticosteroids
- Topical analgesic agents such as capsaicin and methyl salicylate
- Other therapeutic approaches: glucosamine and chondroitin; viscosupplementation (intra-articular injection of hyaluronic acid)

Surgical Management

Use when pain is severe and function is lost.

- Osteotomy
- Joint arthroplasty (replacement)

Nursing Management

Nursing care of the patient with OA is generally the same as the basic care plan for the patient with rheumatic disease (see Arthritis, Rheumatoid). Managing pain and optimizing functional ability are the major goals of nursing intervention, and helping patients understand their disease process and symptom pattern is critical to a plan of care.

- Assist patients with management of obesity (weight loss and an increase in aerobic activity) and other health problems or diseases, if applicable.
- Refer patient for physical therapy or to an exercise program. Exercises such as walking should begin in moderation and increase gradually.
- Provide and encourage use of canes or other assistive devices for ambulation as indicated.

For more information, see Chapter 42 in Hinkle, J. L., & Cheever, K. H. (2014). *Brunner and Suddarth's textbook of medical-surgical nursing* (13th ed.). Philadelphia: Lippincott Williams & Wilkins.

Osteomalacia

Osteomalacia is a metabolic bone disease characterized by inadequate mineralization of bone. The primary defect is a deficiency in activated vitamin D (calcitriol), which promotes calcium absorption from the gastrointestinal tract and facilitates mineralization of bone. Osteomalacia may result from failed calcium absorption (malabsorption) or excessive loss of calcium (celiac disease, biliary tract obstruction, chronic pancreatitis, bowel resection) and loss of vitamin D (liver and kidney disease). Additional risk factors include severe renal insufficiency, hyperparathyroidism, prolonged use of anti-seizure medication, malnutrition, and insufficient vitamin D (e.g., from inadequate dietary intake or inadequate sunlight exposure).

Clinical Manifestations
- Bone pain and tenderness
- Muscle weakness from calcium deficiency
- Waddling or limping gait
- Pathologic fractures
- Skeletal deformities (spinal kyphosis and bowed legs); often, compression of vertebrae, shortening patient's trunk
- Weakness and unsteadiness, presenting risk of falls and fractures

Assessment and Diagnostic Findings
- X-ray studies are conducted, and bone biopsy shows increased osteoid (demineralized bone matrix).
- Laboratory studies show low serum calcium and phosphorus levels, moderately elevated alkaline phosphatase level, and decreased urine calcium and creatinine excretion.

Gerontologic Considerations
Promote adequate intake of calcium and vitamin D and a nutritious diet in disadvantaged older patients. Encourage patient to spend time in the sun. Reduce incidence of fractures with prevention, identification, and management of osteomalacia. When osteomalacia is combined with osteoporosis, the incidence of fracture increases.

Medical Management
Physical, psychological, and pharmaceutical measures are used to reduce the patient's discomfort and pain.

- Underlying cause is corrected when possible (e.g., diet modifications, vitamin D and calcium supplements, sunlight).
- If osteomalacia is caused by malabsorption, increased doses of vitamin D, along with supplemental calcium, are usually prescribed.
- Exposure to sunlight may be recommended.

- If osteomalacia is dietary in origin, a diet with adequate protein and increased calcium and vitamin D is provided.
- Long-term monitoring is undertaken to ensure stabilization or reversal.
- Orthopedic deformities may be treated with braces or surgery (osteotomy).

For more information, see Chapter 42 in Hinkle, J. L., & Cheever, K. H. (2014). *Brunner and Suddarth's textbook of medical-surgical nursing* (13th ed.). Philadelphia: Lippincott Williams & Wilkins.

Osteomyelitis

Osteomyelitis is an infection of the bone. It may occur by extension of soft tissue infections, contiguous focus osteomyelitis (e.g., bone surgery, gunshot wound), or hematogenous (bloodborne) infections spread from other focal points of infection. *Staphylococcus aureus* causes more than 50% of bone infections. Among other pathogenic organisms frequently found are gram-positive organisms that include streptococci and enterococci and gram-negative bacteria that include *Pseudomonas* species. Patients at risk include poorly nourished, older adults; patients who are obese; those with impaired immune systems and chronic illness (e.g., diabetes); and those on long-term corticosteroid therapy or immunosuppressive agents. The condition may be prevented by prompt treatment and management of focal and soft tissue infections.

Clinical Manifestations
- When the infection is bloodborne, onset is sudden, occurring with clinical manifestations of sepsis (e.g., chills, high fever, rapid pulse, and general malaise).
- Extremity becomes painful, swollen, warm, and extremely tender.
- Patient may describe a constant, pulsating pain that intensifies with movement (due to the pressure of collecting pus).
- When osteomyelitis is caused by adjacent infection or direct contamination, no symptoms of sepsis are seen; the area is swollen, warm, painful, and tender to touch.
- Chronic osteomyelitis presents with a nonhealing ulcer that overlies the infected bone with a connecting sinus; this ulcer will intermittently and spontaneously drain pus.

Assessment and Diagnostic Findings

- In acute osteomyelitis, early x-ray films show only soft tissue swelling.
- In chronic osteomyelitis, x-ray films show large, irregular cavities and raised periosteum, sequestra, or dense bone formations.
- Radioisotope bone scans and MRI are performed.
- Blood studies and blood cultures are obtained.

Medical Management

The initial goal is to control and arrest the infective process.

- General supportive measures (e.g., hydration, diet high in vitamins and protein, correction of anemia) should be instituted; affected area is immobilized.
- Blood and wound cultures are performed to identify organisms and select the antibiotic.
- Intravenous antibiotic therapy is given around the clock and continues for three to 6 weeks.
- Antibiotic medication is administered orally (on an empty stomach) when infection appears to be controlled; the medication regimen is continued for up to 3 months.
- Surgical débridement of bone is performed with irrigation; adjunctive antibiotic therapy is maintained.

NURSING PROCESS

The Patient With Osteomyelitis

Assessment

- Assess for risk factors (e.g., older age, diabetes, long-term steroid therapy) and for previous injury, infection, or orthopedic surgery.
- Observe for guarded movement of infected area and generalized weakness due to systemic infection.
- Observe for swelling and warmth of affected area, purulent drainage, and elevated temperature.
- Note that patients with chronic osteomyelitis may have minor temperature elevations, occurring in the afternoon or evening.

Diagnosis

- Acute pain related to inflammation and swelling
- Impaired physical mobility associated with pain, immobilization devices, and weight-bearing limitations

- Risk for extension of infection: bone abscess formation
- Deficient knowledge about treatment regimen

Planning and Goals

Major goals may include relief of pain, improved physical mobility within therapeutic limitations, control and eradication of infection, and knowledge of the treatment regimen.

Nursing Interventions

RELIEVING PAIN

- Immobilize affected part with splint to decrease pain and muscle spasm.
- Monitor neurovascular status of affected extremity.
- Handle affected part with great care to avoid causing pain.
- Elevate affected part to reduce swelling and discomfort.
- Administer prescribed analgesic agents.

IMPROVING PHYSICAL MOBILITY

- Educate the patient on the rationale for activity restrictions (bone is weakened by the infective process).
- Gently move through their range of motion the joints above and below the affected part.
- Encourage activities of daily living within physical limitations.

CONTROLLING INFECTIOUS PROCESS

- Monitor response to antibiotic therapy. Observe intravenous sites for evidence of phlebitis or infiltration. Monitor for signs of superinfection with long-term, intensive antibiotic therapy (e.g., oral or vaginal candidiasis; loose or foul-smelling stools).
- If surgery was necessary, ensure adequate circulation (wound suction, elevation of area, avoidance of pressure on grafted area); maintain immobility as needed; comply with weight-bearing restrictions. Change dressings using aseptic technique to promote healing and prevent cross-contamination.
- Monitor general health and nutrition of patient.
- Provide a balanced diet high in protein to ensure positive nitrogen balance and promote healing; encourage adequate hydration.

PROMOTING HOME- AND COMMUNITY-BASED CARE

Educating Patients About Self-Care

- Advise patient and family to adhere strictly to the therapeutic regimen of antibiotics; stress the prevention of falls or other injuries that could result in fracture.

- Educate patient and family on how to maintain and manage the intravenous access site and intravenous administration equipment.
- Provide in-depth medication education (e.g., drug name, dosage, frequency, administration rate, safe storage and handling, adverse reactions), including need for laboratory monitoring.
- Educate patient to observe for, and report, elevated temperature, drainage, odor, signs of increased inflammation, adverse reactions, and signs of superinfection.

Continuing Care

- Complete a home assessment to determine ability of the patient and family to continue therapeutic regimen.
- Refer for a home care nurse if indicated.
- Monitor patient for response to treatment, signs and symptoms of superinfection, and adverse drug reactions.
- Stress importance of follow-up health care appointments and recommend age-appropriate health screening.

Evaluation

EXPECTED PATIENT OUTCOMES

- Experiences pain relief
- Increases physical mobility
- Shows absence of infection
- Adheres to therapeutic plan

For more information, see Chapter 42 in Hinkle, J. L., & Cheever, K. H. (2014). *Brunner and Suddarth's textbook of medical-surgical nursing* (13th ed.). Philadelphia: Lippincott Williams & Wilkins.

Osteoporosis

Osteoporosis is characterized by reduced bone mass, deterioration of bone matrix, and diminished bone architectural strength. The rate of bone resorption is greater than the rate of bone formation. The bones become progressively porous, brittle, and fragile, and they fracture easily. Multiple compression fractures of the vertebrae result in skeletal deformity (kyphosis). This kyphosis is associated with loss of height. Patients at risk include postmenopausal women and small-framed, nonobese Caucasian women.

Risk factors include inadequate nutrition, inadequate vitamin D and calcium, and lifestyle choices (e.g., smoking, caffeine intake, and alcohol consumption); genetics; and lack of physical activity. Age-related bone loss begins soon after peak bone mass is achieved (in the fourth decade). Withdrawal of estrogens at menopause (or oophorectomy) causes decreased calcitonin and accelerated bone resorption, which continues during menopausal years. Immobility contributes to the development of osteoporosis. Secondary osteoporosis is the result of medications or other conditions and diseases that affect bone metabolism. Specific diseases (e.g., celiac disease, hypogonadism) and medications (e.g., corticosteroids, antiseizure medications) that place patients at risk need to be identified and therapies instituted to reverse the development of osteoporosis.

Assessment and Diagnostic Findings

- Osteoporosis is identified on routine x-ray films when there has been 25% to 40% demineralization.
- Dual-energy x-ray absorptiometry (DEXA; DXA) provides information about spine and hip bone mass and bone mineral density (BMD).
- Laboratory studies (e.g., serum calcium, serum phosphate, serum alkaline phosphatase, urine calcium excretion, urinary hydroxyproline excretion, hematocrit, erythrocyte sedimentation rate [ESR]) and x-ray studies are used to exclude other diagnoses.

🌸 Gerontologic Considerations

Older adults fall frequently as a result of environmental hazards, neuromuscular disorders, diminished senses, diminished cardiovascular responses, and responses to medications. The patient and family need to be included in planning for care and preventive management regimens. For example, the home environment should be assessed for safety and elimination of potential hazards (e.g., scatter rugs, cluttered rooms and stairwells, toys on the floor, pets underfoot). A safe environment can then be created (e.g., well-lit staircases with secure hand rails, grab bars in the bathroom, properly fitting footwear).

Medical Management

- Adequate, balanced diet rich in calcium and vitamin D
- Increased calcium intake during adolescence, young adulthood, and middle age, or a prescribed calcium supplement with meals or beverages high in vitamin C

- Regular, weight-bearing exercise to promote bone formation (20 to 30 minutes of aerobic exercise 3 days per week)
- Other medications: alendronate (Fosamax), risedronate (Actonel), ibandronate (Boniva), and zoledronic acid (Reclast); calcitonin (Miacalcin); selective estrogen receptor modulators (SERMs) such as raloxifene (Evista); teriparatide (Forteo)
- Conservative management of osteoporotic compression fractures of the vertebrae; for patients nonresponsive to first-line approaches to vertebral compression fracture treatment, possibly percutaneous vertebroplasty or kyphoplasty (injection of polymethyl methacrylate bone cement into the fractured vertebra, followed by inflation of a pressurized balloon to restore the shape of the affected vertebra)

NURSING PROCESS

The Patient With a Spontaneous Vertebral Fracture Related to Osteoporosis

Assessment

- To identify risk for, and to recognize, problems associated with osteoporosis, interview patient regarding family history, previous fractures, dietary consumption of calcium, exercise patterns, onset of menopause, use of corticosteroid agents, use of alcohol, smoking, and caffeine intake.
- On physical examination, observe for fracture, kyphosis of thoracic spine, or shortened stature; explore any symptoms the patient is experiencing (e.g., back pain, constipation).

Diagnosis

- Deficient knowledge of osteoporotic process and treatment regimen
- Acute pain related to fracture and muscle spasm
- Risk for bowel elimination related to immobility or development of ileus
- Risk for injury: fracture related to osteoporotic bone

Planning and Goals

Major goals may include knowledge about osteoporosis and the treatment regimen, relief of pain, improved bowel elimination, and absence of additional fractures.

Nursing Interventions

PROMOTING UNDERSTANDING OF OSTEOPOROSIS AND TREATMENT REGIMEN

- Focus on educating patient about the factors influencing the development of osteoporosis, interventions to slow or arrest the process, and measures to relieve symptoms.
- Emphasize the need for sufficient calcium, vitamin D, and weight-bearing exercise to slow the progression of osteoporosis.
- Educate patient about medication therapy and side effects.

RELIEVING PAIN

- Educate patient on relieving back pain through bed rest and use of a firm, nonsagging mattress, knee flexion, intermittent local heat, and back rubs.
- Instruct patient to move the torso as a unit and avoid twisting; encourage good posture and good body mechanics.
- Encourage patient to wear a lumbosacral corset for immobilization and temporary support when out of bed.
- Encourage the patient to gradually resume activities as pain diminishes.

IMPROVING BOWEL ELIMINATION

- Encourage patient to eat a high-fiber diet, increase fluids, and use prescribed stool softeners.
- Monitor patient's intake, bowel sounds, and bowel activity; ileus may develop if the vertebral collapse involves T10 to L2 vertebrae.

PREVENTING INJURY

- Promote physical activity to strengthen muscles, prevent disuse atrophy, and retard progressive bone demineralization.
- Encourage patient to perform isometric exercises to strengthen trunk muscles.
- Encourage walking, good body mechanics, and good posture.
- Urge patient to avoid sudden bending, jarring, and strenuous lifting.
- Encourage outdoor activity in the sunshine to enhance body's ability to produce vitamin D.

Evaluation

EXPECTED PATIENT OUTCOMES

- Acquires knowledge about osteoporosis and treatment regimen
- Achieves pain relief

- Demonstrates normal bowel elimination
- Experiences no new fractures

For more information, see Chapter 42 in Hinkle, J. L., & Cheever, K. H. (2014). *Brunner and Suddarth's textbook of medical-surgical nursing* (13th ed.). Philadelphia: Lippincott Williams & Wilkins.

Otitis Media, Acute

Acute otitis media is an acute infection of the middle ear, usually lasting less than 6 weeks. The pathogens that cause acute otitis media are usually *bacterial or viral* and enter the middle ear after eustachian tube dysfunction; this dysfunction is caused by obstruction related to upper respiratory infections, inflammation of surrounding structures (e.g., rhinosinusitis, adenoid hypertrophy), or allergic reactions (e.g., allergic rhinitis). Bacteria can enter the eustachian tube from contaminated secretions in the nasopharynx and can also enter the middle ear from a tympanic membrane perforation. The disorder is most common in children.

Clinical Manifestations
- Symptoms vary with the severity of the infection and are usually unilateral in adults.
- Pain in and about the ear (otalgia) may be intense and relieved only after spontaneous perforation of the eardrum or after myringotomy.
- Fever, drainage from the ear, and hearing loss occur.
- The tympanic membrane is erythematous and often bulging.
- Conductive hearing loss results from exudate in the middle ear.
- Even if the condition becomes subacute (2 weeks to 3 months) with purulent discharge, permanent hearing loss is rare.

Complications
- Perforation of the tympanic membrane may persist and develop into chronic otitis media.
- Secondary complications involve the mastoid (mastoiditis), damage to the tympanic membrane or ossicles, or formation of a cholesteatoma.

Medical Management
- With early and appropriate broad-spectrum antibiotic therapy, otitis media may clear with no serious sequelae. If drainage occurs, an antibiotic otic preparation may be prescribed.

- Outcome depends on effectiveness of therapy (the prescribed dose of an oral antibiotic and the duration of therapy), the virulence of the bacteria, and the physical status of the patient.

Myringotomy (Tympanotomy)

If mild cases of otitis media are treated effectively, a myringotomy may not be necessary. If it becomes necessary, an incision is made into the tympanic membrane to relieve pressure and to drain serous or purulent fluid from the middle ear. This painless procedure usually takes less than 15 minutes. If episodes of acute otitis media recur and there is no contraindication, a ventilating, or pressure-equalizing, tube may be inserted.

For more information, see Chapter 64 in Hinkle, J. L., & Cheever, K. H. (2014). *Brunner and Suddarth's textbook of medical-surgical nursing* (13th ed.). Philadelphia: Lippincott Williams & Wilkins.

Otitis Media, Chronic

Chronic otitis media results from repeated episodes of acute otitis media, causing irreversible tissue pathology and persistent perforation of the tympanic membrane. Chronic infections of the middle ear cause damage to the tympanic membrane, can destroy the ossicles, and can involve the mastoid.

Clinical Manifestations

- Symptoms may be minimal, with varying degrees of hearing loss and a persistent or intermittent foul-smelling otorrhea (discharge).
- Pain may be present if acute mastoiditis occurs; the postauricular area is tender; erythema and edema may be present.
- Cholesteatoma (sac filled with degenerated skin and sebaceous material) may be present as a white mass behind the tympanic membrane, visible through an otoscope. If untreated, the cholesteatoma will continue to grow and destroy structures of the temporal bone, possibly causing damage to the facial nerve and horizontal canal as well as destruction of other surrounding structures. Auditory tests often show a conductive or mixed hearing loss.

Medical Management

- Careful suctioning and cleansing of the ear are performed under microscopic guidance.

- Antibiotic drops are instilled or antibiotic powder is applied to treat purulent discharge.
- Tympanoplasty procedures (myringoplasty and more extensive types) may be performed to prevent recurrent infection, re-establish middle ear function, close the perforation, and improve hearing.
- Ossiculoplasty may be undertaken to reconstruct the middle ear bones in order to restore hearing.
- Mastoidectomy may be performed to remove cholesteatoma, gain access to diseased structures, and create a dry (non-infected) and healthy ear.

Nursing Management

See "Nursing Process" under Mastoiditis and Mastoid Surgery for additional information.

For more information, see Chapter 64 in Hinkle, J. L., & Cheever, K. H. (2014). *Brunner and Suddarth's textbook of medical-surgical nursing* (13th ed.). Philadelphia: Lippincott Williams & Wilkins.

O

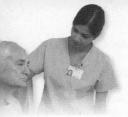

Pancreatitis, Acute

Pancreatitis (inflammation of the pancreas) is a serious disorder that ranges from a mild, self-limited disorder to a severe, rapidly fatal disease that does not respond to any treatment. Acute pancreatitis is commonly described as an autodigestion of the pancreas by the exocrine enzymes it produces, principally trypsin. Eighty percent of patients with acute pancreatitis have the disease as a result of cholelithiasis or sustained alcohol abuse. Other less common causes of pancreatitis include bacterial or viral infection, with pancreatitis occasionally developing as a complication of mumps virus. Many disease processes and conditions have been associated with an increased incidence of pancreatitis, including surgery on or near the pancreas, medications, hypercalcemia, and hyperlipidemia. Acute idiopathic pancreatitis accounts for up to 10% of the cases of acute pancreatitis, and there is a small incidence of hereditary pancreatitis.

Mortality is high because of shock, anoxia, hypotension, or fluid and electrolyte imbalances. Attacks of acute pancreatitis may result in complete recovery, may recur without permanent damage, or may progress to chronic pancreatitis.

Clinical Manifestations
- Severe abdominal pain is the major symptom.
- Pain in the midepigastrium may be accompanied by abdominal distention, a poorly defined, palpable abdominal mass, decreased peristalsis, and vomiting that fails to relieve the pain or nausea.
- Pain is frequently acute in onset (24 to 48 hours after a heavy meal or alcohol ingestion); it may be more severe after meals and unrelieved by antacids.
- Patient appears acutely ill.
- Abdominal guarding occurs; the abdomen may become rigid or boardlike (generally an ominous sign, usually indicating peritonitis)
- Ecchymosis in the flank or around the umbilicus may be seen and may indicate severe hemorrhagic pancreatitis

- Nausea and vomiting, fever, jaundice, mental confusion, and agitation are possible manifestations.
- Hypotension related to hypovolemia and shock may occur.
- Patient may develop tachycardia, cyanosis, and cold, clammy skin.
- Acute renal failure is common.
- Respiratory distress and hypoxia occur.
- Patient may develop diffuse pulmonary infiltrates, dyspnea, tachypnea, and abnormal blood gas values.
- Myocardial depression, hypocalcemia, hyperglycemia, and disseminated intravascular coagulation (DIC) are sometimes seen.

Assessment and Diagnostic Findings

Diagnosis is based on history of abdominal pain, the presence of known risk factors, physical examination findings, and diagnostic findings (increased urine amylase level and white blood cell count [WBC], hypocalcemia, transient hyperglycemia, glucosuria, and elevated serum bilirubin levels in some patients). X-rays of abdomen and chest, ultrasound, contrast-enhanced CT scans, and MRI scans may be performed. Hematocrit and hemoglobin levels are used to monitor the patient for bleeding.

Serum amylase and lipase levels are most indicative (elevated within 24 hours; amylase returns to normal within 48 to 72 hours; lipase remains elevated for longer period). Peritoneal fluid, obtained through paracentesis or peritoneal lavage, is evaluated for increased pancreatic enzymes.

Gerontologic Considerations

The mortality from acute pancreatitis increases with advancing age. Patterns of complications change with age: Younger patients tend to develop local complications, whereas the incidence of multiple organ failure increases with age. Close monitoring of major organ function (e.g., lungs, kidneys) is essential, and aggressive treatment is necessary to reduce mortality in the older adult patient.

Medical Management: Acute Phase

Management of acute pancreatitis is directed toward relieving symptoms and preventing or treating complications.

- Oral intake is withheld to inhibit pancreatic stimulation and secretion of pancreatic enzymes.

- Parenteral nutrition (PN) is administered to the debilitated patient and to those with a prolonged paralytic ileus (more than 48 to 72 hours).
- Nasogastric suction is used to relieve nausea and vomiting and to decrease painful abdominal distention and paralytic ileus.
- Histamine-2 (H_2) receptor antagonists (cimetidine, ranitidine) or, when applicable, proton pump inhibitors (pantoprazole) are given to decrease hydrochloric acid secretion.
- Adequate pain management with parenteral opioid medications, such as morphine, is administered. Antiemetic agents may be prescribed to prevent vomiting.
- Correction of fluid, blood loss, and low albumin levels is necessary to maintain fluid volume and prevent renal failure.
- Antibiotics are administered if infection is present.
- Insulin is necessary if significant hyperglycemia occurs.
- Aggressive respiratory care is provided for pulmonary infiltrates, effusion, and atelectasis.
- Respiratory care may range from close monitoring of arterial blood gases, to use of humidified oxygen, to intubation and mechanical ventilation.
- Biliary drainage (drains and stents) results in decreased pain and increased weight gain.
- Surgical intervention may be performed for diagnosis, drainage, resection, or débridement of an infected, necrotic pancreas.

Medical Management: Postacute Phase
- Oral feedings low in fat and protein are initiated gradually.
- Caffeine and alcohol are eliminated.
- Medications (e.g., thiazide diuretic, corticosteroid, or oral contraceptive agents) are discontinued.
- Follow-up may include ultrasound, x-ray studies, or endoscopic retrograde cholangiopancreatography (ERCP) to determine whether the pancreatitis is resolving and to assess for abscesses and pseudocysts.

Nursing Management

Relieving Pain and Discomfort
- Administer analgesics as prescribed. Current recommendation for pain management is parenteral opioid agents (including morphine), hydromorphone, or fentanyl via patient-controlled analgesia or bolus.

- Frequently assess pain and the effectiveness of the pharmacologic interventions.
- Withhold oral fluids to decrease formation and secretion of secretin.
- Use nasogastric suctioning to remove gastric secretions and relieve abdominal distention; provide frequent oral hygiene and care to decrease discomfort from the nasogastric tube and relieve dryness of the mouth.
- Maintain patient on bed rest to decrease metabolic rate and to reduce secretion of pancreatic enzymes; report increased pain (may be pancreatic hemorrhage or inadequate analgesic dosage).
- Provide frequent and repeated (but simple) explanations about treatment; patient may have clouded sensorium from severe pain, fluid and electrolyte disturbances, and hypoxia.

Improving Breathing Pattern
- Maintain patient in semi-Fowler's position to decrease pressure on diaphragm.
- Change patient's position frequently to prevent atelectasis and pooling of respiratory secretions.
- Assess respiratory status frequently (pulse oximetry, arterial blood gas [ABG] values), and educate patient in techniques of coughing and deep breathing as well as the use of incentive spirometry.

Improving Nutritional Status
- Assess nutritional status and note factors that alter the patient's nutritional requirements (e.g., temperature elevation, surgery, drainage).
- Monitor laboratory test results and daily weights.
- Provide enteral nutrition or PN as prescribed.
- Monitor serum glucose level every 4 to 6 hours.
- Introduce oral feedings gradually as symptoms subside.
- Educate patient to avoid heavy meals and alcoholic beverages.

Maintaining Skin Integrity
- Assess the wound, drainage sites, and skin carefully for signs of infection, inflammation, and breakdown.
- Perform wound care as prescribed and take precautions to protect intact skin from contact with drainage; consult with a wound-ostomy-continence nurse as needed to identify appropriate skin care devices and protocols.

- Turn patient every 2 hours; use of specialty beds may be indicated to prevent skin breakdown.

Monitoring and Managing Complications

Fluid and Electrolyte Disturbances
- Assess fluid and electrolyte status by noting skin turgor and moistness of mucous membranes.
- Weigh daily; measure all fluid intake and output, including urine output, nasogastric secretions, and diarrhea.
- Assess for other factors that may affect fluid and electrolyte status, including increased body temperature and wound drainage.
- Observe for ascites and measure abdominal girth.
- Administer IV fluids and blood or blood products to maintain volume and prevent or treat hypovolemic shock.
- Report decreased blood pressure, reduced urine output, and low serum calcium and magnesium.

Pancreatic Necrosis
- Transfer patient to intensive care unit and closely monitor vital signs, including hemodynamic monitoring.
- Administer prescribed IV fluids, medications, and blood products.
- Assist with supportive management, such as use of a ventilator, preventing additional complications, and providing physical and psychological care.

Shock and Multiple Organ Dysfunction Syndrome (MODS)
- Monitor patient closely for early signs of neurologic, cardiovascular, renal, and respiratory dysfunction.
- Prepare for rapid changes in patient status, treatment, and therapies; respond quickly.
- Inform family of status and progress of patient; allow time with patient.

Promoting Home- and Community-Based Care

Educating Patients About Self-Care
- Provide patient and family with facts and explanations of the acute phase of illness; provide necessary repetition and reinforcement.
- Educate patient about factors implicated in onset of acute pancreatitis, including the need to avoid high-fat foods, heavy meals, and alcohol.

- Offer verbal and written instructions about signs and symptoms and possible complications that should be reported promptly to the health care provider.
- Provide additional explanations on dietary modifications if biliary tract disease is the cause.

Continuing Care
- Refer for home care (often indicated).
- Assess the patient's physical and psychological status and adherence to the therapeutic regimen.
- Assess the home situation and reinforce instructions about fluid and nutrition intake and avoidance of alcohol.
- Provide information about resources and support groups, particularly if alcohol is the cause of acute pancreatitis.

For more information, see Chapter 50 in Hinkle, J. L., & Cheever, K. H. (2014). *Brunner and Suddarth's textbook of medical-surgical nursing* (13th ed.). Philadelphia: Lippincott Williams & Wilkins.

Pancreatitis, Chronic

Chronic pancreatitis is an inflammatory disorder characterized by progressive destruction of the pancreas. Cells are replaced by fibrous tissue with repeated attacks of pancreatitis. The result is obstruction of the pancreatic and common bile ducts and duodenum. In addition, atrophy of the epithelium of the ducts, inflammation, and destruction of the secreting cells of the pancreas occur. Alcohol consumption in Western societies and malnutrition worldwide are the major causes. Excessive and prolonged consumption of alcohol accounts for approximately 70% to 80% of all cases of chronic pancreatitis. The incidence of pancreatitis among alcoholics is 50 times the rate of incidence in the nondrinking population. Smoking is another factor in the development of chronic pancreatitis. Because smoking and drinking are often associated, it is difficult to separate the effects of the alcohol abuse and smoking.

Pathophysiology
Long-term alcohol consumption causes hypersecretion of protein in pancreatic secretions, resulting in protein plugs and calculi within the pancreatic ducts. Alcohol has a direct toxic effect on the cells of the pancreas. Damage is more severe in patients with diets low in protein and very high (or very low) in fat.

Clinical Manifestations

- Attacks of severe upper abdominal and back pain are recurrent, accompanied by vomiting; opioid agents may not provide relief.
- Risk of addiction to opiates is high because of the severe pain.
- There may be continuous severe pain or dull, nagging, constant pain.
- Weight loss is a major problem.
- Altered digestion (malabsorption) of foods (proteins and fats) results in frequent, frothy, and foul-smelling stools with a high fat content (steatorrhea).
- As disease progresses, calcification of the gland may occur and calcium stones may form within the ducts.

Assessment and Diagnostic Findings

- Endoscopic retrograde cholangiopancreatography (ERCP) is the most useful study.
- Various imaging procedures, including MRI, CT scans, and ultrasound, may be useful.
- A glucose tolerance test evaluates pancreatic islet cell function.
- Steatorrhea is best confirmed by laboratory analysis of fecal fat content.

Medical Management

Treatment is directed toward preventing and managing acute attacks, relieving pain and discomfort, and managing exocrine and endocrine insufficiency of pancreatitis.

- Endoscopy to remove pancreatic duct stones, correct strictures, and drain cysts may be effective in selected patients to manage pain and relieve obstruction.
- Pain and discomfort are relieved with analgesic medications; yoga may be an effective nonpharmacologic method for pain reduction and for relief of other coexisting symptoms.
- Patient should avoid alcohol and foods that produce abdominal pain and discomfort. No other treatment will relieve pain if patient continues to consume alcohol.
- Diabetes resulting from dysfunction of pancreatic islet cells is treated with diet, insulin, or oral hypoglycemic agents. Patient and family are taught the danger of severe hypoglycemia related to alcohol use.
- Pancreatic enzyme replacement therapy is instituted for malabsorption and steatorrhea.

- Surgery is performed to relieve abdominal pain and discomfort, restore drainage of pancreatic secretions, and reduce frequency of attacks (pancreaticojejunostomy).
- Minimally invasive procedures to treat chronic pancreatitis may prove to be successful adjuncts in the management of this complex disorder.
- Morbidity and mortality after surgical procedures are high because of patient's poor physical condition before surgery and concomitant occurrence of cirrhosis.

Nursing Management

See "Nursing Management" under Pancreatitis, Acute for treatment guidelines.

For more information, see Chapter 50 in Hinkle, J. L., & Cheever, K. H. (2014). *Brunner and Suddarth's textbook of medical-surgical nursing* (13th ed.). Philadelphia: Lippincott Williams & Wilkins.

Parkinson's Disease

Parkinson's disease is a slowly progressive, degenerative neurologic disorder affecting the brain centers that are responsible for control and regulation of movement. The degenerative, or idiopathic, form of Parkinson's disease is the most common; there is also a secondary form with a known or suspected cause. The cause of the disease is mostly unknown, but research suggests several causative factors (e.g., genetics, atherosclerosis, viral infections, head trauma). The disease usually first appears in the fifth decade of life and is the fourth most common neurodegenerative disease.

Pathophysiology

Parkinson's disease is associated with decreased levels of dopamine, resulting from destruction of pigmented neuronal cells in the substantia nigra, located in the basal ganglia region of the brain. The loss of dopamine stores in this area of the brain results in more excitatory neurotransmitters than inhibitory neurotransmitters, leading to an imbalance that affects voluntary movement. Cellular degeneration causes impairment of the extrapyramidal tracts that control semiautomatic functions and coordinated movements; motor cells of the motor cortex and the pyramidal tracts are not affected. Oxidative stress and protein accumulation may contribute to neuronal death.

Clinical Manifestations

The cardinal signs of Parkinson's disease are tremor, rigidity, bradykinesia (abnormally slow movements), and postural instability.

- Resting tremors manifest as a slow, unilateral turning of the forearm and hand and a pill-rolling motion of the thumb against the fingers; tremors at rest increase with concentration and anxiety.
- Resistance to passive limb movement characterizes muscle rigidity; passive movement may cause the limb to move in jerky increments (lead-pipe or cog-wheel movements); stiffness of the arms, legs, face, and posture are common; involuntary stiffness of passive extremity increases when another extremity is engaged in voluntary active movement.
- Impaired movement: Bradykinesia includes difficulty in initiating, maintaining, and performing motor activities.
- Loss of postural reflexes, shuffling gait, and loss of balance (difficulty pivoting) occur; postural and gait problems place the patient at increased risk for falls.

Other Characteristics

- Autonomic symptoms include excessive and uncontrolled sweating, paroxysmal flushing, orthostatic hypotension, gastric and urinary retention, constipation, and sexual dysfunction.
- Psychiatric changes may include depression, dementia, delirium, and hallucinations; psychiatric manifestations may include personality changes, psychosis, and acute confusion.
- Auditory and visual hallucinations may occur.
- Hypokinesia (abnormally diminished movement) is common.
- As dexterity declines, micrographia (small handwriting) develops.
- A masklike facial expression is noted.
- Dysphonia (soft, slurred, low-pitched, and less audible speech) occurs.

Assessment and Diagnostic Findings

- Patient's history and presence of two of the four cardinal manifestations—tremor, rigidity, bradykinesia, and postural changes—point to this diagnosis.
- Positron emission tomography (PET) and single photon emission computed tomography (SPECT) scanning have

been helpful in understanding the disease and advancing treatment.

- Medical history, presenting symptoms, neurologic examination, and response to pharmacologic management are carefully evaluated when making the diagnosis.

Medical Management

The goal of treatment is to control symptoms and maintain functional independence. No approach prevents disease progression.

Pharmacologic Therapy

- Levodopa (Larodopa) is the most effective agent and the mainstay of treatment; delay start of levodopa as long as possible to avoid on-off syndrome and other adverse effects.
- Though levodopa is the primary treatment agent, nurses caring for patients with Parkinson's disease need a clear understanding of other medications prescribed in addition to levodopa:
  - Anticholinergic agents to control tremor and rigidity
  - Amantadine hydrochloride (Symmetrel), an antiviral agent, to reduce rigidity, tremor, and bradykinesia
  - Dopamine agonists (e.g., pergolide [Permax], bromocriptine mesylate [Parlodel], ropinirole, and pramipexole) used early in disease to postpone the initiation of carbidopa and levodopa therapy, or as secondary therapy after those lose effectiveness
  - Monoamine oxidase inhibitors (MAOIs) to inhibit dopamine breakdown
  - Catechol-O-methyltransferase (COMT) inhibitors to reduce motor fluctuation
  - Antidepressant drugs (tricyclic agents, serotonin-reuptake inhibitors)
  - Antihistamine drugs to allay tremors

Surgical Management

- Deep brain stimulation (DBS) by implanted electrodes can help boost dopamine release or block acetylcholine production in nerve pathways in the brain that cause tremors.
- Surgeries to destroy a part of the thalamus (stereotactic thalamotomy and pallidotomy) to interrupt nerve pathways are rarely used in current practice.
- Transplantation of neural cells from fetal tissue of human or animal source, in order to reestablish normal dopamine release, is still under investigation.

NURSING PROCESS

The Patient With Parkinson's Disease

Assessment

Note how the disease affects the patient's activities of daily living and functional abilities; observe also for degree of disability and functional changes that occur throughout the day, such as responses to medication. Observe the patient for quality of speech, loss of facial expression, swallowing deficits (drooling, poor head control, coughing), tremors, slowness of movement, weakness, forward posture, rigidity, evidence of mental slowness, and confusion. The following questions may facilitate observations:

- Do you have leg or arm stiffness?
- Have you experienced any irregular jerking of your arms or legs?
- Have you ever been "frozen" or rooted to the spot and unable to move?
- Does your mouth water excessively?
- Have you (or others) noticed yourself grimacing or making faces or chewing movements?
- What specific activities do you have difficulty doing?

Diagnosis

- Impaired physical mobility related to muscle rigidity and motor weakness
- Self-care deficits (eating, drinking, dressing, hygiene, and toileting) related to tremor and motor disturbance
- Constipation related to medication and reduced activity
- Imbalanced nutrition: less than body requirements related to tremor, slowness in eating, difficulty in chewing and swallowing
- Impaired verbal communication related to decreased speech volume, slowness of speech, and inability to move facial muscles
- Ineffective coping related to depression and dysfunction due to disease progression

Other nursing diagnoses may include sleep pattern disturbances, deficient knowledge, risk for injury, risk for activity intolerance, disturbed thought processes, and compromised family coping.

Planning and Goals

Patient goals may include improving functional mobility, maintaining independence in activities of daily living (ADLs), achieving adequate bowel elimination, attaining and maintaining acceptable nutritional status, achieving effective communication, and developing positive coping mechanisms.

Nursing Interventions

IMPROVING MOBILITY

- Help patient plan progressive program of daily exercise to increase muscle strength, improve coordination and dexterity, reduce muscular rigidity, and prevent contractures.
- Encourage exercises for joint mobility (e.g., stationary bike, walking).
- Instruct in stretching and range of motion exercises to increase joint flexibility.
- Encourage postural exercises to counter the tendency of the head and neck to be drawn forward and down. Educate patient to walk erect, watch the horizon, use a wide-based gait, swing arms with walking, walk heel–toe, and practice marching to music. Also encourage breathing exercises while walking and frequent rest periods to prevent fatigue or frustration.
- Advise patient that warm baths and massage help relax muscles.

ENHANCING SELF-CARE ACTIVITIES

- Encourage, educate, and support patient during ADLs.
- Modify environment to compensate for functional disabilities; adaptive devices may be useful.
- Enlist assistance of an occupational therapist as indicated.

IMPROVING BOWEL ELIMINATION

- Establish a regular bowel routine.
- Increase fluid intake; eat foods with moderate fiber content.
- Provide raised toilet seat for easier toilet use.

IMPROVING SWALLOWING AND NUTRITION

- Promote swallowing and prevent aspiration by having patient sit in upright position during meals.
- Provide semisolid diet with thick liquids that are easier to swallow.
- Educate patient to place the food on the tongue, close the lips and teeth, lift the tongue up and then back, and swallow;

P

encourage patient to chew first on one side of the mouth and then on the other.
- Remind patient to hold head upright and to make a conscious effort to swallow to control buildup of saliva.
- Monitor patient's weight on a weekly basis.
- Provide supplementary feeding and, as disease progresses, tube feedings.
- Consult a dietitian regarding patient's nutritional needs.

ENCOURAGING USE OF ASSISTIVE DEVICES
- An occupational therapist can assist in identifying appropriate adaptive devices.
- Useful devices may include an electric warming tray that keeps food hot and allows the patient to rest during the prolonged time that it may take to eat; special utensils; a plate that is stabilized, a nonspill cup, and eating utensils.

IMPROVING COMMUNICATION
- Remind patient to face the listener, speak slowly and deliberately, and exaggerate pronunciation of words; a small electronic amplifier is helpful if the patient has difficulty being heard.
- Instruct patient to speak in short sentences and take a few breaths before speaking.
- Enlist a speech therapist to assist the patient.

SUPPORTING COPING ABILITIES
- Encourage faithful adherence to exercise and walking program; point out activities that are being maintained through active participation.
- Provide continuous encouragement and reassurance.
- Assist and encourage patient to set achievable goals.
- Encourage patient to carry out daily tasks to retain independence.

PROMOTING HOME- AND COMMUNITY-BASED CARE
Educating Patients About Self-Care
The education plan should include a clear explanation of the disease and the goal of assisting the patient to remain functionally independent for as long as possible. Make every effort to explain the nature of the disease and its management, to offset disabling anxieties and fears. The patient and family also need to know about the effects and side effects of medications and the importance of reporting side effects to the physician.

Continuing Care
- Acknowledge the stress that the family is under by living with a family member who has disabilities.
- Include caregiver in planning, and counsel caregiver to learn stress reduction techniques; remind caregiver to include others in the caregiving process, obtain periodic relief from responsibilities, and have a yearly health assessment.
- Allow family members to express feelings of frustration, anger, and guilt.
- Remind the patient and family members of the importance of addressing health promotion needs, such as screening for hypertension and stroke risk.

Evaluation

EXPECTED PATIENT OUTCOMES
- Strives toward improved mobility
- Progresses toward self-care
- Maintains bowel function
- Attains improved nutritional status
- Achieves a method of communication
- Copes with effects of Parkinson's disease

For more information, see Chapter 70 in Hinkle, J. L., & Cheever, K. H. (2014). *Brunner and Suddarth's textbook of medical-surgical nursing* (13th ed.). Philadelphia: Lippincott Williams & Wilkins.

Pelvic Infection (Pelvic Inflammatory Disease)

Pelvic inflammatory disease (PID) is an inflammatory condition of the pelvic cavity that may begin with cervicitis and may involve the uterus (endometritis), fallopian tubes (salpingitis), ovaries (oophoritis), pelvic peritoneum, or pelvic vascular system. Each year an estimated 750,000 cases of PID are seen; the true incidence is unknown because some cases are asymptomatic. Risk factors include early age at first intercourse, multiple sexual partners, frequent intercourse, intercourse without condoms, sex with a partner with a sexually transmitted infection (STI), a history of STI, or previous pelvic infection.

Pathophysiology
Infection, which may be acute, subacute, recurrent, or chronic and localized or widespread, is usually caused by bacteria but may be attributed to a virus, fungus, or parasite. Pathogenic

organisms usually enter the body through the vagina, pass through the cervical canal into the uterus, and may proceed to one or both fallopian tubes and ovaries and into the pelvis. Infection most commonly occurs through sexual transmission but also may be caused by invasive procedures such as endometrial biopsy, surgical abortion, hysteroscopy, or insertion of an intra-uterine device (IUD). The most common organisms involved are gonorrhea and chlamydia. The infection is usually bilateral.

Clinical Manifestations

Symptoms may be acute and severe or low-grade and subtle.

- Vaginal discharge, dyspareunia, lower abdominal pelvic pain, and tenderness that occurs after menses may be seen; pain may increase during voiding or defecating.
- Systemic symptoms include fever, general malaise, anorexia, nausea, headache, and possibly vomiting.
- Intense tenderness is noted on palpation of the uterus or movement of cervix (cervical motion tenderness) during pelvic examination.

Complications

- Pelvic or generalized peritonitis, abscesses, strictures, and fallo-pian tube obstruction, which may result in ectopic pregnancy
- Adhesions that eventually may require removal of the uterus, fallopian tubes, and ovaries
- Bacteremia with septic shock
- Chronic pelvic or abdominal pain or recurring PID

Medical Management

Broad-spectrum antibiotic therapy is instituted, with mild to moderate infections being treated on an outpatient basis. If the patient is acutely ill, hospitalization may be required. Indications for hospitalization include surgical emergencies, pregnancy, no clinical response to oral antimicrobial therapy, inability to follow or tolerate an outpatient oral regimen, severe illness (i.e., nausea, vomiting, or high fever), and tubo-ovarian abscess. Once hospitalized, the patient is placed on a regimen of bed rest, IV fluids, and IV antibiotic therapy; vital signs are monitored. Treatment of sexual partners is necessary to prevent reinfection.

Nursing Management

Nursing measures include nutritional support of the patient and administration of antibiotic therapy as prescribed. Vital signs are assessed, as are characteristics of the disorder and the amount of vaginal discharge.

The nurse administers analgesic agents as prescribed for pain relief. Adequate rest and a healthy diet are encouraged. Another nursing intervention is prevention of transmission of infection to others by impeccable hand hygiene and use of barrier precautions and hospital guidelines for disposing of biohazardous articles (e.g., pads).

Promoting Home- and Community-Based Care

Educating Patients About Self-Care

Before discharge, patients are taught self-care measures:

- Inform and encourage the patient to take part in procedures to prevent infecting others and protect herself from reinfection. Use of condoms is essential to prevent infection and sequelae.
- Explain how pelvic infections occur, how they can be controlled and avoided, and their signs and symptoms: abdominal pain, nausea and vomiting, fever, malaise, malodorous purulent vaginal discharge, and leukocytosis.
- Evaluate any pelvic pain or abnormal discharge, particularly after sexual exposure, childbirth, or pelvic surgery.
- Inform patient that intrauterine devices (IUDs) may increase the risk for infection and that antibiotics may be prescribed after the IUD is inserted.
- Instruct patient to use proper perineal care, wiping from front to back.
- Instruct patient to avoid douching, which can reduce natural flora.
- Instruct patient to consult with health care provider if unusual vaginal discharge or odor is noted.
- Educate patient to maintain optimal health with proper nutrition, exercise, weight control, and safer sex practices (e.g., always using condoms before intercourse or any penile-vaginal contact, avoiding multiple sexual partners).
- Advise patient to have a gynecologic examination at least once a year.
- Provide information about signs and symptoms of ectopic pregnancy (pain, abnormal bleeding, faintness, dizziness, and shoulder pain).

For more information, see Chapter 57 in Hinkle, J. L., & Cheever, K. H. (2014). *Brunner and Suddarth's textbook of medical-surgical nursing* (13th ed.). Philadelphia: Lippincott Williams & Wilkins.

Pemphigus

Pemphigus is a group of serious diseases of the skin characterized by the appearance of bullae (blisters) on apparently normal skin and mucous membranes (mouth, vagina). Evidence indicates that pemphigus is an autoimmune disease involving immunoglobulin G (IgG). Today, there are three recognized subsets of these types of IgG-mediated skin disorders, including *pemphigus vulgaris*, *pemphigus foliaceus*, and *paraneoplastic pemphigus*. Pemphigus vulgaris accounts for 70% of these blistering diseases. The diagnosis for these types of disorders is made by histologic examination of a biopsy specimen, usually by a dermatopathologist. Another type of IgG-mediated blistering disorder, called *bullous pemphigoid*, has distinct characteristics that make this disease different from the pemphigus diseases. Bullous pemphigoid is a chronic disease characterized by periodic flare-ups and remission. It is most commonly seen in older adults, with peak incidence at about 65 years of age.

Pathophysiology

Evidence indicates that pemphigus vulgaris is an autoimmune disease where the IgG antibody is directed against specific cell surface antigen in epidermal cells. A blister forms from the antigen–antibody reaction; the level of serum antibody is predictive of disease severity. The condition may be associated with ingestion of penicillin and captopril and with other concomitant autoimmune diseases such as myasthenia gravis. Genetic factors may also play a role, with the highest incidence in those of Jewish or Mediterranean descent. It occurs with equal frequency in men and women in middle and late adulthood.

Clinical Manifestations

- Most patients present with oral lesions appearing as irregularly shaped erosions that are painful, bleed easily, and heal slowly.
- Skin bullae enlarge, rupture, and leave large, painful eroded areas with crusting and oozing.
- A characteristic odor emanates from the bullae and the exuding serum.
- Blistering or sloughing of uninvolved skin occurs when minimal pressure is applied (Nikolsky's sign).
- Eroded skin heals slowly and, eventually, huge areas of the body are involved. Fluid and electrolyte imbalance and hypoalbuminemia may result from loss of fluid and protein.

Assessment and Diagnostic Findings

Diagnosis is confirmed by histologic examination of a biopsy specimen and immunofluorescent examination of the serum, which show circulating pemphigus antibodies. In pemphigus vulgaris, specimens of the blister and surrounding skin demonstrate acantholysis (separation of epidermal cells from each other because of damage to, or an abnormality of, the intracellular substance), and immunofluorescent studies show the presence of intraepidermal IgG.

Medical Management

Goals of therapy are to bring the disease under control as rapidly as possible, prevent loss of serum and development of secondary infection, and promote re-epithelialization of the skin.

- Corticosteroid agents are administered in high doses to control the disease and keep the skin free of blisters. The high dosage level is maintained until remission is apparent. Monitor for serious toxic effects from high-dose corticosteroid therapy.
- Immunosuppressive agents (e.g., azathioprine [Imuran], mycophenolate mofetil [CellCept], cyclophosphamide [Cytoxan]) may be prescribed to help control the disease and reduce the corticosteroid dose. The monoclonal antibody rituximab (Rituxan) is demonstrating promise as an effective therapeutic agent in clinical trials.

NURSING PROCESS

The Patient With Pemphigus or Other Blistering Diseases

Assessment

Disease activity is monitored by examining the skin for the appearance of new blisters as well as signs and symptoms of infection.

Diagnosis

NURSING DIAGNOSES
- Acute pain of oral cavity and skin related to blistering and erosions
- Impaired skin integrity related to ruptured bullae and denuded areas of skin
- Disturbed body image related to appearance of skin

- Risk for infection related to loss of protective barrier of skin and mucous membranes
- Deficient fluid and electrolyte balance related to loss of tissue fluids

Planning and Goals

The major goals may include relief of discomfort from lesions, skin healing, improved body image, absence of infection, and achievement of fluid and electrolyte balance.

Nursing Interventions

RELIEVING ORAL DISCOMFORT

- Provide meticulous oral hygiene for cleanliness and to support regeneration of epithelium.
- Provide frequent chlorhexidine mouthwashes to rinse mouth of debris. Avoid commercial mouthwashes.
- Keep lips moist with petrolatum.
- Use cool mist therapy to humidify environmental air.

ENHANCING SKIN INTEGRITY AND RELIEVING DISCOMFORT

- Provide cool, wet dressings or baths (protective and soothing).
- Premedicate with analgesic agents before skin care is initiated.
- Dry skin carefully and dust with nonirritating powder (e.g., cornstarch).
- Avoid use of tape, which may produce more blisters.
- Keep patient warm to avoid hypothermia.

See "Nursing Process" under Burn Injury for additional information.

PROMOTING A POSITIVE BODY IMAGE

- Demonstrate a warm and caring attitude; allow patient to express anxieties, discomfort, and feelings of hopelessness.
- Educate patient and family regarding the disease.
- Refer to psychological counseling as needed.

MONITORING AND MANAGING POTENTIAL COMPLICATIONS

- Keep skin clean to eliminate debris and dead skin and to prevent infection.
- Unpleasant odor may arise from skin due to a secondary infection.
- Inspect oral cavity for *Candida albicans* infection from high-dose steroid therapy; report if noted.

- Investigate all "trivial" complaints or minimal changes, because corticosteroid agents mask typical symptoms of infection.

> ◤ *Quality and Safety Nursing Alert*
>
> Because infection is the leading cause of death in patients with blistering diseases, meticulous assessment for signs and symptoms of local and systemic infection is required. Seemingly trivial complaints or minimal changes are investigated because corticosteroids can mask or alter typical signs and symptoms of infection.

- Monitor for temperature fluctuations and chills; monitor secretions and excretions for changes suggestive of infection.
- Monitor results of cultures and sensitivities; administer antimicrobial agents as prescribed, and note response to treatment.
- Employ effective hand hygiene techniques; use protective isolation measures and standard precautions.
- Avoid environmental contamination; protective isolation measures and standard precautions are warranted.

PROMOTING FLUID AND ELECTROLYTE BALANCE
- Administer saline infusion for sodium chloride depletion.
- Administer blood component therapy to maintain blood volume, and hemoglobin and plasma protein concentrations if necessary.
- Monitor serum albumin, hemoglobin, hematocrit, and protein levels.
- Encourage adequate oral intake.
- Provide cool, nonirritating fluids for hydration; provide small, frequent feedings of high-protein, high-calorie foods (e.g., oral nutritional supplements, eggnog, milk shakes) and snacks.
- Provide parenteral nutrition if patient cannot eat.

Evaluation

EXPECTED PATIENT OUTCOMES
- Reports relief from painful oral lesions
- Achieves skin healing
- Reports body image has improved

- Remains free of infection and sepsis
- Maintains fluid and electrolyte balance

For more information, see Chapter 61 in Hinkle, J. L., & Cheever, K. H. (2014). *Brunner and Suddarth's textbook of medical-surgical nursing* (13th ed.). Philadelphia: Lippincott Williams & Wilkins.

Peptic Ulcer

A peptic ulcer is an excavation formed in the mucosal wall of the stomach, pylorus, duodenum, or esophagus and is more likely to be in the duodenum rather than in the stomach. It is frequently referred to as a *gastric, duodenal,* or *esophageal ulcer,* depending on its location. The rates of peptic ulcer disease among middle-aged adults have diminished over the last three decades, while the rates among older adults have increased. More adults over age 65 years present to both outpatient and inpatient settings for treatment of peptic ulcers than any other age group.

Peptic ulcers tend to occur singly, but several may be present at one time. Chronic gastric ulcers usually occur in the lesser curvature of the stomach, near the pylorus. Esophageal ulcers occur as a result of the backward flow of hydrochloric acid (HCl) from the stomach into the esophagus (gastroesophageal reflux disease [GERD]). Peptic ulcer has been associated with bacterial infection, such as *Helicobacter pylori* (*H. pylori*). Predisposing factors include family history of peptic ulcer, blood type O, chronic use of nonsteroidal anti-inflammatory drugs (NSAIDs), alcohol ingestion, and excessive smoking; there is an association between peptic ulcers and chronic pulmonary or chronic renal diseases. Zollinger-Ellison syndrome (ZES) involves extreme gastric hyperacidity (hypersecretion of gastric juice), duodenal ulcer, and gastrinomas (islet cell tumors). It can cause severe peptic ulcers, extreme gastric hyperacidity, and gastrin-secreting benign or malignant tumors of the pancreas. *Stress ulcer* is the term given to the acute mucosal ulceration of the duodenal or gastric area that occurs after physiologically stressful events, such as burns, shock, severe sepsis, and multiple organ traumas; these ulcers are clinically different from peptic ulcers. Specific types of ulcers that result from stressful conditions include Curling's ulcers and Cushing's ulcers.

Pathophysiology

Peptic ulcers occur mainly in the gastroduodenal mucosa because this tissue cannot withstand the digestive action of gastric acid (HCl) and pepsin. The erosion is caused by the increased concentration (or activity) of acid–pepsin or by decreased resistance of the mucosa. A damaged mucosa cannot secrete enough mucus to act as a barrier against HCl. The use of NSAIDs inhibits the secretion of mucus that protects the mucosa. Patients with duodenal ulcers secrete more acid than normal, whereas patients with gastric ulcers tend to secrete normal or decreased levels of acid. Damage to the gastroduodenal mucosa results in decreased resistance to bacteria, and thus infection from H. pylori bacteria may occur.

Clinical Manifestations

- Symptoms of an ulcer may last days, weeks, or months and may subside only to reappear without cause. Many patients have asymptomatic ulcers.
- Dull, gnawing pain and a burning sensation in the mid-epigastrium or in the back are characteristic.
- Pain associated with gastric ulcers most commonly occurs immediately after eating, whereas the pain associated with duodenal ulcers most commonly occurs 2 to 3 hours after meals.
- Pain that is relieved by eating or taking an antacid is characteristic of duodenal ulcers.
- Awakening with pain during the night is reported by approximately 50% to 80% of patients with duodenal ulcers; only 30% to 40% of patients with gastric ulcers voice this complaint.
- Other symptoms include pyrosis (heartburn), vomiting (which may relieve severe pain and bloating), constipation or diarrhea, and bleeding (hematemesis or melena).
- Constipation or diarrhea may result from diet and medications.
- Bleeding (15% of patients with gastric ulcers) and tarry stools may occur; a small portion of patients who bleed from an acute ulcer have only very mild symptoms (or none at all).

Assessment and Diagnostic Findings

- Physical examination (epigastric tenderness, abdominal distention)
- Complete blood cell count (CBC) to assess extent of blood loss

P

- Upper endoscopy (preferred; suspicious lesions biopsied for histology and *H. pylori* testing)
- Diagnostic tests: analysis of stool specimens for occult blood; gastric secretory studies; and biopsy and histology with culture to detect *H. pylori* (possible also that serologic testing for *H. pylori* antibodies, stool antigen tests, or a urea breath test will detect *H. pylori*).
- Gastric secretory studies possibly of value in diagnosing achlorhydria and ZES

Medical Management

The goals of treatment are to eradicate *H. pylori* and manage gastric acidity with methods such as medications, lifestyle changes, and surgical intervention.

Pharmacologic Therapy

- Triple therapy used to suppress or eradicate *H. pylori* includes two antibiotics (e.g., metronidazole [Flagyl] or amoxicillin [Amoxil] and clarithromycin [Biaxin]) combined with a proton pump inhibitor (PPI) (e.g., lansoprazole [Prevacid], omeprazole [Prilosec], or rabeprazole [AcipHex]) and bismuth salts (Pepto-Bismol). Quadruple therapy with two antibiotics (metronidazole and tetracycline) plus a PPI and bismuth salts (Pepto-Bismol) is also used.
- H_2-receptor antagonists (in high doses in patients with ZES) are administered to decrease gastric acid secretion; maintenance doses of H_2-receptor antagonists are usually recommended for 1 year.
- PPIs or octreotide (Sandostatin, suppresses gastrin levels) may also be prescribed.
- Duration of treatment depends on location of ulcer.
- Cytoprotective agents (e.g., misoprostol, sucralfate) may be prescribed to protect mucosal cells from acid or NSAIDs.
- Patients at risk for stress ulcers (e.g., patients with head injury or extensive burns) may be treated prophylactically with IV H_2 blockers and cytoprotective agents.

Lifestyle Changes

- Smoking cessation is strongly encouraged because smoking decreases the secretion of bicarbonate into the duodenum, thereby increasing duodenal acidity and significantly inhibiting ulcer repair. Support groups may be helpful.
- Dietary modification may be helpful. Patients should avoid extremes of temperature and consumption of alcohol, coffee

(including decaffeinated coffee), and other caffeinated beverages. Patients should eat three regular meals a day; small, frequent meals are not necessary if antacids or histamine blockers are part of therapy.

Surgical Management

- With the advent of H_2 blockers, surgical intervention is less common.
- If recommended, surgery is usually for intractable ulcers (particularly with ZES for ulcers that fail to heal after 12 to 16 weeks of medical treatment), life-threatening hemorrhage, perforation, or obstruction. Surgical procedures include vagotomy (with or without pyloroplasty) or antrectomy (Billroth I or II).

NURSING PROCESS

The Patient With Peptic Ulcer Disease

Assessment

- Assess pain, its patterns, relationship to meals or sleep, and methods used to relieve it; take a thorough history, including a 72-hour food intake history.
- If patient has vomited, determine how often emesis occurs and whether emesis is bright red or coffee colored in appearance. This helps identify source of the blood. Inquire about any tarry stools.
- Ask patient about usual food habits, alcohol, smoking, and medication use (NSAIDs).
- Obtain a family history of ulcer disease.
- Assess vital signs for indicators of anemia (tachycardia, hypotension).
- Assess for blood in the stools with an occult blood test.
- Palpate abdomen for localized tenderness.

Diagnosis

NURSING DIAGNOSES

- Acute pain related to the effect of gastric acid secretion on damaged tissue
- Anxiety related to coping with an acute disease
- Imbalanced nutrition—less than body requirements—related to changes in diet

P

COLLABORATIVE PROBLEMS/POTENTIAL COMPLICATIONS
- Hemorrhage: upper GI
- Perforation
- Penetration
- Gastric outlet obstruction

Planning and Goals

The major goals for the patient may include relief of pain, reduced anxiety, maintenance of nutritional requirements, knowledge about the management and prevention of ulcer recurrence, and absence of complications.

Nursing Interventions

RELIEVING PAIN AND IMPROVING NUTRITION
- Administer prescribed medications.
- Instruct patient to avoid aspirin and other NSAIDs and avoid alcohol consumption.
- Encourage patient to eat regularly spaced meals in a relaxed atmosphere; obtain regular weights and encourage dietary modifications.
- Encourage relaxation techniques.

REDUCING ANXIETY
- Assess the patient's level of anxiety.
- Explain diagnostic tests and administer medications on schedule.
- Interact in a relaxing manner, help in identifying stressors, and explain effective coping techniques and relaxation methods.
- Encourage family to participate in care, and give emotional support.

MAINTAINING OPTIMAL NUTRITIONAL STATUS
- Assess for weight loss and signs of malnutrition.
- Reinforce importance of adhering to medication regimen and dietary restrictions after recovery from an acute episode.

MONITORING AND MANAGING COMPLICATIONS
Hemorrhage
- Hemorrhage is the most common complication of peptic ulcers; hematemesis or melena may be seen.
- Assess for faintness or dizziness and nausea, before or with bleeding; test stool for occult or gross blood; monitor vital signs frequently (tachycardia, hypotension, and tachypnea).

- Insert an indwelling urinary catheter and monitor intake and output; insert and maintain an IV line for infusing fluid and blood.
- Monitor laboratory values (hemoglobin and hematocrit).
- Insert and maintain a nasogastric (NG) tube and monitor drainage; provide lavage as ordered.
- Monitor oxygen saturation and administer oxygen therapy.
- Treat hypovolemic shock as indicated. (See "Nursing Process" under Shock, Hypovolemic in Section S for additional information.)
- Anticipate necessity of endoscopy to evaluate bleeding and provide targeted endoscopic interventions.
- Arteriography with embolization or surgery may be needed if there is a persistent and coincident gastric ulcer.

Perforation and Penetration
- Note and report symptoms of penetration (back and epigastric pain not relieved by medications that were effective in the past).
- Note and report symptoms of perforation (sudden abdominal pain, referred pain to shoulders, vomiting and collapse [fainting], extremely tender and rigid abdomen, hypotension and tachycardia, or other signs of shock).

Gastric Outlet Obstruction
- Gastric outlet obstruction occurs when the area distal to the pyloric sphincter becomes scarred and stenosed from spasm or edema or from scar tissue that forms when an ulcer alternately heals and breaks down.
- Symptoms include nausea and vomiting, constipation, epigastric fullness, anorexia and, later, weight loss.
- Insert NG tube; residual of more than 400 mL suggests obstruction.
- Treatment may include decompression of the stomach via an NG tube, balloon dilatation of the pylorus via endoscopy, and surgery (vagotomy and antrectomy or gastrojejunostomy and vagotomy).
- See Perioperative Nursing Management for additional information.

PROMOTING HOME- AND COMMUNITY-BASED CARE
Educating Patients About Self-Care
- Assist the patient in understanding the condition and factors that help or aggravate it.
- Educate the patient about prescribed medications, including name, dosage, frequency, and possible side effects. Also

identify medications such as aspirin or other NSAIDs that patient should avoid.
- Instruct patient to avoid foods that may exacerbate symptoms.
- Explain that smoking may interfere with ulcer healing; refer patient to programs to assist with smoking cessation.

Continuing Care
- Educate patient that follow-up supervision is necessary for about 1 year.
- Inform patient that the ulcer could recur and to seek medical assistance if symptoms reappear.
- Inform patient and family that surgery is no guarantee of cure. Discuss possible postoperative sequelae, such as intolerance of specific foods.

Evaluation

Expected Patient Outcomes
- Remains free of pain between meals and at night
- Reports feeling less anxiety
- Maintains weight
- Demonstrates knowledge of self-care activities
- Experiences no complications

For more information, see Chapter 47 in Hinkle, J. L., & Cheever, K. H. (2014). *Brunner and Suddarth's textbook of medical-surgical nursing* (13th ed.). Philadelphia: Lippincott Williams & Wilkins.

Pericarditis (Cardiac Tamponade)

Pericarditis refers to an inflammation of the pericardium, the membranous sac enveloping the heart. It may be primary or may develop in the course of a variety of medical and surgical disorders. Some causes are unknown; others include infection (usually viral, rarely bacterial or fungal), connective tissue disorders, hypersensitivity states, diseases of adjacent structures, neoplastic disease, radiation therapy, trauma, renal disorders, and tuberculosis (TB). Pericarditis also may occur 10 days to 2 months after acute myocardial infarction (Dressler's syndrome).

Pericarditis may be subacute, acute, or chronic and may be classified by the layers of the pericardium becoming attached to each other (adhesive) or by what accumulates in the pericardial sac: serum (serous), pus (purulent), calcium deposits (calcific), clotting proteins (fibrinous), blood (sanguinous), or malignancy (cancer). Frequent or prolonged episodes of pericarditis may lead to thickening and decreased elasticity that restricts the heart's ability to fill properly with blood (constrictive pericarditis). The pericardium may also become calcified, which restricts ventricular contraction. Pericarditis can lead to an accumulation of fluid in the pericardial sac (pericardial effusion) and increased pressure on the heart, leading to cardiac tamponade.

Clinical Manifestations of Pericarditis

- Pericarditis may be asymptomatic. Characteristic symptom is chest pain. Pain, which is felt over the precordium, beneath the clavicle, and in the neck and left scapular region, is aggravated by breathing, turning in bed, and twisting the body; it is relieved by sitting up (or leaning forward).
- The most characteristic sign of pericarditis is a creaky or scratchy friction rub heard most clearly at the left lower sternal border.
- Other signs may include mild fever, increased white blood cell count, anemia, an elevated erythrocyte sedimentation rate (ESR) or C-reactive protein level, nonproductive cough, or hiccups.
- Dyspnea and other signs and symptoms of heart failure (HF) may occur.

Clinical Manifestations of Cardiac Tamponade

- Falling blood pressure, rising venous pressure (distended neck veins), and distant (muffled) heart sounds with pulsus paradoxus
- Shortness of breath, chest tightness, or dizziness
- Anxious, confused, and restless state
- Dyspnea, tachypnea, and precordial pain
- Elevated central venous pressure (CVP)

Assessment and Diagnostic Findings

Diagnosis is based on history, signs, and symptoms; echocardiogram; and 12-lead electrocardiogram (ECG). CT for determining size, shape, and location of pericardial effusions may be used to guide pericardiocentesis. Cardiac magnetic resonance (CMR) may assist with detection of inflammation and adhesions. Occasionally, a video-assisted, pericardioscope-guided biopsy of the pericardium or epicardium is performed.

Medical Management

Objectives of management are to determine the cause, to administer therapy for the specific cause (when known), and to detect signs and symptoms of cardiac tamponade. Bed rest is instituted when cardiac output is impaired until fever, chest pain, and friction rub have disappeared.

Pharmacologic Therapy: Pericarditis

- Analgesics and NSAIDs such as aspirin or ibuprofen (Motrin) may be prescribed to relieve pain and hasten resorption of fluid in rheumatic pericarditis. Colchicine may also be used as an alternative medication.
- Corticosteroid drugs (e.g., prednisone) may be prescribed if the pericarditis is severe or if the patient does not respond to NSAIDs.

Surgical Management: Cardiac Tamponade

- Thoracotomy is performed for penetrating cardiac injuries.
- Pericardiocentesis is undertaken for pericardial fluid removal.
- Pericardial window, a small opening made in the pericardium, may be performed to allow continuous drainage into the chest cavity.
- Surgical removal of the tough, encasing pericardium (pericardiectomy), is performed if indicated.

> ### Quality and Safety Nursing Alert
>
> Nursing assessment skills are key to anticipating and identifying the triad of symptoms of cardiac tamponade: falling arterial pressure, rising venous pressure, and distant heart sounds. Search diligently for a pericardial friction rub.

NURSING PROCESS

The Patient With Pericarditis

Assessment

- Assess pain by observation and evaluation while having patient vary positions to determine precipitating or intensifying factors. (For example, is pain influenced by respiratory movements?)
- Assess pericardial friction rub: A pericardial friction rub is continuous, distinguishing it from a pleural friction rub. Ask patient to hold breath to help in differentiation: audible on

auscultation; synchronous with heartbeat; best heard at the left sternal edge in the fourth intercostal space where the pericardium comes into contact with the left chest wall; scratchy or leathery sound; louder at the end of expiration and may be best heard with patient in sitting position.

- Monitor temperature frequently, because pericarditis causes an abrupt onset of fever in a previously afebrile patient.
- Assess for signs and symptoms of cardiac tamponade, including shortness of breath, chest tightness, or dizziness.
- Observe for signs that the patient is becoming progressively more restless.
- Assess blood pressure; this may reveal a decrease of 10 mm Hg or more in systolic blood pressure during inspiration (pulsus paradoxus). Usually, the systolic pressure decreases and the diastolic pressure remains stable; hence, the pulse pressure narrows. The patient usually has tachycardia, and ECG voltage may be decreased or QRS complexes may alternate in height (electrical alternans). Heart sounds may progress from distant to imperceptible. Blood continues to return to the heart from the periphery but cannot flow into the heart to be pumped back into the circulation. The patient develops jugular vein distention (JVD) and other signs of rising CVP.

Diagnosis

NURSING DIAGNOSIS

Acute pain related to inflammation of the pericardium

COLLABORATIVE PROBLEMS/POTENTIAL COMPLICATIONS
- Pericardial effusion
- Cardiac tamponade

Planning and Goals

The major goals for the patient may include relief of pain and absence of complications.

Nursing Interventions

RELIEVING PAIN
- Advise bed rest or chair rest in a sitting-upright and leaning-forward position.
- Educate patient to resume activities of daily living as chest pain and friction rub abate. If chest pain and friction rub recur, encourage patient to resume bed rest.
- Administer medications; monitor and record responses.

MONITORING AND MANAGING POTENTIAL COMPLICATIONS

- Observe for pericardial effusion, which can lead to cardiac tamponade: arterial pressure falls; systolic pressure falls while diastolic pressure remains stable; pulse pressure narrows; heart sounds progress from being distant to imperceptible.
- Observe for neck vein distention and other signs of rising CVP.
- Notify physician immediately on observing any of the aforementioned symptoms, and prepare for diagnostic echocardiography and pericardiocentesis. Reassure patient and continue to assess and record signs and symptoms until physician arrives.

Evaluation

EXPECTED PATIENT OUTCOMES

- Is pain-free
- Experiences no complications

For more information, see Chapters 28 and 29 in Hinkle, J. L., & Cheever, K. H. (2014). *Brunner and Suddarth's textbook of medical-surgical nursing* (13th ed.). Philadelphia: Lippincott Williams & Wilkins.

Perioperative Nursing Management

As techniques to perform surgery change with improved technology and expertise, some surgeries have become less invasive and thereby less debilitating. The increased use of minimally invasive surgery—surgical procedures that use specialized instruments inserted into the body either through natural orifices or through small incisions—enable many surgeries to be performed on an outpatient basis. Surgery, whether elective or emergent, remains a complex, stressful experience. Even healthy patients having outpatient surgery may experience unanticipated complications during otherwise benign procedures.

The perioperative period standards encompass the domains of behavioral response, physiologic response, and patient safety and are used as guides toward development of nursing diagnoses, interventions, and plans, assuring the best outcomes. Perioperative nursing, which spans the entire surgical experience, consists of three phases: **preoperative** (which begins when the decision to proceed with surgical intervention is made until the time of transfer to the operating room [OR]),

intraoperative (which begins with the transfer to the OR until admission to the postanesthesia care unit [PACU]), and **postoperative** (which begins with admission to the PACU through discharge and follow-up).

Preoperative Concerns

Many patients enter the hospital 90 minutes prior to surgery and have necessary medical assessments and analyses preceding the surgical intervention. The surgical period is followed by a recovery period typically lasting a few hours in the PACU, and the patient may return home for recuperation the same day. For more invasive procedures, or when comorbidities exist, the patient may have laboratory studies completed prior to admission and may be required to be admitted to the hospital for a number of days postoperatively for physiotherapy, monitoring, and evaluation.

Traumatic and emergency surgery most often result in prolonged hospital stays. Patients who are acutely ill or undergoing major surgery and patients with concurrent medical disorders may require supportive supplementary care from other medical disciplines within the hospital setting. Regardless of the surgical setting, all patients require a comprehensive, preoperative nursing assessment, patient education, and nursing interventions to prepare for surgery.

Gerontologic Considerations

The hazards of surgery for older adults are proportional to the number and severity of coexisting morbidities and the nature and duration of the operative procedure. The underlying principle that guides the preoperative assessment, surgical care, and postoperative care is that older adults have less physiologic reserve (i.e., the ability of an organ to return to normal after a disturbance in its equilibrium) than younger patients. Sensory limitations, such as impaired vision or hearing and reduced tactile sensitivity, frequently interact with the postoperative environment.

Bariatric Patients

Bariatrics has to do with patients who are obese; like age, obesity increases the risk and severity of complications associated with surgery. Fatty tissues are especially susceptible to infection, and wound infections are more common in the obese patient. These patients tend to have shallow respirations when supine, increasing the risk of hypoventilation and postoperative pulmonary complications.

Patients With Disabilities

Special considerations for patients with mental or physical disabilities include the need for appropriate assistive devices, modifications in preoperative education, and additional assistance with and attention to positioning or transferring. Ensuring the security of assistive devices is important as well, because these devices are expensive and require time to replace if lost.

NURSING PROCESS

The Preoperative Patient

Assessment

PREOPERATIVE ASSESSMENT
- Obtain a health history, including chronic medical conditions, use of tobacco products, alcohol use, and use of illicit drugs.
- Perform a physical examination to establish vital signs and a database for future comparisons.
- Determine the existence of any allergies, previous allergic reactions, any sensitivities to medications or foods, and past adverse reactions to these agents; report a history of allergies, particularly bronchial asthma, to the anesthesiologist.
- Assess for allergies to latex by inquiring about allergies or adverse reactions to kiwi, avocado, bananas, or blowing up balloons (any of which may suggest latex allergy).

> ⚑ *Quality and Safety Nursing Alert*
>
> A latex allergy can manifest as a rash, asthma, or full anaphylactic shock.

- During the physical examination, note significant physical findings such as signs of physical abuse, pressure ulcers, edema, or abnormal breath sounds that further describe the patient's overall condition.
- Obtain and document medication history; include dosage and frequency of prescribed and over-the-counter (OTC) preparations, including supplements and herbal preparations.

> ◣ *Quality and Safety Nursing Alert*
>
> The possible adverse interactions of some medications require the nurse to assess and document the patient's use of prescription medications, OTC medications (especially aspirin), herbal agents, and the frequency with which medications are used. The nurse must clearly communicate this information to the anesthesiologist or anesthetist.

- Assess patient's usual activity level, including regular aerobic activity.
- Determine nutritional needs on the basis of patient's height and weight, body mass index (BMI), and waist circumference. Nutrition deficiencies should be corrected before surgery; assess hydration status.
- Assess mouth for dental caries, dentures, and partial plates. Decayed teeth or dental prostheses may become dislodged during intubation for anesthetic delivery and occlude the airway.
- Assess medical history for presence of any chronic conditions (e.g., asthma, chronic obstructive pulmonary disease [COPD], diabetes, recent corticosteroid therapy, uncontrolled thyroid disorders, immune disorders) that may be additional risk factors.
- Determine the extent and role of patient's support systems.
- Assess patient's readiness to learn; elicit patient concerns that can have a bearing on the surgical experience.
- Identify the ethnic or religious groups to which the patient relates and the customs and beliefs the patient holds about illness and health care providers.
- Monitor patients who are obese for abdominal distention, phlebitis, and cardiovascular, endocrine, hepatic, and biliary diseases, which occur more readily in the obese.
- Be alert for a history of drug or alcohol abuse when obtaining the patient's history; remain patient, ask frank questions, and maintain a nonjudgmental attitude.
- Investigate any abnormalities in baseline vital signs.

ASSESSMENT: AMBULATORY SURGERY
- Obtain the health history of the ambulatory or same-day surgical patient by telephone interview, at preadmission testing, or on admission to the preoperative area.

- Ask about health history, allergies, medications (including OTC or supplements), the extent of preoperative preparation, and psychosocial and demographic factors.
- Complete the physical assessment the day of surgery.

GERONTOLOGIC CONSIDERATIONS FOR ASSESSMENT

Because older adults have less physiologic reserve (cardiac, renal, and hepatic function and GI activity) than younger patients, monitor the older person undergoing surgery for subtle clues that indicate underlying problems. Ensure older patients have their glasses and any other assistive devices to support sensory deficits. Also monitor older adults for dehydration, hypovolemia, and electrolyte imbalances, which can be a significant problem in this population. The depletion of fluids and electrolytes following bowel preparation can result in dehydration and chemical imbalances, even among healthy surgical patients.

Diagnosis

NURSING DIAGNOSES

- Anxiety related to the surgical experience (anesthesia, pain) and the outcome of surgery
- Risk for ineffective therapeutic management regimen related to deficient knowledge of preoperative procedures and protocols and postoperative expectations
- Fear related to perceived threat of the surgical procedure and separation from support system
- Deficient knowledge related to the surgical process

Planning and Goals

The preoperative surgical patient's major goals may include relief of preoperative anxiety, adequate nutrition and fluids, optimal respiratory and cardiovascular status, optimal hepatic and renal function, mobility and active body movement, spiritual comfort, and knowledge of preoperative preparations and postoperative expectations.

Nursing Interventions

PROVIDING PREOPERATIVE PATIENT EDUCATION

- Educate each patient as an individual, with consideration for any unique concerns or learning needs; use written instructions, audiovisual resources, and contact numbers for follow-up information.

- Begin educational discussions as soon as possible, starting in the physician's office and continuing during the preadmission visit and through arrival in the OR.
- During the preadmission visit, arrange for the patient to meet and ask questions of the perianesthesia nurse, view audiovisuals, and review written materials. Include descriptions of the procedures and explanations of the sensations the patient will experience. Provide a telephone number for patient to call if questions arise closer to the date of surgery.
- Reinforce information about the presence of drainage tubes or other types of equipment to help the patient adjust during the postoperative period. If mechanical ventilation is expected, discuss this prior to surgery.
- Inform the patient when family and friends will be able to visit after surgery and that a spiritual advisor will be available if desired.

EDUCATING THE AMBULATORY SURGICAL PATIENT
- Educational concepts in previous sections should be covered as relevant to the patient.
- Assess preoperative educational needs and educate the patient if there are deficiencies. For the same-day or ambulatory surgical patient, discuss discharge and follow-up home care.
- Identify the individual who will drive the patient home.
- Answer questions and describe what to expect.
- Tell the patient when and where to report, what to bring (e.g., insurance card, list of medications and allergies), what to leave at home (e.g., jewelry, watch, medications, contact lenses), and what to wear (e.g., loose-fitting, comfortable clothes; flat shoes).
- During the last preoperative phone call, remind the patient not to eat or drink as directed; brushing teeth is permitted, but no fluids should be swallowed.

OBTAINING INFORMED CONSENT
- Reinforce information provided by surgeon.
- Ask patient to describe the planned surgery in his or her own words to assess patient's comprehension.
- Notify physician if patient needs additional information to make his or her decision.
- Ascertain that the appropriate consent form has been signed before administering psychoactive premedication.

- Arrange for a responsible family member or legal guardian to be available to give consent when the patient is a minor or is unconscious or incompetent; an emancipated minor (married or independently earning own living) may sign his or her own surgical consent form.

> ▶ *Quality and Safety Nursing Alert*
>
> The signed consent form is placed on the patient's medical record and accompanies the patient to the OR.

REDUCING ANXIETY AND FEAR: PROVIDING PSYCHOSOCIAL SUPPORT

- Be a good listener, be empathetic, and provide information that helps alleviate concerns.
- During preliminary contacts, give the patient opportunities to ask questions and to become acquainted with those who might be providing care during and after surgery.
- Acknowledge patient concerns or worries about impending surgery by listening and communicating therapeutically.
- Explore any fears with patient, and arrange for the assistance of other health professionals if required.
- Educate patient regarding cognitive strategies that may be useful for relieving tension, overcoming anxiety, and achieving relaxation, including imagery, distraction, or optimistic affirmations.

MAINTAINING PATIENT SAFETY

- Protecting patients from injury is one of the major roles of the perioperative nurse.
- Adherence to recommended practices and patient safety goals as set out by the Association of Perioperative Registered Nurses (AORN) and the Joint Commission is crucial.

MANAGING NUTRITION AND FLUIDS

- Provide nutritional support as ordered to correct any nutrient deficiency before surgery, ensuring that the patient has sufficient protein for tissue repair.
- Instruct patient that oral intake of food or water should be withheld 8 to 10 hours before the operation (most common), unless physician allows clear fluids up to 3 to 4 hours before surgery. Review specific dietary requirements based on individual patient's circumstance.
- In dehydrated patients, and especially in older patients, encourage fluids by mouth, as ordered, before surgery, and administer IV fluids as ordered.

- Monitor the patient with a history of chronic alcoholism for malnutrition and other systemic problems that increase the surgical risk, as well as for alcohol withdrawal (delirium tremens up to 72 hours after alcohol withdrawal).

Promoting Optimal Respiratory and Cardiovascular Status

- Urge patient to stop smoking 2 months before surgery (or at least 24 hours before).
- Educate patient about effective coughing and deep breathing exercises and how to use an incentive spirometer if indicated. Demonstrate proper splinting to support surgical area during coughing.
- In the patient with cardiovascular disease, avoid sudden changes of position, prolonged immobilization, hypotension or hypoxia, and overloading of the circulatory system with fluids or blood.

Supporting Hepatic and Renal Function

- If the patient has a disorder of the liver, carefully assess various liver function tests and acid–base status.
- Frequently monitor blood glucose levels of the patient with diabetes before, during, and after surgery.
- Report to the anesthesiologist and surgeon the patient's use of steroid medications for any purpose during the preceding year; monitor patient for signs of adrenal insufficiency.

Promoting Mobility and Active Body Movement

- Explain the rationale for frequent position changes after surgery (to improve circulation, prevent venous stasis, and promote optimal respiratory function) and show patient how to turn from side to side and assume the lateral position without causing pain or disrupting IV lines, drainage tubes, or other apparatus.
- Discuss any special position patient will need to maintain after surgery (e.g., adduction or elevation of an extremity) and the importance of maintaining as much mobility as possible despite restrictions.
- Instruct patient in exercises of the extremities, including extension and flexion of the knee and hip joints (similar to bicycle riding while lying on the side); foot rotation (tracing the largest possible circle with the great toe); and range of motion of the elbow and shoulder.
- Use proper body mechanics and instruct patient to do the same. Maintain patient's body in proper alignment when patient is placed in any position.

Introducing Pain Management and Cognitive Coping Strategies

- Introduce concept of pain scale and encourage patient to take prescribed pain medication as needed.
- Educate patients in cognitive strategies that may be useful for relieving tension, overcoming anxiety, decreasing fear, and achieving relaxation including imagery, distraction, optimistic self-recitation, or music.
- Encourage patient to take medications as frequently as prescribed during the initial postoperative period for pain relief.
- Before surgery, discuss with patient the use of oral analgesic agents and assess patient's interest and willingness to participate in pain relief methods.

Respecting Spiritual and Cultural Beliefs

- Help patient obtain spiritual help if he or she requests it; respect and support the beliefs of each patient.
- Ask whether the patient's spiritual advisor knows about the impending surgery.
- When assessing pain, remember that some cultural groups are unaccustomed to expressing feelings openly. Individuals from some cultural groups may not make direct eye contact with others; this lack of eye contact is not avoidance or a lack of interest but a sign of respect.
- Listen carefully to the patient, especially when obtaining the history. Correct use of communication and interviewing skills can help the nurse acquire invaluable information and insight. Remain unhurried, understanding, and caring.

Preparing the Bowel for Surgery

- If ordered preoperatively, administer or instruct the patient to take the antibiotic and a cleansing enema or laxative the evening before surgery and repeat it the morning of surgery.
- Have the patient use the toilet or bedside commode, rather than the bedpan, for evacuation of the enema, unless the patient's condition presents some contraindication.

Preparing the Skin for Surgery

- Instruct patient to use detergent–germicide for several days at home (if the surgery is not an emergency).
- If hair is to be removed, remove it immediately before the operation using electric clippers.
- Dress patient in a hospital gown that is left untied and open in the back.
- To ensure the correct site, the surgical site is typically marked by the patient and the surgeon prior to the procedure.

Immediately Preoperative Nursing Interventions

- Verify the identity of the patient and the patient's understanding of the expected surgical procedure.
- Cover patient's hair completely with a disposable paper cap; if patient has long hair, it may be braided; hairpins are removed.
- Inspect patient's mouth and remove dentures or plates.
- Remove jewelry, including wedding rings; if patient objects, securely fasten the ring with tape.
- Give all articles of value, including dentures, jewelry, and prosthetic devices, to family members or, if needed, label articles clearly with patient's name and store in a safe place according to agency policy.
- Assist patients (except those with urologic disorders) to void immediately before going to the operating room.
- Administer pre-anesthetic medication as ordered and keep the patient in bed with the side rails raised. Observe patient for any untoward reaction to the medications. Keep the immediate surroundings quiet to promote relaxation.

> ### Quality and Safety Nursing Alert
>
> Patient safety is the priority throughout the perioperative period but especially when administering prescribed pre-anesthetic medications. Pre-anesthetic medications can affect the central nervous system, causing changes in the patient's level of alertness and thus placing the patient at risk for injury.

- Check and verify all critical elements on preoperative checklist.

TRANSPORTING PATIENT TO OPERATING ROOM

- Send the completed preoperative checklist and the medical chart with patient to OR; attach signed surgical consent form and all laboratory reports and nurses' records, noting at the front of the chart in a prominent place any unusual last-minute observations that may have a bearing on the anesthesia or surgery.
- Take the patient to the preoperative holding area, greet by name, and position comfortably on the stretcher or bed. Keep the area quiet, avoiding unpleasant sounds or conversation.
- Use of a standard process or procedure to verify patient identification, the surgical procedure, and the surgical site is imperative to maximize patient safety.

Quality and Safety Nursing Alert

Someone should be with the preoperative patient at all times to ensure safety and provide reassurance (verbally as well as nonverbally by facial expression, manner, or the warm grasp of a hand).

 Gerontologic Considerations

Maintain a safe environment for the older patient with sensory limitations such as impaired vision or hearing and reduced tactile sensitivity. Initiate protective measures for the older patient with arthritis, which may affect mobility and comfort. Use adequate padding for tender areas. Move patient slowly and protect bony prominences from prolonged pressure. Provide gentle massage to promote circulation. Take added precautions when moving an older patient, because decreased perspiration leads to dry, itchy, fragile skin that is easily abraded. Apply a lightweight cotton blanket as a cover when an older patient is moved to and from the OR, because decreased subcutaneous fat makes older people more susceptible to temperature changes. Provide the older patient with an opportunity to express fears; this enables patient to gain some peace of mind and a sense of being understood.

ATTENDING TO THE FAMILY'S NEEDS

- Assist the family to the surgical waiting room, where the surgeon may meet the family after surgery.
- Reassure the family that they should not judge the seriousness of an operation by the length of time the patient is in the OR.
- Inform those waiting to see the patient after surgery that the patient may have certain equipment or devices in place (e.g., IV lines, indwelling urinary catheter, nasogastric [NG] tube, suction bottles, oxygen lines, monitoring equipment, and blood transfusion lines).
- When the patient returns to the room, provide explanations regarding the frequent postoperative observations.

Evaluation

EXPECTED PATIENT OUTCOMES

- Reports decreased fear and anxiety
- Voices understanding of surgical intervention
- Displays no evidence of preoperative complications

Postoperative Nursing Management

The postoperative period extends from the time the patient leaves the OR until the last follow-up visit with the surgeon (as short as a day or two or as long as several months). During the postoperative period, nursing care focuses on reestablishing the patient's physiologic equilibrium, alleviating pain, preventing complications, and educating the patient about self-care. Careful assessment and immediate intervention assist the patient in returning to optimal function quickly, safely, and as comfortably as possible. Ongoing care in the community through home care, telephone follow-up, and clinic or office visits promotes an uncomplicated recovery.

Postanesthesia care in some hospitals and ambulatory surgical centers is divided into three phases. Phase I, the immediate recovery phase, requires intensive nursing care. In phase II, the patient is prepared for self-care or care in the hospital or an extended care setting. In phase III, the patient is prepared for discharge.

Nursing Management in the Postanesthesia Care Unit

Patients still under anesthesia or recovering from it are placed in the PACU, formerly called the *postanesthesia recovery room*, which is located adjacent to the ORs. Patients may be in the PACU for as long as 4 to 6 hours or for as little as 1 to 2 hours. In some cases, the patient is discharged to home directly from this unit. Documentation of information and events germane to admission to the PACU care includes the following:

- Medical diagnosis, type of surgery performed, and location of surgical site
- Patient's age and general condition, airway patency, vital signs
- Anesthetic and other medications used (e.g., opioid drugs and other analgesics, muscle relaxants, antibiotic agents)
- Any problems that occurred in the OR that might influence postoperative care (e.g., extensive hemorrhage, shock, cardiac arrest)
- Fluid administered, estimated blood loss and replacement
- Any tubing, drains, catheters, or other supportive aids
- Specific information about which the surgeon, anesthesiologist, or anesthetist wishes to be notified
- Pathology encountered (if malignancy, whether the patient or family has been informed)

The nursing management objectives for the patient in the PACU are to provide care until the patient has recovered from the effects of anesthesia (i.e., until return of motor and sensory functions), is oriented, has stable vital signs, and shows no evidence of hemorrhage.

Role of PACU Nurse

Initial Assessment of the Patient Admitted to PACU

The nurse who admits the patient to the PACU reviews essential information with the anesthesiologist or anesthetist and any other licensed member of the OR team. Oxygen is administered, monitoring equipment is applied, and an immediate baseline physiologic assessment is conducted.

Maintaining a Patent Airway

- Obtain frequent assessments of the patient's oxygen saturation, pulse volume and regularity, depth and nature of respirations, skin color, level of consciousness, and ability to respond to commands; in some cases, end-tidal carbon dioxide ($ETCO_2$) levels are monitored as well.
- Assess airway patency, provide supplemental oxygen, and assess respiratory rate and depth, ease of respirations, oxygen saturation, and breath sounds.
- Prolonged anesthesia may result in relaxation that extends to the muscles of the pharynx so that when the patient is supine, the lower jaw and the tongue fall backward and the air passages become obstructed. This is called *hypopharyngeal obstruction* and can cause decreased oxygen saturation scores and, within minutes, a blue, dusky skin color (cyanosis).

> ### Quality and Safety Nursing Alert
>
> The treatment of hypopharyngeal obstruction involves tilting the head back and pushing forward on the angle of the lower jaw, as if to push the lower teeth in front of the upper. This maneuver pulls the tongue forward and opens the air passages.

Maintaining Cardiovascular Stability

- Check the surgical site for drainage or hemorrhage; secure connections for all drainage tubes and monitoring lines.
- Note IV fluids or medications currently infusing, and check against orders.
- Monitor vital signs and assess the patient's general physical status at least every 15 minutes, including assessment of cardiovascular function with the preceding assessments.

- Promote cardiovascular stability with prevention, prompt recognition, and treatment of hemorrhage, hypertension, dysrhythmias, hypotension, and shock.
- Inspect surgical site for bleeding; if bleeding is evident, a sterile gauze pad and a pressure dressing are applied, and the site of the bleeding is elevated to level of the heart, if possible.

> ⚑ *Quality and Safety Nursing Alert*
>
> A systolic blood pressure of less than 90 mm Hg is usually considered immediately reportable. However, the patient's preoperative or baseline blood pressure is used to make informed postoperative comparisons. A previously stable blood pressure that shows a downward trend of 5 mm Hg at each 15-minute reading should also be reported.

Relieving Anxiety and Pain

- Based on the patient's physiologic status, manage pain and provide psychological support in an effort to relieve the patient's fears and concerns.
- Opioid analgesic medications are administered mostly by IV in the PACU.
- Interventions to control postoperative nausea and vomiting (PONV) are best implemented at first report.

> ⚑ *Quality and Safety Nursing Alert*
>
> At the slightest indication of nausea, the patient is turned completely to one side to promote mouth drainage and prevent aspiration of vomitus, which can cause asphyxiation and death.

- Identify factors that increase risk for PONV (general anesthesia, female gender, nonsmoker, history of PONV, and history of motion sickness).

🌣 *Gerontologic Considerations for the PACU*

Special attention is given to keeping the older patient warm, because older patients are more susceptible to hypothermia. The patient's position is changed frequently to stimulate respirations and to promote circulation and comfort. Changes associated with the aging process, the prevalence of chronic diseases, alteration in fluid and nutrition status, and the increased use of medications result in the need for postoperative vigilance. Slower recovery from anesthesia for older adults is common due to the prolonged time to eliminate sedatives and anesthetic agents.

Postoperative confusion and delirium may occur in up to half of all older patients. Acute confusion may be caused by pain, altered pharmacokinetics of analgesic agents, hypotension, fever, hypoglycemia, fluid loss, fecal impaction, urinary retention, anemia, hypoxia, blood loss, and electrolyte imbalance and may be avoided by providing adequate hydration, reorientation to the environment, and careful assessment and titration of sedation and analgesia.

Determining Readiness for Discharge From the PACU

Usually the following measures are used to determine the patient's readiness for discharge from the PACU:

- Adequate respiratory function
- Adequate oxygen saturation level as compared with baseline
- Stable blood pressure
- Nausea and vomiting under control
- Adequate control of pain

Nursing Management: Discharge From Same-Day Surgery

Because patients in an ambulatory surgical center are most often discharged directly to home, expert patient education, including discharge planning, is necessary.

- Verify that the patient can be transported home safely by a responsible person.
- Inform the patient and caregiver (i.e., family member or friend) about expected outcomes and immediate postoperative changes anticipated in the patient's capacity for self-care.
- Provide written instructions about wound care, activity and dietary recommendations, medication, and follow-up visits to the same-day surgery unit or the surgeon. Provide caregiver with verbal and written instructions about what to watch for in the patient and about the actions to take if complications occur.
- Give prescriptions to patient, provide the nurse's or surgeon's telephone number, and encourage patient and caregiver to call if questions arise. Follow-up telephone calls from the nurse or surgeon may be used to assess patient's progress and to answer any questions.

- Instruct patient to limit activity for 24 to 48 hours (avoid driving a vehicle, drinking alcoholic beverages, or performing tasks that require energy or skill); to consume fluids as desired; and to consume smaller than normal amounts of food.
- Caution patient not to make important decisions at this time because the medications, anesthesia, and surgery may affect thinking ability.
- Refer patient for home care as indicated (older adults or frail patients, those who live alone, and patients with other health care problems that may interfere with self-care or resumption of usual activities).

Promoting Home- and Community-Based Care

- The home care nurse assesses the patient's physical status (e.g., respiratory and cardiovascular status, adequacy of pain management, surgical incision) and the patient's and family's ability to adhere to the recommendations given at the time of discharge. Previous instructions, including the necessity of follow-up, are reinforced as needed.
- The home care nurse may assess the surgical site; change surgical dressings or catheters or educate the patient or family about how to do so; monitor the patency of a drainage system; administer medications or educate the patient and family about how to do so; and assess for surgical complications.
- The home care nurse determines whether any additional services are needed and assists the patient and family to arrange for them (needed supplies, resources or support groups the patient may want to contact).

NURSING PROCESS

The Hospitalized Postoperative Patient

The nurse anticipates the arrival of the postoperative patient on the hospital unit and prepares the patient's room by assembling the necessary equipment and supplies: IV pole, drainage receptacle holder, emesis basin, tissues, disposable pads (Chux), blankets, and postoperative charting forms.

Assessment

- Receive report from the PACU nurse containing baseline data, including demographic data, medical diagnosis, procedure performed, comorbid conditions, unexpected intraoperative events, estimated blood loss, type and amount of fluids received, medications administered for pain, whether patient has voided, information patient and family have received about patient's condition, and specific information about which the surgeon, anesthesiologist, or anesthetist wishes to be notified.

- Review the postoperative orders, admit patient to unit, perform an initial assessment, and attend to patient's immediate needs.
- During the first hours after surgery, interventions focus on helping the patient recover from the effects of anesthesia, performing frequent assessments, monitoring for complications, managing pain, and implementing measures to promote self-care, successful management of the therapeutic regimen, discharge to home, and full recovery.
- In the initial hours after admission to the clinical unit, adequate ventilation, hemodynamic stability, incisional pain, surgical site integrity, nausea and vomiting, neurologic status, and spontaneous voiding are primary concerns.

> ### Quality and Safety Nursing Alert
>
> Unless indicated more frequently, record the pulse, blood pressure, and respirations every 15 minutes for the first hour and every 30 minutes for the next 2 hours. Thereafter, they are measured less frequently if they remain stable. Monitor patient's temperature every 4 hours for the first 24 hours.

Diagnosis

NURSING DIAGNOSES

Based on the assessment data, major nursing diagnoses may include the following:

- Risk for ineffective airway clearance related to depressed respiratory function, pain, and bed rest
- Decreased cardiac output related to shock, hemorrhage, or hypovolemia
- Acute pain related to surgical incision
- Impaired skin integrity related to surgical incision and drains
- Ineffective thermoregulation related to surgical environment and anesthetic agents
- Risk for imbalanced nutrition—less than body requirements—related to decreased intake and increased need for nutrients secondary to surgery

- Risk for constipation related to effects of medications, surgery, dietary change, and immobility
- Risk for urinary retention related to anesthetic agents
- Risk for activity intolerance related to generalized weakness secondary to surgery
- Risk for injury related to surgical procedure or positioning or anesthetic agents
- Risk for falls due to decreased consciousness or impairments to mobility
- Anxiety related to surgical procedure
- Risk for ineffective management of therapeutic regimen after discharge (care, dietary restrictions, activity recommendations, medications, follow-up care, or signs and symptoms of complications).

COLLABORATIVE PROBLEMS/POTENTIAL COMPLICATIONS

Based on the assessment data, potential complications may include the following:

- Venous thromboembolism (including deep vein thrombosis [DVT] or pulmonary embolism)
- Hematoma or hemorrhage
- Infection (wound sepsis)
- Wound dehiscence or evisceration

Planning and Goals

The major goals for the patient include optimal respiratory function, relief of pain, optimal cardiovascular function, increased activity tolerance, unimpaired wound healing, maintenance of body temperature, and maintenance of nutritional balance. Further goals include resumption of usual pattern of bowel and bladder elimination, identification of any perioperative positioning injury, acquisition of sufficient knowledge to manage self-care after discharge, and absence of complications.

Nursing Interventions

PREVENTING RESPIRATORY COMPLICATIONS

- Check the orders for and apply supplemental oxygen. Assess respiratory rate and depth, ease of respirations, oxygen saturation, and breath sounds.
- Risk for hypoxemia is increased in patients who have undergone major (particularly abdominal) surgery, are obese, or have pre-existing pulmonary problems. Hypoxemia is detected by pulse oximetry that measures blood oxygen saturation.

- Encourage patient to turn frequently, take deep breaths, and cough, and to use the incentive spirometer at least every 2 hours.
- Carefully assist patient to splint an abdominal or thoracic incision site to help patient overcome the fear that the exertion of coughing might open the incision.

> ▶ *Quality and Safety Nursing Alert*

Coughing is contraindicated in patients who have head injuries or who have undergone intracranial surgery, eye surgery, or plastic surgery.

- Administer pain medications to permit more effective coughing and deep breathing; suction patient as needed.
- Encourage early ambulation as soon as possible.

PROMOTING CARDIAC OUTPUT
- On patient's arrival in the clinical unit, observe the surgical site for bleeding, type and integrity of dressing, and drains (e.g., Penrose, Hemovac, and Jackson-Pratt).
- Monitor cardiovascular stability by assessing patient's mental status; vital signs; cardiac rhythm; skin temperature, color, and moisture; and urine output.
- Assess patency of all IV lines and ensure that the correct fluids are administered at the prescribed rate.
- Frequently assess output from wound drainage systems and amount of bloody drainage on the surgical dressing. Mark and time spots of drainage on dressings; immediately report excess drainage or fresh blood to surgeon.
- Reinforce dressing with sterile gauze bandages and record the time. Do not change initial dressing; surgeon will usually wish to be present.
- Monitor electrolyte, hemoglobin, and hematocrit levels.

ASSESSING AND MANAGING PAIN
- Assess pain level using a verbal or visual analog scale and assess the characteristics of the pain within the context of the individual patient's situation. (For example, patient's tolerance for pain may depend on the incision site, the nature of the surgical procedure, the extent of surgical trauma, the type of anesthesia, and route of administration.)
- Discuss options in pain relief measures with patient to determine the best medication. Assess effectiveness of medication

periodically, beginning 30 minutes after administration (sooner if given intravenously).

- Administer medication at prescribed intervals or, if ordered as needed, before pain becomes severe or unbearable. Risk of addiction is negligible with use of opioid agents for short-term pain control.
- Educate patient and family in the operation of patient-controlled analgesia.
- Provide other pain relief measures (e.g., changing patient's position, using distraction, applying cool washcloths to the face, and rubbing the back with a soothing lotion) to relieve general discomfort temporarily.

CARING FOR WOUNDS

- Inspect surgical site for approximation of wound edges, integrity of sutures or staples, redness, discoloration, warmth, swelling, unusual tenderness, or drainage.
- Assess area around wound for localized reactions to tape or trauma from tight bandages.
- Maintain adequate records of output from drains and dressings.
- Usually the first dressing change is performed by surgical team. Dressing changes should be performed at times to minimize patient discomfort (e.g., away from mealtimes or with visitors present).
- Hand hygiene is essential prior to any dressing changes. Assemble all needed supplies, and then proceed with dressing change using aseptic techniques.
- Remove old tape and dressing. Clean the surgical site based on surgeon's preference for skin cleanser. Dispose of old dressing and cleansing materials in designated biomedical waste container.
- Observe the surgical site for any drainage, redness, swelling, or bruising.
- Change to a fresh set of gloves and apply clean dressing with appropriate tape or occlusive material to hold the dressing in place.
- Provide patient education by reviewing steps for dressing changes and answering any questions.

MAINTAINING NORMAL BODY TEMPERATURE

- Monitor body system function and vital signs with temperature every 4 hours for the first 24 hours and every shift thereafter.

- Report signs of hyperthermia or hypothermia to physician. Hypothermia is a particular risk in older patients and those with lengthy surgeries.
- Maintain the room at a comfortable temperature and provide blankets to prevent chilling.
- Monitor patient for cardiac dysrhythmias.
- Make effort to identify malignant hyperthermia and to treat it early.

ASSESSING MENTAL STATUS

- Assess mental status (level of consciousness, speech, and orientation) and compare to preoperative baseline; change may be related to anxiety, pain, medications, oxygen deficit, or hemorrhage.
- Assess for possible causes of discomfort, such as tight, drainage-soaked bandages or distended bladder.
- Address sources of discomfort and report signs of complications to surgeon for immediate treatment.
- Assess neurovascular status; have patient move the hand or foot distal to the surgical site through a full range of motion, ensuring that all surfaces have intact sensation and assessing peripheral pulses.

MANAGING GI FUNCTION AND
RESUMING NUTRITION

- If in place, maintain NG tube and monitor patency and drainage.
- Provide symptomatic therapy, including antiemetic medications for nausea and vomiting.
- Administer phenothiazine medications as prescribed for severe, persistent hiccups.
- Assist patient to return gradually to normal dietary intake, at a pace set by patient (liquids first; then soft foods, such as gelatin, custard, milk, and creamed soups, added gradually; then soft and solid foods).
- Auscultate for bowel sounds. Paralytic ileus and intestinal obstruction are potential postoperative complications that occur more frequently in patients undergoing intestinal or abdominal surgery. See specific GI disorders for discussion of treatment.
- Encourage patient to turn frequently and ambulate as soon as possible to minimize postoperative abdominal distention. Early ambulation, improved dietary intake, and a stool

softener (if prescribed) promote bowel elimination, thereby decreasing risk of constipation.

- Arrange for patient to consult with the dietitian to plan appealing, high-protein meals that provide sufficient fiber, calories, and vitamins. Nutritional supplements, such as Ensure® or Sustacal, may be recommended.
- Instruct patient to take multivitamins, iron, and vitamin C supplements postoperatively if prescribed.
- Constipation is common after surgery owing to decreased mobility, decreased oral intake, and opioid analgesic medications. Early ambulation, improved dietary intake, and a stool softener (if prescribed) promote bowel elimination. If there is no bowel movement by the second or third postoperative day, the physician should be notified for additional interventions (e.g., laxative or other tests or intervention).

Managing Voiding

- Assess for bladder distention and urge patient to void on his or her arrival in the unit and frequently thereafter. (Patient should void within 8 hours of surgery.)
- Obtain order for catheterization before the end of the 8-hour time limit if patient has an urge to void and cannot, or if the bladder is distended and no urge is felt or patient cannot void.
- Initiate methods to encourage the patient to void (e.g., letting water run, applying heat to perineum).
- Warm the bedpan to reduce discomfort and automatic tightening of muscles and urethral sphincter.
- For the patient who complains of not being able to use the bedpan, assist to use a commode or stand or sit to void (males), unless contraindicated.
- Take safeguards to prevent the patient from falling or fainting due to loss of coordination from medications or orthostatic hypotension.
- Note the amount of urine voided (report less than 30 mL per hour) and palpate the suprapubic area for distention or tenderness or use a portable ultrasound device to assess residual volume.
- Intermittent catheterization may be prescribed every 4 to 6 hours until patient can void spontaneously and postvoid residual is less than 100 mL.

Encouraging Activity

- Have patient perform as much routine hygiene care as possible on first postoperative day (setting up patient to bathe with a bedside wash basin, or, if possible, assisting patient to bathroom to sit at a chair at the sink).

- Encourage most surgical patients to ambulate as soon as possible.
- Remind patient of the importance of early mobility in preventing complications (helps overcome fears).
- Anticipate and avoid orthostatic hypotension (postural hypotension: 20 mm Hg fall in systolic blood pressure or 10 mm Hg fall in diastolic blood pressure; weakness, dizziness, and fainting).
- Assess patient's feelings of dizziness and his or her blood pressure first in the supine position, after patient sits up, again after patient stands, and 2 to 3 minutes later.
- Assist patient to change position gradually; encourage the patient to splint the incision when applicable. If patient becomes dizzy, return patient to supine position and delay his or her getting out of bed for several hours.
- When patient gets out of bed, remain at patient's side to give physical support and encouragement.
- Take care not to tire patient.
- Initiate and encourage patient to perform bed exercises to improve circulation (range of motion to arms, hands and fingers, feet, and legs; leg flexion and leg lifting; abdominal and gluteal contraction).
- Encourage frequent position changes early in the postoperative period to stimulate circulation. Avoid positions that compromise venous return (raising the knee gatch or placing a pillow under the knees, sitting for long periods, and dangling the legs with pressure at the back of the knees).
- Apply antiembolism stockings and assist patient in early ambulation. Check postoperative activity orders before getting patient out of bed. Then have patient sit on the edge of bed for a few minutes initially; advance to ambulation as tolerated.

Encouraging Activity in Older Adults

Be aware that older adults are at increased risk for orthostatic hypotension secondary to age-related changes in vascular tone.

MAINTAINING A SAFE ENVIRONMENT

- Initially, patients recovering from anesthesia should have bed in lowest position with three bed rails up.
- Assess patient's level of consciousness and orientation; provide assistive devices (e.g., glasses or hearing aid) as soon as possible.

- Provide education for patient and family about call light and ensure call light is secured within easy reach for patient. Remind patient to call for assistance.
- Use of restraints should be avoided; agency policy on the use of restraints must be consulted and followed.
- If patient has had surgery of the lower extremities or will require a mobility aid (i.e., walker, crutches) at home, a physical therapist may be involved the first time patient gets out of bed.

PROVIDING EMOTIONAL SUPPORT TO THE PATIENT AND FAMILY

- Provide reassurance and information regarding the patient's diagnosis and surgery and explain hospital routines and what to expect in the time before discharge. Spend time listening to and addressing patient's and family's concerns.
- Informing patients when they will be able to drink fluids or eat, when they will be allowed to get out of bed, and when tubes and drains will be removed helps them gain a sense of control and participation in recovery and engages them in the plan of care.
- Modify the environment as necessary to promote rest and relaxation by providing privacy, reducing noise, adjusting lighting, providing seating for family members, and encouraging a supportive atmosphere.

MONITORING AND PREVENTING POSTOPERATIVE COMPLICATIONS

Venous thromboembolism (VTE). Monitor for symptoms of VTE, which may be a pain or a cramp in the calf elicited on ankle dorsiflexion (Homans' sign); pain and tenderness may be followed by a painful swelling of the entire leg and may be accompanied by a slight fever and sometimes chills and perspiration. Pulmonary embolism (PE) is another potential complication due to VTE. Avoid using blanket rolls, pillow rolls, or any form of elevation that can constrict vessels under the knees. Even prolonged "dangling" (having the patient sit on the edge of the bed with legs hanging over the side) can be dangerous and is not recommended in susceptible patients. Encourage early ambulation and adequate hydration (offer juices and water throughout the day).

Hematoma. A hematoma is concealed bleeding that occurs beneath the skin at the surgical site and usually stops spontaneously with clot formation. If it is small, the clot will be absorbed and need not be treated. If the clot is large, the wound usually bulges somewhat, and healing will be delayed unless the clot is removed. The surgical site may be re-opened and the clot evacuated, the wound may be packed with gauze and heal by granulation, or a secondary closure may be performed.

Infection (wound sepsis). Infection (wound sepsis) is a localized infection of the surgical site. Infection may not be evident until postoperative day 5; signs and symptoms of wound infection include increased pulse rate and temperature; an elevated white blood cell count; wound swelling, warmth, tenderness, or discharge; and incisional pain. *Staphylococcus aureus* accounts for many postoperative wound infections. Infections are treated with antibiotic medications, and surgeon may remove one or more sutures or staples in the incision to insert a drain.

Wound dehiscence and evisceration. Wound dehiscence (disruption of surgical incision or wound) and evisceration (protrusion of wound contents) are serious surgical complications, particularly when they involve abdominal incisions or wounds. These complications result from sutures giving way, from infection or, more frequently, from marked distention or strenuous cough. They may also occur because of increasing age, anemia, poor nutritional status, obesity, malignancy, jaundice, diabetes, use of steroid medications, and other factors.

> ### Quality and Nursing Alert
>
> If disruption of a wound occurs, the patient is placed in the low Fowler's position and instructed to lie quietly. These actions minimize protrusion of body tissues. The protruding coils of intestine are covered with sterile dressings moistened with sterile saline solution, and the surgeon is notified at once.

Gerontologic Considerations

Older adult patients recover more slowly, have longer hospital stays, and are at greater risk for development of postoperative complications. Delirium, pneumonia, decline in functional ability, exacerbation of comorbid conditions, pressure ulcers, decreased oral intake, GI disturbance, and falls are all threats to recovery in the older adult. Other problems confronting the older adult postoperative patient, such as pneumonia, altered bowel function, DVT, weakness, and functional decline, often can be prevented by early and progressive ambulation. Prolonged sitting positions are avoided as they promote venous stasis in the lower extremities. In addition to monitoring and managing physiologic recovery of the older adult, the nurse identifies and addresses psychosocial needs. The older adult may require much encouragement and support to resume activities, and the pace may be slow. Sensory deficits may require frequent repetition of instructions, and decreased physiologic reserve may necessitate frequent rest periods. The older adult may require extensive discharge planning to coordinate both professional and family care providers.

PROMOTING HOME- AND COMMUNITY-BASED CARE

Continuing Care

Community-based services are frequently necessary after surgery. Older patients, patients who live alone, patients without family support, and patients with preexisting chronic illness or disabilities are often in greatest need. Planning for discharge involves arranging early during the acute care hospitalization for necessary services for wound care, drain management, catheter care, infusion therapy, and physical or occupational therapy. During home care visits, the nurse assesses the patient's surgical incision, respiratory and cardiovascular status, adequacy of pain management, fluid and nutritional status, and progress in returning to preoperative status and evaluates the patient's and family's ability to manage all the components of care at home. The patient and family are instructed about signs and symptoms to be reported to the surgeon. In addition, the nurse provides information about how to obtain needed supplies and suggests resources or support groups.

Evaluation

EXPECTED PATIENT OUTCOMES

- Maintains optimal respiratory function
- Indicates that pain is decreased in intensity
- Increases activity as prescribed
- Experiences wound healing without complication
- Maintains body temperature within normal limits
- Resumes oral intake
- Reports resumption of usual bowel elimination and voiding pattern
- Is free of injury
- Reports decreased anxiety
- Acquires knowledge and skills necessary to manage therapeutic regimen
- Experiences no complications

For more information, see Chapters 17, 18, and 19 in Hinkle, J. L., & Cheever, K. H. (2014). *Brunner and Suddarth's textbook of medical-surgical nursing* (13th ed.). Philadelphia: Lippincott Williams & Wilkins.

Peripheral Arterial Occlusive Disease

Peripheral arterial occlusive disease (peripheral arterial occlusive disease [PAD]) is an arterial insufficiency of the extremities found more often in men and predominantly in the legs. The age of onset and the severity are influenced by the type and number of atherosclerotic risk factors present. Obstructive lesions are predominantly confined to segments of the arterial system extending from the aorta below the renal arteries to the popliteal artery.

Clinical Manifestations
- Intermittent claudication, the hallmark of PAD, is insidious and described as aching, cramping, fatigue, or weakness and is relieved with rest. Patient may report increased pain with ambulation; pain commonly occurs distal to the area of occlusion.
- Coldness or numbness in the extremities may accompany intermittent claudication.
- Rest pain is persistent, aching, or boring and is usually present in distal extremities with severe disease.
- Elevation or horizontal placement of the extremity aggravates the pain; lowering the extremity to a dependent position reduces pain.
- Extremities may be cool and exhibit pallor on elevation or a ruddy, cyanotic color when in a dependent position.
- Skin and nail changes, ulcerations, gangrene, and muscle atrophy may be evident.
- Bruits may be auscultated, and peripheral pulses may be diminished or absent.
- Inequality of pulses between extremities or absence of a normally palpable pulse is a sign of PAD.
- Nails may be thickened and opaque and the skin shiny, atrophic, and dry, with sparse hair growth.

Assessment and Diagnostic Findings
The diagnosis of PAD may be made using continuous wave (CW) Doppler and ankle-brachial index (ABI) tests, treadmill testing for claudication, duplex ultrasonography, or other imaging studies previously described.

Medical Management
- Walking programs help to reduce symptoms and improve walking durations.

- Weight reduction and smoking cessation further improve activity tolerance.
- Arm-ergometer exercise training effectively improves physical fitness, central cardiorespiratory function, and walking capacity in patients with PAD claudication symptoms.

Pharmacologic Therapy
- Pentoxifylline (Trental) and cilostazol (Pletal) are approved for the treatment of symptomatic claudication.
- Antiplatelet agents such as aspirin or clopidogrel (Plavix) are used to prevent the formation of thromboemboli.
- Statin therapy can be used in some patients to reduce the incidence of new intermittent claudication symptoms; however, statin therapy has not improved overall mortality rates in patients without known vascular risks.

Surgical Management
Surgery is reserved for treatment of severe and disabling claudication or when the limb is at risk for amputation because of tissue necrosis and may include endarterectomy, bypass grafts (synthetic or autologous), and vein grafts.

Nursing Management

Maintaining Circulation Postoperatively
The primary objective in postoperative management of patients who have had vascular procedures is to maintain adequate circulation through the arterial repair.

- Check pulses, Doppler assessment, color and temperature, capillary refill, and sensory and motor function of the affected extremity and compare with those of the other extremity; record values initially every 15 minutes and then at progressively longer intervals.
- Perform Doppler evaluation of the vessels distal to the bypass graft for all patients after vascular surgery because it is more sensitive than palpation for pulses.
- Monitor ABI every 8 hours for the first 24 hours and then once daily until discharge.
- Notify surgeon immediately if a peripheral pulse disappears; this may indicate thrombotic occlusion of the graft.

Monitoring and Managing Potential Complications
- Monitor urine output (more than 30 mL per hour), central venous pressure, mental status, and pulse rate and volume to permit early recognition and treatment of fluid imbalances.

- Monitor for bleeding at the surgical site and the area of anastamosis.
- Instruct patient to avoid leg crossing and prolonged extremity dependence.
- Educate patient to perform leg elevation and to exercise limbs while in bed to reduce edema.
- Monitor for compartment syndrome (severe limb edema, pain, and decreased sensation).

Promoting Home- and Community-Based Care

- Assess patient's ability to manage independently or, if necessary, the availability of a support network (family and friends) to assist with daily activities.
- Determine patient's motivation to make lifestyle changes needed with chronic disease.
- Assess patient's knowledge and ability to assess for postoperative complications, such as infection, occlusion of graft, and decreased blood flow.
- Inquire whether patient wants to stop smoking and encourage all efforts to do so; provide local resources to assist the patient's smoking cessation.

For more information, see Chapter 30 in Hinkle, J. L., & Cheever, K. H. (2014). *Brunner and Suddarth's textbook of medical-surgical nursing* (13th ed.). Philadelphia: Lippincott Williams & Wilkins.

P | Peritonitis

Peritonitis, inflammation of the serous lining of the abdominal cavity (peritoneum), is usually the result of bacterial infection; the organisms come from diseases of the GI tract or, in women, the internal reproductive organs. It may occur secondary to a fungal or mycobacterial infection. It can also result from external sources, such as injury, trauma, or an inflammation from an extraperitoneal organ such as the kidney. Other common causes of peritonitis are appendicitis, perforated ulcer, diverticulitis, and bowel perforation; peritonitis may be associated with abdominal surgical procedures and peritoneal dialysis.

Pathophysiology

Peritonitis is caused by leakage of contents from abdominal organs into the abdominal cavity, usually as a result of inflammation, infection, ischemia, trauma, or tumor perforation. The most common bacteria implicated are *Escherichia coli* (*E. coli*), *Klebsiella*, *Proteus*, *Pseudomonas*, and *Streptococcus*. As bacterial proliferation begins, the tissues become edematous, and exudation of fluid develops in a short time. Fluid in the peritoneal cavity becomes turbid with increasing amounts of protein, white blood cells, cellular debris, and blood. The immediate response of the intestinal tract is hypermotility, soon followed by paralytic ileus with an accumulation of air and fluid in the bowel. Inflammation and paralytic ileus are the direct effects of the infection; intestinal obstruction from bowel adhesions may develop. Sepsis is the major cause of death from peritonitis (shock, from sepsis or hypovolemia).

Clinical Manifestations
Clinical features depend on the location and extent of inflammation.

- Diffuse pain becomes constant, localized, and more intense near the site of the inflammatory process.
- Pain is aggravated by movement.
- Affected area of the abdomen becomes extremely tender and distended, and muscles become rigid.
- Rebound tenderness and paralytic ileus may be present.
- Anorexia, nausea, and vomiting occur, and peristalsis is diminished.
- Temperature and pulse increase; hypotension may develop.

Assessment and Diagnostic Findings
- Complete blood cell counts (elevated leukocytes; possibly low hemoglobin and hematocrit if blood loss has occurred)
- Serum electrolytes (may show altered potassium, sodium, and chloride)
- Abdominal x-rays, ultrasound, CT scan, and peritoneal aspiration with culture and sensitivity studies
- MRI possibly useful for diagnosis of intra-abdominal abscesses

Medical Management
Fluid, colloid, and electrolyte replacement with an isotonic solution is the major focus of medical management. Hypovolemia occurs because massive amounts of fluid and electrolytes move from the intestinal lumen into the peritoneal cavity and deplete the fluid in the vascular space. Analgesic agents are administered for pain; antiemetic medications are administered

for nausea and vomiting. Intestinal intubation with nasogastric [NG] tubes and suction are used to relieve abdominal distention. Oxygen therapy by nasal cannula or mask is instituted to improve ventilatory function. Occasionally, airway intubation and ventilatory assistance are required. Massive antibiotic therapy may be instituted. If peritonitis is caused by peritoneal dialysis (PD), prompt antibiotic therapy is crucial. If the peritonitis does not respond to the therapy in 5 days, the PD catheter should be removed. Surgical objectives include removal of infected material: Surgery is directed toward excision (appendix), resection (intestine), repair (perforation), or drainage (abscess). The two most common postoperative complications are wound evisceration and abscess formation. Any suggestion from the patient that an area of the abdomen is tender, painful, or "feels as if something just gave way" must be reported. The sudden occurrence of serosanguineous wound drainage strongly suggests wound dehiscence.

Nursing Management

- Monitor the patient's blood pressure by arterial line if shock is present.
- Frequently monitor central venous or pulmonary artery pressures, as well as urine output.
- Provide ongoing assessment of pain, GI function, and fluid and electrolyte balance.
- Assess nature of pain, location in the abdomen, and changes in location.
- Administer analgesic medication and position for comfort (e.g., on side with knees flexed to decrease tension on abdominal organs).
- Record intake and output, as well as central venous and pulmonary artery pressures.
- Administer and monitor IV fluids closely; NG intubation may be necessary.
- Observe for decrease in temperature and pulse rate, softening of the abdomen, return of peristaltic sounds, and passage of flatus and bowel movements, which indicate peritonitis is subsiding.
- Increase food and oral fluids gradually, and decrease parenteral fluid intake when peritonitis subsides.
- Observe and record character of drainage from postoperative wound drains if inserted; take care to avoid dislodging drains.

- Postoperatively, prepare patient and family for discharge; educate the patient regarding care of incision and drains if still in place at discharge.
- Refer for home care if necessary.

For more information, see Chapter 48 in Hinkle, J. L., & Cheever, K. H. (2014). *Brunner and Suddarth's textbook of medical-surgical nursing* (13th ed.). Philadelphia: Lippincott Williams & Wilkins.

Pharyngitis, Acute

Acute pharyngitis, commonly referred to as a "sore throat," is a sudden painful inflammation of the pharynx caused mostly by viral infections, with bacterial infections accounting for the remainder of cases. When group A streptococci cause acute pharyngitis, the condition is known as *strep throat*. The inflammatory response results in pain, fever, vasodilation, edema, and tissue damage, manifested by redness and swelling in the tonsillar pillars, uvula, and soft palate. Uncomplicated viral infections usually subside within 3 to 10 days. Pharyngitis caused by more virulent bacteria is a more severe illness because of dangerous complications (e.g., sinusitis, otitis media, peritonsillar abscess, mastoiditis, and cervical adenitis). In rare cases, the infection may lead to bacteremia, pneumonia, meningitis, rheumatic fever, and nephritis.

Clinical Manifestations
- Fiery-red pharyngeal membrane and tonsils
- Lymphoid follicles swollen and freckled with white-purple exudate
- Cervical lymph nodes enlarged and tender
- Fever, malaise, and sore throat
- Hoarseness

Assessment and Diagnostic Findings
- Swab specimens obtained from posterior pharynx and tonsils (tongue not included)
- Rapid antigen detection test (RADT) for streptococcus used with professional clinical evaluation
- Backup culture of negative RADT

Medical Management
Viral pharyngitis is treated with supportive measures, whereas antibiotic agents are used to treat pharyngitis caused by

bacteria: penicillin (5 days) for group A streptococci and cephalosporins and macrolides (from 3 to 10 days) for patients with penicillin allergies or erythromycin resistance. In addition, a liquid or soft diet is recommended during the acute stage. In severe instances, IV fluids are administered if the patient cannot swallow. If the patient can swallow, he or she is encouraged to drink at least 2 to 3 L of fluid daily.

Analgesic medications (e.g., aspirin or acetaminophen [Tylenol]) can be given at 4- to 6-hour intervals; if required, acetaminophen with codeine can be taken three or four times daily.

Nursing Management

- Encourage bed rest during febrile stage of illness; encourage frequent rest periods once patient is up and about.
- Instruct patient about signs and symptoms that warrant prompt contact with the primary care provider including dyspnea, drooling, inability to swallow, and inability to fully open the mouth.
- Instruct patient about secretion precautions (e.g., disposing of used tissues properly) to prevent spread of infection and to replace his or her toothbrush.
- Examine patient's skin once or twice daily for possible rash because acute pharyngitis may precede some other communicable disease (e.g., rubella).
- Administer warm saline gargles or irrigations (105°F to 110°F [40.6°C to 43.3°C]) to ease pain. Also instruct patient regarding purpose and technique for warm gargles (as warm as patient can tolerate) to promote maximum effectiveness.
- Apply an ice collar for symptomatic relief.
- Perform mouth care to prevent fissures of lips and inflammation in the mouth.
- Permit gradual resumption of activity.
- Advise patient of importance of taking the full course of antibiotic therapy.
- Inform patient and family of symptoms to watch for, signs that may indicate development of complications, including nephritis and rheumatic fever.

For more information, see Chapter 22 in Hinkle, J. L., & Cheever, K. H. (2014). *Brunner and Suddarth's textbook of medical-surgical nursing* (13th ed.). Philadelphia: Lippincott Williams & Wilkins.

Pharyngitis, Chronic

Chronic pharyngitis is a persistent inflammation of the pharynx common in adults who work or live in dusty surroundings, use their voice to excess, suffer from chronic cough, and habitually use alcohol and tobacco. Three types are recognized: **hypertrophic**, a general thickening and congestion of the pharyngeal mucous membranes; **atrophic**, a late stage of type 1; and **chronic granular**, marked by numerous swollen lymph follicles of the pharyngeal wall.

Clinical Manifestations
- Constant sense of irritation or fullness in the throat
- Mucus that collects in the throat and is expelled by coughing
- Intermittent postnasal drip
- Difficulty in swallowing

Medical Management
- Treatment is based on symptom relief, avoidance of exposure to irritants, and correction of any upper respiratory, pulmonary, or cardiac condition that might be responsible for chronic cough.
- Nasal sprays or medications containing ephedrine sulfate or phenylephrine are used to relieve nasal congestion.
- Antihistamine decongestant medications, such as pseudoephedrine or brompheniramine/pseudoephedrine, may be used with a history of allergic rhinitis.
- Aspirin (for patients older than 20 years) or acetaminophen may be recommended to control inflammation and relieve discomfort.
- Tonsillectomy may be an effective option, if consideration is given to morbidity and complications relating to the surgery.

Nursing Management
- Recommend avoidance of alcohol, tobacco, secondhand smoke, exposure to cold, and environmental and occupational pollutants. Wearing a disposable mask may decrease exposure to pollutants.
- Encourage patient to drink plenty of fluids and to gargle with warm salt water to relieve throat discomfort. Using lozenges may help to keep the throat moist.

For more information, see Chapter 22 in Hinkle, J. L., & Cheever, K. H. (2014). *Brunner and Suddarth's textbook of medical-surgical nursing* (13th ed.). Philadelphia: Lippincott Williams & Wilkins.

Pheochromocytoma

A pheochromocytoma is a tumor (usually benign) that originates from the chromaffin cells of the adrenal medulla. In 90% of patients, the tumor arises in the medulla; in the remaining patients, it occurs in the extra-adrenal chromaffin tissue located in or near the aorta, ovaries, spleen, or other organs. The tumor may occur at any age, but peak incidence is between 40 and 50 years; it affects men and women equally and has familial tendencies. Ten percent of the tumors are bilateral, and 10% are malignant. Although uncommon, it is one cause of hypertension that is usually cured by surgery, but without detection and treatment it is usually fatal.

Clinical Manifestations

- Triad of symptoms is headache, diaphoresis, and palpitations in the patient with hypertension.
- Hypertension (intermittent or persistent) and other cardiovascular disturbances are common.
- Other symptoms may include tremor, headache, flushing, and anxiety.
- Hyperglycemia may result from conversion of liver and muscle glycogen to glucose due to epinephrine secretion; insulin may be required to maintain normal blood glucose levels.

Symptoms of Paroxysmal Form of Pheochromocytoma

- Acute, unpredictable attacks, lasting seconds or several hours, during which patient is extremely anxious, tremulous, and weak; usually abrupt onset of symptoms and slow subsidence
- Headache, vertigo, blurring of vision, tinnitus, air hunger, and dyspnea
- Polyuria, nausea, vomiting, diarrhea, abdominal pain, and feeling of impending doom
- Palpitations and tachycardia
- Life-threatening blood pressure elevation (more than 250/150 mm Hg), which can cause such severe complications as cardiac dysrhythmias, dissecting aneurysm, stroke, and acute renal failure
- Postural hypotension (decrease in systolic blood pressure, lightheadedness, dizziness on standing)

Assessment and Diagnostic Findings

- The signs associated with the "five Hs"—hypertension, headache, hyperhidrosis (excessive sweating), hypermetabolism, and hyperglycemia—are assessed.
- Measurements of urine and plasma levels of catecholamines and metanephrine ([MN], a catecholamine metabolite) and vanillylmandelic acid [VMA] or free catecholamines are the most direct and conclusive tests for overactivity of the adrenal medulla.
- Total plasma catecholamine (epinephrine and norepinephrine) concentration is measured with the patient supine and at rest for 30 minutes.
- A clonidine suppression test may be performed if the results of plasma and urine tests of catecholamines are inconclusive.
- Imaging studies (e.g., CT and MRI scans, ultrasonography, ^{131}I-metaiodobenzylguanidine [MIBG] scintigraphy) are used to localize the pheochromocytoma and to determine whether more than one tumor is present.
- Function of other endocrine glands is evaluated.

Medical Management

- Bed rest with the head of the bed elevated is recommended.
- The patient may be moved to the intensive care unit for close monitoring of ECG changes and careful administration of alpha-adrenergic blocking agents (e.g., phentolamine [Regitine]), sometimes in tandem with a beta-adrenergic blocker (e.g., propranalol [Inderal]). Smooth muscle relaxants (e.g., sodium nitroprusside [Nipride]) may be added to lower the blood pressure quickly.
- Preoperatively, the patient may begin treatment with a low dose of an alpha-adrenergic blocker (phenoxybenzamine [Dibenzyline]) 10 to 14 days (or longer) prior to surgery.
- Treatment is surgical removal of the tumor, usually with adrenalectomy; hypertension usually subsides with treatment. Patient preparation includes control of blood pressure and blood volumes, which is typically carried out over 4 to 7 days.
- Patient is hydrated before, during, and after surgery.
- Postoperative corticosteroid replacement is required as a long-term medication after bilateral adrenalectomy.
- Careful attention is directed toward monitoring and treating hypotension and hypoglycemia.
- Several days after surgery, urine and plasma levels of catecholamines and their metabolites are measured to determine whether the surgery was successful.

Nursing Management

- Monitor ECG changes, arterial pressures, fluid and electrolyte balance, and blood glucose levels.
- Monitor for a hypertensive crisis, which may result from manipulation of the tumor during surgical excision; this causes a release of stored epinephrine and norepinephrine, with marked increases in blood pressure and changes in heart rate.
- Encourage patient to schedule follow-up appointments to ensure that pheochromocytoma does not recur undetected.
- Inform patient about the potential for adverse effects of the medications, which include orthostasis, nasal stuffiness, increased fatigue, and retrograde ejaculation in men.
- Educate the patient about the purpose of corticosteroid agents, the medication schedule, and the risks of skipping doses or abruptly stopping administration of the doses.
- Educate the patient and family about how to measure the patient's blood pressure and when to notify the physician about changes in blood pressure.
- Encourage patient to begin a high-sodium diet on the second or third day after the introduction of an alpha-adrenergic blocking agent.
- Provide verbal and written instructions on collecting 24-hour urine specimen.
- Refer for home care nurse if indicated.
- Give encouragement and support, because patient may be fearful of repeated attacks.
- Educate patient on the importance of periodic checkups owing to high risk of hypertension recurrence, especially in young patients.

For more information, see Chapter 52 in Hinkle, J. L., & Cheever, K. H. (2014). *Brunner and Suddarth's textbook of medical-surgical nursing* (13th ed.). Philadelphia: Lippincott Williams & Wilkins.

Pituitary Tumors

Approximately 95% of pituitary tumors are benign. The tumors may be primary or secondary and functional or nonfunctional. Functional tumors secrete pituitary hormones, whereas nonfunctional tumors do not. The location and effects of these tumors on hormone production by target organs can be life threatening. Pituitary tumors are of three principal types, representing an overgrowth of eosinophilic cells, basophilic cells (hyperadrenalism), or chromophobic cells (cells with no affinity for either eosinophilic or basophilic stains).

Clinical Manifestations

Eosinophilic Tumors Developing Early in Life
- Gigantism: Patient may be more than 7 feet tall and large in all proportions.
- Patient is weak and lethargic, hardly able to stand.

Eosinophilic Tumors Developing in Adulthood
- Acromegaly (excessive skeletal growth of the feet, hands, superciliary ridge, molar eminences, nose, and chin)
- Enlargement of every tissue and organ of the body
- Severe headaches and visual disturbances because the tumors exert pressure on the optic nerves
- Loss of color discrimination, diplopia (double vision), or blindness of a portion of the field of vision
- Decalcification of the skeleton, muscular weakness, and endocrine disturbances, similar to those occurring in hyperthyroidism

Basophilic Tumors
Cushing's syndrome: masculinization and amenorrhea in females, truncal obesity, hypertension, osteoporosis, and polycythemia.

Chromophobic Tumors (90% of Pituitary Tumors)
- Obesity and somnolence
- Fine, scanty hair; dry, soft skin; a pasty complexion; and small bones
- Headaches, loss of libido, and visual defects progressing to blindness
- Polyuria, polyphagia, lowering of the basal metabolic rate, and subnormal body temperature

Assessment and Diagnostic Findings
- History and physical examination (visual field assessment)
- CT and MRI scans
- Measurements of hormones of target organs (e.g., thyroid, adrenal)

Medical Management of Pituitary Tumors and Acromegaly

- Surgical removal of the pituitary tumor (hypophysectomy) through a transsphenoidal approach is the treatment of choice.
- Stereotactic radiation therapy is used to deliver external-beam radiation therapy to the tumor with minimal effect on normal tissue.
- Conventional radiation therapy and the use of bromocriptine (dopamine agonist) and octreotide (somatostatin analogue) inhibit production or release of growth hormone.
- Hypophysectomy is used to surgically remove primary tumors.

For more information, see Chapter 52 in Hinkle, J. L., & Cheever, K. H. (2014). *Brunner and Suddarth's textbook of medical-surgical nursing* (13th ed.). Philadelphia: Lippincott Williams & Wilkins.

Pleural Effusion

Pleural effusion, a collection of fluid in the pleural space, is usually secondary to other diseases (e.g., heart failure, tuberculosis, pneumonia, pulmonary infections, nephrotic syndrome, connective tissue disease, pulmonary embolus, and neoplastic tumors). The effusion can be relatively clear fluid (a transudate or an exudate), or it can be bloody or purulent. Pleural fluid accumulates due to an imbalance in hydrostatic or oncotic pressures (transudate) or as a result of inflammation by bacterial products or tumors (exudate).

Clinical Manifestations

Some symptoms are caused by the underlying disease. Pneumonia causes fever, chills, and pleuritic chest pain. Malignant effusion may result in dyspnea and coughing. The size of the effusion, the speed of its formation, and the underlying lung disease determine the severity of symptoms.

- Small to moderate effusion: dyspnea possibly absent
- Large effusion: shortness of breath to acute respiratory distress
- Decreased or absent breath sounds, decreased fremitus, and a dull, flat sound on percussion over areas of fluid, and tracheal deviation away from the affected side

Assessment and Diagnostic Findings

- Physical examination
- Chest x-rays (lateral decubitus)
- Chest CT scan

- Thoracentesis
- Pleural fluid analysis (culture, Gram stain, acid-fast bacillus stain, red and white blood cell counts, chemistry, cytology, and pH)
- Pleural biopsy

Medical Management

Objectives of treatment are to discover the underlying cause; to prevent reaccumulation of fluid; and to relieve discomfort, dyspnea, and respiratory compromise. Specific treatment is directed at the underlying cause.

- Thoracentesis is performed to remove fluid, collect specimen for analysis, and relieve dyspnea and respiratory compromise.
- Chest tube placement and connection to water-seal drainage or suction may be necessary for drainage and lung re-expansion.
- With chemical pleurodesis, drugs are instilled into the pleural space. This promotes adhesion formation, which essentially obliterates the pleural space and prevents further accumulation of fluid.
- Other treatment modalities include surgical pleurectomy (insertion of a small catheter attached to a drainage bottle) or implantation of a pleuroperitoneal shunt.

Nursing Management

- Provide adequate analgesia prior to procedure. (This is a *very* painful procedure).
- Support medical regimen: Prepare and position the patient for thoracentesis and offer support throughout the procedure.
- Send thoracentesis fluid for laboratory testing as appropriate.
- Monitor chest tube drainage and water-seal system; record the amount of drainage at prescribed intervals.
- Administer nursing care related to the underlying cause of the pleural effusion. See "Nursing Process" or "Nursing Management" under the applicable disorder heading in this handbook for more information.
- Assist the patient in pain relief, including positioning the patient to assume positions that are least painful with frequent turning.
- Administer analgesic medication as prescribed and evaluate pain level.
- If the patient is an outpatient with a pleural catheter for drainage, educate the patient and family about management and care of the catheter and drainage system.

For more information, see Chapter 23 in Hinkle, J. L., & Cheever, K. H. (2014). *Brunner and Suddarth's textbook of medical-surgical nursing* (13th ed.). Philadelphia: Lippincott Williams & Wilkins.

Pleurisy

Pleurisy refers to inflammation of both the visceral and parietal pleurae. Pleurisy may develop in conjunction with pneumonia or an upper respiratory tract infection, tuberculosis, or collagen disease; after chest trauma, pulmonary infarction, or pulmonary embolism; as a result of primary or metastatic cancer; and after thoracotomy. When inflamed, pleural membranes rub together, resulting in a severe, sharp, knifelike pain intensified on inspiration.

Clinical Manifestations
- Pain usually occurs on one side and worsens with deep breathing, coughing, or sneezing.
- Pain is minimal or absent when the breath is held and is localized or radiates to the shoulder or abdomen.
- As pleural fluid develops, pain decreases.

Assessment and Diagnostic Findings
- Auscultation for pleural friction rub
- Chest x-rays
- Sputum analysis
- Thoracentesis for pleural fluid examination
- Pleural biopsy (less common)

Medical Management
Objectives of treatment are to discover the underlying condition causing the pleurisy and to relieve the pain.

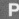

- Monitor patient for signs and symptoms of pleural effusion: shortness of breath, pain, assumption of a position that decreases pain, and decreased chest wall excursion.
- Prescribed analgesic agents, such as nonsteroidal anti-inflammatory drugs, may relieve pain to allow deep breathing and effective coughing.
- Topical applications of heat or cold are provided for symptomatic relief.
- An intercostal nerve block is done for severe pain.

Nursing Management
- Enhance comfort by turning the patient frequently on affected side to splint chest wall.
- Educate the patient to use hands or pillow to splint rib cage while coughing.

For more information, see Chapter 23 in Hinkle, J. L., & Cheever, K. H. (2014). *Brunner and Suddarth's textbook of medical-surgical nursing* (13th ed.). Philadelphia: Lippincott Williams & Wilkins.

Pneumonia

Pneumonia is an inflammation of the lung parenchyma caused by various microorganisms, including bacteria, mycobacteria, fungi, and viruses. Pneumonias can be classified into four types: community-acquired pneumonia (CAP), health care–associated pneumonia (HCAP), hospital-acquired pneumonia (HAP), and ventilator-associated pneumonia (VAP). Subcategories of the HCAP are those with immunocompromised host and aspiration pneumonia. Overlap is seen in the way specific pneumonias are classified, because they may occur in differing settings. Those at risk for pneumonia often have chronic underlying disorders, severe acute illness, a suppressed immune system from disease or medications, immobility, and other factors that interfere with normal lung protective mechanisms. Older adults are also at high risk.

Pathophysiology

An inflammatory reaction can occur in the alveoli, producing an exudate that interferes with the diffusion of oxygen and carbon dioxide, thus affecting both ventilation and perfusion. Bronchospasm may also occur if the patient has reactive airway disease. *Lobar pneumonia* is the term used if a substantial portion of one or more lobes is involved. Bronchopneumonia, the most common form, is distributed in a patchy fashion originating within the bronchi and extending to the adjacent surrounding lung parenchyma. Pneumonia has multiple risk factors based on pathogen type, including penicillin-resistant and drug-resistant pneumococci, enteric gram-negative bacteria, and *Pseudomonas aeruginosa*.

Clinical Manifestations

Signs and symptoms vary depending on the type, causal organism, and presence of underlying disease. The clinical signs and symptoms of a viral pneumonia are often difficult to distinguish from those of a bacterial pneumonia.

- Sudden chills and rapidly rising fever (38.5°C to 40.5°C [101°F to 105°F])
- Pleuritic chest pain aggravated by deep breathing and coughing
- In a severely ill patient, marked tachypnea (25 to 45 breaths/min), shortness of breath, and use of accessory muscles
- A relative bradycardia for the amount of fever, suggesting viral infection, mycoplasma infection, or infection with a *Legionella* organism

- Other signs: nasal congestion, sore throat, headache, low-grade fever, pleuritic pain, myalgia, rash, and pharyngitis; after a few days, expectoration of mucoid or mucopurulent sputum.
- Severe pneumonia: flushed cheeks, lips, and nail beds, demonstrating central cyanosis
- Orthopnea (patient preferring to be propped up or sitting in bed leaning forward)
- Poor appetite, diaphoretic, and easily tired
- Sputum purulent, rusty, blood-tinged, viscous, or green, depending on etiologic agent
- Signs and symptoms of pneumonia dependent on a patient's underlying condition (e.g., different signs possibly occurring in patients with conditions such as cancer and in those undergoing treatment with immunosuppressive agents, which decrease the resistance to infection)

Assessment and Diagnostic Findings

- Primarily history, physical examination
- Chest x-rays, blood culture, and sputum examination
- Nasotracheal or orotracheal suctioning or bronchoscopy in patients who cannot expectorate or induce sputum specimen

Medical Management

Pharmacologic Therapy

- Antibiotics are prescribed based on results of culture and sensitivity and antibiotic guidelines (resistance patterns, prevalence of causative organisms, risk factors, inpatient or outpatient setting, cost and availability of antibiotic agents must be considered).
- Supportive treatment includes hydration, antipyretics, antitussive medications, antihistamines, or nasal decongestants.
- Bed rest is recommended until infection shows signs of clearing.
- Oxygen therapy is given for hypoxemia.
- Respiratory support includes high inspiratory oxygen concentrations, endotracheal intubation, and mechanical ventilation.
- Treatment of shock, respiratory failure, or pleural effusion, if needed.
- For groups at high risk for CAP, pneumococcal vaccination is advised.

Gerontologic Considerations

Pneumonia in older adult patients may occur as a primary diagnosis or as a complication of a chronic disease. Pulmonary infections in older people frequently are difficult to treat and result in a mortality rate higher than that in younger people. General deterioration, weakness, abdominal symptoms, anorexia, confusion, tachycardia, and tachypnea may signal the onset of pneumonia. The diagnosis of pneumonia may be missed because the classic symptoms of cough, chest pain, sputum production, and fever may be absent or masked in older adults. Also, the presence of some signs may be misleading. Abnormal breath sounds, for example, may be caused by microatelectasis that occurs as a result of decreased mobility, decreased lung volumes, or other respiratory function changes. Chest x-rays may be needed to differentiate chronic heart failure (HF) from pneumonia as the cause of clinical signs and symptoms.

Supportive treatment includes hydration (with caution and with frequent assessment because of the risk of fluid overload in older adults); supplemental oxygen therapy; and assistance with deep breathing, coughing, frequent position changes, and early ambulation. To reduce or prevent serious complications of pneumonia in older adults, vaccination against pneumococcal and influenza infections is recommended.

P

NURSING PROCESS

The Patient With Pneumonia

Assessment

- Assess the patient for fever, chills, night sweats; pleuritic-type pain, fatigue, tachypnea, use of accessory muscles for breathing, bradycardia or relative bradycardia, coughing, and purulent sputum.
- Monitor the patient for the following: changes in temperature and pulse; amount, odor, and color of secretions; frequency and severity of cough; degree of tachypnea or shortness of breath; changes in physical assessment findings (primarily assessed by inspecting and auscultating the chest); and changes in the chest x-ray findings.

- Assess older adult patients for unusual behavior, altered mental status, dehydration, excessive fatigue, and concomitant HF.

Diagnosis

NURSING DIAGNOSES

- Ineffective airway clearance related to copious tracheobronchial secretions
- Fatigue and activity intolerance related to impaired respiratory function
- Risk for deficient fluid volume related to fever and a rapid respiratory rate
- Imbalanced nutrition: less than body requirements
- Deficient knowledge about treatment regimen and preventive health measures

COLLABORATIVE PROBLEMS/POTENTIAL COMPLICATIONS

- Continuing symptoms after initiation of therapy
- Sepsis and septic shock
- Respiratory failure
- Atelectasis
- Pleural effusion
- Confusion

Planning and Goals

The major goals for the patient may include improved airway patency, increased activity, maintenance of proper fluid volume, maintenance of adequate nutrition, an understanding of the treatment protocol and preventive measures, and absence of complications.

Nursing Interventions

IMPROVING AIRWAY PATENCY

- Encourage hydration: fluid intake (2 to 3 L per day) to loosen secretions.
- Provide humidified air using high-humidity face mask.
- Encourage patient to cough effectively, providing correct positioning to induce a cough.
- Perform chest physiotherapy; monitor patient for cough and sputum after completion.
- Encourage deep breathing with incentive spirometry.
- Provide nasotracheal suctioning if necessary.
- Provide appropriate method of oxygen therapy.

- Monitor effectiveness of oxygen therapy with pulse oximetry or arterial blood gas (ABG).

PROMOTING REST AND CONSERVING ENERGY

- Encourage the debilitated patient to rest and avoid over-exertion and possible exacerbation of symptoms.
- Patient should assume a comfortable position to promote rest and breathing (e.g., semi-Fowler's position) and should change positions frequently to enhance secretion clearance and pulmonary ventilation and perfusion.
- Instruct outpatients not to overexert themselves and to engage in only moderate activity during the initial phases of treatment.

PROMOTING FLUID INTAKE AND MAINTAINING NUTRITION

- Encourage fluids (at least 2 L per day minimum with electrolytes and calories).
- Administer IV fluids and nutrients, if necessary.
- Encourage small, frequent meals.

PROMOTING PATIENTS' KNOWLEDGE

- Instruct patient on cause of pneumonia, management of symptoms, signs and symptoms that should be reported to the physician or nurse, and the need for follow-up.
- Explain treatments in a simple manner and using appropriate language; provide written instructions and information and alternative formats for patients with hearing or vision loss.
- Repeat instructions and explanations as needed.

MONITORING AND PREVENTING POTENTIAL COMPLICATIONS

Continuing Symptoms After Initiation of Therapy

- Monitor for continuing symptoms of pneumonia (patients usually begin to respond to treatment within 24 to 48 hours after antibiotic therapy is initiated).
- Monitor for changes in physical status (deterioration of condition or resolution of symptoms) and for persistent recurrent fever, which may be a result of medication allergy (signaled possibly by a rash); medication resistance, or slow response (greater than 48 hours) of the susceptible organism to therapy; pleural effusion; or pneumonia caused by an unusual organism.
- Monitor for other complications such as septic shock, multiple organ dysfunction syndrome, and atelectasis.

P

Shock and Respiratory Failure
- Assess for signs and symptoms of septic shock and respiratory failure (e.g., evaluate vital signs, pulse oximetry, and hemodynamic monitoring parameters).
- Assess for atelectasis and pleural effusion.

Pleural Effusion
- Assist with thoracentesis, and monitor patient for pneumothorax after procedure.
- Monitor for pneumothorax or recurrence of pleural effusion.

Confusion
- Monitor for confusion or cognitive changes.
- Assess for and correct underlying factors: hypoxemia, fever, dehydration, sleep deprivation, or developing sepsis.

PROMOTING HOME- AND COMMUNITY-BASED CARE

Educating Patients About Self-Care
- Instruct patient to continue taking a full course of antibiotics as prescribed; educate the patient about their proper administration and potential side effects.
- Instruct patient about symptoms that require contacting the primary provider: difficulty breathing, worsening cough, recurrent/increasing fever, and medication intolerance.
- Advise patient to increase activities gradually after fever subsides.
- Advise patient that fatigue and weakness may linger.
- Encourage breathing exercises to promote lung expansion and clearing.
- Encourage follow-up chest x-rays and physical examination.
- Encourage patient to stop smoking, if necessary.
- Instruct patient to avoid stress, fatigue, sudden changes in temperature, and excessive alcohol intake, all of which lower resistance to pneumonia.
- Review principles of adequate nutrition and rest.

Continuing Care
- Refer patient for home care to facilitate adherence to therapeutic regimen, as indicated.
- Recommend influenza vaccine to all patients at risk.

Evaluation

Expected patient outcomes may include the following:
- Demonstrates improved airway patency, as evidenced by adequate oxygenation by pulse oximetry or ABG analysis,

normal temperature, normal breath sounds, and effective coughing

- Rests and conserves energy by limiting activities and remaining in bed while symptomatic and then slowly increasing activities
- Maintains adequate hydration, as evidenced by an adequate fluid intake and urine output and normal skin turgor
- Consumes adequate dietary intake, as evidenced by maintenance or increase in body weight without excess fluid gain
- Verbalizes increased knowledge about management strategies
- Complies with management strategies
- Exhibits no complications
- Exhibits acceptable vital signs, pulse oximetry, and ABG measurements
- Reports productive cough that diminishes over time
- Has absence of signs or symptoms of sepsis, septic shock, respiratory failure, or pleural effusion
- Remains oriented and aware of surroundings
- Maintains or increases weight
- Complies with treatment protocol and prevention strategies

For more information, see Chapter 23 in Hinkle, J. L., & Cheever, K. H. (2014). *Brunner and Suddarth's textbook of medical-surgical nursing* (13th ed.). Philadelphia: Lippincott Williams & Wilkins.

Pneumothorax and Hemothorax

Any organ or structure within the chest is potentially susceptible to traumatic penetration, including the chest wall, lung and pleura, tracheobronchial system, esophagus, diaphragm, major thoracic blood vessels, and heart and other mediastinal structures. Common injuries include pneumothorax and cardiac tamponade.

Pneumothorax occurs when the parietal or visceral pleura is breached and the pleural space is exposed to positive atmospheric pressure. Normally, the pressure in the pleural space is negative or subatmospheric; this negative pressure is required to maintain lung inflation. When either pleura is breached, air enters the pleural space, and the lung or a portion of it collapses. Hemothorax is the collection of blood in the chest cavity because of torn intercostal vessels or laceration of the lungs injured through trauma. Often, both blood and air are found in the chest cavity (hemopneumothorax).

Types of Pneumothorax

Simple Pneumothorax

A simple, or spontaneous, pneumothorax occurs when air enters the pleural space through a breach of either the parietal or visceral pleura. Most commonly, this occurs as air enters the pleural space through the rupture of a bleb or a bronchopleural fistula. A spontaneous pneumothorax may occur in an apparently healthy person in the absence of trauma owing to rupture of an air-filled bleb, or blister, on the surface of the lung, allowing air from the airways to enter the pleural cavity. It may be associated with diffuse interstitial lung disease and severe emphysema.

Traumatic Pneumothorax

A traumatic pneumothorax occurs when air escapes from a laceration in the lung itself and enters the pleural space or from a wound in the chest wall. It may result from blunt trauma (e.g., rib fractures), penetrating chest or abdominal trauma (e.g., stab wounds or gunshot wounds), or diaphragmatic tears. Traumatic pneumothorax may occur during invasive thoracic procedures (i.e., thoracentesis, transbronchial lung biopsy, insertion of a subclavian line) in which the pleura is inadvertently punctured or with barotrauma from mechanical ventilation. A traumatic pneumothorax resulting from major injury to the chest is often accompanied by hemothorax. Open pneumothorax is one form of traumatic pneumothorax. It occurs when a wound in the chest wall is large enough to allow air to pass freely in and out of the thoracic cavity with each attempted respiration.

> ◣ *Quality and Safety Nursing Alert*
>
> Traumatic open pneumothorax calls for emergency interventions. Stopping the flow of air through the opening in the chest wall is a life-saving measure.

Tension Pneumothorax

A tension pneumothorax occurs when air is drawn into the pleural space and is trapped with each breath. Tension builds up in the affected pleural space, causing lung collapse. The heart, great vessels, and trachea shift toward the unaffected side of the chest (called a *mediastinal shift*), which is life-threatening. Both respiratory and circulatory function are compromised and may cause pulseless electrical activity.

Clinical Manifestations

Signs and symptoms associated with pneumothorax depend on its size and cause:

- Pain with sudden onset may be pleuritic.
- Small/uncomplicated pneumothorax causes chest discomfort and tachypnea.
- Large pneumothorax signals acute respiratory distress with total lung collapse.
- Anxiety, dyspnea, air hunger, use of accessory muscles, and central cyanosis from severe hypoxemia may occur.
- In a simple pneumothorax, the trachea is midline, expansion of the chest is decreased, breath sounds may be diminished or absent, and percussion of the chest may reveal normal sounds or hyperresonance depending on the size of the pneumothorax.
- In a tension pneumothorax, the trachea is shifted away from the affected side, chest expansion may be decreased or fixed in a hyperexpansion state, breath sounds are diminished or absent, and percussion to the affected side is hyper-resonant. The clinical picture is one of air hunger, agitation, increasing hypoxemia, central cyanosis, hypotension, tachycardia, and profuse diaphoresis.

Medical Management

The treatment goal is to evacuate air or blood from the pleural space.

- For pneumothorax, a small chest tube is inserted near the second intercostal space.
- For hemothorax, a large-diameter chest tube is inserted, usually in the fourth or fifth intercostal space at the midaxillary line.
- For excessive bleeding from the chest tube, autotransfusion is begun by taking the patient's own blood drained from the chest, filtering it, and then transfusing it back into the patient's vascular system.
- Traumatic open pneumothorax is plugged (petroleum gauze); patient is asked to inhale and strain against a closed glottis to re-expand the lung and eject air from the thorax until the chest tube is inserted and connected to water-seal drainage. Antibiotics are usually prescribed to combat infection from contamination.
- If more than 1,500 mL of blood is aspirated initially by thoracentesis (or is the initial chest tube output) or if chest tube

output continues at greater than 200 mL per hour, chest wall is opened surgically (thoracotomy). Urgency is determined by the degree of respiratory compromise.

- An emergency thoracotomy may also be performed in the emergency department if a cardiovascular injury secondary to chest or penetrating trauma is suspected.
- Patients with possible tension pneumothorax should immediately be given a high concentration of supplemental oxygen to treat the hypoxemia, and pulse oximetry should be used to monitor oxygen saturation.
- In an emergency situation, a tension pneumothorax can be decompressed or quickly converted to a simple pneumothorax by inserting a large-bore needle (14-gauge) at the second intercostal space, midclavicular line on the affected side. A chest tube is then inserted and connected to suction to remove the remaining air and fluid, re-establish the negative pressure, and re-expand the lung.

For more information, see Chapter 23 in Hinkle, J. L., & Cheever, K. H. (2014). *Brunner and Suddarth's textbook of medical-surgical nursing* (13th ed.). Philadelphia: Lippincott Williams & Wilkins.

Polycythemia

Polycythemia is an increased volume of red blood cells. The hematocrit is elevated by more than 55% in males or more than 50% in females. Polycythemia is classified as either primary or secondary.

Secondary Polycythemia

Secondary polycythemia is caused by excessive production of erythropoietin. This may occur in response to a reduced amount of oxygen (which acts as a hypoxic stimulus), as in cases of heavy cigarette smoking, chronic obstructive pulmonary disease (COPD), cyanotic heart disease, or nonpathologic conditions such as living at a high altitude. It can also result from certain hemoglobinopathies (e.g., hemoglobin Chesapeake), in which the hemoglobin has an abnormally high affinity for oxygen, or it can occur from a neoplasm, such as renal cell carcinoma. Secondary polycythemia can also occur from neoplasms (e.g., renal cell carcinoma) that stimulate erythropoietin production.

Polycythemia Vera (Primary)

Polycythemia vera, or primary polycythemia, is a proliferative disorder of the myeloid stem cells. The bone marrow is hypercellular, and the erythrocyte, leukocyte, and platelet counts in the peripheral blood are elevated. Diagnosis is based on an elevated erythrocyte mass, a normal oxygen saturation level, and often an enlarged spleen. The erythropoietin level may not be as low as would be expected with an elevated hematocrit.

Clinical Manifestations

- Ruddy complexion and splenomegaly
- Increased blood volume leading to headache, dizziness, tinnitus, fatigue, paresthesias, and blurred vision
- Increased blood viscosity leading to angina, claudication, dyspnea, and thrombophlebitis
- Elevated blood pressure and uric acid levels
- Erythromelalgia (a burning sensation in the fingers and toes)

 Quality and Safety Nursing Alert

Patients with neutropenia often do not exhibit classic signs of infection. Fever is the most common indicator of infection, yet it is not always present, particularly if the patient is taking corticosteroid agents.

Medical Management

Management of secondary polycythemia involves treatment of the primary problem. If the cause cannot be corrected, phlebotomy may be necessary to reduce hypervolemia and hyperviscosity.

The objective of management is to reduce the high red blood cell mass.

- Phlebotomy is performed repeatedly to keep the hemoglobin within normal range; iron supplements are avoided.
- Chemotherapeutic agents are used to suppress marrow function (may increase risk for leukemia).
- Anagrelide (Agrylin) may be used to inhibit platelet aggregation and control the thrombocytosis related to polycythemia vera.
- Interferon-alpha-2b (IntronA) is the most effective treatment for managing the pruritus associated with polycythemia vera.

- Antihistamines may be administered to control pruritus (not very effective).
- Allopurinol is used to prevent attacks of gout when the uric acid level is elevated.

Nursing Management

- Assess risk factors for thrombotic complications and educate patient in ways to recognize signs and symptoms of thrombosis.
- Discourage sedentary behavior, crossing the legs, and wearing tight or restrictive clothing (particularly stockings); this will reduce the likelihood of deep vein thrombosis.
- Advise patient to avoid aspirin and medications containing aspirin (if patient has a history of bleeding).
- Advise patient to minimize alcohol intake and avoid iron (and vitamins containing iron).
- Suggest a cool or tepid bath for pruritus, along with cocoa butter–based lotions and bath products to relieve itching.

For more information, see Chapter 33 in Hinkle, J. L., & Cheever, K. H. (2014). *Brunner and Suddarth's textbook of medical-surgical nursing* (13th ed.). Philadelphia: Lippincott Williams & Wilkins.

Prostatitis

Prostatitis is an inflammation of the prostate gland that is often associated with lower urinary tract symptoms and symptoms of sexual discomfort and dysfunction. It is the most common urologic diagnosis in men younger than 50 years and is also a common diagnosis after 50 years of age.

Pathophysiology

Prostatitis may be caused by infectious agents (bacteria, fungi, mycoplasma) or other conditions (e.g., urethral stricture, benign prostatic hyperplasia). The microorganisms colonize the urinary tract and ascend to the prostate, ultimately causing infection; the causal pathogen is usually the same in recurrent infections; *Escherichia coli* is the most commonly isolated organism. There are four types of prostatitis: acute bacterial prostatitis (type I), chronic bacterial prostatitis (type II), chronic prostatitis/chronic pelvic pain syndrome (CP/CPPS; type III, most common), and asymptomatic inflammatory prostatitis (type IV).

Clinical Manifestations

- Sudden onset of fever, dysuria, perineal prostatic pain, and severe lower urinary tract symptoms (dysuria, frequency, urgency, hesitancy, and nocturia) occur.
- Approximately 5% of cases of type I prostatitis (acute prostatitis) progress to type II prostatitis (chronic bacterial prostatitis); patients with type II disease are typically asymptomatic between episodes.
- Patients with type III prostatitis often have no bacteria in the urine in the presence of genitourinary pain.
- Patients with type IV prostatitis are usually diagnosed incidentally during a workup for infertility, an elevated prostate-specific antigen (PSA) test, or evaluation for other disorders.

Assessment and Diagnostic Findings

- Urinalysis including microscopy, urine culture and sensitivities
- Complete blood cell count (if patient is acutely ill)
- Electrolyte panel, including blood urea nitrogen (BUN; if symptoms of urinary obstruction or retention)
- Additional imaging studies (if significant voiding dysfunction is present)

Medical Management

The goal of treatment is to eradicate the causal organisms. Specific treatment is based on the type of prostatitis and on the results of culture and sensitivity testing of the urine. Hospital admission may be necessary for patients with unstable vital signs, sepsis, or intractable pelvic pain, those who are frail or immunosuppressed, or those who have diabetes or renal insufficiency.

Pharmacologic Management

If bacteria are cultured from the urine, antibiotic medications, including trimethoprim-sulfamethoxazole (TMP-SMZ) or a fluoroquinolone (e.g., ciprofloxacin [Cipro]), may be prescribed, and continuous therapy with low-dose antibiotic agents may be used to suppress the infection. If the patient is afebrile and has a normal urinalysis, anti-inflammatory agents may be used; alpha-adrenergic blocker therapy (e.g., tamsulosin [Flomax]) may be prescribed to promote bladder and prostate relaxation. Supportive, nonpharmacologic therapies may be prescribed (e.g., biofeedback, pelvic floor training, physical therapy, sitz baths, stool softeners).

Nursing Management

- Administer antibiotics as prescribed.
- Recommend comfort measures: analgesics, sitz baths for 10 to 20 minutes several times daily.
- Encourage fluids to satisfy thirst but do not "force" them, because effective drug levels must be maintained in urine.
- Instruct patient to avoid foods and drinks that have diuretic action or increase prostatic secretions, including alcohol, coffee, tea, chocolate, cola, and spices.
- Advise patient to avoid sitting for long periods to minimize discomfort.

Promoting Home- and Community-Based Care

Educating Patients About Self-Care

- Encourage patient to continue self-care activities at home, including sitz baths, avoiding foods or liquids with diuretic activity, avoiding sexual arousal or intercourse during periods of acute inflammation, and avoiding sitting for long periods of time
- Provide education regarding importance of completing entire course of therapy.
- If IV antibiotic medications will be given at home, educate family and patient regarding correct and safe administration; arrange for home care nurse if necessary.
- Advise patient and family that medical follow-up will be required from 6 months to 1 year.
- Educate patient to recognize signs and symptoms of a urinary tract infection and to seek appropriate care.

For more information, see Chapter 59 in Hinkle, J. L., & Cheever, K. H. (2014). *Brunner and Suddarth's textbook of medical-surgical nursing* (13th ed.). Philadelphia: Lippincott Williams & Wilkins.

Pruritus

Pruritus (itching) is one of the most common dermatologic complaints. Although it usually is due to primary skin disease, pruritus may also reflect systemic internal disease, such as diabetes; renal, hepatic, thyroid, or blood disorders; or cancer. Pruritus may be caused by certain oral medications (aspirin, antibiotic agents, hormones, opioid medications), contact with irritating agents (soaps, chemicals), or prickly heat (miliaria).

Pruritus may also be a side effect of radiation therapy, a reaction to chemotherapy, or a symptom of infection.

Gerontologic Considerations

Pruritus may occur in older adults as a result of dry skin; however, older adults are also more likely to have a systemic illness that triggers pruritus. They are at higher risk for occult malignancy and are more likely than younger people to be taking multiple medications. All of these factors increase the incidence of pruritus in older adults.

Pathophysiology

Scratching the itchy area causes the inflamed cells and nerve endings to release histamine, which produces more pruritus and, in turn, a vicious itch–scratch cycle. Scratching can result in altered skin integrity, with excoriation, redness, raised areas (wheals), infection, or changes in pigmentation.

Clinical Manifestations

- Itching and scratching, often more severe at night (itch–scratch–itch cycle)
- Excoriations, redness, raised areas on the skin (wheals), as a result of scratching
- Usually more severe at night
- Infections or changes in pigmentation
- Debilitating itching, in severe cases

Assessment and Diagnostic Findings

- Thorough physical examination of the skin and history to identify underlying cause of the pruritus (e.g., hay fever, allergy, recent medication change, change of cosmetics or soaps)
- Identification of signs of infection and environmental clues (i.e., warm, dry air or irritating bed linens)

Medical Management

The cause of pruritus needs to be identified and treated. The patient is advised to avoid washing with soap and hot water.

- Bath oils (Lubath or Alpha Keri) are prescribed, except for older adult patients or those with impaired balance, who should not add oil to the bath because of the danger of slipping.
- Warm baths with a mild soap, followed by application of a bland emollient to the moist skin, can control xerosis (dry skin).

- Applying a cold compress, ice cube, or cool agents that contain menthol and camphor (which constrict blood vessels) may also help relieve pruritus.

Pharmacologic Therapy

- Topical anesthetic agents (e.g., lidocaine, prilocaine) or capsaicin cream (Capzasin) may be useful in providing localized relief.
- Topical corticosteroid medications are prescribed to decrease itching secondary to inflammatory conditions.
- Oral antihistamine medications (diphenhydramine [Benadryl] or hydroxyzine [Atarax]) may be used; other nonsedating antihistamine agents are not helpful.
- Tricyclic antidepressant drugs (doxepin [Sinequan]) may be prescribed when pruritus is of neuropsychogenic origin.
- Selective serotonin reuptake inhibitor (SSRI) antidepressant drugs (e.g., fluoxetine [Prozac], sertraline [Zoloft]) may be effective, but results from studies to date are inconclusive.

Nursing Management

- Reinforce reasons for the prescribed therapeutic regimen.
- Remind patient to use tepid (not hot) water, to shake off excess water, and to blot between intertriginous areas (body folds) with a towel.
- Advise patient to avoid rubbing vigorously with towel, which overstimulates skin, causing more itching.
- Lubricate skin with an emollient that traps moisture (most effective immediately after bathing).
- Advise patient to avoid situations that cause vasodilation (warm environment, ingestion of alcohol, or hot foods and liquids).
- Keep room cool and humidified.
- Advise patient to wear soft cotton clothing next to skin and to avoid activities that result in perspiration.
- Instruct patient to avoid scratching and to trim nails short to prevent skin damage and infection.
- When the underlying cause of pruritus is unknown and further testing is required, explain each test and the expected outcome.

For more information, see Chapter 61 in Hinkle, J. L., & Cheever, K. H. (2014). *Brunner and Suddarth's textbook of medical-surgical nursing* (13th ed.). Philadelphia: Lippincott Williams & Wilkins.

Psoriasis

Psoriasis is a common, chronic, noninfectious, inflammatory disease of the skin characterized by the appearance of silvery plaques, most often over the elbows, knees, scalp, lower back, and buttocks. Bilateral symmetry often exists. Psoriasis may be associated with asymmetric rheumatoid factor–negative arthritis of multiple joints. An exfoliative psoriatic state may develop in which the disease progresses to involve the total body surface (erythrodermic psoriatic state). Onset may occur at any age, with a median age of 28 years; it is more prevalent in women, in Caucasians, and among persons who are obese. Psoriasis has a tendency to improve and then recur throughout life.

Pathophysiology

Current evidence supports an immunologic basis for psoriasis. The epidermis becomes infiltrated by activated T cells and cytokines, resulting in vascular engorgement and proliferation of keratinocytes, with resulting epidermal hyperplasia (overgrowth of the epidermis). These epidermal cells tend to improperly retain their nuclei, crippling their ability to release lipids that encourage cellular adhesion. This results in rapid turnover of poorly matured cells that do not adhere well to one another, resulting in the classic presentation of plaquelike lesions that have a silvery, scaly, flaky appearance.

Clinical Manifestations

Symptoms range from a cosmetic annoyance to a physically disabling and disfiguring affliction.

- Lesions appear as red, raised patches of skin covered with silvery scales.
- If scales are scraped away, the dark red base of lesion is exposed, with multiple bleeding points.
- Patches are dry and may itch.
- The condition may involve nail pitting, discoloration, crumbling beneath the free edges, and separation of the nail plate.

Complications

Asymmetric rheumatoid factor–negative arthritis of multiple joints occurs in up to 30% of people with psoriasis. Other complications such as spondylarthropathies, including psoriatic arthritis, may be seen. In addition, exfoliative dermatitis, also called *erythroderma*, may result from psoriasis.

Psychological complications from psoriasis should also be recognized. Psoriasis may cause despair and frustration; observers may stare, comment, ask embarrassing questions, or even avoid the person. The condition can eventually exhaust resources, interfere with work, and negatively affect many aspects of life. Teenagers are especially vulnerable to its psychological effects.

Assessment and Diagnostic Findings
- Presence of classic plaque-type lesions (which change histologically, progressing from early to chronic plaques)
- Signs of nail and scalp involvement and positive family history
- Biopsy of little diagnostic value

Medical Management
Goals of management are to slow the rapid turnover of epidermis, to promote resolution of the psoriatic lesions, and to control the natural cycles of the disease. There is no known cure. The therapeutic approach should be understandable, cosmetically acceptable, and not too disruptive of lifestyle.

First, any precipitating or aggravating factors are addressed. An assessment is made of lifestyle, because psoriasis is significantly affected by stress. The most important principle of psoriasis treatment is gentle removal of scales (baths that include oils, coal tar preparations, and a soft brush used to scrub the psoriatic plaques). After bathing, the application of emollient creams containing alpha-hydroxy acids (Lac-Hydrin, Penederm) or salicylic acid will continue to soften thick scales. Three types of therapy are standard: topical therapy, photochemotherapy, and systemic therapy.

Topical Therapy
- Topical treatment is used to slow the overactive epidermis.
- Topical corticosteroid therapy acts to reduce inflammation; occlusive dressings increase the effectiveness of topical corticosteroids.
- Medications include tar preparations (e.g., coal tar topical [Balnetar]), alpha-hydroxy or salicylic acid, and corticosteroid agents. Calcipotriene (Dovonex; not recommended for use by older adult patients because of their more fragile skin, or in pregnant or lactating women), tazarotene (Tazorac), and vitamin D are additional nonsteroidal agents. Medications may take the form of lotions, ointments, pastes, creams, and shampoos.

Photochemotherapy

Photochemotherapy (also known as *phototherapy*) using narrow-band ultraviolet B (UVB) therapy may be helpful for patients who do not respond well to topical treatments. It is generally more effective when administered as ultraviolet A in conjunction with a photosensitizing oral agent (PUVA) such as psoralens.

Systemic Therapy

- Systemic cytotoxic preparations, such as methotrexate, have long been used successfully in treating extensive psoriasis that fails to respond to other forms of therapy.
- Cyclosporine (Neoral), a cyclic peptide used to prevent rejection of transplanted organs, has shown some success in treatment of severe, therapy-resistant cases of psoriasis.
- The newest line of treatments for psoriasis includes a group called biologic agents because of their derivation from immunomodulators and bioengineered proteins (such as antibodies or recombinant cytokines) and their targeted action directly on the T cells. Examples of these are infliximab (Remicade), ustekinumab (Stelara), etanercept (Enbrel), and adalimumab (Humira). Each has a slightly different mechanism and all have significant side effects, making close monitoring essential.

Nursing Management

Assessment

Assessment focuses on how the patient is coping with the skin condition, the appearance of "normal" skin, and the appearance of skin lesions.

- Examine areas especially affected: elbows, knees, scalp, gluteal cleft, and all nails for small pits.
- Assess the impact of the disease on the patient and the coping strategies used for conducting normal activities and interactions with family and friends.
- Reassure patient that the condition is not infectious, is not a reflection of poor personal hygiene, and is not skin cancer.
- Create an environment in which the patient feels comfortable discussing important quality-of-life issues related to his or her psychosocial and physical response to this chronic illness.

Nursing Interventions

Promoting Understanding

- Explain with sensitivity that there is no cure and that life-time management is necessary; the disease process can usually be controlled.
- Review pathophysiology of psoriasis and factors that provoke it: any irritation or injury to the skin (cut, abrasion, sunburn), any current illness, emotional stress, unfavorable environment (cold), and drugs (caution patient about non-prescription medication).
- Review and explain treatment regimen to ensure compliance; provide patient education materials in addition to face-to-face discussions.

Enhancing Skin Integrity

- Advise patient not to pick or scratch areas.
- Encourage patient to prevent the skin from drying out; dry skin causes psoriasis to worsen.
- Inform patient that water should not be too hot and skin should be dried by patting with a towel.
- Educate patient about using bath oil or emollient cleansing agent for sore and scaling skin.

Improving Self-Concept and Body Image

Introduce coping strategies and suggestions for reducing or coping with stressful situations, thus facilitating a more positive outlook and acceptance of the disease.

Monitoring and Managing Complications

- Note joint discomfort and evaluate further for psoriatic arthritis.
- Educate patient about care and treatment and need for compliance.
- Consult a rheumatologist to assist in the diagnosis and treatment of the arthropathy.

Promoting Home- and Community-Based Care

Educating Patients About Self-Care

- Provide patient with educational materials to reinforce face-to-face discussions about treatment guidelines and other considerations.

- Advise patient that topical corticosteroid preparations on face and around eyes predispose to cataract development. Follow strict guidelines to avoid overuse.
- Educate patient to avoid exposure to sun when undergoing PUVA treatments; if exposure is unavoidable, the skin must be protected with sunscreen and clothing, and sunglasses should be worn.
- Remind patient to schedule ophthalmic examinations on a regular basis.
- Advise female patients of childbearing age that PUVA therapy is teratogenic (can cause fetal defects). They may want to consider using contraceptives during therapy.
- If indicated, refer patient to a mental health professional who can help to ease emotional strain and give support.
- Encourage patient to join a support group and to contact the National Psoriasis Foundation for information.

For more information, see Chapter 61 in Hinkle, J. L., & Cheever, K. H. (2014). *Brunner and Suddarth's textbook of medical-surgical nursing* (13th ed.). Philadelphia: Lippincott Williams & Wilkins.

Pulmonary Arterial Hypertension

Pulmonary hypertension is a general term used to describe a hemodynamic state defined as a resting mean pulmonary artery pressure at or above 25 mm Hg. Pulmonary arterial hypertension (PAH), a type of pulmonary hypertension, is characterized by elevations in pulmonary arterial pressure, pulmonary vascular resistance, and secondary right heart ventricular failure. PAH may be suspected in a patient with dyspnea on exertion; however, it is difficult to measure pulmonary pressures noninvasively. Previously, patients were classified as having primary or secondary PAH; however, patients currently are classified by the World Health Organization (WHO) into five groups based on the mechanism. Conditions such as collagen vascular disease, congenital heart disease, anorexigenic medications (specific appetite depressants), chronic use of stimulants, portal hypertension, and HIV infection increase the risk of PAH in susceptible patients.

Pathophysiology
Vascular injury occurs with endothelial dysfunction and vascular smooth muscle dysfunction, which leads to disease

progression (vascular smooth muscle hypertrophy, adventitial and intimal proliferation [thickening of the wall], and advanced vascular lesion formation). When the pulmonary vascular bed is destroyed or obstructed, its ability to handle the blood volume received is impaired. The increased blood flow increases the pulmonary artery pressure and pulmonary vascular resistance and pressure (hypertension). This increases the workload of the right ventricle, leading to right ventricular hypertrophy (enlargement and dilation) and, eventually, right-sided heart failure (HF).

Clinical Manifestations
- Dyspnea, the main symptom, is noticed first with exertion and then at rest.
- Substernal chest pain is common.
- Weakness, fatigability, syncope, and occasional hemoptysis may occur.
- Signs of right-sided HF (peripheral edema, ascites, distended neck veins, liver engorgement, crackles, heart murmur) are noted.
- Anorexia and abdominal pain in the right upper quadrant may also occur.
- PaO_2 is decreased (hypoxemia).
- ECG changes (right ventricular hypertrophy) are seen, with right axis deviation; tall, peaked P waves in inferior leads; tall anterior R waves; and ST-segment depression or T-wave inversion anteriorly.

Assessment and Diagnostic Findings
Complete diagnostic evaluation includes a history, physical examination, chest x-ray, pulmonary function studies, ECG, echocardiogram (to estimate the pulmonary artery systolic pressure as well as to assess atrial and ventricular sizes, thickness, and function), ventilation–perfusion scan, sleep studies, autoantibody tests (to identify diseases of collagen vascular origin), HIV tests, liver function testing, and cardiac catheterization. Right heart catheterization is necessary to confirm the diagnosis of PAH and accurately assess the hemodynamic abnormalities: PAH is confirmed with a mean pulmonary artery pressure greater than 25 mm Hg.

Medical Management
The goal of treatment is to manage the underlying condition related to PAH of known cause. Most patients with PAH do not have hypoxemia at rest but require supplemental oxygen with exercise. Therapies are tailored to the patient's individual

situation, functional New York Heart Association class, and specific needs, and include diuretics, oxygen, anticoagulation, digoxin, and exercise training. Oxygen therapy reverses vasoconstriction and reduces the PAH in a relatively short time.

Pharmacologic Therapy

- Anticoagulation should be considered for patients at risk for intrapulmonary thrombosis.
- Digoxin may improve right ventricular ejection fraction in some patients and may help to control heart rate; however, patients must be monitored closely for potential complications.
- Different classes of medications are used to treat pulmonary hypertension; these include calcium channel blockers, phosphodiesterase-5 inhibitors (e.g., sildenafil [Revatio, Viagra]), endothelin antagonists (e.g., bosentan [Tracleer]), and prostanoids (e.g., epoprostenol [Flolan], treprostinil [Remodulin], and iloprost [Ventavis]). The choice of therapeutic agents is based on the severity of the disease.
- A small number of patients with pulmonary hypertension respond favorably to acute vasodilation and do well with a calcium channel blocking agent. Calcium channel blockers have a significant advantage over other medications taken to treat PAH in that they may be taken orally and are generally less costly.
- The oral medications sildenafil (Revatio, Viagra), tadalafil (Cialis, Adcirca), and vardenafil (Levitra) are potent, specific phosphodiesterase-5 inhibitors that degrade cyclic 3′,5′-guanosine monophosphate (cGMP) and promote pulmonary vasodilation.
- Endothelin receptor antagonists such as bosentan (Tracleer) are potent vasodilators and improve exercise ability. Other selective endothelin receptor antagonists include sitaxsentan (Thelin) and ambrisentan (Letairis).
- Prostanoids mimic the effect of the prostaglandin and relax the vascular smooth muscle. Prostanoids used to treat PAH include epoprostenol (Flolan), treprostinil (Remodulin), and iloprost (Ventavis); however, these have limitations owing to a short half-life.

Surgical Management

Lung transplantation remains an option for all eligible patients whose disease is refractory to medical therapy. Bilateral lung or heart-lung transplantation is the procedure of choice. Atrial septostomy may be considered for selected patients.

Nursing Management

- Identify patients at high risk for developing pulmonary hypertension (e.g., those with chronic obstructive pulmonary disease, pulmonary emboli, congenital heart disease, and mitral valve disease).
- Be alert for signs and symptoms of PAH.
- Administer prescribed oxygen therapy appropriately.
- Inform and instruct patient and family about home oxygen supplementation.
- For patients treated with prostanoids, educate patient and family about the need for central venous access (epoprostenol) and subcutaneous infusion (treprostinil) as well as proper administration and dosing of the medication, pain at the injection site, and potential severe side effects.
- Address emotional and psychosocial aspects of this disease with the patient.

For more information, see Chapter 23 in Hinkle, J. L., & Cheever, K. H. (2014). *Brunner and Suddarth's textbook of medical-surgical nursing* (13th ed.). Philadelphia: Lippincott Williams & Wilkins.

Pulmonary Edema, Acute

Pulmonary edema is the abnormal accumulation of fluid in the interstitial spaces of the lungs that diffuses into the alveoli; it can be categorized as cardiogenic or noncardiogenic in origin. Cardiogenic pulmonary edema is an acute event that results from left ventricular failure. With increased resistance to left ventricular filling, blood backs up into the pulmonary circulation. The patient quickly develops pulmonary edema, sometimes called *flash pulmonary edema,* from the blood volume overload in the lungs. Pulmonary edema can also be caused by noncardiac disorders, such as renal failure and other conditions that cause the body to retain fluid. Noncardiogenic pulmonary edema can also occur as a result of damage of the pulmonary capillary lining due to direct injury to the lung (e.g., chest trauma, aspiration, smoke inhalation), hematogenous injury (e.g., sepsis, pancreatitis, multiple transfusions, cardiopulmonary bypass), or injury plus elevated hydrostatic pressures. The pathophysiology is similar to that seen in heart failure, in that the left ventricle cannot handle the volume overload and so blood volume and pressure build up in the left atrium. The rapid increase in atrial pressure results in an acute increase in pulmonary venous pressure, which produces an increase in hydrostatic pressure that forces fluid out of the pulmonary capillaries into the interstitial spaces and alveoli. Lymphatic drainage of the excess fluid is ineffective.

Clinical Manifestations

- As a result of decreased cerebral oxygenation, the patient becomes increasingly restless and anxious.
- Along with a sudden onset of breathlessness and a sense of suffocation, the patient's hands become cold and moist, the nail beds become cyanotic (bluish), and the skin turns ashen (gray).
- The pulse is weak and rapid, and the neck veins are distended.
- Incessant coughing may occur, producing increasing quantities of foamy sputum.
- As pulmonary edema progresses, the patient's anxiety and restlessness increase; the patient becomes confused, then stuporous.
- Breathing is rapid, noisy, and moist sounding; the patient's oxygen saturation is significantly decreased.
- The patient, nearly suffocated by the blood-tinged, frothy fluid filling the alveoli, is literally drowning in secretions. The situation demands emergent action.

Assessment and Diagnostic Findings

- Patient's airway and breathing are assessed to determine the severity of respiratory distress.
- Abrupt onset of signs of left-sided HF (e.g., crackles on auscultation of the lungs) may occur without evidence of right-sided HF (e.g., no jugular venous distention [JVD], no dependent edema).
- Laboratory tests include electrolytes, blood urea nitrogen (BUN), creatinine, and CBC.
- Chest x-ray reveals increased interstitial markings and extent of edema.
- Pulse oximetry is used to assess arterial blood gas (ABG) levels.

Medical Management

Goals of medical management are to reduce volume overload, improve ventricular function, and increase respiratory exchange using a combination of oxygen and medication therapies.

Oxygenation

- Oxygen in concentrations adequate to relieve hypoxia and dyspnea (e.g., non-rebreather mask)

- Oxygen by noninvasive intermittent or continuous positive pressure if signs of hypoxemia persist
- Endotracheal intubation and mechanical ventilation if respiratory failure occurs
- Positive end-expiratory pressure (PEEP)
- Monitoring of pulse oximetry and ABGs

Pharmacologic Therapy
- Diuretic agents (e.g., furosemide) to produce a rapid diuretic effect
- Vasodilator drugs such as IV nitroglycerin or nitroprusside (Nipride), which may enhance symptom relief

Nursing Management
- Assist with administration of oxygen; be prepared for intubation and mechanical ventilation if necessary.
- Position patient upright (in bed if necessary) with legs dangling over the side of bed.
- Provide psychological support by reassuring patient. Use touch to convey a sense of concrete reality. Because the patient is in an unstable condition, remain with the patient.
- Give frequent, simple, concise information about what is being done to treat the condition and the expected results.
- Monitor effects of medications. Observe patient for large amount of urine after diuretics are given, excessive respiratory depression, hypotension, and vomiting. Keep a morphine antagonist available (e.g., naloxone hydrochloride) if morphine has been given. Insert and maintain an indwelling catheter if ordered or provide bedside commode.
- The patient receiving continuous IV infusions of vasoactive medications requires ECG monitoring and frequent measurement of vital signs.

For more information, see Chapters 23 and 29 in Hinkle, J. L., & Cheever, K. H. (2014). *Brunner and Suddarth's textbook of medical-surgical nursing* (13th ed.). Philadelphia: Lippincott Williams & Wilkins.

Pulmonary Embolism

Pulmonary embolism (PE) refers to the obstruction of the pulmonary artery or one of its branches by a thrombus (or thrombi) that originates somewhere in the venous system or in the right side of the heart. Deep venous thrombosis (DVT), a related condition, refers to thrombus formation in the deep veins, usually in the calf or thigh, but sometimes in the arm, especially in patients with peripherally inserted central catheters. DVT is discussed in detail in Vein Disorders in Section V. *Venous thromboembolism* (VTE) is a term that includes both DVT and PE. PE is a common disorder and often is associated with trauma, surgery (orthopedic, major abdominal, pelvic, gynecologic), pregnancy, heart failure, age older than 50 years, hypercoagulable states, and prolonged immobility; it also may occur in apparently healthy people. The outcome in acute PE is dependent on the presence of preexisting comorbidities and the extent of hemodynamic compromise.

Pathophysiology

Most commonly, PE is due to a blood clot or thrombus and gas exchange is impaired in the lung mass supplied by the obstructed vessel. Although that area continues to be ventilated, it receives little or no blood flow. This results in localized vasoconstriction and an increase in pulmonary vascular resistance that compounds the ventilation–perfusion imbalance. Massive PE is a life-threatening emergency; death commonly occurs within 1 hour after the onset of symptoms.

Clinical Manifestations

Symptoms depend on the size of the thrombus and the area of the pulmonary artery occlusion.

- Dyspnea is the most common symptom. Tachypnea is the most frequent sign.
- Chest pain is common, usually sudden in onset and pleuritic in nature; it can be substernal and may mimic angina pectoris or a myocardial infarction.
- Anxiety, fever, tachycardia, apprehension, cough, diaphoresis, hemoptysis, syncope, shock, and sudden death may occur.
- The clinical picture may mimic that of bronchopneumonia or HF.
- In atypical instances, PE causes few signs and symptoms, whereas in other instances, it mimics various other cardiopulmonary disorders.
- Obstruction of the pulmonary artery results in pronounced dyspnea, sudden substernal pain, rapid and weak pulse, shock, syncope, and sudden death.

Assessment and Diagnostic Findings
- Initial clinical assessment focuses on the clinical probability of risk, clinical history, symptoms, signs, and testing.
- Because the symptoms of acute PE can vary from few to severe, a diagnostic workup is performed to rule out other diseases.
- The initial diagnostic workup may include chest x-ray, ECG, pulse oximetry, arterial blood gas (ABG) analysis, and ventilation–perfusion ($\dot{V}/\dot{Q}$) scan.
- Frequent ECG abnormalities include sinus tachycardia and T-wave inversions in leads V_1 to V_4.
- Pulmonary angiography is considered the best method for diagnosing PE; however, it may not be feasible, cost-effective, or easily performed, especially with critically ill patients.
- Spiral CT scan of the lung, D-dimer assay (blood test for evidence of blood clots), and pulmonary arteriogram may be warranted.

Prevention
- Ambulation or active leg exercises in patients on bed rest to prevent DVT
- Anticoagulant therapy for patients whose hemostasis is adequate and who are undergoing major elective abdominal or thoracic surgery

See additional guidelines for prevention and treatment of VTE under Vein Disorders in Section V.

Medical Management
The immediate objective is to stabilize the cardiopulmonary system.

- Nasal oxygen is administered immediately to relieve hypoxemia, respiratory distress, and central cyanosis; severe hypoxemia may necessitate emergent endotracheal intubation and mechanical ventilation.
- IV infusion lines are inserted to establish routes for medications or fluids that will be needed.
- For hypotension not responsive to fluids, prompt initiation of vasopressor therapy is recommended (dobutamine, dopamine, or norepinephrine).
- A perfusion scan, hemodynamic measurements, and evaluation of hypoxemia (via pulse oximetry or ABG determinations) are performed. Spiral (helical) CT or pulmonary angiography may be performed.

- The ECG is monitored continuously for dysrhythmias and right ventricular failure, which may occur suddenly.
- Blood is drawn for serum electrolytes, complete blood cell count, and coagulation studies.
- If the patient has suffered massive embolism and is hypotensive, an indwelling urinary catheter is inserted to monitor urinary output.
- Small doses of IV morphine or sedatives are administered to relieve patient anxiety, to alleviate chest discomfort, to improve tolerance of the endotracheal tube, and to ease adaptation to the mechanical ventilator, if necessary.

Pharmacologic Therapy

Treatment of a nonmassive PE has three phases: initial phase, early maintenance phase, and long-term secondary prevention phase.

Anticoagulation Therapy

- Low-molecular-weight heparin (LMWH) and fondaparinux (Arixtra) are the cornerstones of therapy, but IV unfractionated heparin (IVUH) may be used in the initial phase.
- The early maintenance stage usually consists of overlapping regimens of heparin or fondaparinux for 3 to 5 days with a vitamin K antagonist (e.g., warfarin [Coumadin]).
- Long-term maintenance for 3 to 6 months after an embolic event may include warfarin.
- Other heparinoids may also be used for PE. These include enoxaparin, fondaparinux (Arixtra), dalteparin (Fragmin), inzaparin (Innohep), lepirudin (Refludan), and argatroban (Novastan).
- Patients must continue to use some form of anticoagulation for at least 3 to 6 months after the embolic event.
- Major side effects are bleeding anywhere in the body and anaphylactic reaction resulting in shock or death. Other side effects include fever, abnormal liver function, and allergic skin reaction.

Thrombolytic (Fibrinolytic) Therapy

- Anticoagulant use is stopped prior to administration of a thrombolytic agent.
- International normalized ratio (INR), partial thromboplastin time (PTT), hematocrit, and platelet counts are obtained before thrombolytic therapy is started.
- Thrombolytic (fibrinolytic) therapy with recombinant tissue plasminogen activator (tPA) may include urokinase,

streptokinase, and alteplase. It is reserved for PE affecting a significant area and causing hemodynamic instability.

- Bleeding is a significant side effect; nonessential invasive procedures are avoided.

Surgical Management

- Embolectomy can be performed using transvenous catheters or surgical removal.
- A surgical embolectomy must be performed by the cardiovascular surgical team because of the necessity of cardiopulmonary bypass.
- Multiple techniques to remove the embolus via transvenous catheters are available including suction and rheolytic or rotational embolectomies with or without insertion of an inferior vena caval (IVC) filter (e.g., Greenfield).

Nursing Management

Minimizing the Risk of PE

The nurse must have a high degree of suspicion for PE in all patients but particularly in those with conditions predisposing to a slowing of venous return.

Preventing Thrombus Formation

- Encourage early ambulation and active and passive leg exercises.
- Instruct patient to move legs in a "pumping" exercise.
- Advise patient to avoid prolonged sitting, immobility, and constrictive clothing.
- Do not permit dangling of legs and feet in a dependent position.
- Instruct patient to place feet on floor or chair and to avoid crossing legs.
- Do not leave IV catheters in veins for prolonged periods.

Monitoring Anticoagulant and Thrombolytic (Fibrinolytic) Therapy

- Advise bed rest, monitor vital signs every 2 hours, and limit invasive procedures.
- Measure INR or activated PTT every 3 to 4 hours after thrombolytic (fibrinolytic) infusion is started, to confirm activation of fibrinolytic systems.
- Perform only essential ABG studies on upper extremities, with manual compression of puncture site for at least 30 minutes.

> ▰ *Quality and Safety Nursing Alert*
>
> Because of the prolonged clotting time, only essential arterial punctures or venipunctures are performed in patients who have received thrombolytic (fibrinolytic) agents; manual pressure is applied to any puncture site for at least 30 minutes. Pulse oximetry is used to monitor changes in oxygenation. The thrombolytic (fibrinolytic) infusion is discontinued immediately if uncontrolled bleeding occurs.

Minimizing Chest Pain, Pleuritic
- Place patient in semi-Fowler's position; turn and reposition frequently.
- Administer analgesic medications as prescribed for severe pain.

Managing Oxygen Therapy
- Assess the patient frequently for signs of hypoxemia, and monitor the pulse oximetry values.
- Assist patient with deep breathing and incentive spirometry.
- If necessary for management of secretions, possibly use nebulizer therapy or percussion and postural drainage.

Alleviating Anxiety
- Encourage patient to express feelings and concerns.
- Answer questions concisely and accurately.
- Explain therapy and describe how to recognize untoward effects early.

Monitoring for Complications
Be alert for the potential complication of cardiogenic shock or right ventricular failure subsequent to the effect of PE on the cardiovascular system.

Providing Postoperative Nursing Care
- Measure pulmonary arterial pressure and urinary output.
- Assess insertion site of arterial catheter for hematoma formation and infection.
- Maintain blood pressure to ensure perfusion of vital organs; this is crucial.
- Encourage isometric exercises, antiembolism stockings, and walking when patient is permitted out of bed. Elevate foot of bed when patient is resting.
- Discourage sitting; hip flexion compresses large veins in the legs.

Promoting Home- and Community-Based Care

Educating Patients About Self-Care

- Before discharge and at follow-up clinic or home visits, educate the patient in ways to prevent recurrence and which signs and symptoms should alert the patient to seek medical attention.
- Educate the patient to look for bruising and bleeding when taking anticoagulant agents and to avoid bumping into objects. Advise patient to use a toothbrush with soft bristles to prevent gingival bleeding and to avoid use of sharps (e.g., razors, knives); electric razors are preferred.
- Instruct patient not to take aspirin (an anticoagulant medication) and other nonsteroidal anti-inflammatory medications (NSAIDs) or antihistamine drugs while taking warfarin sodium (Coumadin).
- Advise patient to check with physician before taking any medication, including over-the-counter drugs.
- Advise patient to continue wearing antiembolism stockings as long as directed.
- Instruct patient to avoid laxatives, which affect vitamin K absorption; vitamin K promotes coagulation. Educate the patient to avoid regular consumption of foods high in vitamin K (e.g., green leafy and cruciferous vegetables).
- Instruct patient to avoid sitting with legs crossed or for prolonged periods.
- Recommend that patient change position regularly when traveling, walk occasionally, and exercise legs and ankles actively.
- Advise patient to drink plenty of liquids.
- Instruct patient to report dark, tarry stools immediately.
- Recommend that patient wear identification stating that he or she is taking anticoagulant agents.

For more information, see Chapters 23 and 30 in Hinkle, J. L., & Cheever, K. H. (2014). *Brunner and Suddarth's textbook of medical-surgical nursing* (13th ed.). Philadelphia: Lippincott Williams & Wilkins.

Pyelonephritis, Acute

Pyelonephritis, an upper urinary tract infection (UTI), is a bacterial infection of the renal pelvis, tubules, and interstitial tissue of one or both kidneys. Causes involve either the upward spread of bacteria from the bladder or spread from systemic sources reaching the kidney via the bloodstream. An incompetent ureterovesical valve or obstruction occurring in the urinary tract increases the susceptibility of the kidneys to infection. Bladder tumors, strictures, benign prostatic hyperplasia, and urinary stones are some potential causes of obstruction that can lead to infections. Pyelonephritis may be acute or chronic.

Clinical Manifestations
- Chills, fever, leukocytosis, bacteriuria, and pyuria may be present.
- Low back pain, flank pain, nausea and vomiting, headache, malaise, and painful urination are common findings.
- Patient may have pain and tenderness in the area of the costovertebral angle.
- Symptoms of lower urinary tract involvement, such as urgency and frequency, are common.

Assessment and Diagnostic Findings
- Ultrasound or CT scan
- An IV pyelogram may be indicated with pyelonephritis if functional and structural renal abnormalities are suspected.
- Urine culture and sensitivity tests
- Radionuclide imaging with gallium or indium-111 labeled–white blood cells (WBCs) if other studies are not conclusive

Medical Management
Acute uncomplicated pyelonephritis is most often treated on an outpatient basis; a 2-week course of antibiotics is recommended. Commonly prescribed agents include some of the same medications prescribed for the treatment of UTIs. Pregnant women may be hospitalized for 2 or 3 days of parenteral antibiotic therapy. Oral antibiotic agents may be prescribed once the patient is afebrile and showing clinical improvement. After the initial antibiotic regimen, the patient may need antibiotic therapy for up to 6 weeks if a relapse occurs. A follow-up urine culture is obtained 2 weeks after completion of antibiotic therapy to document clearing of the infection. Hydration with oral or parenteral fluids is essential in all patients with UTIs when there is adequate kidney function.

Nursing Management
- If patient is hospitalized, encourage fluids (3 to 4 L per day) unless contraindicated.
- Monitor and record intake and output.

P

- Assess body temperature every 4 hours and administer antipyretic and antibiotic agents as prescribed.
- Educate patient regarding preventive measures and early recognition of symptoms.
- Stress the importance of taking antimicrobial medications exactly as prescribed, along with the need for keeping follow-up appointments.

For more information, see Chapter 55 in Hinkle, J. L., & Cheever, K. H. (2014). *Brunner and Suddarth's Textbook of Medical-Surgical Nursing* (13th ed.). Philadelphia: Lippincott Williams & Wilkins.

Pyelonephritis, Chronic

Repeated bouts of acute pyelonephritis may lead to chronic pyelonephritis. Complications of chronic pyelonephritis include end-stage renal disease (from progressive loss of nephrons secondary to chronic inflammation and scarring), hypertension, and formation of kidney stones (from chronic infection with urea-splitting organisms).

Clinical Manifestations
- Patient usually has no symptoms of infection unless an acute exacerbation occurs.
- Fatigue, headache, and poor appetite may occur.
- Polyuria, excessive thirst, and weight loss may result.
- Persistent and recurring infection may produce progressive scarring resulting in renal failure.

Assessment and Diagnostic Findings
- Assess prior history of pyelonephritis.
- IV urography
- Measurement of blood urea nitrogen (BUN), creatinine levels, and creatinine clearance

Medical Management
Long-term use of prophylactic antimicrobial therapy to eradicate bacteria in the urine may help limit recurrence of infections and renal scarring. Impaired renal function alters the excretion of antimicrobial agents and necessitates careful monitoring of renal function, especially if the medications are potentially toxic to the kidneys.

Nursing Management

- If patient is hospitalized, encourage fluids (3 to 4 L per day) unless contraindicated.
- Monitor and record intake and output.
- Assess body temperature every 4 hours and administer antipyretic and antibiotic agents as prescribed.
- Educate patient and family about preventive measures and early recognition of symptoms.
- Stress the importance of taking antimicrobial medications exactly as prescribed, along with the need for keeping follow-up appointments.

For more information, see Chapter 55 in Hinkle, J. L., & Cheever, K. H. (2014). *Brunner and Suddarth's Textbook of Medical-Surgical Nursing* (13th ed.). Philadelphia: Lippincott Williams & Wilkins.

P

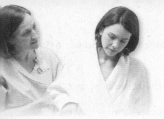

Raynaud's Phenomenon and Other Acrosyndromes

Raynaud's phenomenon is a form of intermittent arteriolar vasoconstriction that results in coldness, pain, and pallor of the fingertips or toes. Primary or idiopathic Raynaud's (Raynaud's disease) occurs in the absence of an underlying disease. Secondary Raynaud's (Raynaud's syndrome) occurs in association with an underlying disease, usually a connective tissue disorder, such as systemic lupus erythematosus, rheumatoid arthritis, scleroderma, trauma, or obstructive arterial lesions. Raynaud's phenomenon is most common in women between the ages of 16 and 40 years, and it occurs more frequently in cold climates and during the winter. Acrocyanosis was previously thought to be a variant of Raynaud's phenomenon because both are aggravated by cold climates and during emotional stress and present with blue discoloration of the fingers and hyperhidrosis (excessive sweating).

The prognosis for patients with Raynaud's phenomenon varies; some slowly improve, some become progressively worse, and others show no change. Raynaud's symptoms may be so mild that treatment is not required. However, secondary Raynaud's is characterized by vasospasm and fixed blood vessel obstructions that may lead to ischemia, ulceration, and gangrene. Acrocyanosis is a poorly understood phenomenon that may be benign, requiring little or no treatment, or may result in chronic pain and ulcerations.

Clinical Manifestations

- Classic Raynaud's reveals pallor brought on by sudden vasoconstriction followed by cyanosis followed by hyperemia (exaggerated reflow) due to vasodilation with a resultant red color (rubor); the progression follows the characteristic color change: white, blue, red.
- Numbness, tingling, and burning pain occur as color changes.
- Involvement tends to be bilateral and symmetric and may involve toes and fingers.

- In acrocyanosis, there are persistent skin color changes, symmetry and absence of paroxysmal pallor, marked clamminess, and hyperhidrosis of the hands and feet, which tend to worsen in warmer climates while the color changes improve.

Medical Management

Avoiding the particular stimuli (e.g., cold, tobacco) that provoke vasoconstriction is a primary factor in controlling Raynaud's phenomenon. Calcium channel blockers (nifedipine [Procardia], amlodipine [Norvasc]) may be effective in relieving symptoms. Sympathectomy (interrupting the sympathetic nerves by removing the sympathetic ganglia or dividing their branches) may help some patients. Avoiding cold and trauma as well as implementing measures to protect extremities from these stressors are the primary focus of treatment for acrocyanosis.

Nursing Management

- Instruct patient to avoid situations that may be stressful or unsafe.
- Advise patient to minimize exposure to cold, remain indoors as much as possible, and wear protective clothing when outdoors during cold weather.
- Reassure patient that serious complications (e.g., gangrene and amputation) are not usual.
- Emphasize the importance of avoiding all forms of nicotine (smoking cessation without use of nicotine patches); assist in finding support group.
- Advise patient to handle sharp objects carefully to avoid injuring the fingers.
- Inform patient about postural hypotension that may result from medications.

For more information, see Chapter 30 in Hinkle, J. L., & Cheever, K. H. (2014). *Brunner and Suddarth's textbook of medical-surgical nursing* (13th ed.). Philadelphia: Lippincott Williams & Wilkins.

Renal Failure, Acute

Renal failure results when the kidneys are unable to remove metabolic waste and perform their regulatory functions. Acute kidney injury (AKI) is a rapid loss of renal function due to damage to the kidneys. Three major categories of AKI are:

- Prerenal: hypoperfusion (as from volume depletion disorders), extreme vasodilation, or impaired cardiac performance

- Intrarenal: parenchymal damage to the glomeruli or kidney tubules, as from burns, crush injuries, infections, transfusion reaction or nephrotoxicity (which may lead to acute tubular necrosis [ATN])
- Postrenal: urinary tract obstruction, as from calculi, tumor, strictures, prostatic hyperplasia, or blood clots

AKI is an increase in serum creatinine of 50% or greater above baseline (normal creatinine being less than 1.0 mg/dL).

Clinical Stages
- Initiation period: The initial insult and oliguria occur.
- Oliguric period (urine volume less than 400 mL per day): Uremic symptoms first appear and hyperkalemia may develop.
- Diuresis period: Urine output gradually increases, signaling the beginning of glomerular filtration's recovery. Laboratory values stabilize and start to decrease.
- Recovery period: Renal function improves (may take 3 to 12 months).

Clinical Manifestations
- Critical illness and lethargy are seen, with persistent nausea, vomiting, and diarrhea.
- Skin and mucous membranes are dry.
- Central nervous system manifestations include drowsiness, headache, muscle twitching, and seizures.
- Urine output is scanty to normal; urine may be bloody with low specific gravity.
- Steady rise in blood urea nitrogen (BUN) may occur depending on the degree of catabolism; serum creatinine values increase (greater than 1.0 mg/dL) with disease progression.
- Hyperkalemia may lead to dysrhythmias and cardiac arrest.
- Progressive acidosis, increase in serum phosphate concentrations, and low serum calcium levels may be noted.
- Anemia occurs from blood loss due to uremic GI lesions, reduced red blood cell life span, and reduced erythropoietin production.

Assessment and Diagnostic Findings
- Urine output measurements (oliguria: less than 0. 5 mL/kg per hour; nonoliguria: greater than 800 mL per day; or anuria: less than 50 mL per day)
- Hematuria possible; low specific gravity of urine (as compared with a normal value of 1.010 to 1.025)

- Classification using the RIFLE (risk, injury, failure, loss and end-stage kidney disease) criteria for AKI from the Acute Dialysis Quality Initiative group
- Prerenal azotemia: decreased amount of sodium in the urine (less than 20 mEq/L) and normal urinary sediment.
- Intrarenal azotemia: usually, urinary sodium levels greater than 40 mEq/L with urinary casts and other cellular debris
- Renal ultrasonography and CT and MRI scans
- BUN, creatinine, and electrolyte analyses, including hyperkalemia and metabolic acidosis

Gerontologic Considerations

About half of all patients who develop AKI during hospitalization are older than 60 years. The etiology of AKI in older adults includes prerenal causes, such as dehydration; intrarenal causes, such as nephrotoxic agents (e.g., medications, contrast agents); and complications of major surgery. Suppression of thirst, enforced bed rest, lack of access to drinking water, and confusion all contribute to the older adult patient's failure to consume adequate fluids and may lead to dehydration, further compromising already decreased renal function.

AKI in the older adult is often seen in the community setting. Nurses in the ambulatory setting also need to be aware of the risk. All medications need to be monitored for potential side effects that could result in damage to the kidney, either through reduced circulation or nephrotoxicity. Outpatient procedures that require fasting or a bowel preparation may cause dehydration and therefore require careful monitoring.

Prevention

AKI has a high mortality rate that ranges from 40% to 90%, mortality being influenced by the following factors: increased age, comorbid conditions, preexisting kidney and vascular diseases, and respiratory failure. Thus, adherence to AKI prevention procedures is essential.

- Provide adequate hydration to patients at risk for dehydration.
- Prevent and treat shock promptly with blood and fluid replacement.
- Monitor central venous and arterial pressures as well as hourly urine output.
- Treat hypotension promptly.
- Continually assess renal function (urine output, laboratory values) as appropriate.

- Take precautions to ensure appropriate administration of blood products.
- Prevent and treat infections promptly.
- Pay special attention to wounds, burns, or other precursors of sepsis.
- To prevent infections from ascending in the urinary tract, give meticulous care to patients with indwelling catheters. Remove catheters as soon as possible.
- To prevent toxic drug effects, closely monitor dosage, duration of use, and blood levels of all medications metabolized or excreted by the kidneys.

Medical Management

Treatment objectives are to restore normal chemical balance and prevent complications until renal tissues are repaired and renal function is restored. Possible causes of damage are identified and treated.

- Fluid balance is managed on the basis of daily weight, serial measurements of central venous pressure, serum and urine concentrations, fluid losses, blood pressure, and clinical status. Fluid excesses are treated with mannitol, furosemide (Lasix), or ethacrynic acid (Edecrin) to initiate diuresis and prevent or minimize subsequent renal failure.
- Blood flow is restored to the kidneys with the use of IV fluids, albumin, or blood product transfusions.
- Dialysis (hemodialysis, hemofiltration, or peritoneal dialysis) is started to prevent complications, including hyperkalemia, metabolic acidosis, pericarditis, and pulmonary edema.
- Cation-exchange resins , such as sodium polystyrene sulfonate (Kayexelate), are given orally or by retention enema.
- IV dextrose 50%, insulin, and calcium replacement are administered to the patient who is hemodynamically unstable (low blood pressure, changes in mental status, dysrhythmia).
- Shock and infection are treated if present.
- Arterial blood gases are monitored when severe acidosis is present.
- Sodium bicarbonate is used to elevate plasma pH.
- If respiratory problems develop, ventilatory measures are started.
- Phosphate-binding agents are used to control elevated serum phosphate concentrations.
- Replacement of dietary proteins is individualized to provide the maximum benefit and minimize uremic symptoms.
- Caloric requirements are met with high-carbohydrate feedings or parenteral nutrition (PN).

- Foods and fluids containing potassium and phosphorus are restricted.
- Blood chemistries are evaluated to determine amount of sodium, potassium, and water replacement during the oliguric phase.
- After the diuretic phase, a high-protein, high-calorie diet is given with gradual resumption of activities.

Nursing Management
- Monitor for complications; assist in emergency treatment of fluid and electrolyte imbalances.
- Assess progress and response to treatment; provide physical and emotional support.
- Keep family informed about condition; this helps them understand the treatments and provides psychological support.
- Continue to provide nursing care indicated for the primary disorder (e.g., burns, shock, trauma, obstruction of the urinary tract).

Monitoring Fluid and Electrolyte Balance
- Monitor serum electrolyte levels and physical indicators of these complications during all phases of disorder.
- Screen parenteral fluids, all oral intake, and all medications for hidden sources of potassium.
- Monitor cardiac function and musculoskeletal status for signs of hyperkalemia.
- Pay careful attention to fluid intake (IV medications should be administered in the smallest volume possible), urine output, apparent edema, distention of the jugular veins, alterations in heart sounds and breath sounds, and increased difficulty in breathing.
- Maintain accurate records of intake and output and daily weight.
- Immediately report indicators of deteriorating fluid and electrolyte status. Prepare for emergency treatment of hyperkalemia. Prepare patient for dialysis as indicated to correct fluid and electrolyte imbalances.

R

Quality and Safety Nursing Alert

Hyperkalemia is the most immediate, life-threatening imbalance seen in AKI. Parenteral fluids, all oral intake, and all other medications are screened carefully to ensure that sources of potassium are not inadvertently administered or consumed.

Reducing Metabolic Rate
- Reduce exertion and metabolic rate with bed rest during most acute stage.
- Prevent or treat fever and infection promptly.

Promoting Pulmonary Function
- Assist patient to move, turn, cough, and take deep breaths frequently.
- Encourage and assist patient to move and turn.

Preventing Infection
- Practice asepsis when working with invasive lines and catheters.
- Avoid using an indwelling catheter if possible.

Providing Skin Care
- Perform meticulous skin care.
- Bathe the patient with cool water, turn patient frequently, keep the skin clean and well moisturized, and keep fingernails trimmed; this will provide for patient comfort and will prevent skin breakdown.

Providing Psychosocial Support
- Support patient and family during hemodialysis, peritoneal dialysis (PD), or continuous renal replacement therapy (CCRT); do not overlook psychological needs and concerns.
- Explain rationale of treatment to patient and family. Repeat explanations and clarify answers as needed.
- Encourage family to touch and converse with patient during dialysis.
- Continually assess patient for complications of AKI and its precipitating causes.

For more information, see Chapter 54 in Hinkle, J. L., & Cheever, K. H. (2014). *Brunner and Suddarth's textbook of medical-surgical nursing* (13th ed.). Philadelphia: Lippincott Williams & Wilkins.

Renal Failure, Chronic
(End-Stage Kidney Disease)

When a patient has sustained enough kidney damage to require renal replacement therapy on a permanent basis, the patient has moved into the final stage of chronic kidney disease, also referred to as *chronic renal failure (CRF)* or *end-stage kidney disease (ESKD)*.

The rate of decline in renal function and progression of ESKD is related to the underlying disorder, the urinary excretion of protein, and the presence of hypertension. The disease tends to progress more rapidly in patients who excrete significant amounts of protein (or have elevated blood pressure) than in patients without these conditions.

Clinical Manifestations

- Cardiovascular: peripheral neuropathy, hypertension, pitting edema (feet, hands, sacrum), periorbital edema, pericardial friction rub, engorged neck veins, pericarditis, pericardial effusion, pericardial tamponade, hyperkalemia, hyperlipidemia
- Integumentary: gray-bronze skin color; dry; flaky skin; severe pruritus; ecchymosis; purpura; thin, brittle nails; coarse, thinning hair
- Pulmonary: crackles; thick, tenacious sputum; depressed cough reflex; pleuritic pain; shortness of breath; tachypnea; Kussmaul-type respirations; uremic pneumonitis
- GI: ammonia odor to breath; metallic taste; mouth ulcerations and bleeding; anorexia; nausea and vomiting; hiccups; constipation or diarrhea; bleeding from GI tract
- Neurologic: weakness and fatigue, confusion, inability to concentrate, disorientation, tremors, seizures, asterixis, restlessness of legs, burning of soles of feet, behavioral changes
- Musculoskeletal: muscle cramps, loss of muscle strength, renal osteodystrophy, bone pain, fractures, foot drop
- Reproductive: amenorrhea, testicular atrophy, infertility, decreased libido
- Hematologic: anemia, thrombocytopenia

Assessment and Diagnostic Findings

Decreased glomerular filtration rate (GFR) and creatinine clearance; sodium and water retention; metabolic acidosis; anemia; elevated serum phosphate level and decreased serum calcium level; increase in parathyroid hormone.

Complications

Potential complications of ESKD that necessitate a collaborative approach to care include the following:

- Hyperkalemia due to decreased excretion, metabolic acidosis, catabolism, and excessive intake (diet, medications, fluids)
- Pericarditis, pericardial effusion, and pericardial tamponade due to retention of uremic waste products and inadequate dialysis

- Hypertension due to sodium and water retention, and malfunction of the renin–angiotensin–aldosterone system
- Anemia due to decreased erythropoietin production, decreased RBC life span, bleeding in the GI tract from irritating toxins and ulcer formation, and blood loss during hemodialysis
- Bone disease and metastatic and vascular calcifications due to retention of phosphorus, low serum calcium levels, abnormal vitamin D metabolism, and elevated aluminum levels

🍂 Gerontologic Considerations

Diabetes, hypertension, chronic glomerulonephritis, interstitial nephritis, and urinary tract obstruction are the causes of ESKD in the older adult. The symptoms of other disorders (heart failure, dementia) can mask the symptoms of renal disease and delay or prevent diagnosis and treatment. The patient often complains of signs and symptoms of nephrotic syndrome, such as edema and proteinuria. The older adult patient may develop nonspecific signs of disturbed renal function, and fluid and electrolyte imbalances. Hemodialysis and peritoneal dialysis have been used effectively in older adult patients. Concomitant disorders have made transplantation a less common treatment for the older adult. Conservative management, including nutritional therapy, fluid control, and medications (such as phosphate binders), may be used if dialysis or transplantation is not suitable.

Medical Management

Goals of management are to retain kidney function and maintain homeostasis for as long as possible. All factors that contribute to ESKD and those that are reversible (e.g., obstruction) are identified and treated. Management is accomplished primarily with medications and diet therapy. Dialysis may be needed to decrease uremic waste in the blood and to control electrolyte balance.

Pharmacologic Management

Complications can be prevented or delayed by administering prescribed, phosphate-binding agents, calcium supplements, antihypertensive and cardiac medications, antiseizure medications, and erythropoietin (Epogen).

- Hyperphosphatemia and hypocalcemia are treated with medications that bind dietary phosphorus in the GI tract (e.g., calcium carbonate, calcium acetate, sevelamer hydrochloride); all binding agents must be administered with food.

- Hypertension is managed by intravascular volume control and antihypertensive medication.
- Heart failure and pulmonary edema are treated with fluid restriction, low-sodium diet, diuretics, inotropic agents (e.g., digoxin or dobutamine), and dialysis.
- Metabolic acidosis is treated, if necessary, with sodium bicarbonate supplements or dialysis.
- Patient is observed for early evidence of neurologic abnormalities (e.g., slight twitching, headache, delirium, or seizure activity); IV diazepam (Valium) or phenytoin (Dilantin) is administered to control seizures.
- Anemia is treated with recombinant human erythropoietin (Epogen); hemoglobin and hematocrit are monitored frequently.
- Heparin is adjusted as necessary to prevent clotting of dialysis lines during treatments.
- Supplementary iron may be prescribed.
- Blood pressure and serum potassium levels are monitored.

Nutritional Therapy
- Dietary intervention is needed, with careful regulation of protein intake, of fluid intake to balance fluid losses, and of sodium intake, as well as some restriction of potassium.
- Adequate intake of calories and vitamins is ensured. Calories are supplied with carbohydrates and fats to prevent wasting.
- Protein is restricted; allowed protein must be of high biologic value (dairy products, eggs, meats).
- Fluid allowance is 500 to 600 mL of fluid or more than the previous day's 24-hour urine output.
- Vitamin supplements are given.

Dialysis
The patient with increasing symptoms of renal failure is referred to a dialysis and transplantation center early in the course of progressive renal disease. Dialysis is usually initiated when the patient cannot maintain a reasonable lifestyle with conservative treatment.

Nursing Management
- Assess fluid status and identify potential sources of imbalance.
- Implement a dietary program to ensure proper nutritional intake within the limits of the treatment regimen.

- Promote positive feelings by encouraging increased self-care and greater independence.
- Provide explanations and information to the patient and family concerning ESKD, treatment options, and potential complications.
- Provide emotional support.

Promoting Home- and Community-Based Care

Educating Patients About Self-Care

- Provide ongoing explanations and information to patient and family concerning ESKD, including treatment options and potential complications; monitor the patient's progress and compliance with the treatment regimen.
- Refer patient for dietary counseling and assist with nutritional planning.
- Educate patient about how to check the vascular access device for patency and instruct in appropriate precautions, such as avoiding venipuncture and the taking of blood pressure measurements on the arm with the access device.
- Educate patient and family regarding the problems to report: signs of worsening renal failure, hyperkalemia, access problems.

Continuing Care

- Stress the importance of follow-up examinations and treatment.
- Refer patient to home care nurse for continued monitoring and support.
- Reinforce the dietary restrictions required, including fluid, sodium, potassium, and protein restriction.
- Remind the patient about the need for health promotion activities and health screening.

For more information, see Chapter 54 in Hinkle, J. L., & Cheever, K. H. (2014). *Brunner and Suddarth's textbook of medical-surgical nursing* (13th ed.). Philadelphia: Lippincott Williams & Wilkins.

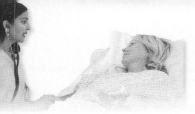

Seborrheic Dermatoses

Seborrhea is an excessive production of sebum (secretion of sebaceous glands). Seborrheic dermatitis has a genetic predisposition; hormones, nutritional status, infection, and emotional stress influence its course. Remissions and exacerbations of this condition are the norm; however, the condition is chronic.

Pathophysiology

Seborrheic dermatitis is a chronic inflammatory disease of the skin with a predilection for areas that are well supplied with sebaceous glands or that lie between folds of the skin, where the bacterial count is high. Areas most often affected are the face, scalp, cheeks, ears, axillae, and various skin folds.

Clinical Manifestations

Two forms of seborrheic dermatitis can occur: oily and dry. Either form may start in childhood with fine scaling of the scalp or other areas and continue throughout life.

Oily Form
• Moist or greasy patches of sallow skin, with or without scaling
• Slight erythema (redness), predominantly on the forehead, nasolabial fold, beard area, and scalp, and between adjacent skin surfaces in the regions of the axillae, groin, and breasts
• Small pustules or papulopustules on trunk, resembling acne

Dry Form
• Flaky desquamation of the scalp (dandruff) with profuse fine, powdery scales
• May be asymptomatic in mild forms of the disease
• Scaling often accompanied by pruritus, leading to scratching and secondary infections and excoriation

Medical Management

Because there is no known cure for seborrhea, the objectives of therapy are to control the disorder and allow the skin to repair itself. Treatment measures include the following:

- Administer topical corticosteroid cream to body and face; use with caution near eyes.
- Aerate skin and carefully clean creases or folds to prevent candidal yeast infection; evaluate patients with persistent candidiasis for diabetes.
- Shampoo hair daily (or at least three times weekly) with medicated (antiseborrheic) shampoos. Two or three different types of shampoos are used in rotation to prevent the seborrhea from becoming resistant to a particular shampoo; shampoo must be left on for 5 to 10 minutes to be effective.

Nursing Management
- Advise patient to avoid external irritants, excess heat, and perspiration; rubbing and scratching prolong the disorder.
- Educate patient to avoid secondary infections by airing the skin and keeping skin folds clean and dry.
- Reinforce instructions for using medicated shampoos; frequent shampooing is contrary to some cultural practices—be sensitive to these differences when instructing the patient about home care.
- Caution patient that seborrheic dermatitis is a chronic problem that tends to reappear. The goal is to keep it under control.
- Encourage patient to adhere to treatment program.
- Treat patients with sensitivity and an awareness of their need to express their feelings, especially when they become discouraged by the disorder's effect on body image.

For more information, see Chapter 61 in Hinkle, J. L., & Cheever, K. H. (2014). *Brunner and Suddarth's textbook of medical-surgical nursing* (13th ed.). Philadelphia: Lippincott Williams & Wilkins.

Seizures

Seizures are episodes of abnormal motor, sensory, autonomic, or psychic activity (or a combination of these) that result from a sudden, excessive discharge from cerebral neurons. A part or all of the brain may be involved. The International League Against Epilepsy (ILAE) differentiates between three main seizure types: generalized, focal, and unknown seizures. *Generalized seizures* occur in, and rapidly engage, bilaterally distributed networks. *Focal seizures* are thought to originate within one hemisphere in the brain. *Unknown seizures*, which include epileptic spasms, are so termed because of incomplete data, but this is not considered a classification.

Pathophysiology

The specific causes of seizures are varied and can be categorized as genetic in origin, due to a structural or metabolic condition, or the cause may be yet unknown. Causes of seizures include the following:

- Cerebrovascular disease
- Hypoxemia of any cause, including vascular insufficiency
- Fever (childhood)
- Head injury
- Hypertension
- Central nervous system infections
- Metabolic and toxic conditions (e.g., renal failure, hyponatremia, hypocalcemia, hypoglycemia, pesticide exposure)
- Brain tumor
- Drug and alcohol withdrawal
- Allergies

Clinical Manifestations

- Generalized seizures often involve both hemispheres of the brain, causing both sides of the body to react.
  - Generalized tonic–clonic contraction: Intense rigidity of the entire body may occur, followed by alternating muscle relaxation and contraction of diaphragm; chest muscles may produce a characteristic epileptic cry; tongue is often chewed; patient is incontinent of urine and feces; after 1 or 2 minutes, the convulsive movements begin to subside; the patient relaxes and lies in deep coma, breathing noisily. The respirations at this point are chiefly abdominal. In the postictal state (after the seizure), patient is confused and difficult to arouse and may sleep for hours; patient may have headache, sore muscles, fatigue, and depression.
- Focal seizures have no natural classification. Clinical manifestations include impairment of consciousness or awareness or other dyscognitive features, localization, and progression of ictal events.

Assessment and Diagnostic Findings

- History to determine type of seizures, their frequency and severity, and the factors that precipitate them, including the following:
  - Circumstances before the seizure (visual, auditory, or olfactory stimuli; tactile stimuli; emotional or psychological disturbances; sleep; hyperventilation)

S

- Occurrence of an aura (a premonitory or warning sensation, which may be visual, auditory, or olfactory)
- Patient's initial movements in the seizure—where the movement or the stiffness begins, conjugate gaze position, and the position of the head at the beginning of the seizure (may provide clues regarding seizure origin in the brain)
- Areas of the body involved (turn back bedding to expose patient)
- Size of both pupils and whether the eyes are open; whether eyes or head turned to one side
- Presence or absence of automatisms (involuntary motor activity, such as lip smacking or repeated swallowing); incontinence of urine or stool
- Duration of each phase of the seizure; unconsciousness, if present, and its duration; any obvious paralysis or weakness of arms or legs after the seizure
- Inability to speak after the seizure; movements at the end of the seizure
- Whether the patient sleeps afterward; cognitive status (confused or not confused) after the seizure
- MRI, electroencephalography (EEG), and single-photon emission CT (SPECT: useful for identifying the epileptogenic zone so that the area in the brain giving rise to seizures can be removed surgically)
- Video recording of seizures, taken simultaneously with EEG telemetry; useful in determining the type of seizure, as well as its duration and magnitude

Nursing Management

Nursing Care During a Seizure

A major responsibility of the nurse is to observe and record the sequence of signs. The nature of the seizure usually indicates the type of treatment required. Prevent injury and support the patient, not only physically but also psychologically (e.g., anxiety, embarrassment, fatigue, and depression).

- Provide privacy and protect the patient from curious onlookers.
- Ease the patient to the floor, if possible.
- Protect the head from striking a hard surface by using a pad.
- Loosen constrictive clothing.
- Push aside any furniture that may injure the patient during the seizure.
- If the patient is in bed, remove pillows and raise side rails.

- If an aura precedes the seizure, insert an oral airway to reduce the possibility of the patient biting the tongue or cheek.
- Do not attempt to pry open jaws that are clenched in a spasm or insert anything into the mouth. Broken teeth and injury to the lips and tongue may result from such action.
- No attempt should be made to restrain the patient during the seizure, because muscular contractions are strong and restraint can produce injury.
- If possible, place the patient on one side with head flexed forward, which allows the tongue to fall forward and facilitates drainage of saliva and mucus. If available, use suction to clear secretions.

Nursing Care After a Seizure

- Document events leading to the seizure, during the seizure, and after the seizure and actions taken to prevent complications (e.g., aspiration, injury).
- Prevent hypoxia, vomiting, and pulmonary aspiration. To prevent complications, place the patient in the side-lying position to facilitate drainage of oral secretions; suction, if needed, to maintain a patent airway and prevent aspiration.
- Maintain seizure precautions: keep suction equipment ready, with a suction catheter and oral airway; place bed in a low position with two to three side rails up and padded.
- Assist in reorienting patient on awakening.
- If the patient becomes agitated after a seizure (postictal), use persuasion and gentle restraint to assist him or her in staying calm.

For more information, see Chapter 66 in Hinkle, J. L., & Cheever, K. H. (2014). *Brunner and Suddarth's textbook of medical-surgical nursing* (13th ed.). Philadelphia: Lippincott Williams & Wilkins.

S

Sexually Transmitted Infections

A sexually transmitted infection (STI) is a collective term to describe diseases acquired through sexual contact with an infected person. STIs are the most common infectious diseases in the United States and are epidemic in most parts of the world. STIs have severe health consequences; they represent a financial burden estimated to be as high as $17 billion per year. Because of perceived stigma and possible threat to emotional relationships, people with symptoms of STIs are often reluctant to seek health care in a timely fashion. STIs may progress without symptoms, and a delay in diagnosis and treatment is potentially harmful because the risk of complications for the infected person (and the risk of transmission to others) increases over time. Infection with one STI suggests the possibility of infection with other diseases as well (e.g., human immunodeficiency virus [HIV]). See the Sexually Transmitted Infections and Their Routes of Transmission table.

Sexually Transmitted Infections and Their Routes of Transmission

Disease	Route(s) of Transmission
Chancroid, *Lymphogranuloma venereum*, and *Granuloma inguinale*	Sexual
Chlamydia	Sexual
Cytomegalovirus (CMV)	Sexual, less intimate contact
Gonorrhea	Sexual, perinatal
Hepatitis B (HBV)	Sexual, percutaneous, perinatal
Hepatitis C (HCV)	Percutaneous, probably sexual, probably perinatal
Herpes simplex	Sexual
HIV infection/AIDS	Sexual, percutaneous, perinatal
Human papillomavirus (HPV)	Sexual
Syphilis	Sexual, perinatal

Pathophysiology

Portals of entry of STI-causing microorganisms and sites of infection include the skin and mucosal linings of the urethra, cervix, vagina, rectum, and oropharynx. STIs can be acquired in utero from an infected mother. Symptoms are variable based on the infecting organism and may mimic other diagnoses; diagnostic screening for patients in specific risk groups is recommended by the Centers for Disease Control and Prevention (CDC).

Prevention

Education about prevention of STIs includes discussion of risk factors and behaviors that can lead to infection. The most recommended educational strategies involve using straightforward language and personal testimonials for targeted audiences, as well as conducting presentations in trusted establishments (e.g., churches, health care facilities). The use of condoms to provide a protective barrier from transmission of STI-related organisms has been broadly promoted; however, the use of condoms has been shown to reduce but not *eliminate* the risk of transmission of HIV and other STIs. Therefore, the term *safer sex* (rather than *safe sex*) is more appropriate when promoting condom use.

Syphilis

Syphilis is an acute and chronic infectious disease caused by the spirochete *Treponema pallidum*. The primary, secondary, and tertiary stages reflect the time from infection and the clinical manifestations observed in that period; these stages form the basis for treatment decisions.

- *Primary syphilis* occurs 2 to 3 weeks after initial inoculation. A painless lesion at the site of infection is called a *chancre* and usually resolves within 3 to 12 weeks.
- *Secondary syphilis* occurs when the hematogenous spread of organisms from the original chancre leads to generalized infection. The rash of secondary syphilis occurs about 2 to 8 weeks after the chancre and involves the trunk and the extremities, including the palms of the hands and the soles of the feet. Generalized signs of infection may include lymphadenopathy, arthritis, meningitis, hair loss, fever, malaise, and weight loss.
- *Tertiary syphilis* is the final stage in the natural history of the disease; between 20% and 40% of those affected have no symptoms. Tertiary syphilis presents as a slowly progressive, inflammatory disease with the potential to affect multiple organs. The most common manifestations at this level are aortitis and neurosyphilis, as evidenced by dementia, psychosis, paresis, stroke, or meningitis.

Assessment and Diagnostic Findings

- Clinical history and physical examination
- Laboratory evaluations: important because syphilis can mimic other diseases
- Direct identification of the spirochete from a chancre
- Serologic tests such as nontreponemal or reagin tests (e.g., Venereal Disease Research Laboratory [VDRL] or the rapid plasma reagin circle card test [RPR-CT]); treponemal tests, such as the fluorescent treponemal antibody (FTA-ABS) and the microhemagglutination test (MHA-TP)

Medical Management

Medical treatment includes antibiotic treatment of both the patient and the patient's sexual contacts. Since syphilis is a reportable communicable disease, patients diagnosed with syphilis must be reported to the state or local public health department to ensure community follow-up. Treatment guidelines established by the CDC are updated on a regular basis. Recommendations provide special guidelines for treatment in the setting of pregnancy, allergy, HIV infection, pediatric infection, congenital infection, and neurosyphilis.

Pharmacologic Therapy
- Antibiotic agents are used to treat all stages of syphilis.
- Penicillin G benzathine intramuscularly in a single dose is the medication of choice for early syphilis or early latent syphilis of less than 1 year's duration; doxycycline can be substituted if the patient has allergies to penicillin.
- Late latent or latent syphilis of unknown duration should receive three antibiotic injections at 1 week intervals.

Nursing Management
In any health care facility, a mechanism must be in place to ensure that all patients diagnosed with a reportable STI are reported to the state or local public health department to ensure community follow-up. The public health department is responsible for identification of sexual contacts, contact notification, and contact screening. Lesions of primary and secondary syphilis may be highly infective. Gloves are worn when direct contact with lesions is likely, and hand hygiene is performed after gloves are removed.

Chlamydia and Gonorrhea
Chlamydia trachomatis and *Neisseria gonorrhoeae* are the most commonly reported infectious diseases in the United States. Patients infected with *N. gonorrhoeae* often become infected with *C. trachomatis*. Chlamydia causes about 2.5 million infections every year in the United States; it is most commonly found in young, sexually active people with more than one partner and is transmitted through sexual intercourse. The greatest risk of *C. trachomatis* infection occurs in young women between 15 and 19 years of age and can result in serious complications, including pelvic infection, an increased risk for ectopic pregnancy, and infertility. Gonorrhea is also a major cause of pelvic inflammatory disease (PID), tubal infertility, ectopic pregnancy, and chronic pelvic pain.

Clinical Manifestations
- Patient may be asymptomatic.
- The most frequent symptoms of chlamydia in women include mucopurulent cervicitis with exudates in the endocervical

canal; they may have dyspareunia, dysuria, bleeding, or symptoms of urinary tract infection or vaginitis.

- When present in men, symptoms may include penile discharge and a burning sensation during urination; the patient may also report painful, swollen testicles with *N. gonorrhoeae* infection.

Complications

- In women, PID, ectopic pregnancy, endometritis, and infertility may occur; inflamed cervix from chlamydia can leave a woman more vulnerable to HIV transmission from an infected partner. Other complications include conjunctivitis and perihepatitis. If a pregnant woman is infected with chlamydia, stillbirth, neonatal death, and premature labor may occur.
- In men, epididymitis, a painful disease that may lead to infertility, may result from infection with either bacterium.
- In either gender, arthritis or bloodstream infection may be caused by *N. gonorrhoeae*.

Assessment and Diagnostic Findings

Assess for fever, discharge (urethral, vaginal, or rectal), and signs of arthritis.

- For *N. gonorrhoeae*: Gram stain (appropriate only for male urethral samples), culture, and nucleic acid amplification tests (NAATs)
- For *C. trachomatis*: samples taken from the anal canal and pharynx for both genders, endocervical samples for women, and urethral samples for men; Gram stain, direct fluorescent antibody test, and NAAT testing
- CDC recommendation: annual chlamydia testing for all pregnant women, sexually active women younger than 25 years, and older women with a new sexual partner or multiple partners

Medical Management

Because patients are often infected with both *N. gonorrhoeae* and *C. trachomatis*, the CDC recommends dual therapy even if only gonorrhea has been laboratory proven. CDC guidelines should be used to determine alternative therapy for the patient who is pregnant or allergic or who has a complicated chlamydial infection. The CDC updates STI therapy recommendations regularly because of growing problems with bacterial antibiotic resistance patterns and drug shortages. Serologic testing for syphilis and HIV should be offered to patients with gonorrhea or chlamydia, because any STI increases the risk of other STIs.

Nursing Management

- Ensure patients diagnosed with gonorrhea and chlamydia are reported to the appropriate public health agency; educate the patient about the necessity to treat all sexual partners.
- Educate adolescents and young adults about sexual health by reinforcing the importance of abstinence, limiting the number of sexual partners, and using condoms for barrier protection.

NURSING PROCESS

The Patient With a Sexually Transmitted Infection

Assessment

- Ask the patient to describe the onset and progression of symptoms, including the location of any lesion and a description of drainage, if occurring. Clarify why information is needed.
- Clarify any unfamiliar terms used by either the patient or nurse.
- Protecting confidentiality is important when discussing sexual issues; use a systematic collection of data using the five Ps: partners, prevention of pregnancy, protection from STIs, practices, past history of STIs.
- Describe the public health notification process and resources that are available to assist sexual partners or infants and children.
- Physical examination includes looking for rashes, lesions, drainage, discharge, or swelling; palpate inguinal nodes to assess for tenderness and swelling; inspect the mouth (while wearing gloves) for signs of inflammation or exudate; women are examined for abdominal or uterine tenderness.

Diagnosis

NURSING DIAGNOSES

- Knowledge deficit about the disease and risk for spread of infection
- Anxiety related to anticipated stigmatization and to prognosis and complications
- Nonadherence to treatment regimen

COLLABORATIVE PROBLEMS/POTENTIAL COMPLICATIONS

Based on assessment data, potential complications that may develop include the following:

- Ectopic pregnancy
- Infertility
- Transmission of infection to fetus, resulting in congenital abnormalities and other outcomes
- Neurosyphilis
- Gonococcal meningitis
- Gonococcal arthritis
- Syphilitic aortitis
- HIV-related complications

Planning and Goals

Major goals are increased patient understanding of the natural history and treatment of the infection, reduction in anxiety, increased compliance with therapeutic and preventive goals, and absence of complications.

Nursing Interventions

INCREASING KNOWLEDGE AND PREVENTING SPREAD OF DISEASE

- Provide education about STIs, causative agents, mode of transmission, and prevention of the spread of STIs to others.
- Stress the importance of completing therapy as prescribed and the need to report any side effects or symptom progression. Reiterate that continued sexual exposure to the same person may lead to reinfection unless the partner has been treated.
- Encourage patient to discuss any reasons for resistance to condom use.

REDUCING ANXIETY

- Encourage patient to discuss any anxieties and fear associated with diagnosis, treatment, or prognosis.
- Provide individualized educational plan that includes reassurance; assist patient in planning discussion with partner.
- If indicated, consider referral to social worker to assist the patient with difficult discussions.

INCREASING COMPLIANCE

- An open discussion about STI information in group settings (e.g., an outpatient obstetric setting) or in a one-to-one setting facilitates patient education.
- Factual explanation of causes, consequences, treatments, prevention, and responsibilities can reduce discomfort and dispel misinformation.

- Referrals to appropriate agencies can complement individual educational efforts and ensure that later questions or uncertainties can be addressed by experts.

MONITORING AND MANAGING POTENTIAL COMPLICATIONS

Infertility and Increased Risk of Ectopic Pregnancy
STIs may lead to PID and, subsequently, increased risk of ectopic pregnancy and infertility.

Congenital Infections
All STIs can be transmitted to infants in utero or at the time of birth. Complications of congenital infection can range from localized infection (e.g., throat infection with *N. gonorrhoeae*), to congenital abnormalities (e.g., stunting of growth or deafness from congenital syphilis), to life-threatening disease (e.g., congenital herpes simplex virus).

Neurosyphilis, Gonococcal Meningitis, Gonococcal Arthritis, and Syphilitic Aortitis
STIs can cause disseminated infection. The central nervous system may be infected, as seen in cases of neurosyphilis or gonococcal meningitis. Gonorrhea that infects the skeletal system may result in gonococcal arthritis. Syphilis can infect the cardiovascular system by forming vegetative lesions on the mitral or aortic valves.

Complications Related to Human Immunodeficiency Virus
HIV infection leads to the profound immunosuppression characteristic of AIDS. Among the complications of HIV infection are many opportunistic infections, including those due to *Pneumocystis jiroveci*, *Cryptococcus neoformans*, cytomegalovirus, and *Mycobacterium avium*. See Acquired Immunodeficiency Syndrome (HIV Infection) in section A for more information.

Evaluation

EXPECTED PATIENT OUTCOMES
- Exhibits knowledge about STIs and their transmission
- Demonstrates a less anxious demeanor
- Complies with treatment
- Achieves effective treatment
- Reports for follow-up examinations, if necessary
- Is free of complications

For more information, see Chapter 71 in Hinkle, J. L., & Cheever, K. H. (2014). *Brunner and Suddarth's textbook of medical-surgical nursing* (13th ed.). Philadelphia: Lippincott Williams & Wilkins.

Shock, Anaphylactic

Anaphylactic shock is caused by a severe allergic reaction when patients who have already produced antibodies to a foreign substance (antigen) are subsequently exposed to the antigen and then develop a systemic antigen–antibody reaction: specifically, an IgE-mediated response.

Risk Factors
- Prior history of an allergic reaction
- Previous adverse drug reaction
- Known allergies to iodine or seafood (increased risk for contrast dye reactions)

Pathophysiology
The antigen–antibody reaction provokes mast cells to release potent vasoactive substances, such as histamine and bradykinin, and activates inflammatory cytokines causing widespread vasodilation and capillary permeability. The most common triggers are foods (especially peanuts), medications, and insects.

Anaphylaxis has three defining characteristics:

- Acute onset of symptoms
- Two or more of the following conditions: respiratory compromise, decreased BP, gastrointestinal distress, and skin or mucosal irritation
- Cardiovascular compromise

Clinical Manifestations
Signs and symptoms present within 5 to 30 minutes of exposure to the antigen; however, occasionally reactions may be seen hours later.

- Headache
- Lightheadedness
- Nausea, vomiting, acute abdominal pain or discomfort
- Pruritus
- Feelings of impending doom
- Diffuse erythema and generalized flushing
- Difficulty breathing (laryngeal edema), bronchospasm
- Cardiac dysrhythmias
- Hypotension

Severe anaphylaxis includes the following:

- Rapid onset of hypotension
- Neurologic compromise
- Respiratory distress
- Cardiac arrest

Medical Management
- Identify and remove causative agent (e.g., antibiotic).
- Ensure adequate IV lines are available early.
- Administer medications to restore vascular tone.
- Manage fluids in light of massive fluid shifts.
- Provide emergency support of basic life functions.
- Provide cardiopulmonary resuscitation if cardiac and/or respiratory arrest is imminent or has occurred.
- Endotracheal intubation may be required to establish an adequate airway.

Pharmacologic Therapy
- Intramuscular epinephrine (vasoconstrictive)
- Diphenhydramine (antihistamine; reduces capillary permeability)
- Nebulized medications to relieve histamine-induced bronchospasm (e.g., albuterol)

Nursing Management
- Aid in prevention by assessing for allergies and previous allergic reactions (e.g., medications, blood products, foods, contrast agents, iodine, seafood, latex).
- Observe patient for symptoms when administering a new medication, particularly with the following: antibiotics, beta-blockers, angiotensin inhibitors (angiotensin converting enzyme inhibitors [ACE-Is]), angiotensin receptor blockers (ARBs), aspirin (ASA), and nonsteroidal anti-inflammatory drugs (NSAIDs).
- Prepare to administer epinephrine intramuscularly in the event of an anaphylactic reaction.
- Educate patient and family on how to avoid future exposure to antigens, how to recognize an anaphylactic reaction, and how to administer emergency medications.

For more information, see Chapter 14 in Hinkle, J. L., & Cheever, K. H. (2014). *Brunner and Suddarth's textbook of medical-surgical nursing* (13th ed.). Philadelphia: Lippincott Williams & Wilkins.

Shock, Cardiogenic

Cardiogenic shock occurs when the heart's ability to contract and to pump blood is impaired and the supply of oxygen is inadequate for the heart and tissues. The causes of cardiogenic shock are known as either *coronary* or *noncoronary*. Coronary cardiogenic shock is more common than noncoronary cardiogenic shock and is seen most often in patients with acute myocardial infarction (MI). Noncoronary causes of cardiogenic shock are related to conditions that stress the myocardium (e.g., severe hypoxemia, acidosis, hypoglycemia, hypocalcemia, and tension pneumothorax) and conditions that result in ineffective myocardial function (e.g., cardiomyopathies, valvular damage, cardiac tamponade, dysrhythmias).

Clinical Manifestations

- Classic signs include low blood pressure (BP) and a rapid, weak pulse.
- Dysrhythmias are common.
- Angina can be present.
- Hemodynamic instability can occur.
- Patient complains of fatigue and may express feelings of doom.

Medical Management

Goals of medical treatment include limiting further myocardial damage, preserving the healthy myocardium, and improving cardiac function by increasing cardiac contractility, decreasing ventricular afterload, or both. In general, these goals are met by increasing oxygen supply to the heart muscle while reducing oxygen demands.

- The underlying cause of cardiogenic shock must be corrected.
- First-line treatment includes administering supplemental oxygen, controlling chest pain, administering fluids, and administering vasoactive medications (e.g., dobutamine, nitroglycerin, dopamine) and antiarrhythmic medications.
- Monitoring to be performed includes hemodynamic monitoring (e.g., arterial line or multilumen pulmonary artery [PA] catheter) and laboratory marker monitoring for ventricular dysfunction such as brain-type natriuretic peptide (BNP) and biomarkers of cardiac muscle damage (e.g., creatine kinase isoenzyme with MB bands [CK-MB] and cardiac troponin-I [cTn-I]). Inflammatory cytokine markers (e.g., C-reactive protein [CRP] and procalcitonin levels) may be obtained.

S

- Mechanical cardiac support may be necessary (e.g., cardio-pulmonary resuscitation, intra-aortic balloon pump therapy [IABP], or a left ventricular assist device [LVAD]).
- Coronary cardiogenic shock may be treated with thrombolytic/fibrinolytic therapy, a percutaneous coronary intervention, coronary artery bypass graft surgery, or IABP therapy.
- Noncoronary cardiogenic shock may be treated with cardiac valve replacement, correction of dysrhythmia, correction of acidosis and electrolyte disturbances, or treatment of the tension pneumothorax.
- If cardiogenic shock was related to cardiac arrest, targeted temperature management (therapeutic hypothermia) may be used after resuscitation to actively lower the core temperature (e.g., 32° to 34°C [89.6° to 93.2°F]) to preserve neurologic function.

Nursing Management

Prevention
- Early on, identify patients at risk for cardiogenic shock.
- Promote adequate oxygenation of the heart muscle, and decrease cardiac workload (e.g., conserve energy, relieve pain, administer oxygen).

Hemodynamic Monitoring
- Monitor hemodynamic and cardiac status: Maintain arterial lines, PA catheters, and electrocardiogram (ECG) equipment.
- Anticipate need for medications, IV fluids, and other equipment.
- Document and promptly report changes in hemodynamic, cardiac, and pulmonary status.

Medication and Fluid Administration
Provide for safe and accurate administration of IV fluids and medications (e.g., ionotropic–chronotropic agents and vasodilators).

> **Quality and Safety Nursing Alert**
>
> A fluid bolus should never be given rapidly, because rapid fluid administration in patients with cardiac failure may result in acute pulmonary edema.

- Monitor for desired effects and side effects (e.g., decreased BP after administering morphine or nitroglycerin, bleeding at arterial and venous puncture sites).

- Monitor urine output, blood urea nitrogen, and serum creatinine levels to detect any decrease in renal function.

Intra-Aortic Balloon Counterpulsation
- Provide ongoing timing adjustments of the balloon pump for maximum effectiveness.
- Perform frequent checks of neurovascular status of lower extremities, particularly to the leg on the side of IABP insertion.

Safety and Comfort
Take an active role in ensuring patient's safety and comfort and in reducing anxiety including administering pain medication to relieve chest pain, preventing infection at catheter insertion sites, and proper positioning to promote effective breathing.

For more information, see Chapter 14 in Hinkle, J. L., & Cheever, K. H. (2014). *Brunner and Suddarth's textbook of medical-surgical nursing* (13th ed.). Philadelphia: Lippincott Williams & Wilkins.

Shock, Hypovolemic

Hypovolemic shock, the most common type of shock, is characterized by decreased intravascular volume. Hypovolemic shock can be caused by external fluid losses, as in traumatic blood loss, or by internal fluid shifts, as in severe dehydration, severe edema, or ascites. Decreased blood volume results in decreased venous return and subsequent decreased ventricular filling, decreased stroke volume and cardiac output, and decreased tissue perfusion.

🍂 Gerontologic Considerations
In older adult patients, dehydration may be the cause of hypovolemic shock.

Clinical Manifestations
- Fall in venous pressure, rise in peripheral resistance, tachycardia
- Cold, moist skin, pallor, thirst, and diaphoresis
- Altered sensorium, oliguria, metabolic acidosis, and tachypnea
- Most dependable criterion: level of arterial blood pressure (BP)

Medical Management
Goals of treatment are to restore intravascular volume, redistribute fluid volume, and correct the underlying cause as

quickly as possible. If the patient is hemorrhaging, bleeding is stopped by applying pressure or by surgery. Diarrhea and vomiting are treated with medications.

Fluid and Blood Replacement

- At least two large-gauge IV lines are inserted to administer fluid, medications, and blood. If an IV catheter cannot be quickly obtained, an intraosseous (IO) catheter may be used for access in the sternum, legs, arms, or pelvis to facilitate rapid fluid replacement.
- Lactated Ringer's solution, colloids (e.g., albumin, hetastarch), or 0.9% sodium chloride solution (normal saline) are administered to restore intravascular volume.
- If hypovolemia is primarily due to blood loss, the American College of Surgeons recommends administration of 3 mL of crystalloid solution for each milliliter of estimated blood loss.
- Blood products are used only if other alternatives are unavailable or blood loss is extensive and rapid.

Redistribution of Fluids

Positioning the patient properly assists fluid redistribution. A modified Trendelenburg position is recommended in hypovolemic shock. Elevation of the legs promotes the return of venous blood.

Pharmacologic Therapy

If fluid administration fails to reverse hypovolemic shock, vasoactive medications that prevent cardiac failure are given. Medications are also administered to reverse the cause of the dehydration (e.g., insulin for diabetes or desmopressin acetate [DDAVP] for diabetes insipidus).

Nursing Management

- Closely monitor patients at risk for fluid deficits (younger than 1 year or older than 65 years).
- Assist with fluid replacement before intravascular volume is depleted.
- Ensure safe administration of prescribed fluids and medications and document effects.
- Reduce fear and anxiety about the need for an oxygen mask by giving patient explanations and frequent reassurance.
- Monitor and promptly report signs of complications and effects of treatment. Monitor patient closely for adverse effects.

- Monitor for cardiovascular overload, signs of difficulty breathing, and pulmonary edema: hemodynamic pressure, vital signs including temperature, arterial blood gases, serum lactate levels, hemoglobin and hematocrit levels, bladder pressure monitoring, and fluid intake and output.
- Monitor for changes in respiratory status: Acute coronary syndrome (ACS) is also a possible complication of excessive fluid resuscitation and may initially present with respiratory symptoms.

Gerontologic Considerations
The risk of these complications is increased in older adults and in patients with preexisting cardiac disease.

For more information, see Chapter 14 in Hinkle, J. L., & Cheever, K. H. (2014). *Brunner and Suddarth's textbook of medical-surgical nursing* (13th ed.). Philadelphia: Lippincott Williams & Wilkins.

Shock, Neurogenic

Neurogenic shock is a shock state resulting from loss of sympathetic tone, causing relative hypovolemia.

Risk Factors
- Spinal cord injury
- Spinal anesthesia
- Nervous system damage
- Depressant action of medications
- Hypoglycemia

Pathophysiology
Sympathetic stimulation causes vascular smooth muscle to constrict, and parasympathetic stimulation causes vascular smooth muscle to relax or dilate. Vasodilation occurs as a result of a loss of balance between parasympathetic and sympathetic stimulation. The overriding parasympathetic stimulation that occurs with neurogenic shock causes a drastic decrease in the patient's systemic vascular resistance and bradycardia. Inadequate BP, despite an adequate blood volume, results in the insufficient perfusion of tissues and cells that is common to all shock states.

Clinical Manifestations
Symptoms are consistent with signs of parasympathetic stimulation:

- Dry, warm skin
- Bradycardia

Medical Management
- Restore sympathetic tone (e.g., stabilizing spinal injury or repositioning patient with spinal anesthesia).
- Specific treatment depends on the cause of the shock.

Nursing Management
- Elevate head of the bed at least 30 degrees for spinal or epidural anesthesia.
- Immobilize patient if spinal cord injury is suspected to prevent further damage.
- Assess for lower-extremity pain, redness, tenderness, or warmth that may suggest formation of a venous thromboembolism.
- Provide passive range of motion to promote circulation.
- Use pneumatic compression devices combined with antithrombotic agents (e.g., low-molecular-weight heparin).
- Assess for signs of internal bleeding.

For more information, see Chapter 14 in Hinkle, J. L., & Cheever, K. H. (2014). *Brunner and Suddarth's textbook of medical-surgical nursing* (13th ed.). Philadelphia: Lippincott Williams & Wilkins.

Shock, Septic

Septic shock, the most common type of circulatory shock, is caused by widespread infection or sepsis and is the leading cause of death in noncoronary ICU patients. Gram-negative bacteria are the most common pathogens. Other infectious agents, such as gram-positive bacteria (increasingly) and viruses and fungi, can also cause septic shock.

Risk Factors

Risk factors for septic shock include the increased use of invasive procedures and indwelling medical devices; the increased number of antibiotic-resistant microorganisms; and the increasingly older population. Other patients at risk are those with malnutrition or immunosuppression, those with chronic illness (e.g., diabetes, hepatitis), and those undergoing surgical and other invasive procedures, especially patients who have emergency surgery or multiple surgeries.

🍁 Gerontologic Considerations
Older adult patients are at particular risk for sepsis because of decreased physiologic reserves and an aging immune system.

Pathophysiology

Gram-negative bacteria traditionally have been the most commonly implicated microorganisms in septic shock. However, gram-positive bacteria, viruses, and fungi can also cause septic shock. Microorganism invasion causes an immune response. This immune response activates biochemical cytokines and mediators associated with an inflammatory response and produces a variety of effects leading to shock. Increased capillary permeability results in fluid loss from the capillaries. Capillary instability and vasodilation causes inadequate perfusion of oxygen and interferes with the transport of nutrients to the tissues and cells. Proinflammatory and anti-inflammatory cytokines released during the inflammatory response activate the coagulation system, which begins to form clots regardless of whether bleeding is present. This results in microvascular occlusions that further disrupt cellular perfusion but also in an inappropriate consumption of clotting factors. Sepsis is an evolving process, with neither clearly definable clinical signs and symptoms nor predictable progression.

Clinical Manifestations

In the early stage of septic shock:

- BP possibly remaining within normal limits (or hypotensive but responsive to fluids)
- Elevated heart and respiratory rates
- High cardiac output with vasodilation
- Hyperthermia (febrile) with warm, flushed skin, bounding pulses
- Urinary output normal or decreased
- Gastrointestinal status compromised (e.g., nausea, vomiting, diarrhea, or decreased gastric motility)
- Subtle changes in mental status (e.g., confusion or agitation)
- Elevations in white blood cell (WBC) count, C-reactive protein (CRP), and procalcitonin levels

As sepsis progresses:

- Low cardiac output with vasoconstriction
- BP dropping; not responsive to fluids or vasoactive medications
- Skin cool and pale with delayed capillary refill
- Temperature normal or below normal
- Heart and respiratory rates rapid
- Anuria and multiple organ dysfunction progressing to failure

S

🍂 Gerontologic Considerations

Septic shock may be manifested by atypical or confusing clinical signs. Suspect septic shock in any older adult who develops an unexplained acute confused state, tachypnea, or hypotension.

Medical Management

- Early assessments and identification of source helps to guide interventions.
- Blood, sputum, urine, wound drainage specimens, and tips of indwelling catheters are collected to identify and eliminate the cause of infection prior to initiating antibiotic therapy.
- Potential routes of infection are eliminated (IV lines rerouted if necessary). Abscesses are drained, and necrotic areas are débrided.
- Fluid replacement is instituted, including fluid challenges with crystalloids or colloids.
- Monitor BP, central venous pressure (CVP), urine output, and serum lactate levels to assess effectiveness of fluid resuscitation.

Pharmacologic Therapy

- Broad-spectrum antibiotics are started ideally within first hour of treatment.
- Vasopressor agents and/or ionotropic agents may be required to improve tissue perfusion and provide support for myocardium.
- Packed red blood cells support oxygen delivery and transport to the tissues.
- Neuromuscular blockade agents as well as sedation agents reduce metabolic demands and provide comfort to the patient.
- Deep vein thrombosis prophylaxis with low-dose unfractionated heparin or low-molecular-weight heparin, in combination with mechanical prophylaxis (e.g., sequential compression devices [SCDs]) should be initiated.
- Stress ulcer prophylaxis (e.g., H_2 blocking agents, proton pump inhibitors) should be added.

Nutritional Therapy

- Aggressive nutritional supplementation (high protein) is used within 24 to 48 hours after ICU admission.
- Enteral feedings are preferred.

Nursing Management

Identify patients at risk for sepsis and septic shock.

 Quality and Safety Nursing Alert

Nurses should identify patients who are at particular risk for sepsis and septic shock (i.e., older adults and immuno-suppressed patients and those with extensive trauma, burns, or diabetes), keeping in mind that these high-risk patients may not develop typical or classic signs of infection and sepsis. For example, confusion may be the first sign of infection and sepsis in older adult patients.

- Carry out all invasive procedures with correct aseptic technique after careful hand hygiene.
- Monitor IV lines, arterial and venous puncture sites, surgical incisions, trauma wounds, urinary catheters, and pressure ulcers for signs of infection.
- Implement interventions to prevent ventilator-associated pneumonia and pressure ulcers.
- Reduce patient's temperature when ordered for temperatures higher than 40°C (104°F) or if the patient is uncomfortable by administering acetaminophen or applying a hypothermia blanket; monitor closely for shivering.
- Administer prescribed IV fluids and medications.
- Monitor and report blood levels (peak and trough antibiotic levels, procalcitonin, CRP, blood urea nitrogen, and creatinine levels; WBC; hemoglobin and hematocrit levels; platelet count; coagulation studies).
- Monitor hemodynamic status, fluid intake and output, and nutritional status.
- Monitor daily weights and serum albumin and prealbumin levels to determine daily protein requirements.

For more information, see Chapter 14 in Hinkle, J. L., & Cheever, K. H. (2014). *Brunner and Suddarth's textbook of medical-surgical nursing* (13th ed.). Philadelphia: Lippincott Williams & Wilkins.

Spinal Cord Injury

Spinal cord injuries (SCIs) are a major health problem. Most SCIs result from motor vehicle crashes. Other causes include falls, violence (primarily from gunshot wounds), and recreational sporting activities. Half of the victims are between 16 and 30 years of age; most are male. Another risk factor is substance abuse (alcohol and drugs). There is a high frequency of associated injuries and medical complications. The vertebrae most frequently involved in SCIs are the fifth, sixth, and seventh cervical vertebrae (C5–C7), the 12th thoracic vertebra (T12), and the first lumbar vertebra (L1). These vertebrae are the most susceptible because there is a greater range of mobility in the vertebral column in these areas. Damage to the spinal cord ranges from: (1) transient concussion (patient recovers fully), to (2) contusion, laceration, and compression of the cord substance (either alone or in combination), to (3) complete transection of the cord (paralysis below the level of injury). Injury can be categorized as primary (usually permanent) or secondary (nerve fibers swell and disintegrate as a result of ischemia, hypoxia, edema, and hemorrhagic lesions). Whereas a primary injury is permanent, a secondary injury may be reversible if treated within 4 to 6 hours of the initial injury. The type of injury refers to the extent of injury to the spinal cord itself.

Incomplete spinal cord lesions are classified according to the area of spinal cord damage: central, lateral, anterior, or peripheral. A complete SCI can result in paraplegia (paralysis of the lower body) or tetraplegia (formerly *quadriplegia*—paralysis of all four extremities).

Clinical Manifestations

The consequences of SCI depend on the type and level of injury of the cord.

Neurologic Level

The neurologic level refers to the lowest level at which sensory and motor functions are normal. Signs and symptoms include the following:

- Total sensory and motor paralysis below the neurologic level
- Loss of bladder and bowel control (usually with urinary retention and bladder distention)
- Loss of sweating and vasomotor tone
- Marked reduction of BP from loss of peripheral vascular resistance
- Acute pain in back or neck (if patient is conscious and can report); possible fear that the neck or back is broken

Respiratory Problems

- Related to compromised respiratory function; severity depends on level of injury
- Acute respiratory failure: leading cause of death in high cervical cord injury

Assessment and Diagnostic Findings

Detailed neurologic examination, x-ray examinations (lateral cervical spine x-rays), CT, and MRI, are common assessment and diagnostic tools. ECG is also commonly used, as bradycardia and asystole are frequent findings in acute spinal injuries.

Complications

Spinal shock, a serious complication of SCI, is a sudden depression of reflex activity in the spinal cord (areflexia) below the level of injury. The muscles innervated by the cord segment situated below the level of the lesion become completely paralyzed and flaccid, and the reflexes are absent. BP and heart rate fall as vital organs are affected. Parts of the body below the level of the cord lesion are paralyzed and left without sensation.

Emergency Management

- Immediate patient management at the accident scene is crucial. Improper handling can cause further damage and loss of neurologic function.
- Consider that any victim of a motor vehicle crash, a diving or contact sports injury, a fall, or any direct trauma to the head and neck has an SCI until it is ruled out.
- Initial care includes rapid assessment, immobilization, extrication, stabilization or control of life-threatening injuries, and transportation to an appropriate medical facility.
- Maintain patient in an extended position (not sitting); no body part should be twisted or turned.
- The standard of care is referral to a regional spinal injury center or trauma center for treatment in first 24 hours.

Medical Management

Acute Phase

Goals of management are to prevent further SCI and to observe for symptoms of progressive neurologic deficits. The patient is resuscitated as necessary, and oxygenation and cardiovascular stability are maintained. High-dose corticosteroid drugs (methylprednisolone) may be administered to counteract spinal cord edema, though this is no longer the standard of care because studies suggest it offers only slight benefit.

Oxygen is administered to maintain a high arterial PaO_2. Extreme care is taken to avoid flexing or extending the neck if endotracheal intubation is necessary. Diaphragm pacing (electrical stimulation of the phrenic nerve) may be considered for patients with high cervical spine injuries. Surgically implanted, intramuscular diaphragm pacing techniques may be used.

SCI requires immobilization, reduction of dislocations, and stabilization of the vertebral column. The cervical fracture is reduced and the cervical spine aligned with a form of skeletal traction (using skeletal tongs, calipers, or the halo-vest technique). Weights are hung freely so as not to interfere with the traction.

Early surgery reduces the need for traction. The goals of surgical treatment are to preserve neurologic function by removing pressure from the spinal cord and to provide stability.

Management of Complications

Spinal and Neurogenic Shock

- Intestinal decompression is used to treat bowel distention and paralytic ileus caused by depression of reflexes. This loss of sympathetic innervation causes a variety of other clinical manifestations, including neurogenic shock signaled by decreased cardiac output, venous pooling in the extremities, and peripheral vasodilation.
- Patient who does not perspire on paralyzed portion of body requires close observation for early detection of an abrupt onset of fever.
- Special attention is paid to the respiratory system (may not be enough intrathoracic pressure to cough effectively). Special problems include decreased vital capacity, decreased oxygen levels, and pulmonary edema.
- Chest physiotherapy and suctioning are implemented to help clear pulmonary secretions. Patient is monitored for respiratory complications (respiratory failure, pneumonia).

> ▶ *Quality and Safety Nursing Alert*
>
> The patient's vital organ functions and body defenses must be supported and maintained until spinal and neurogenic shock abates and the neurologic system has recovered from the traumatic insult; this can take up to 4 months.

Deep Vein Thrombosis and Other Complications

- Patient is observed for deep vein thrombosis (DVT), a complication of immobility (e.g., pulmonary embolism [PE]). Symptoms include pleuritic chest pain, anxiety, shortness of breath, and abnormal blood gas values.
- Low-dose anticoagulation therapy is initiated to prevent DVT and PE, along with the use of anti-embolism stockings or pneumatic compression devices. A permanent indwelling filter may be placed in the vena cava to prevent dislodged clots (emboli) from migrating to the lungs and causing PE.
- Patient is monitored for autonomic hyperreflexia (characterized by pounding headache, profuse sweating, nasal congestion, piloerection [gooseflesh], bradycardia, and hypertension).
- Constant surveillance is maintained for signs and symptoms of pressure ulcers and infection (urinary, respiratory, local infection at pin sites).

> *Quality and Safety Nursing Alert*
>
> **The calves or thighs should never be massaged because of the danger of dislodging an undetected thromboembolus.**

NURSING PROCESS

The Patient With Acute SCI

Assessment

- Observe breathing pattern; assess strength of cough; auscultate lungs.
- Monitor patient closely for any changes in motor or sensory function and for symptoms of progressive neurologic damage.
- Test motor ability by asking patient to spread fingers, squeeze examiner's hand, and move toes or turn the feet.
- Evaluate sensation by pinching the skin or touching it lightly with a tongue blade, starting at shoulder and working down both sides; patient's eyes should be closed. Ask patient where sensation is felt.
- Assess for spinal shock.
- Palpate lower abdomen for signs of urinary retention and overdistention of the bladder.
- Assess for gastric dilation and paralytic ileus due to atonic bowel.

- Monitor temperature; hyperthermia may result owing to autonomic disruption.

Diagnosis

NURSING DIAGNOSES

- Ineffective breathing patterns and airway clearance related to weakness (or paralysis) of abdominal and intercostal muscles, and inability to clear secretions
- Impaired physical mobility related to motor and sensory impairment
- Disturbed sensory perception related to immobility and sensory loss
- Risk for impaired skin integrity related to immobility or sensory loss
- Impaired urinary elimination related to patient's inability to void spontaneously
- Constipation related to presence of atonic bowel as a result of autonomic disruption
- Acute pain and discomfort related to treatment and prolonged immobility
- Autonomic dysreflexia related to uninhibited sympathetic response of the nervous system following SCI

COLLABORATIVE PROBLEMS/POTENTIAL COMPLICATIONS

- Venous thromboembolism (DVT, PE)
- Orthostatic hypotension
- Autonomic hyperreflexia

Planning and Goals

Major patient goals may include improved breathing pattern and airway clearance; improved mobility; improved sensory and perceptual awareness; maintenance of skin integrity; relief of urinary retention; improved bowel function; promotion of comfort; and absence of complications.

Nursing Interventions

PROMOTING ADEQUATE BREATHING AND AIRWAY CLEARANCE

- Detect potential respiratory failure by observing patient, measuring vital capacity, and monitoring oxygen saturation through pulse oximetry and arterial blood gas values.
- Prevent retention of secretions and resultant atelectasis with early and vigorous attention to clearing bronchial and pharyngeal secretions.

- Suction with caution, because this procedure can stimulate the vagus nerve, producing bradycardia and cardiac arrest.
- Initiate chest physical therapy and assisted coughing to mobilize secretions if the patient cannot cough effectively.
- Supervise breathing exercises to increase strength and endurance of inspiratory muscles, particularly the diaphragm.
- Ensure proper humidification and hydration to maintain thin secretions.
- Assess for signs of respiratory infection: cough, fever, and dyspnea.
- Monitor respiratory status frequently.

IMPROVING MOBILITY
- Maintain proper body alignment at all times.
- Reposition the patient frequently and assist patient out of bed as soon as the spinal column is stabilized.
- Apply splints (various types) to prevent footdrop, and apply trochanter rolls to prevent external rotation of the hip joints; reapply every 2 hours.
- Patients with lesions above the midthoracic level may tolerate changes in position poorly; monitor BP when position is changed.
- Do not turn a patient who is not on a rotating specialty bed, unless physician indicates that it is safe to do so.
- Perform passive range of motion exercises as soon as possible after injury to avoid complications such as contractures and atrophy.
- Provide a full range of motion at least four or five times daily to toes, metatarsals, ankles, knees, and hips.
- For patients who have a cervical fracture without neurologic deficit, reduction in traction followed by rigid immobilization for 6 to 8 weeks restores skeletal integrity. These patients are allowed to move gradually to an erect position. Apply a neck brace or molded collar when the patient is mobilized after traction is removed.

PROMOTING ADAPTATION TO DISTURBED SENSORY PERCEPTION
- Stimulate the area above the level of the injury through touch, aromas, flavorful food and beverages, conversation, and music.
- Provide prism glasses to enable patient to see from supine position.
- Encourage use of hearing aids, if applicable.

- Provide emotional support; teach patient strategies to compensate for, or cope with, sensory deficits.

MAINTAINING SKIN INTEGRITY
- Change patient's position every 2 hours and inspect the skin, particularly under cervical collar.
- Assess for redness or breaks in skin over pressure points; check perineum for soilage; observe catheter for adequate drainage; assess general body alignment and comfort.
- Wash skin every few hours with a mild soap, rinse well, and blot dry. Keep pressure-sensitive areas well lubricated and soft with oil or lotion.
- Educate patient about pressure ulcers and encourage participation in preventive measures.

MAINTAINING URINARY ELIMINATION
- Perform intermittent catheterization to avoid overstretching the bladder and infection. If this is not feasible, insert an indwelling catheter.
- Show family members how to catheterize and encourage them to participate in this facet of care.
- Educate patient in recording fluid intake, voiding pattern, amounts of residual urine after catheterization, characteristics of urine, and any unusual feelings.

IMPROVING BOWEL FUNCTION
- Monitor reactions to gastric intubation.
- Provide a high-calorie, high-protein, high-fiber diet. Food amount may be gradually increased after bowel sounds resume.
- Administer prescribed stool softener to counteract effects of immobility and analgesic agents, and institute a bowel program as early as possible.

PROVIDING COMFORT MEASURES
- Reassure patient in halo traction that he or she will adapt to steel frame (i.e., feeling caged in and hearing noises).
- Cleanse pin sites daily and observe for redness, drainage, and pain; observe for loosening. If one of the pins becomes detached, stabilize the patient's head in a neutral position and have someone notify the neurosurgeon; keep a torque screwdriver readily available.
- Inspect the skin under the halo vest for excessive perspiration, redness, and skin blistering, especially on the bony

prominences. Open vest at the sides to allow torso to be washed. Do not allow vest to become wet; do not use powder inside vest.

MONITORING AND MANAGING POTENTIAL COMPLICATIONS

Thrombophlebitis

Refer to "Medical Management" under Vein Disorders in Section V.

Orthostatic Hypotension

Reduce frequency of hypotensive episodes by administering prescribed vasopressor medications. Provide anti-embolism stockings and abdominal binders; allow time for slow position changes and use tilt tables as appropriate. Close monitoring of vital signs before and during position changes is essential.

Autonomic Hyperreflexia

- Perform a rapid assessment to identify and alleviate the cause of autonomic hyperreflexia and remove the stimulating trigger.
- Place patient immediately in sitting position to lower BP.
- Catheterize the patient to empty bladder immediately.
- Examine rectum for fecal mass. Apply topical anesthetic for 10 to 15 minutes before removing fecal mass.
- Examine skin for areas of pressure, irritation, or breaks.
- As prescribed, administer a ganglionic blocking agent such as hydralazine hydrochloride (Apresoline) if the foregoing measures do not relieve hypertension and excruciating headache.
- Label chart clearly and visibly, noting the risk for autonomic hyperreflexia.
- Educate patient in prevention and management measures. Inform patient with lesion above T6 that hyperreflexic episode can occur years after initial injury.

PROMOTING HOME- AND COMMUNITY-BASED CARE

Educating Patients About Self-Care

- Shift emphasis from ensuring that patient is stable and free of complications to specific assessment and planning for independence and the skills necessary for activities of daily living.
- Initially, focus patient education on the injury and its effects on mobility, dressing, and bowel, bladder, and sexual function. As the patient and family acknowledge the consequences of the injury and the resulting disability, broaden the focus of education to address issues necessary for the patient

to carry out the tasks of daily living and take charge of his or her life.

Continuing Care

- Support and assist patient and family in assuming responsibility for increasing care; provide assistance in dealing with psychological impact of SCI and its consequences.
- Coordinate management team and serve as liaison with rehabilitation centers and home care agencies.
- Reassure female patients with SCI that pregnancy is not contraindicated and fertility is relatively unaffected but that pregnant women with acute or chronic SCI pose unique management challenges.
- Refer for home care nursing support as indicated or desired.
- Refer patient to mental health care professional as indicated.

Evaluation

EXPECTED PATIENT OUTCOMES

- Demonstrates improvement in gas exchange and clearance of secretions
- Moves within limits of dysfunction and demonstrates completion of exercises within functional limitations
- Demonstrates adaptation to sensory and perceptual alterations
- Demonstrates optimal skin integrity
- Regains urinary bladder function
- Regains bowel function
- Reports absence of pain and discomfort
- Is free of complications

For more information, see Chapter 68 in Hinkle, J. L., & Cheever, K. H. (2014). *Brunner and Suddarth's textbook of medical-surgical nursing* (13th ed.). Philadelphia: Lippincott Williams & Wilkins.

S

Stroke, Hemorrhagic

Hemorrhagic strokes account for 15% to 20% of cerebrovascular disorders and are primarily caused by intracranial or subarachnoid hemorrhage, with bleeding into the brain tissue, the ventricles, or the subarachnoid space. Primary intracerebral hemorrhage from a spontaneous rupture of small vessels accounts for approximately 80% of hemorrhagic strokes and is caused chiefly by uncontrolled hypertension. Subarachnoid hemorrhage results from a ruptured intracranial aneurysm (a weakening in the arterial wall) in about half the cases. The cerebral arteries most commonly affected by an aneurysm are the internal carotid artery (ICA), anterior cerebral artery (ACA), anterior communicating artery (ACoA), posterior communicating artery (PCoA), posterior cerebral artery (PCA), and middle cerebral artery (MCA). Secondary intracerebral hemorrhages are associated with arteriovenous malformations (AVMs), intracranial aneurysms, intracranial neoplasms, or certain medications (e.g., anticoagulant drugs, amphetamines).

Pathophysiology

The pathophysiology of hemorrhagic stroke depends on the cause and type of cerebrovascular disorder. Symptoms are produced when a primary hemorrhage, aneurysm, or AVM presses on nearby cranial nerves or brain tissue or, more dramatically, when an aneurysm or AVM ruptures, causing subarachnoid hemorrhage (hemorrhage into the cranial subarachnoid space). Normal brain metabolism is disrupted by any of the following factors: exposure of the brain to extravascular blood, by an increase in intracranial pressure (ICP) owing to the increased extravascular blood volume that compresses and injures brain tissue, or by secondary ischemia resulting from the reduced blood flow and vasospasm that frequently accompany subarachnoid hemorrhage.

Risk Factors

Nonmodifiable
- Advanced age (older than 55 years)
- Cerebral amyloid angiopathy
- Gender (male)

Modifiable or Treatable
- Hypertension
- Excessive alcohol consumption
- AVMs (younger patients), intracranial aneurysms, intracranial neoplasms
- Certain medications (e.g., anticoagulant drugs, amphetamines, illicit drug use)
- Atherosclerosis

Clinical Manifestations
- Sudden severe headache (if conscious)
- Vomiting
- Early sudden changes in level of consciousness
- Possibly focal seizures (due to frequent brain stem involvement)

- Neurologic deficits including motor, sensory, cranial nerve, cognitive, and other functions similar to ischemic stroke
- Sudden severe headache, loss of consciousness for a variable period of time; pain and rigidity of neck and spine, characteristic of an intracranial aneurysm rupture or AVM
- Possibly visual disturbances (visual loss, diplopia, ptosis) if oculomotor nerve is involved
- Tinnitus, dizziness or hemiparesis also possible
- May see other neurologic deficits similar to those seen in ischemic stroke
- Severe bleeding, which may result in coma and death

Assessment and Diagnostic Findings
- History and complete physical and neurologic examination
- CT or MRI scan
- Cerebral angiography (confirms diagnosis of intracranial aneurysm or AVM)
- Lumbar puncture (only if CT negative and no evidence of ICP)
- Toxicology screen for patients younger than 40 years

Prevention
Help patients alter risk factors for stroke; encourage patient to control hypertension, maintain a healthy weight, follow a healthy diet (including modest alcohol consumption), and exercise daily.

Complications
Immediate complications of a hemorrhagic stroke include cerebral hypoxia, decreased cerebral blood flow, and extension of the area of injury. Subsequent complications include rebleeding or hematoma expansion; cerebral vasospasm, resulting in cerebral ischemia; acute hydrocephalus (prevents resorption of cerebrospinal fluid [CSF]); and seizures.

Medical Management
The goals of medical treatment for hemorrhagic stroke are to allow the brain to recover from the initial insult (bleeding), to prevent or minimize the risk of rebleeding, and to prevent or treat complications. Management may consist of bed rest with sedation to prevent agitation and stress, management of vasospasm, and surgical or medical treatment to prevent rebleeding. If the bleeding is caused by anticoagulation with warfarin, the international normalized ratio (INR) may be corrected with fresh-frozen plasma and vitamin K. Reversing the anticoagulation effect of the newer anticoagulant agents is more complicated. Prophylactic measures to prevent venous

thromboembolism are instituted, including sequential compression devices (or anti-embolism stockings).

Pharmacologic Therapy

- Seizures are treated with antiepileptic drugs such as phenytoin (Dilantin).
- Hyperglycemia should also be treated.
- Analgesic agents are given for head and neck pain.
- Antihypertensive medications are given to control hypertension.

Surgical Management

- Indications for surgery include signs of worsening neurologic exam, increased ICP, or signs of brain stem compression.
- Surgery may prevent bleeding in an unruptured aneurysm or prevent further bleeding in an already ruptured aneurysm by isolating the aneurysm with a ligature or a clip across its neck. The aneurysm can be reinforced by wrapping it with some substance to provide support and induce scarring.
- Surgical evacuation is most frequently accomplished via a craniotomy.
- Endovascular techniques may be used in selected patients to occlude the blood flow from the artery that feeds the aneurysm with coils, or other techniques may be used to occlude the aneurysm itself. For large or wide aneurysms, a stentlike device may be used to divert the blood flow away from the aneurysm.
- Postoperative complications include psychological symptoms (disorientation, amnesia, Korsakoff's syndrome, personality changes); intraoperative embolization or artery rupture; postoperative artery occlusion; fluid and electrolyte disturbances (from dysfunction of the neurohypophyseal system); and gastrointestinal bleeding.

S

NURSING PROCESS

The Patient Recovering From a Hemorrhagic Stroke

Assessment

- Altered level of consciousness or responsiveness, ability to speak, and orientation
- Sluggish pupillary reactions to light and ocular position
- Motor and sensory deficits
- Cranial nerve deficits (extraocular eye movements, facial droop, presence of ptosis)
- Speech difficulties and visual disturbance

- Headache and nuchal rigidity or other neurologic deficits
- Ongoing assessments for any impairment in performance of patient's daily activities.

Diagnosis

NURSING DIAGNOSES

- Ineffective tissue perfusion (cerebral) related to bleeding or vasospasm
- Anxiety related to illness or medically imposed restrictions (aneurysm precautions)

COLLABORATIVE PROBLEMS/POTENTIAL COMPLICATIONS

- Vasospasm
- Seizures
- Hydrocephalus
- Rebleeding
- Hyponatremia

Planning and Goals

The major goals for the patient (and family) may include improved cerebral tissue perfusion, relief of anxiety, and absence of complications.

Nursing Interventions

OPTIMIZING CEREBRAL TISSUE PERFUSION

- Monitor for changes in neurologic deterioration; record assessments via neurologic flow record.
- Perform hourly checks of blood pressure, pulse, level of consciousness (an indicator of cerebral perfusion), pupillary responses, and motor function.
- Monitor respiratory status, because a reduction in oxygen in areas of the brain with impaired autoregulation increases the chance of a cerebral infarction.
- Implement aneurysm precautions, including providing a nonstimulating environment; plan care to prevent increases in ICP and minimize risk of further bleeding by providing pain relief and minimizing anxiety.
- Increase head of bed to 15 to 30 degrees to promote venous drainage and decrease ICP.
- Avoid any straining or Valsalva maneuvers; any activity requiring exertion is contraindicated.
- Dim lighting is helpful, because photophobia (visual intolerance of light) is common; external stimuli are kept

to a minimum, including no television, no radio, and no reading.

- Avoid caffeinated beverages.
- Stool softeners and mild laxatives are prescribed to prevent constipation; no enemas are permitted.
- Administer all personal care, including feeding and bathing, to prevent any exertion that might increase the blood pressure.

Relieving Anxiety

- Keep sensory stimulation to a minimum; reorient frequently to help maintain orientation.
- Keep patient well informed of the plan of care; provide appropriate reassurances to help relieve fears and anxiety.
- Include family in discussions of care and support family members.

Monitoring and Managing Potential Complications

- Vasospasm: Assess for signs of vasospasm, including intensified headaches, a decrease in level of responsiveness (confusion, disorientation, lethargy), or evidence of aphasia or partial paralysis. Administer the calcium channel blocker nimodipine (Nimotop) for prevention of vasospasm; fluid volume expanders may also be prescribed.
- Seizures: Should a seizure occur, maintaining the airway and preventing injury are the primary goals. Medication therapy is initiated at this time.
- Hydrocephalus: Hydrocephalus can occur within the first 24 hours (acute) after subarachnoid hemorrhage or several days (subacute) to several weeks (delayed) later. Symptoms vary according to the time of onset and may be nonspecific. Acute hydrocephalus is characterized by sudden onset of stupor or coma and is managed with a ventriculostomy drain to decrease ICP; symptoms of subacute and delayed hydrocephalus include gradual onset of drowsiness, behavioral changes, and ataxic gait. A ventriculoperitoneal (VP) shunt is placed for chronic hydrocephalus.
- Rebleeding: Hypertension is the most serious and modifiable risk factor. Aneurysm rebleeding occurs most frequently during the first 2 weeks after the initial hemorrhage, is considered a major complication, and is confirmed by CT scan. Symptoms of rebleeding include sudden severe headache, nausea, vomiting, decreased level of consciousness, and neurologic deficit.

- Hyponatremia: Hyponatremia occurs in 50% of patients with subarachnoid hemorrhage and must be identified as early as possible. The patient is then evaluated for syndrome of inappropriate antidiuretic hormone (SIADH) or cerebral salt-wasting syndrome. Treatment most often is with IV hypertonic 3% saline.

PROMOTING HOME- AND COMMUNITY-BASED CARE

Educating Patients About Self-Care

- Review with patient and family principles of care and rationale for restrictions required in the acute phase.
- Encourage patient to resume as much self-care as possible; provide assistive devices as indicated. Modifications of the home may be required.
- Provide education to patient and family regarding causes of hemorrhagic stroke, possible consequences, relevant medical or surgical treatments, and the importance of interventions taken to prevent and detect complications.
- Educate family to support patient and give positive reinforcement.

Continuing Care

- Assess and address obvious needs and deficits after the hemorrhagic stroke.
- Remind patient and family of importance of following recommendations to prevent further hemorrhagic stroke and of keeping follow-up appointments with health care providers to monitor for risk factors.
- Review signs and symptoms of specific complications.
- Identify safety measures to prevent falls.
- Educate patient and family about medications, including name, dosing regimens, and side effects; identify any barriers to accessing medications and obtain referrals to resolve barriers.
- Refer to home health care agency as needed.

Evaluation

EXPECTED PATIENT OUTCOMES

- Demonstrates stable neurologic status and normal respiratory patterns
- Reports reduced anxiety level
- Is free of complications

For more information, see Chapter 67 in Hinkle, J. L., & Cheever, K. H. (2014). *Brunner and Suddarth's textbook of medical-surgical nursing* (13th ed.). Philadelphia: Lippincott Williams & Wilkins.

Stroke, Ischemic

An ischemic stroke (also referred to as a *cerebrovascular accident* [CVA] or "*brain attack*") is a sudden loss of brain function resulting from a disruption of the blood supply to a part of the brain. Stroke is the primary cerebrovascular disorder in the United States.

Pathophysiology

A stroke is an upper motor neuron lesion and results in loss of voluntary control over motor movements. Strokes are usually hemorrhagic (15%) or ischemic (nonhemorrhagic) (85%). Ischemic strokes are categorized according to their cause: large artery thrombotic strokes (20%), small penetrating artery thrombotic strokes (25%), cardiogenic embolic strokes (20%), cryptogenic strokes (30%), and other strokes (5%). Cryptogenic strokes have no known cause, and other strokes result from causes such as illicit drug use, coagulopathies, migraine, and spontaneous dissection of the carotid or vertebral arteries. The result is an interruption in the blood supply to the brain, causing temporary or permanent loss of movement, thought, memory, speech, or sensation. Early interventions in the ischemic process with medications such as tissue plasminogen activator (t-PA) and medications that protect the brain from secondary injury (called *neuroprotective agents*) can limit the extent of secondary brain injury caused by a stroke.

Risk Factors

Nonmodifiable
- Advanced age (older than 55 years)
- Gender (male)
- Race (African American)

Modifiable or Treatable
- Hypertension
- Atrial fibrillation
- Hyperlipidemia
- Obesity
- Smoking
- Diabetes
- Asymptomatic carotid stenosis and valvular heart disease (e.g., endocarditis, prosthetic heart valves)

- Sickle cell diseases
- Periodontal disease
- Chronic inflammatory conditions (e.g., systemic lupus erythematosus and rheumatoid arthritis)

Clinical Manifestations

General signs and symptoms include numbness or weakness of face, arm, or leg (especially on one side of body); confusion or change in mental status; trouble speaking or understanding speech; visual disturbances; loss of balance or coordination; dizziness; difficulty walking; or sudden, severe headache.

Motor Loss

- Disturbance of voluntary motor control on one side of the body, possibly reflecting damage to the upper motor neurons on the opposite side of the brain
- Hemiplegia, hemiparesis
- Flaccid paralysis and loss of, or decrease in, the deep tendon reflexes (initial clinical feature), followed by reappearance (after 48 hours) of deep reflexes and abnormally increased muscle tone (spasticity)

Communication Loss

- Dysarthria (difficulty speaking)
- Dysphasia (impaired speech) or aphasia (loss of speech)
- Apraxia (inability to perform a previously learned action)

Perceptual Disturbances and Sensory Loss

- Visual-perceptual dysfunctions (homonymous hemianopia [loss of half of the visual field])
- Disturbances in visual–spatial relations (perceiving the relation of two or more objects in spatial areas), frequently seen in patients with right hemispheric damage
- Sensory losses: slight impairment of touch, or more severe with loss of proprioception; difficulty in interrupting visual, tactile, and auditory stimuli; agnosias (loss of the ability to recognize previously familiar objects perceived by one of the senses)

Cognitive Impairment and Psychological Effects

- Frontal lobe damage: Learning capacity, memory, or other higher cortical intellectual functions may be impaired. Such dysfunction may be reflected in a limited attention span, difficulties in comprehension, forgetfulness, and lack of motivation.

S

- Depression, other psychological problems: Emotional lability, hostility, frustration, resentment, and lack of cooperation may be seen.

Assessment and Diagnostic Findings
- Medical history; complete physical and neurologic examination; airway patency assessment, including gag or cough reflex
- Noncontrast CT scan
- 12-lead ECG and carotid ultrasound
- CT angiography or MRI and angiography
- Transcranial Doppler flow studies
- Transthoracic or transesophageal echocardiography
- Xenon-enhanced CT scan
- Single photon emission CT (SPECT) scan

Prevention
- Help patient alter risk factors for stroke; encourage patient to quit smoking, maintain a healthy weight, follow a healthy diet (including modest alcohol consumption), and exercise daily.
- Prepare and support patient through carotid endarterectomy.
- Administer anticoagulant agents as prescribed (e.g., low-dose aspirin therapy).

Medical Management
Prompt diagnosis and treatment is essential to preserving brain function. Patients who have experienced a transient ischemic attack (TIA) or stroke should have medical management for secondary prevention. Underlying modifiable or treatable conditions should be addressed and managed (e.g., atrial fibrillation is treated with dose-adjusted warfarin for anticoagulation). Initial interventions to treat ischemic stroke include thrombolytic agents, which are used to dissolve the blood clot that is blocking blood flow to the brain, and anticoagulant administration.

Pharmacologic Therapy
- Recombinant t-PA is administered, unless contraindicated; monitor for bleeding.
- Anticoagulation therapy (IV heparin or low-molecular-weight heparin) is initiated.
- Management of increased intracranial pressure (ICP) involves the use of osmotic diuretics, maintaining $PaCO_2$ at 30 to 35 mm Hg, and positioning the patient to avoid hypoxia (elevate the head of bed to promote venous drainage and to lower increased ICP).

Surgical Management

- Hemicraniectomy may be performed for increased ICP from brain edema in a very large stroke.
- Intubation with an endotracheal tube is used to establish a patent airway, if necessary.
- Continuous hemodynamic monitoring should be instituted. (The goals for blood pressure remain controversial for a patient who has not received thrombolytic therapy; antihypertensive treatment may be withheld unless the systolic blood pressure exceeds 220 mm Hg or the diastolic blood pressure exceeds 120 mm Hg.)
- Neurologic assessment is undertaken to determine whether the stroke is evolving and whether other acute complications are developing.
- The main surgical procedure for selected patients with TIAs and mild stroke is carotid endarterectomy (CEA); carotid stenting, with or without angioplasty, is a less invasive procedure that is used for selected patients with severe stenosis.

Management of Complications

- In the case of decreased cerebral blood flow, institute pulmonary care, maintenance of a patent airway, and administration of supplemental oxygen as needed.
- Monitor for urinary tract infections, cardiac dysrhythmias, and complications of immobility.
- Monitor for hyperglycemia and treat if blood glucose is greater than 140 mg/dL.

NURSING PROCESS

The Patient Recovering From an Ischemic Stroke

Assessment

DURING ACUTE PHASE (1 TO 3 DAYS)

Weigh patient (used to determine medication dosages) and maintain a neurologic flow sheet to reflect the following nursing assessment parameters:

- Change in level of consciousness or responsiveness, ability to speak, and orientation
- Presence or absence of voluntary or involuntary movements of the extremities: muscle tone, body posture, and head position

- Eye opening, comparative size of pupils and pu[pillary reac]tions to light, and ocular position
- Color of face and extremities; temperature and m[oisture of] skin
- Quality and rates of pulse and respiration; arterial bl[ood gas] levels, body temperature, and arterial pressure
- Volume of fluids ingested or administered and volum[e of] urine excreted per 24 hours
- Signs of bleeding
- Blood pressure maintained within normal limits

POSTACUTE PHASE
Assess the following functions:

- Mental status (memory, attention span, perception, orientation, affect, speech and language)
- Sensation and perception (patient's awareness of pain and temperature usually decreased)
- Motor control (upper and lower extremity movement), swallowing ability, nutritional and hydration status, skin integrity, activity tolerance, and bowel and bladder function
- Continued focus on impairment of function in patient's daily activities

Diagnosis

NURSING DIAGNOSES

- Impaired physical mobility related to hemiparesis, loss of balance and coordination, spasticity, and brain injury
- Acute pain related to hemiplegia and disuse
- Deficient self-care (bathing, hygiene, toileting, dressing, grooming, and feeding) related to stroke sequelae
- Disturbed sensory perception (kinesthetic, tactile, or visual) related to altered sensory reception, transmission, or integration
- Impaired swallowing
- Impaired urinary elimination related to flaccid bladder, detrusor instability, confusion, or difficulty in communicating
- Disturbed thought processes and impaired verbal communication related to brain damage
- Risk for impaired skin integrity related to hemiparesis or hemiplegia, and decreased mobility
- Interrupted family processes related to catastrophic illness and caregiving burdens
- Sexual dysfunction related to neurologic deficits or fear of failure

S

POTENTIAL COMPLICATIONS

d flow due to increased ICP

ery to the brain

Goals

ls for the patient (and family) may include im-
ity, avoidance of shoulder pain, achievement of
ef of sensory and perceptual deprivation, preven-
ration, continence of bowel and bladder, improved
ocesses, achieving a form of communication, main-
kin integrity, restored family functioning, improved
unction, and absence of complications. Goals are af-
ed by knowledge of what the patient was like before the
roke.

Nursing Interventions

IMPROVING MOBILITY AND PREVENTING JOINT DEFORMITIES

- Position to prevent contractures; use measures to relieve pressure, assist in maintaining good body alignment, and prevent compressive neuropathies.
- Apply a splint at night to prevent flexion of affected extremity.
- Prevent adduction of the affected shoulder with a pillow placed in the axilla.
- Elevate affected arm to prevent edema and fibrosis.
- Position fingers so that they are barely flexed; place hand in slight supination. If upper extremity spasticity is noted, do not use a hand roll; a dorsal wrist splint may be used.
- Change patient's position every 2 hours; place patient in a prone position for 15 to 30 minutes several times a day; use pillows between legs for lateral turns to maintain proper alignment.

ESTABLISHING AN EXERCISE PROGRAM

- Provide full range of motion four or five times daily to maintain joint mobility, help patient regain motor control, prevent contractures in the paralyzed extremity, prevent further deterioration of the neuromuscular system, and enhance circulation. If tightness occurs in any area, perform range of motion exercises more frequently.
- Exercise is helpful in preventing venous stasis, which may predispose the patient to thrombosis and pulmonary embolus.

- Observe for signs of pulmonary embolus or excessive cardiac workload during exercise period (e.g., shortness of breath, chest pain, cyanosis, and increasing pulse rate).
- Supervise and support patient during exercises; plan frequent, short periods of exercise; encourage patient to exercise unaffected side at intervals throughout the day.
- Quadriceps muscle setting and gluteal setting exercises are started early to improve the muscle strength needed for walking.

PREPARING FOR AMBULATION
- Start an active rehabilitation program when consciousness returns (and all evidence of bleeding is gone).
- Educate patient to maintain balance in a sitting position and then to balance while standing (use a tilt table if needed).
- Begin patient walking as soon as standing balance is achieved; use parallel bars and have wheelchair available in anticipation of possible dizziness.
- Keep training periods for ambulation short and frequent.

> **Quality and Safety Nursing Alert**
>
> Initiate a full rehabilitation program, even for older adult patients.

PREVENTING SHOULDER PAIN
- Never lift patient by the flaccid shoulder or pull on the affected arm or shoulder.
- Use proper patient movement and positioning (e.g., flaccid arm on a table or pillows when patient is seated, use of sling when ambulating).
- Range of motion exercises are beneficial, but avoid overstrenuous arm movements.
- Elevate patient's arm and hand to prevent dependent edema of the hand; administer analgesic agents as indicated.

ENHANCING SELF-CARE
- Encourage personal hygiene activities as soon as the patient can sit up; select suitable self-care activities that can be carried out with one hand.
- Help patient to set realistic goals; add a new task daily.
- As a first step, encourage patient to carry out all self-care activities on the unaffected side.

- Make sure patient does not neglect affected side; provide assistive devices as indicated.
- Improve morale by making sure patient is fully dressed during ambulatory activities.
- Assist with dressing activities (e.g., clothing with Velcro closures; put garment on the affected side first); keep environment uncluttered and organized.
- Provide emotional support and encouragement to prevent fatigue and discouragement.

RELIEVING DISCOMFORT
Administer analgesic agents to help manage poststroke pain, including amitriptyline (Elavil); antiseizure medications lamotrigine (Lamictal) and pregabalin (Lyrica) are good alternatives for patients who cannot tolerate amitriptyline.

MANAGING VISUAL-PERCEPTUAL DIFFICULTIES
- Approach patient with a decreased field of vision on the side where visual perception is intact; place all visual stimuli on this side.
- Educate patient to turn and look in the direction of the defective visual field to compensate for the loss; make eye contact with patient and draw attention to affected side.
- Increase natural or artificial lighting in the room; provide eyeglasses to improve vision.
- Remind patient with hemianopsia about the other side of the body; place extremities so that patient can see them.

ASSISTING WITH NUTRITION
- A swallow assessment should be performed as soon as possible after the patient's arrival in the emergency department, prior to any oral intake.
- Observe patient for paroxysms of coughing, food dribbling out or pooling in one side of the mouth, food retained for long periods in the mouth, or nasal regurgitation when swallowing liquids.
- Consult with speech therapist to evaluate gag reflexes; assist in educating patient in alternate swallowing techniques, advise patient to take smaller boluses of food, and inform patient of foods that are easier to swallow; provide thicker liquids or pureed food as indicated.
- Have patient sit upright, preferably on chair, when eating and drinking; advance diet as tolerated.
- Prepare for enteral feedings through a tube if indicated; elevate the head of bed during feedings, check tube position

before feeding, administer feeding slowly, and ensure that cuff of tracheostomy tube is inflated (if applicable); monitor and report excessive retained or residual feeding.

ATTAINING BLADDER AND BOWEL CONTROL

- Perform intermittent sterile catheterization during period of loss of sphincter control, bladder atony, or spasticity.
- Analyze voiding pattern and offer urinal or bedpan on patient's voiding schedule.
- Assist the male patient to an upright posture for voiding.
- Provide high-fiber diet and adequate fluid intake (2 to 3 L per day) to prevent constipation, unless contraindicated.
- Establish a regular time (after breakfast) for toileting.

IMPROVING THOUGHT PROCESSES

- Reinforce structured training program using cognitive-perceptual retraining, visual imagery, reality orientation, and cueing procedures to compensate for losses.
- Support patient: Observe performance and progress, give positive feedback, convey an attitude of confidence and hopefulness; provide other interventions as used for improving cognitive function after a head injury.

IMPROVING COMMUNICATION

- Anticipate communication disturbances in patients who are paralyzed on the right side. Broca's area (area of brain responsible for speech) is so close to the left motor area that a disturbance in the motor area often affects the speech area.
- Jointly establish goals, with patient taking an active part.
- Make the atmosphere conducive to communication, remaining sensitive to patient's reactions and needs and responding to them in an appropriate manner; treat patient as an adult.
- Provide strong emotional support and understanding to allay anxiety; avoid completing patient's sentences.
- Be consistent in schedule, routines, and repetitions. A written schedule, checklists, and audiotapes may help with memory and concentration; a communication board may be used. Computer-based communication software that runs on tablets may be helpful.
- Maintain patient's attention when talking to him or her, speak slowly, and give one instruction at a time; allow patient time to process. Use of gestures may enhance comprehension.
- Talk to aphasic patients when providing care activities to provide social contact.

S

MAINTAINING SKIN INTEGRITY
- Frequently assess skin for signs of breakdown, with emphasis on bony areas and dependent body parts.
- Employ pressure-relieving devices; continue regular turning and positioning (every 2 hours minimally); minimize shear and friction when positioning.
- Keep skin clean and dry, gently massage healthy dry skin, and maintain adequate nutrition.

IMPROVING FAMILY COPING
- Provide counseling and support to family.
- Involve others in patient's care; provide education about stress management techniques and maintenance of personal health for family coping.
- Give family information about the expected outcome of the stroke and counsel family members to avoid doing things for patient that he or she can do.
- Develop attainable goals for patient at home by involving the total health care team, patient, and family.
- Encourage everyone to approach patient with a supportive and optimistic attitude, focusing on abilities that remain; explain to family that emotional lability usually improves with time.

HELPING THE PATIENT COPE WITH SEXUAL DYSFUNCTION
- Perform sensitive, in-depth assessment to determine sexual history before and after the stroke.
- Interventions for patient and partner focus on providing relevant information, education, reassurance, adjustment of medications, counseling regarding coping skills, suggestions for alternative sexual positions, and a means of sexual expression and satisfaction.

PROMOTING HOME- AND COMMUNITY-BASED CARE
Educating Patients About Self-Care
- Encourage patient to resume as much self-care as possible; provide assistive devices as indicated.
- Advise family that patient may tire easily, become irritable and upset by small events, and show less interest than usual in daily events.
- Provide patient with information to attend community-based "stroke clubs," so as to provide a feeling of belonging and fellowship with others.
- Encourage patient to continue with hobbies, recreational and leisure interests, and contact with friends to prevent social isolation.

Continuing Care

- Have occupational therapist make a home assessment and make recommendations to help patient become more independent.
- Coordinate care provided by numerous health care professionals; help family plan aspects of care.
- Physical therapy can be beneficial at home or in an outpatient program.
- Make referral for home speech therapy. Encourage family involvement. Provide family with practical instructions to help patient between speech therapy sessions.
- Discuss patient's depression with physician, including possible need for antidepressant therapy.

Evaluation

EXPECTED PATIENT OUTCOMES

- Achieves improved mobility
- Reports absence of shoulder pain
- Achieves self-care; performs hygiene care; uses adaptive equipment
- Demonstrates techniques to compensate for the discomfort of sensory deficits, such as turning the head to see people or objects
- Demonstrates safe swallowing
- Achieves normal bowel and bladder elimination
- Participates in cognitive improvement program
- Demonstrates improved communication
- Maintains intact skin without breakdown
- Develops alternative approaches to sexual expression

In addition, family members demonstrate a positive attitude and effective coping mechanisms.

For more information, see Chapter 67 in Hinkle, J. L., & Cheever, K. H. (2014). *Brunner and Suddarth's textbook of medical-surgical nursing* (13th ed.). Philadelphia: Lippincott Williams & Wilkins.

S

Syndrome of Inappropriate Antidiuretic Hormone Secretion

Excessive antidiuretic hormone (ADH) secretion from the pituitary gland, even in the face of subnormal serum osmolality, is known as the *syndrome of inappropriate antidiuretic hormone secretion* (SIADH). Patients with SIADH cannot excrete a dilute urine or retain fluids and subsequently develop a sodium deficiency known as *dilutional hyponatremia*. SIADH is often of nonendocrine origin; for instance, the syndrome may occur in patients with bronchogenic carcinoma, in which malignant lung cells synthesize and release ADH. Other causes include severe pneumonia, pneumothorax, other disorders of the lungs, and malignant tumors that affect other organs. Disorders of the central nervous system (head injury, brain surgery or tumor, or infection) are thought to produce SIADH by direct stimulation of the pituitary gland. Some medications (vincristine, diuretic agents, phenothiazines, tricyclic antidepressant medications) and nicotine have been implicated in SIADH. These medications either directly stimulate the pituitary gland or increase the sensitivity of renal tubules to circulating ADH.

Medical Management
SIADH is generally managed by eliminating the underlying cause (if possible) and restricting fluid intake. Diuretics are used with fluid restriction to treat severe hyponatremia. Diuretics such as furosemide (Lasix) may be used along with fluid restriction if severe hyponatremia is present.

Nursing Management
- Monitor fluid intake and output, daily weight, urine and blood chemistries, and neurologic status.
- Provide supportive measures and explanations of procedures and treatments to assist patient to deal with this disorder.

For more information, see Chapter 52 in Hinkle, J. L., & Cheever, K. H. (2014). *Brunner and Suddarth's textbook of medical-surgical nursing* (13th ed.). Philadelphia: Lippincott Williams & Wilkins.

S

Systemic Lupus Erythematosus

Systemic lupus erythematosus (SLE) is a chronic, inflammatory autoimmune collagen disease that affects nearly every organ in the body. SLE results from disturbed immune regulation that causes an exaggerated production of autoantibodies.

Pathophysiology
This disturbance is brought about by some combination of genetic, hormonal (as evidenced by the usual onset during the childbearing years), and environmental factors (exposure

to a virus, sunlight, stress, or diet). Certain medications, such as hydralazine (Apresoline), procainamide (Pronestyl), isoniazid or INH (Nydrazid), chlorpromazine (Thorazine), and some antiseizure medications, have been implicated in chemical or drug-induced SLE. Specifically, B cells and T cells both contribute to the immune response in SLE. B cells are instrumental in promoting the onset and flares of the disease.

Clinical Manifestations
Onset is insidious or acute. SLE can go undiagnosed for many years. The clinical course is one of exacerbations and remissions.

- Systemic symptoms include fever, fatigue, weight loss and, possibly, arthritis and pleurisy.
- Musculoskeletal system: Arthralgias and arthritis (synovitis) are common presenting features; joint swelling, tenderness, and pain on movement are common, accompanied by morning stiffness.
- Integumentary system: Several different types are seen (e.g., subacute cutaneous lupus erythematosus [SCLE], discoid lupus erythematosus [DLE]). A butterfly rash across the bridge of the nose and cheeks occurs in more than half of patients and may be a precursor to systemic involvement. Lesions worsen during exacerbations (flares) and may be provoked by sunlight or artificial ultraviolet light. Oral ulcers may involve buccal mucosa or hard palate; papular, erythematous, and purpuric lesions may occur on fingertips, elbows, toes, and extensor surfaces of forearms (or on lateral sides of the hands) and may progress to necrosis.
- Cardiovascular system: Pericarditis is the most common clinical cardiac manifestation. Women who have SLE are also at risk for early atherosclerosis.
- Renal system: Nephritis, referred to as *lupus nephritis*, occurs; high serum creatinine levels and hypertension are seen.
- Neurologic: Neuropsychiatric presentations are varied and frequent and generally are demonstrated by subtle changes in behavior or cognitive ability.

Assessment and Diagnostic Findings
Diagnosis is based on a complete history, physical examination, and blood tests. No single laboratory test confirms SLE. Blood testing reveals moderate to severe anemia, thrombocytopenia,

leukocytosis, or leukopenia and positive antinuclear antibodies. Other diagnostic immunologic tests support, but do not confirm, the diagnosis. Inspect the skin for erythematous rash, hyperpigmentation, or depigmentation. Auscultate for pericardial friction rub and assess for abnormal lung sounds. The antinuclear antibody (ANA) test is positive in more than 95% of patients with SLE.

Medical Management

Treatment includes management of acute and chronic disease. Goals of treatment include preventing progressive loss of organ function, reducing the likelihood of acute disease, minimizing disease-related disabilities, and preventing complications from therapy. Monitoring is performed to assess disease activity and therapeutic effectiveness.

Pharmacologic Therapy

- Nonsteroidal anti-inflammatory drugs (NSAIDs) are used with corticosteroid agents to minimize corticosteroid requirements.
- Corticosteroid medications are used topically for cutaneous manifestations.
- IV administration of corticosteroid drugs is an alternative to traditional high-dose oral use.
- Cutaneous, musculoskeletal, and mild systemic features of SLE are managed with antimalarial drugs.
- Immunosuppressive agents are generally reserved for the most serious forms of SLE that have not responded to conservative therapies.
- Belimumab (Benlysta), a human antibody that specifically recognizes and binds to B-lymphocyte stimulator, is administered to reduce disease activity and flares.

Nursing Management

The nursing care of the patient with SLE is generally the same as that for the patient with rheumatic disease (see "Nursing Management" under Arthritis, Rheumatoid). The primary nursing diagnoses address fatigue, impaired skin integrity, disturbed body image, and deficient knowledge.

- Be sensitive to the psychological reactions of the patient due to the changes and the unpredictable course of SLE; encourage participation in support groups, which can provide disease information, daily management tips, and social support.

- Educate patient to avoid sun and ultraviolet light exposure and to use sunscreen or protective clothing.
- Because of the increased risk of involvement of multiple organ systems, educate patients about the importance of routine periodic screenings and health promotion activities.
- Refer to dietitian if necessary.
- Educate patient about the importance of continuing prescribed medications, and address the changes and potential side effects that are likely to occur with their use.
- Remind the patient of the importance of monitoring because of the increased risk of systemic involvement, including renal and cardiovascular effects.

For more information, see Chapter 39 in Hinkle, J. L., & Cheever, K. H. (2014). *Brunner and Suddarth's textbook of medical-surgical nursing* (13th ed.). Philadelphia: Lippincott Williams & Wilkins.

S

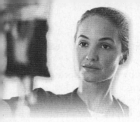

Thrombocytopenia

Thrombocytopenia (low platelet count) is the most common cause of abnormal bleeding.

Pathophysiology

Thrombocytopenia can result from decreased production of platelets within the bone marrow, from increased destruction of platelets, or increased consumption of platelets (e.g., the use of platelets in clot formation). Decreased platelet production can be a result of hematologic malignancies, myelodysplastic syndromes, metastatic involvement of bone marrow from solid tumors, certain anemias, toxins, medications, infections, chronic alcohol abuse, chemotherapy, chronic liver disease, radiation, and delayed engraftment after stem cell transplantation. Causes of increased destruction of platelets include immune thrombocytopenic purpura, lupus erythematosus, malignant lymphoma, chronic lymphocytic leukemia, medications, infections (bacteremia, sepsis, postviral), and splenic sequestration. Causes of increased platelet consumption include disseminated intravascular coagulation (DIC), major bleeding, severe pulmonary embolism/thrombosis, intravascular devices (e.g., intra-aortic balloon pump, cardiac assist devices), or extracorporeal circulation (e.g., hemofiltration, extracorporeal lung assist).

Clinical Manifestations

- With platelet count below 50,000/mm^3: bleeding and petechiae
- With platelet count below 20,000/mm^3: petechiae, along with nasal and gingival bleeding, excessive menstrual bleeding, and excessive bleeding after surgery or dental extractions
- With platelet count below 5,000/mm^3: spontaneous, potentially fatal central nervous system hemorrhage or gastrointestinal hemorrhage

Assessment and Diagnostic Findings

- Bone marrow aspiration and biopsy are helpful if platelet deficiency is secondary to decreased production.

- Increased megakaryocytes (the cells from which platelets originate) and normal or even increased platelet production in bone marrow can occur, when platelet destruction is the cause
- Screen for hepatitis B and C as these can cause thrombocytopenia

Medical Management

The management of secondary thrombocytopenia is usually treatment of the underlying disease. Platelet transfusions are used to raise platelet count and stop bleeding or prevent spontaneous hemorrhage if platelet production is impaired; if excessive platelet destruction is the cause, the patient is treated as indicated for immune thrombocytopenic purpura. For some patients, a splenectomy can be therapeutic, although it may not be an option for other patients (e.g., patients in whom the enlarged spleen is due to portal hypertension related to cirrhosis).

Nursing Management

Consider the cause of thrombocytopenia, likely duration and overall condition of patient when selecting nursing interventions. Interventions focus on preventing injury (e.g., use soft toothbrush and electric razors, minimize needlestick procedures, and educate about fall prevention for older adult or frail patients), stopping or slowing bleeding (e.g., pressure, cold), and administering medications and platelets as ordered as well as patient education. See "Nursing Management" under Immune Thrombocytopenic Purpura in Section I for additional information.

For more information, see Chapter 33 in Hinkle, J. L., & Cheever, K. H. (2014). *Brunner and Suddarth's textbook of medical-surgical nursing* (13th ed.). Philadelphia: Lippincott Williams & Wilkins.

T

Thyroid Storm (Thyrotoxic Crisis)

Thyroid storm (thyrotoxic crisis) is a form of severe hyperthyroidism, usually of abrupt onset and manifested by cardiac dysrhythmias, fever, and neurologic impairment that frequently appears as delirium. Thyroid storm is a life-threatening condition that is usually precipitated by one or more of the following: stress (such as with an injury), infection, surgery, tooth extraction, insulin reaction, diabetic ketoacidosis, pregnancy, digitalis intoxication, abrupt withdrawal of antithyroid drugs, extreme emotional stress, or vigorous palpation of the thyroid. These factors precipitate thyroid storm in the partially controlled or completely untreated patient with hyperthyroidism. Untreated thyroid storm is almost always fatal but, with proper treatment, the mortality rate can be reduced substantially.

Clinical Manifestations
- High fever (hyperpyrexia) above 38.5°C (101.3°F)
- Extreme tachycardia (more than 130 bpm)
- Exaggerated symptoms of hyperthyroidism with disturbances of a major system, such as gastrointestinal (weight loss, diarrhea, abdominal pain) or cardiovascular (edema, chest pain, dyspnea, palpitations)
- Altered neurologic or mental state, which frequently appears as delirium psychosis, somnolence, or coma

Medical Management
Immediate objectives are to reduce body temperature and heart rate and prevent vascular collapse.

- A hypothermia mattress or blanket, ice packs, a cool environment, and acetaminophen (Tylenol) are used.
- Humidified oxygen is administered to improve tissue oxygenation and meet high metabolic demands, and respiratory status is monitored by arterial blood gas analysis or pulse oximetry.
- Intravenous fluids containing dextrose are administered to replace glycogen stores.
- Hydrocortisone is given to treat shock or adrenal insufficiency.
- Propylthiouracil (PTU) or methimazole is given to impede formation of thyroid hormone.
- Iodine is administered to decrease output of thyroxine (T_4) from thyroid gland.
- Sympatholytic agents are given for cardiac problems. Propranolol, combined with digitalis, has been effective in reducing cardiac symptoms.

> **Quality and Safety Nursing Alert**
>
> Salicylates are not used in the management of thyroid storm because they displace thyroid hormone from binding proteins and worsen the hypermetabolism.

Nursing Management

Observe patient carefully and provide aggressive and supportive nursing care during and after the acute stage of illness. Care provided for the patient with hyperthyroidism is the basis for nursing management of patients with thyroid storm.

For more information, see Chapter 52 in Hinkle, J. L., & Cheever, K. H. (2014). *Brunner and Suddarth's textbook of medical-surgical nursing* (13th ed.). Philadelphia: Lippincott Williams & Wilkins.

Thyroiditis, Acute

Thyroiditis (inflammation of the thyroid) can be acute, subacute, or chronic. Each type is characterized by inflammation, fibrosis, or lymphocytic infiltration of the thyroid gland. Acute thyroiditis is a rare disorder caused by infection of the thyroid gland. The causes are bacteria (*Staphylococcus aureus* most common), fungi, mycobacteria, or parasites. Subacute cases may be granulomatous thyroiditis (de Quervain's thyroiditis) or painless thyroiditis (silent thyroiditis or subacute lymphocytic thyroiditis). Acute thyroiditis can occur in the postpartum period and is thought to be an autoimmune reaction.

Clinical Manifestations

Acute Thyroiditis
- Anterior neck pain and swelling; fever; dysphagia; and dysphonia
- Pharyngitis or pharyngeal pain
- Warmth, erythema, and tenderness of the thyroid gland

Subacute Thyroiditis
- Myalgias, pharyngitis, low-grade fever, and fatigue, which progress to a painful swelling in the anterior neck that lasts 1 to 2 months and then disappears spontaneously without residual effect
- Symmetrical enlargement of thyroid, which may be painful
- Unilateral or bilateral tenderness
- Overlying skin often reddened and warm
- Possibly difficult and uncomfortable swallowing
- Irritability, nervousness, insomnia, and weight loss (manifestations of hyperthyroidism) common
- Possibly chills and fever
- Painless thyroiditis: possibly symptoms of hyperthyroidism or hypothyroidism

T

Medical Management

Acute Thyroiditis

- Antimicrobial agents and fluid replacement
- Surgical incision and drainage if abscess is present

Subacute Thyroiditis

- Control of inflammation; nonsteroidal anti-inflammatory drugs (NSAIDs) to relieve neck pain
- Beta-blocking agents to control symptoms of hyperthyroidism
- Oral corticosteroid drugs to relieve pain and reduce swelling; do not usually affect the underlying cause
- Follow-up monitoring
- Painless thyroiditis: treatment directed at symptoms; recommended annual follow-up to determine patient's need for treatment of subsequent hypothyroidism

For more information, see Chapter 52 in Hinkle, J. L., & Cheever, K. H. (2014). *Brunner and Suddarth's textbook of medical-surgical nursing* (13th ed.). Philadelphia: Lippincott Williams & Wilkins.

Thyroiditis, Chronic (Hashimoto's Thyroiditis)

Chronic lymphocytic thyroiditis, also known as *Hashimoto's disease*, occurs most frequently in women aged 30 to 50 years. The most common cause of hypothyroidism in adults is autoimmune thyroiditis, in which the immune system attacks the thyroid gland. Diagnosis is based on the histologic appearance of the inflamed gland. The chronic forms usually are not accompanied by pain, pressure symptoms, or fever, and thyroid activity is usually normal or low. Cell-mediated immunity may play a significant role in the pathogenesis of chronic thyroiditis. A genetic predisposition also appears to be significant in its etiology. If untreated, the disease slowly progresses to hypothyroidism.

Clinical Manifestations

- Multiple nodules, mild tenderness, diffuse goiter with irregular surface; rubbery or firm, occasionally tender pyramidal lobe; possibly hard fibrous variant
- Fatigue, sluggishness, pale skin, constipation, and increased sensitivity to cold

Medical Management

Objectives of treatment are to reduce the size of the thyroid gland and to prevent hypothyroidism.

- Thyroid hormone therapy is prescribed to reduce thyroid activity and production of thyroglobulin.
- Thyroid hormone is given when hypothyroid symptoms are present.
- Surgery is performed when pressure symptoms persist.

For more information, see Chapter 52 in Hinkle, J. L., & Cheever, K. H. (2014). *Brunner and Suddarth's textbook of medical-surgical nursing* (13th ed.). Philadelphia: Lippincott Williams & Wilkins.

Toxic Epidermal Necrolysis and Stevens-Johnson Syndrome

Toxic epidermal necrolysis (TEN) and Stevens-Johnson syndrome (SJS) are potentially fatal acute skin disorders and the most severe forms of erythema multiforme. Risk factors include immunosuppression (including those with HIV or acquired immunodeficiency syndrome [AIDS]).

Pathophysiology

The mechanism leading to TEN seems to be a cell-mediated cytotoxic reaction. TEN and SJS are characterized by widespread erythema and macule formation, with blister formation resulting in epidermal detachment, sloughing, and erosion formation. These diseases are believed to be one and the same but manifest along a spectrum of reactions, with TEN being most severe. Both conditions are most commonly triggered by medications in adults, whereas infections are the most common precipitant in children. Antibiotics, antiseizure agents, NSAIDs, and allopurinol (Zyloprim) are the medications most commonly implicated. The complete body surface may be involved, with widespread areas of erythema and blisters. Sepsis and keratoconjunctivitis are possible complications.

Clinical Manifestations

- Initial signs are conjunctival burning or itching, cutaneous tenderness, fever, headache, cough, sore throat, extreme malaise, and myalgias (e.g., aches and pains).
- Rapid onset of erythema follows, involving much of the skin surface and mucous membranes; large, flaccid bullae appear in

some areas; in other areas, large sheets of epidermis are shed, exposing underlying dermis; fingernails, toenails, eyebrows, and eyelashes may all be shed, along with surrounding epidermis.

- Excruciatingly tender skin and loss of skin lead to a weeping surface similar to that of a total-body, partial-thickness burn; this condition was previously referred to as *scalded skin syndrome*.
- In severe cases of mucosal involvement, there may be danger of damage to the larynx, bronchi, and esophagus from ulcerations.

Complications
- Keratoconjunctivitis, sepsis, and multiple organ dysfunction syndrome (MODS) are potential complications.
- Keratoconjunctivitis can impair vision and result in conjunctival retraction, scarring, and corneal lesions.
- Sepsis and MODS can be life threatening.

Assessment and Diagnostic Findings
- Careful physical examination, particularly of the skin
- History of medication use, with particular attention to medications known to precipitate TEN or SJS used within the 4 weeks prior to the onset of illness
- Complete blood cell count (may show leukopenia and normochromic, normocytic anemia)
- Skin biopsy to confirm diagnosis

Medical Management
Treatment goals include control of fluid and electrolyte balance, prevention of sepsis, and prevention of ophthalmic complications. The mainstay of treatment is supportive care.

- All medications implicated as precipitating TEN or SJS are discontinued immediately.
- If possible, patient is treated in a regional burn center.
- Surgical débridement or hydrotherapy is initially used to remove involved skin.
- Tissue samples from the nasopharynx, eyes, ears, blood, urine, skin, and unruptured blisters are used to identify pathogens.
- Intravenous crystalloid fluids are prescribed to maintain fluid and electrolyte balance using parameters similar to those used for burn patients.
- Thermoregulation, wound care, and pain management guidelines for patients with burns are implemented.

- Systemic corticosteroid drugs (e.g., methylprednisolone [Solu-Medrol]) are given early in the disease process, although this therapy is somewhat controversial.
- Administration of intravenous immunoglobulin (IVIG) may provide rapid improvement and skin healing; the immunosuppressive agents cyclosporine (Neoral) or cyclophosphamide (Cytoxan) may also be effective.
- Skin is protected with topical agents; topical antibacterial and anesthetic agents are used to prevent wound sepsis.
- Temporary biologic dressings (pigskin, amniotic membrane) or plastic semipermeable dressings (Vigilon) are applied.
- Meticulous oropharyngeal and eye care is essential when there is severe involvement of mucous membranes and eyes.

NURSING PROCESS

The Patient With Toxic Epidermal Necrolysis

Assessment

- Inspect appearance and extent of skin involvement. Monitor blister drainage for amount, color, and odor.
- Inspect oral cavity for blistering and erosive lesions daily. Determine patient's ability to swallow and drink fluids, as well as to speak normally.
- Assess eyes daily for itching, burning, and dryness.
- Monitor vital signs, paying special attention to fever, respiratory status, and secretions.
- Assess high fever, tachycardia, and extreme weakness and fatigue. Indicate the process of epidermal necrosis, increased metabolic needs, and possible gastrointestinal and respiratory mucosal sloughing.
- Monitor urine volume, specific gravity, and color.
- Inspect intravenous insertion sites for local signs of infection.
- Record daily weight.
- Question patient about fatigue and pain levels.
- Assess level of anxiety and coping mechanisms; identify new, effective coping skills.

Diagnosis

NURSING DIAGNOSES

- Impaired tissue integrity (oral, eye, and skin) related to epidermal shedding

T

- Deficient fluid volume and electrolyte losses related to loss of fluids from denuded skin
- Risk for imbalanced body temperature (hypothermia) related to heat loss, secondary to skin loss
- Acute pain related to denuded skin and oral lesions
- Anxiety related to patient's physical appearance and prognosis

COLLABORATIVE PROBLEMS/POTENTIAL COMPLICATIONS
- Sepsis
- Conjunctival retraction, scars, and corneal lesions

Planning and Goals

Major goals may include skin and oral tissue healing, fluid balance, prevention of heat loss, relief of pain, reduced anxiety, and absence of complications.

Nursing Interventions

MAINTAINING SKIN AND MUCOUS MEMBRANE INTEGRITY
- Take special care to avoid friction involving the skin when moving the patient in bed; check skin after each position change to ensure that no new denuded areas have appeared.
- Apply prescribed topical agents to reduce wound bacteria.
- Apply warm compresses gently, if prescribed, to denuded areas.
- Use topical antibacterial agent in conjunction with hydrotherapy; monitor treatment and encourage patient to exercise extremities during hydrotherapy.
- Perform oral hygiene carefully. Use prescribed chlorhexidine mouthwashes, anesthetics, or coating agents frequently to rid mouth of debris, soothe ulcerative areas, and control odor. Inspect oral cavity frequently and note changes. Apply petrolatum to lips.

PROMOTING FLUID AND ELECTROLYTE BALANCE
- Observe vital signs, urine output, and mental status; assess for signs of hypovolemia.
- Evaluate laboratory tests and report abnormal results.
- Weigh patient daily.
- Provide enteral nourishment or, if necessary, parenteral nutrition.
- Record intake and output and daily calorie count.

PREVENTING HYPOTHERMIA
- Maintain patient's comfort and body temperature with cotton blankets, ceiling-mounted heat lamps, or heat shields.

- Work rapidly and efficiently, when large wounds are exposed, to minimize shivering and heat loss.
- Monitor patient's temperature carefully and frequently.

RELIEVING PAIN
- Assess the patient's pain, its characteristics, factors that influence the pain, and the patient's behavioral responses.
- Administer prescribed analgesic agents and observe for pain relief and side effects.
- Administer analgesic agents before painful treatments.
- Provide explanations and speak calmly to patient during treatments to allay anxiety, which may intensify pain.
- Provide measures to promote rest and sleep; provide emotional support and reassurance to achieve pain control.
- Instruct in self-management techniques for pain relief, such as progressive muscle relaxation and imagery.

REDUCING ANXIETY
- Assess emotional state (anxiety, fear of dying, and depression); reassure patient that these reactions are normal.
- Give support, be honest, and offer hope that the situation will improve. Listen to patient's concerns.
- Encourage patient to express feelings to someone he or she trusts.
- Provide emotional support during the long recovery period by referring patient to psychiatric nurse, chaplain, psychologist, or psychiatrist.

MONITORING AND MANAGING POTENTIAL COMPLICATIONS
- Sepsis: Monitor vital signs and note changes to allow early detection of infection. Maintain strict asepsis. Wear sterile gloves and practice excellent hand hygiene when carrying out procedures. If a large portion of the body is involved, place patient in private room with reverse isolation. Visitors with illnesses should not visit the patient.
- Conjunctival retraction, scars, and corneal lesions: Inspect eyes for progression of disease to keratoconjunctivitis (itching, burning, and dryness). Applying a cool, damp cloth over the eyes may relieve burning sensations. Administer eye lubricant. Use eye patches. Encourage patient to avoid rubbing eyes. Document and report progression of symptoms.

PROMOTING HOME- AND COMMUNITY-BASED CARE
Educating Patients About Self-Care
- Involve patient and family during procedures such as wound care and dressing changes that will need to be continued at home.

- Educate patient and family about pain management, nutrition, measures to increase mobility, and prevention of complications (including preventing infection).
- Provide written instructions about required procedures and techniques.
- Assist family in procuring necessary supplies for home care (e.g., sterile dressing supplies).

Continuing Care
- Some patients may require a rehabilitation center prior to returning home.
- Home care nurses can coordinate services from outpatient health care team (e.g., physical and occupational therapy); provide ongoing assessment to identify complications; monitor adherence to treatment plan; and assess patient's adaptation to home care environment.
- Make referrals to community agencies as appropriate.

Evaluation

EXPECTED PATIENT OUTCOMES
- Achieves increasing skin and oral tissue healing
- Attains fluid and electrolyte balance
- Attains thermoregulation
- Achieves pain relief
- Reports less anxiety
- Exhibits absence of complications, such as sepsis and impaired vision

For more information, see Chapter 61 in Hinkle, J. L., & Cheever, K. H. (2014). *Brunner and* Suddarth's *textbook of medical-surgical nursing* (13th ed.). Philadelphia: Lippincott Williams & Wilkins.

T

Transient Ischemic Attack

A transient ischemic attack (TIA) is a transient neurologic deficit typically lasting less than 1 hour. A TIA is manifested by a sudden loss of motor, sensory, or visual function. A TIA may serve as a warning of impending stroke; approximately 15% of all strokes are preceded by a TIA. Lack of evaluation and subsequent treatment of a patient who has experienced previous TIAs may result in a stroke and irreversible deficits.

Pathophysiology
The neurologic symptoms result from temporary ischemia (impairment of blood flow) to a specific region of the brain, but when brain imaging is performed, there is no evidence of ischemia or infarction. Symptoms may include changes in behavior, speech, gait, memory, or movement.

Risk Factors
Risk factors for ischemic stroke are also a factor in TIAs.

Clinical Manifestations
- Sudden loss of neurologic function similar to that seen in a stroke, which resolves within an hour; may be focal or generalized, including weakness or numbness of the face, arm, or leg, particularly on one side; confusion, trouble speaking or understanding; trouble seeing out of one or both eyes; trouble walking, dizziness, loss of balance or coordination; and headache with no known cause.
- Symptoms may last only minutes to less than 1 hour.

Assessment and Diagnostic Findings
- History and complete physical and neurologic examination are conducted; interviews with witnesses are particularly important as the patient may not remember the event.
- Alternate diagnoses (e.g., hypoglycemia) that may cause similar symptoms should be ruled out prior to making a diagnosis of TIA.
- CT or MRI scan is performed; additional studies recommended for ischemic stroke may be considered based on presenting symptoms and history.

Prevention
Help patients alter risk factors for stroke; encourage patient to control hypertension, maintain a healthy weight, follow a healthy diet (including modest alcohol consumption), and exercise daily.

Medical Management
The goals of medical treatment for TIAs are to allow the brain to recover from the initial insult and to prevent or minimize the risk of stroke or additional TIAs. Management may consist of controlling modifiable risk factors (e.g., hypertension or atrial fibrillation) and mild anticoagulation medications.

Pharmacologic Therapy
Antihypertensive medications are given to control hypertension. Anticoagulant agents (typically low-dose aspirin initially) are used for anticoagulation.

Nursing Management

See additional information under "Nursing Process" in Stroke, Ischemic, and Stroke, Hemorrhagic in Section S.

For more information, see Chapter 67 in Hinkle, J. L., & Cheever, K. H. (2014). *Brunner and Suddarth's textbook of medical-surgical nursing* (13th ed.). Philadelphia: Lippincott Williams & Wilkins.

Trigeminal Neuralgia (*Tic Douloureux*)

Trigeminal neuralgia, a condition affecting the fifth cranial nerve, is characterized by unilateral paroxysms of shooting, stabbing, or burning pain in the area innervated by any of the three trigeminal nerve branches (but most commonly the second and third branches). The pain ends as abruptly as it starts and is described as a unilateral shooting and stabbing sensation. The unilateral nature of the pain is an important feature. Associated involuntary contraction of the facial muscles can cause sudden closing of the eye or twitching of the mouth—hence the former name, *tic douloureux* (painful twitch). Trigeminal neuralgia occurs most often around age 50; those in whom the condition is diagnosed at an earlier age should be assessed for multiple sclerosis (MS). Pain-free intervals may last minutes, hours, days, or longer. With advancing years, the painful episodes tend to become more frequent and agonizing. The patient lives in constant fear of attacks.

Pathophysiology

Although the cause is not certain, vascular compression and pressure are suggested causes. The disorder occurs more commonly in women and in people with MS as compared with the general population.

Clinical Manifestations

- Paroxysms are aroused by any stimulation of terminals of the affected nerve branches (e.g., washing the face, shaving, brushing teeth, eating, and drinking). Patients may avoid these activities (behavior provides a cue to diagnosis).
- Drafts of cold air and direct pressure against the nerve trunk may cause pain.
- Trigger points are areas where the slightest touch immediately starts a paroxysm.

Assessment and Diagnostic Findings

Diagnosis is based on characteristic behavior: avoiding stimulating trigger point areas (e.g., trying not to touch or wash the face, shave, chew, or do anything else that might cause an attack).

Medical Management

Pharmacologic Therapy

Antiseizure agents, such as carbamazepine (Tegretol), reduce transmission of impulses at certain nerve terminals and relieve pain in most patients. Carbamazepine is given with meals. The patient is observed for side effects, including nausea, dizziness, drowsiness, and aplastic anemia. Serious drug reactions are more common in patients of Asian ancestry. The patient is monitored for bone marrow depression during long-term therapy. Gabapentin (Neurontin) and baclofen (Lioresal) are also used to treat pain. If pain control is still not achieved, phenytoin (Dilantin) may be used as adjunctive therapy.

Surgical Management

For microvascular decompression of the trigeminal nerve, an intracranial approach (craniotomy) is used. Percutaneous radiofrequency produces a thermal lesion on the trigeminal nerve. Although immediate pain relief is experienced, dysesthesia of the face and loss of the corneal reflex may occur. Use of stereotactic MRI for identification of the trigeminal nerve, followed by gamma knife radiosurgery, is being used at some medical centers. Percutaneous balloon microcompression disrupts large myelinated fibers in all three branches of the trigeminal nerve.

Nursing Management

- Assist patient to recognize the factors that trigger excruciating facial pain (e.g., hot or cold food or water, jarring motions). Instruct patient in ways to lessen these discomforts by using cotton pads and room-temperature water to wash face.
- Instruct patient to rinse mouth after eating if brushing teeth causes pain, and to perform personal hygiene during pain-free intervals.
- Advise patient to take food and fluids at room temperature, to chew on unaffected side, and to ingest soft foods.
- Recognize that anxiety, depression, and insomnia often accompany chronic painful conditions, and use appropriate interventions and referrals.

- Provide postoperative care by performing neurologic checks to assess facial motor and sensory deficits.
- Instruct patient not to rub the eye if the surgery results in sensory deficits to the affected side of the face, because pain will not be felt if injury occurs. Assess the eye for irritation or redness. Insert artificial tears, if prescribed, to prevent dryness to affected eye.
- Caution patient not to chew on the affected side until numbness diminishes. Observe patient carefully for any difficulty in eating and swallowing foods of different consistencies.

For more information, see Chapter 69 in Hinkle, J. L., & Cheever, K. H. (2014). *Brunner and Suddarth's textbook of medical-surgical nursing* (13th ed.). Philadelphia: Lippincott Williams & Wilkins.

Tuberculosis, Pulmonary

Tuberculosis (TB), an infectious disease primarily affecting the lung parenchyma, is most often caused by *Mycobacterium tuberculosis*. It is spread by airborne transmission of respiratory droplets, and infection can occur in almost any part of the body, including the meninges, kidney, bones, and lymph nodes. The initial infection usually occurs 2 to 10 weeks after exposure. The patient may then develop active disease because of a compromised or inadequate immune system response. The active process may be prolonged and characterized by long remissions when the disease is arrested, only to be followed by periods of renewed activity. Active disease also may occur with reinfection and activation of dormant bacteria. Reactivation TB represents 90% of adult cases in the non–HIV-infected population. TB is a worldwide public health problem that is closely associated with poverty, malnutrition, overcrowding, substandard housing, and inadequate health care. Mortality and morbidity rates continue to rise.

TB is transmitted by a person with active pulmonary disease expelling the organisms in respiratory secretions. A susceptible person inhales the droplets and becomes infected, most commonly occurring in the lungs. Bacteria are transmitted to the alveoli and multiply. An inflammatory reaction results in exudate in the alveoli and bronchopneumonia, granulomas, and fibrous tissue. Onset is usually insidious.

Risk Factors
- Close contact with someone who has active TB
- Immunocompromised status (e.g., older adults, cancer, corticosteroid therapy, and HIV)
- Injection drug use and alcoholism
- Inadequate health care (e.g., individuals who are homeless or impoverished, minorities, children, and young adults)
- Preexisting medical conditions, including diabetes, chronic renal failure, silicosis, and malnourishment
- Immigration from countries with a high incidence of TB (e.g., Haiti, southeast Asia)
- Institutionalization (e.g., long-term care facilities, prisons)
- Living conditions (i.e., in overcrowded, substandard housing)
- Occupation (e.g., health care workers, particularly those performing high-risk activities)

Clinical Manifestations
- Insidious onset of low-grade fever, cough, night sweats, fatigue, and weight loss
- Nonproductive cough, which may progress to mucopurulent sputum with hemoptysis
- Possible presence of symptoms for weeks or months
- Extrapulmonary disease, which is found more commonly in patients infected with HIV.

Assessment and Diagnostic Findings
- TB skin test (Mantoux test); QuantiFERON-TB Gold (QFT-G), QuantiFERON-TB Gold in-tube test (QFT-GIT), T-SPOT TB test (T-Spot), and Xpert MTB/RIF test
- Chest x-ray
- Sputum smear for acid-fast bacillus (AFB) followed by culture if smear is positive
- Additional assessments, including complete history and physical examination and drug susceptibility, if test results are positive

🍂 Gerontologic Considerations
Older adult patients may have atypical manifestations, such as unusual behavior or disturbed mental status, fever, anorexia, and weight loss. Older adult patients usually present with less pronounced symptoms than younger patients. TB is increasingly encountered in the nursing home population. In many older adults, the TB skin test produces no reaction and may need to be repeated in 1 to 2 weeks.

Medical Management

Pulmonary TB is treated primarily with antituberculosis agents for 6 to 12 months. A prolonged treatment duration is necessary to ensure eradication of the organisms and to prevent relapse.

Pharmacologic Therapy

Recommended treatment guidelines for newly diagnosed cases of pulmonary TB have two phases: an initial treatment phase (daily medications for 8 weeks) and a continuation phase (an additional 4 to 7 months).

- Treatment in the initial phase includes a daily multiple medication regimen of the first-line medications plus vitamin B_6. The continuation phase of treatment includes isoniazid (INH [Nydrazid]) and rifampin (Rifadin) or INH and rifapentine.
- First-line medications include INH (Nydrazid), rifampin (Rifadin), pyrazinamide (PZA), and ethambutol (Myambutol) daily for 8 weeks and continuing for up to 4 to 7 months. Combinations such as INH and rifampin (Rifamate), or INH, PZA, and rifampin (Rifater) and medications administered twice per week (e.g., rifapentine [Priftin]) are available to help improve patient adherence; however, these are costly.
- Second-line medications include capreomycin (Capastat), ethionamide (Trecator), para-aminosalicylate sodium, and cycloserine (Seromycin).
- INH is also used as a prophylactic measure for people who are at risk for TB.

Nursing Management

Promoting Airway Clearance

- Encourage increased fluid intake.
- Instruct the patient about the best position to facilitate airway drainage.

Promoting Adherence to Treatment Regimen

- Explain that TB is a communicable disease and that taking medications is the most effective way of preventing transmission.
- Educate the patient about medications, schedule, interactions, and side effects; monitor for side effects of anti-TB medications, including avoidance of alcohol and certain foods that interact with INH (e.g., tuna, aged cheeses, red wine, soy, yeast extracts).

- Educate the patient about the risk of drug resistance if the medication regimen is not strictly and continuously followed.
- Carefully monitor vital signs and observe for spikes in temperature or changes in the patient's clinical status.
- Educate caregivers of a patient who is not hospitalized to monitor the patient's temperature and respiratory status; report any changes in the patient's respiratory status to the primary health care provider.

Promoting Activity and Adequate Nutrition

- Plan a progressive activity schedule with the patient to increase activity tolerance and muscle strength.
- Devise a complementary plan to encourage adequate nutrition. A nutritional regimen of small, frequent meals and nutritional supplements may be helpful in meeting daily caloric requirements.
- Identifying facilities (e.g., shelters, soup kitchens, Meals on Wheels) that provide meals in the patient's neighborhood may increase the likelihood that the patient with limited resources and energy will have access to a more nutritious intake.

Preventing Transmission of TB Infection

- Carefully instruct the patient about important hygiene measures, including mouth care, covering the mouth and nose when coughing and sneezing, proper disposal of tissues, and hand hygiene.
- Report any cases of TB to the health department so that people who have been in contact with the affected patient during the infectious stage can undergo screening and possible treatment, if indicated.
- Educate the patient about the risk of spreading TB to other parts of the body (spread or dissemination of TB infection to nonpulmonary sites of the body is known as *miliary TB*).
- Carefully monitor the patient for miliary TB: Monitor vital signs and observe for spikes in temperature as well as changes in renal and cognitive function; few physical signs may be elicited on physical examination of the chest but, at this stage, the patient has a severe cough and dyspnea. Treatment of miliary TB is the same as for pulmonary TB.

For more information, see Chapter 23 in Hinkle, J. L., & Cheever, K. H. (2014). *Brunner and Suddarth's textbook of medical-surgical nursing* (13th ed.). Philadelphia: Lippincott Williams & Wilkins.

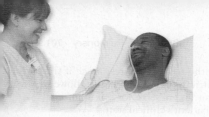

Ulcerative Colitis

Ulcerative colitis (UC) is a recurrent ulcerative and inflammatory disease of the mucosal and submucosal layers of the colon and rectum. The prevalence of UC is highest in Caucasians and people of Jewish heritage. It is a serious disease, accompanied by systemic complications and a high mortality rate; approximately 5% of patients with UC develop colon cancer. The disease is classified as mild, severe, or fulminant, depending on the severity of the symptoms. UC is one of the diseases in the group of diseases collectively referred to as inflammatory bowel disease (IBD).

Pathophysiology

UC affects the superficial mucosa of the colon and is characterized by multiple ulcerations, diffuse inflammations, and desquamation (or shedding) of the colonic epithelium, with alternating periods of exacerbation and remission. Bleeding occurs from the ulceration, and the mucosa becomes edematous and inflamed, with continuous lesions and abscesses. The disease process usually begins in the rectum and spreads proximally to involve the entire colon. Eventually, the bowel narrows, shortens, and thickens because of muscular hypertrophy and fat deposits. Because the inflammatory process is not transmural (i.e., it affects the inner lining only), fistulas, obstruction, and fissures are uncommon in UC.

Clinical Manifestations

- Predominant symptoms: diarrhea, passage of mucus and pus, left lower quadrant abdominal pain, intermittent tenesmus, and rectal bleeding
- Bleeding mild to severe, with resultant pallor, anemia, and fatigue
- Anorexia, weight loss, fever, vomiting, dehydration, cramping, and feeling an urgent need to defecate (may pass 10 to 20 liquid stools daily)
- Hypocalcemia possible
- Rebound tenderness in right lower quadrant

- Skin lesions (e.g., erythema nodosum), eye lesions (uveitis), joint abnormalities (e.g., arthritis), and liver disease

Assessment and Diagnostic Findings

- Assessment for tachypnea, tachycardia, hypotension, fever, and pallor
- Assessment of nutritional status and level of hydration
- Abdominal examination for bowel sounds, distention, and tenderness
- Stool examination for parasites and other microbes to rule out dysentery; stool occult blood test
- Abdominal x-rays, CT, MRI, ultrasound
- Sigmoidoscopy or colonoscopy and barium enema
- Blood studies (low hematocrit and hemoglobin, high white blood cell count, decreased albumin level, electrolyte imbalance); elevated antineutrophil cytoplasmic antibody levels common

Medical Management

Medical treatment for both Crohn's disease and UC is aimed at reducing inflammation, suppressing inappropriate immune responses, providing rest for a diseased bowel so that healing may take place, improving quality of life, and preventing or minimizing complications. Most patients have long periods of well-being interspersed with short intervals of illness. Management depends on the disease location, severity, and complications.

Nutritional Therapy

- Initial therapy consists of diet and fluid management with oral fluids; low-residue, high-protein, high-calorie diets; supplemental vitamin therapy; and iron replacement.
- Fluid and electrolyte balance may be corrected by IV therapy.
- Additional treatment measures include smoking cessation and avoiding foods that exacerbate symptoms, such as milk and cold foods.
- Parenteral nutrition (PN) may be provided as indicated.

Pharmacologic Therapy

- Sedative, antidiarrheal, and antiperistaltic medications
- Aminosalicylates: sulfasalazine (Azulfidine); effective for mild or moderate inflammation
- Sulfa-free aminosalicylates (e.g., mesalamine [Asacol, Pentasa]): effective in preventing and treating recurrence of inflammation

U

- Antibiotic agents (e.g., metronidazole [Flagyl]): for secondary infections, particularly for purulent complications such as abscesses, perforation, and peritonitis
- Corticosteroid drugs (e.g., oral: prednisone; parenteral: hydrocortisone [Solu-Cortef]; topical: budesonide [Entocort])
- Immunomodulator agents (e.g., azathioprine [Imuran], mercaptopurine [6-MP], methotrexate [MTX], cyclosporine [Neoral])
- Biologic agents (e.g., infliximab [Remicade], adalimumab [Humira], certolizumab pegol [Cimzia], and natalizumab [Tysabri])

Nonadherence is a major issue associated with pharmacologic treatment of inflammatory bowel disease (IBD).

Surgical Management

When nonsurgical measures fail to relieve the severe symptoms of inflammatory bowel disease, surgery may be recommended. The most common indications for surgery are medically intractable disease, poor quality of life, or complications from the disease or its treatment. A common procedure performed for strictures of the small intestines is laparoscope-guided strictureplasty. In some cases, a small bowel resection is performed. In cases of severe Crohn's disease of the colon, a total colectomy and ileostomy may be the procedure of choice. A newer option may be intestinal transplantation, especially for children and young adults who have lost intestinal function because of the disease. At least 25% of patients with UC eventually have total colectomies. Proctocolectomy with ileostomy (i.e., complete excision of colon, rectum, and anus) is recommended when the rectum is severely diseased. If the rectum can be preserved, restorative proctocolectomy with ileal pouch–anal anastomosis (IPAA) is the procedure of choice for UC; IPAA is also the procedure of choice for familial adenomatous polyposis. Fecal diversions may be needed.

U NURSING PROCESS

The Patient With Inflammatory Bowel Disease

Both regional enteritis (Crohn's disease) and UC are categorized as inflammatory bowel diseases. The *Nursing Assessment Findings in Ulcerative Colitis and Regional Enteritis* box lists assessment findings that help distinguish one from the other.

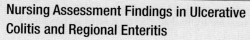

Nursing Assessment Findings in Ulcerative Colitis and Regional Enteritis

Ulcerative Colitis

- Dominant sign is rectal bleeding.
- Distended abdomen with rebound tenderness may be present.

Regional Enteritis

- Most prominent symptom is intermittent pain associated with diarrhea that does not decrease with defecation.
- Pain is usually localized in the right lower quadrant.
- Abdominal tenderness noted on palpation.
- Periumbilical regional pain suggests involvement of terminal ileum.

Assessment

- Determine the onset, duration, and characteristics of abdominal pain; the presence of diarrhea or fecal urgency, straining at stool (tenesmus), nausea, anorexia, or weight loss; and family history.
- Explore dietary pattern, including amounts of alcohol, caffeine, and nicotine products used daily or weekly.
- Determine bowel elimination patterns, including character, frequency, and presence of blood, pus, fat, or mucus.
- Inquire about allergies or food intolerances, especially to milk (lactose).
- Ask about sleep pattern disturbances if diarrhea or pain occurs at night.

Diagnosis

NURSING DIAGNOSES

- Diarrhea related to inflammatory process
- Acute pain related to increased peristalsis and gastrointestinal inflammation
- Deficient fluid volume related to anorexia, nausea, and diarrhea
- Imbalanced nutrition, less than body requirements, related to dietary restrictions, nausea, and malabsorption

- Activity intolerance related to generalized weakness
- Anxiety related to impending surgery
- Ineffective individual coping related to repeated episodes of diarrhea
- Risk for impaired skin integrity related to malnutrition and diarrhea
- Risk for ineffective self–health management of therapeutic regimen, related to insufficient knowledge concerning process and management of disease

COLLABORATIVE PROBLEMS/POTENTIAL COMPLICATIONS
- Electrolyte imbalance
- Cardiac dysrhythmias related to electrolyte imbalances
- Gastrointestinal bleeding with fluid volume loss
- Perforation of bowel

Planning and Goals

Major goals may include attainment of normal bowel elimination patterns; relief of abdominal pain and cramping; prevention of fluid volume deficit; maintenance of optimal nutrition and weight; avoidance of fatigue; reduction of anxiety; promotion of effective coping; absence of skin breakdown; increased knowledge about the disease process and self–health management; and avoidance of complications.

Nursing Interventions

MAINTAINING NORMAL ELIMINATION PATTERNS
- Identify any relationship between diarrhea and certain foods, activities, or emotional stressors; identify any precipitating factors.
- Identify the characteristics and frequency of the bowel movements.
- Provide ready access to bathroom, commode, or bedpan; keep environment clean and odor-free.
- Administer antidiarrheal agents as prescribed, and record frequency and consistency of stools after therapy has started.
- Encourage bed rest to decrease peristalsis.

RELIEVING PAIN
- Describe character of pain (dull, burning, or cramplike) and its onset, pattern, and medication relief.
- Administer anticholinergic medications 30 minutes before a meal to decrease intestinal motility.

- Give analgesic agents as prescribed; reduce pain by position changes, local application of heat (as prescribed), diversional activities, and prevention of fatigue.

MAINTAINING FLUID INTAKE
- Record intake and output, including wound or fistula drainage.
- Monitor weight daily.
- Assess for signs of fluid volume deficit: dry skin and mucous membranes, decreased skin turgor, oliguria, fatigue, decreased temperature, increased hematocrit, elevated urine specific gravity, and hypotension.
- Encourage oral intake; monitor IV flow rate.
- Initiate measures to decrease diarrhea: dietary restrictions, stress reduction, and antidiarrheal agents.

MAINTAINING OPTIMAL NUTRITION
- Use PN when symptoms are severe and patient is intolerant of enteral nutrition; continue use of PN if patient is expected to remain intolerant for more than 1 or 2 weeks.
- Record fluid intake and output and daily weights during PN therapy; test for glucose every 6 hours.
- Give oral elemental feedings (high in protein and low in fat and residue) after PN therapy; note intolerance (e.g., vomiting, diarrhea, distention).
- Provide small, frequent, low-residue feedings if oral foods are tolerated.
- Restrict activities to conserve energy, reduce peristalsis, and reduce calorie requirements.

PROMOTING REST
- Recommend intermittent rest periods during the day; schedule or restrict activities to conserve energy and reduce metabolic rate. Activity restrictions may need to be modified on a day-to-day basis.
- Encourage activity within limits; advise bed rest with active or passive exercises for a patient who is febrile, has frequent stools, or is bleeding.
- If the patient cannot perform active exercises, perform passive exercises and joint range of motion for the patient.

REDUCING ANXIETY
Rapport can be established by being attentive and displaying a calm, confident manner; allow time for the patient to ask

U

questions and express feelings. Tailor information about impending surgery to patient's level of understanding and desire for detail; pictures and illustrations help explain the surgical procedure and help the patient visualize what a stoma looks like. Careful listening and sensitivity to nonverbal indicators of anxiety (e.g., restlessness, tense facial expressions) are helpful.

ENHANCING COPING MEASURES
- Understanding and emotional support from the nurse are essential; remember that patients respond to stress in a variety of ways (e.g., anger, denial, self-isolation) that may alienate others.
- Develop a relationship with the patient that supports all attempts to cope with stressors of anxiety, discouragement, and depression.
- Implement stress reduction measures such as relaxation techniques, visualization, breathing exercises, and biofeedback.
- Refer to professional counseling if needed.

PREVENTING SKIN BREAKDOWN
- Examine skin, especially perianal skin.
- Provide perianal care, including the use of a skin barrier, after each bowel movement.
- Give immediate care to reddened or irritated areas over bony prominences.
- Use pressure-relieving devices to avoid skin breakdown.
- Consult with a wound-ostomy-continence nurse as indicated.

MONITORING AND MANAGING POTENTIAL COMPLICATIONS
- Monitor serum electrolyte levels; administer replacements.
- Report dysrhythmias or change in level of consciousness (LOC) immediately.
- Monitor rectal bleeding and give blood and volume expanders.
- Monitor blood pressure; obtain laboratory blood studies; administer vitamin K as prescribed.
- Monitor for indications of perforation: acute increase in abdominal pain, rigid abdomen, vomiting, or hypotension.
- Monitor for signs of obstruction and toxic megacolon: abdominal distention; decreased or absent bowel sounds; change in mental status; fever; tachycardia; hypotension; dehydration; and electrolyte imbalances.

PROMOTING HOME- AND COMMUNITY-BASED CARE

Educating Patients About Self-Care

- Assess need for additional information about medical management (medications, diet) and surgical interventions.
- Provide information about nutritional management (bland, low-residue, high-protein, high-calorie, and high-vitamin diet) during an acute phase.
- Give rationale for using corticosteroid, anti-inflammatory, antibacterial, antidiarrheal, and antispasmodic medications.
- Emphasize importance of taking medications as prescribed and not abruptly discontinuing regimen.
- Review ileostomy care as necessary. Obtain patient education information from the Crohn's & Colitis Foundation of America; a patient skills education program is available through the American College of Surgeons.

Continuing Care

- Refer for home care nurse if nutritional status is compromised and patient is receiving PN.
- Explain that disease can be controlled and patient can lead a healthy life between exacerbations.
- Instruct about medications and the need to take them on schedule while at home. Recommend use of medication reminders (containers that separate pills according to day and time).
- Encourage patient to rest as needed and modify activities according to energy levels during a flare-up. Advise patient to limit tasks that impose strain on the lower abdominal muscles and to sleep close to bathroom because of frequent diarrhea. Suggest room deodorizers for odor control.
- Encourage patient to keep a record of foods that irritate bowel and to eliminate them from diet. Recommend intake of eight glasses of water per day.
- Provide support for prolonged nature of disease because of the strain on family life and financial resources. Arrange for individual and family counseling as indicated.
- Provide time for patient to express fears and frustrations.

Evaluation

EXPECTED PATIENT OUTCOMES

- Reports decrease in frequency of diarrheal stools
- Experiences less pain
- Maintains fluid volume balance; tolerates small, frequent feedings without diarrhea

- Attains optimal nutrition
- Avoids fatigue
- Reports feeling less anxious
- Copes successfully with diagnosis
- Maintains skin integrity
- Acquires an understanding of the disease process
- Recovers without complications

For more information, see Chapter 48 in Hinkle, J. L., & Cheever, K. H. (2014). *Brunner and Suddarth's textbook of medical-surgical nursing* (13th ed.). Philadelphia: Lippincott Williams & Wilkins.

Unconscious Patient

Unconsciousness is an altered level of consciousness (LOC) in which the patient is unresponsive to, and unaware of, environmental stimuli, usually for a short duration. **Coma** is a clinical state—an unarousable unresponsive condition—in which the patient is unaware of self or the surrounding environment for prolonged periods (days to months, or even years). **Akinetic mutism** is a state of unresponsiveness to the environment in which the patient makes no voluntary movement. A **persistent vegetative state** is one in which the unresponsive patient resumes sleep–wake cycles after coma but is devoid of cognitive or affective mental function. In a **minimally conscious state**, the patient produces inconsistent but reproducible signs of awareness. **Locked-in syndrome** results from a lesion affecting the pons and results in paralysis and the inability to speak; however, vertical eye movements and lid elevation remain intact and are used to indicate responsiveness. The causes of unconsciousness may be neurologic (head injury, stroke), toxicologic (drug overdose, alcohol intoxication), or metabolic (hepatic or renal failure, diabetic ketoacidosis).

Assessment and Diagnostic Findings

- Neurologic examination (CT, MRI, positron emission tomography [PET], electroencephalography [EEG], single photon emission CT [SPECT]) to identify cause of loss of consciousness
- Laboratory tests: analysis of blood glucose, electrolytes, serum ammonia, and liver function tests; blood urea nitrogen (BUN)

levels; serum osmolality; calcium level; partial thromboplastin time and prothrombin time
- Other studies to evaluate serum ketones, alcohol and drug concentrations, and arterial blood gases

Medical Management

The first priority is a patent and secure airway (intubation or tracheostomy). Then circulatory status (carotid pulse, heart rate and impulse, blood pressure) is assessed and adequate oxygenation maintained. An IV line is established to maintain fluid balance status, and nutritional support is provided (feeding tube or gastrostomy). Neurologic care is based on specific pathology. Other measures include drug therapy and measures to prevent complications.

NURSING PROCESS

The Unconscious Patient

Assessment

- Assess level of responsiveness (consciousness) using the Glasgow Coma Scale. Assess also the patient's ability to respond verbally. Evaluate pupil size, equality, and reaction to light; note movement of eyes.
- Assess for spontaneous, purposeful, or nonpurposeful responses: decorticate posturing (arms flexed, adducted, and internally rotated, and legs in extension) or decerebrate posturing (extremities extended and reflexes exaggerated).
- Rule out paralysis or stroke as cause of flaccidity.
- Examine respiratory status, eye signs, reflexes, and body functions (circulation, respiration, elimination, fluid and electrolyte balance) in a systematic manner.

Diagnosis

NURSING DIAGNOSES
- Ineffective airway clearance, related to inability to clear respiratory secretions
- Risk for fluid volume deficit, related to inability to ingest fluids
- Risk for nutritional imbalance, related to inability to ingest food
- Impaired oral mucous membranes, related to mouth breathing, absence of pharyngeal reflex, and inability to ingest fluids

- Risk for impaired skin integrity, related to immobility or restlessness
- Impaired tissue integrity of cornea, related to diminished or absent corneal reflex
- Ineffective thermoregulation, related to damage to hypothalamic center
- Impaired urinary elimination (incontinence or retention), related to impairment in neurologic sensing and control
- Bowel incontinence, related to impairment in neurologic sensing and control; also related to changes in nutritional delivery methods
- Disturbed health maintenance, related to neurologic impairment
- Interrupted family processes, related to health crisis

COLLABORATIVE PROBLEMS/POTENTIAL COMPLICATIONS
- Respiratory distress or failure
- Pneumonia
- Aspiration
- Pressure ulcer
- Venous thromboembolism (VTE)
- Contractures

Planning and Goals

Goals of care for an unconscious patient may include maintenance of a clear airway, protection from injury, attainment of fluid volume balance, achievement of intact oral mucous membranes, maintenance of normal skin integrity, absence of corneal irritation, attainment of effective thermoregulation, effective urinary elimination, bowel continence, accurate perception of environmental stimuli, maintenance of intact family or support system, and absence of complications.

Nursing Interventions

MAINTAINING THE AIRWAY

- Establish an adequate airway and ensure ventilation.
- Position patient in a lateral or semiprone position; do not allow patient to remain on back.
- Remove secretions to reduce danger of aspiration; elevate head of bed to a 30-degree angle to prevent aspiration; provide frequent suctioning; provide oral hygiene with ventilation before and after suctioning to prevent hypoxia.

- Promote pulmonary hygiene with chest physiotherapy and postural drainage.
- Auscultate chest every 8 hours to detect adventitious breath sounds or absence of breath sounds.
- Maintain patency of endotracheal tube or tracheostomy; monitor arterial blood gases; maintain ventilator settings.

PROTECTING THE PATIENT

- Provide padded side rails for protection; keep two rails in the raised position during the day and three at night.
- Prevent injury from invasive lines and equipment and identify other potential sources of injury: restraints, tight dressings, environmental irritants, damp bedding or dressings, and tubes and drains.
- Protect the patient's dignity and privacy; act as the patient's advocate.

> ### Quality and Safety Nursing Alert
>
> If the patient begins to emerge from unconsciousness, every measure that is available and appropriate for calming and quieting the patient should be used. Any form of restraint is likely to be countered with resistance, leading to self-injury or to a dangerous increase in intracranial pressure (ICP). Therefore, physical restraints should be avoided if possible; a written prescription must be obtained if their use is essential for the patient's well-being.

MAINTAINING FLUID BALANCE AND MANAGING NUTRITIONAL NEEDS

- Assess for hydration status: Examine tissue turgor and mucous membranes, assess intake and output trends, and analyze laboratory data.
- Meet fluid needs by giving required IV fluids and then nasogastric or gastrostomy feedings.
- Give IV fluids and blood transfusions slowly if patient has an intracranial condition.
- Never give oral fluids to a patient who cannot swallow; insert feeding tube for administration of enteral feedings.

PROVIDING MOUTH CARE

- Inspect mouth for dryness, inflammation, and crusting; cleanse and rinse carefully to remove secretions and crusts and keep membranes moist; apply petrolatum to lips.

- Assess sides of mouth and lips for ulceration if patient has an endotracheal tube. Move tube to opposite side of mouth daily.
- If the patient is intubated and mechanically ventilated, good oral care is also necessary; recent evidence shows that antiseptic care with chlorhexidine, or routine toothbrushing and pharmacologic moisturizers, significantly decreases ventilator-associated pneumonia.

MAINTAINING SKIN AND JOINT INTEGRITY

- Follow a regular schedule of turning and repositioning to prevent breakdown and necrosis of the skin and to provide kinesthetic, proprioceptive, and vestibular stimulation. Avoid dragging or pulling the patient up in bed.
- Give passive exercise of extremities to prevent contractures; use a splint or foam boots to prevent footdrop and eliminate pressure on toes.
- Keep hip joints and legs in proper alignment with supporting trochanter rolls.
- Position arms in abduction, fingers lightly flexed, and hands in slight supination; assess heels of feet for pressure areas.
- Specialty beds, such as fluidized or low-air-loss beds, may be used to decrease pressure on bony prominences.

PRESERVING CORNEAL INTEGRITY

- Cleanse eyes with cotton balls moistened with sterile normal saline to remove debris and discharge.
- Instill artificial tears every 2 hours, as prescribed.
- Use cold compresses as prescribed for periorbital edema after cranial surgery. Avoid contact with cornea.
- Use eye patches cautiously because of potential for further corneal abrasions.

MAINTAINING BODY TEMPERATURE

- Adjust environment to promote normal body temperature.
- Use prescribed measures to treat hyperthermia: Remove bedding, except light sheet; give acetaminophen as prescribed; give cools sponge baths, use hypothermia blanket; monitor frequently to assess response to therapy.

> **Quality and Safety Nursing Alert**

Take rectal or tympanic (unless contraindicated) body temperature.

PREVENTING URINARY RETENTION
- Palpate or scan bladder at intervals to detect urinary retention.
- Insert indwelling catheter if there are signs of urinary retention; observe for fever and cloudy urine; inspect urethral orifice for drainage.
- Use external penile catheter (condom catheter) for male patients and absorbent pads for female patients, if patient can urinate spontaneously.
- Initiate bladder training program as soon as patient is conscious.
- Monitor frequently for skin irritation and breakdown; implement appropriate skin care.

PROMOTING BOWEL FUNCTION
- Evaluate abdominal distention by listening for bowel sounds and measuring abdominal girth.
- Monitor number and consistency of bowel movements; perform rectal examination for signs of fecal impaction; patient may require enema every other day to empty lower colon.
- Administer stool softeners and glycerin suppositories as indicated.

PROMOTING SENSORY STIMULATION
- Provide continuing sensory stimulation (e.g., auditory, visual, olfactory, gustatory, tactile, and kinesthetic activities) to help patient overcome profound sensory deprivation.
- Make efforts to maintain usual day and night patterns of activity and sleep; orient patient to time and place every 8 hours.
- Touch and talk to patient; encourage family and friends to do the same; avoid making any negative comments about the patient's status in his or her presence. Avoid overstimulating patient.
- Explain to family that periods of agitation may be a sign of increasing patient awareness of the environment.
- If possible, introduce sounds from patient's usual environment by means of audiotape and videotape.
- Read favorite books and provide familiar radio and television programs to enrich environment.
- Structured sensory stimulation may improve outcome.

MEETING THE FAMILY'S NEEDS
- Reinforce and clarify information about patient's condition to permit family members to mobilize their own adaptive capacities.

U

- Encourage venting of feelings and concerns.
- Support family in decision-making process concerning post-hospital management and placement or end-of-life care.

MONITORING AND MANAGING POTENTIAL COMPLICATIONS

- Monitor vital signs and respiratory function for signs of respiratory failure or distress.
- Assess for adequate red blood cells to carry oxygen; assess complete blood cell count and arterial blood gases.
- Initiate chest physiotherapy and suctioning to prevent respiratory complications, such as pneumonia.
- To decrease the incidence of pneumonia, perform oral care interventions for patients receiving mechanical ventilation.
- If pneumonia develops, obtain culture specimens to identify organism for selection of appropriate antibiotic.
- Monitor for evidence of impaired skin integrity and implement strategies to prevent skin breakdown and pressure ulcers.
- Address factors that contribute to impaired skin integrity and undertake strategies to promote healing if pressure ulcers do develop.
- Monitor for signs and symptoms of VTE, which may manifest as a deep vein thrombosis or pulmonary embolism.

Evaluation

EXPECTED PATIENT OUTCOMES

- Maintains clear airway and demonstrates appropriate breath sounds
- Experiences no injuries
- Attains or maintains adequate fluid balance
- Attains or maintains healthy oral mucous membranes
- Maintains normal skin integrity
- Has no corneal irritation
- Attains or maintains thermoregulation
- Has no urinary retention
- Has no diarrhea or fecal impaction
- Receives appropriate sensory stimulation
- Has family members who cope with crisis
- Avoids other complications

For more information, see Chapter 66 in Hinkle, J. L., & Cheever, K. H. (2014). *Brunner and Suddarth's textbook of medical-surgical nursing* (13th ed.). Philadelphia: Lippincott Williams & Wilkins.

Urolithiasis (Nephrolithiasis)

Urolithiasis and nephrolithiasis refer to stones (calculi) in the urinary tract and kidney, respectively. The problem occurs predominantly in the third to fifth decades and affects men more often than women; about half of patients with a single renal stone have another episode within 5 years.

Pathophysiology

Stones are formed in the urinary tract when the urinary concentration of substances such as calcium oxalate, calcium phosphate, and uric acid increases. Stones vary in size from minute granular deposits to the size of an orange. Factors that favor formation of stones include infection, urinary stasis, hypercalcemia, and periods of immobility, all of which slow renal drainage and alter calcium metabolism. Uric acid stones (5% to 10% of all stones) may be seen in patients with gout or myeloproliferative disorders; predisposing factors for struvite stones include neurogenic bladder, foreign bodies, and recurrent urinary tract infections (UTIs). Additional risk factors include polycystic disease, horseshoe kidneys, chronic strictures, medullary sponge diseases, inflammatory bowel disease and certain medications. Ureteral colic is mediated by prostaglandin E, a substance that increases ureteral contractility and renal blood flow and that leads to increased intraureteral pressure and pain.

Clinical Manifestations

Manifestations depend on the presence of obstruction, infection, and edema. Symptoms range from mild to excruciating pain and discomfort.

Stones in Renal Pelvis

- Intense, deep ache in costovertebral region
- Hematuria and pyuria
- Pain originating in the renal area that radiates anteriorly and downward toward bladder in female and toward testes in male
- Acute pain, nausea, vomiting, costovertebral area tenderness (renal colic)
- Abdominal discomfort, diarrhea

Ureteral Colic (Stones Lodged in Ureter)

- Acute, excruciating, colicky, wavelike pain, radiating down the thigh to the genitalia

- Frequent desire to void, but little urine passed; usually contains blood because of the abrasive action of the stone (known as ureteral colic)

Stones Lodged in Bladder
- Symptoms of irritation associated with UTI and hematuria
- Urinary retention, if stone obstructs bladder neck
- Possible urosepsis if infection is present with stone

Assessment and Diagnostic Findings
- Diagnosis is confirmed by x-rays of the kidneys, ureters, and bladder (KUB) or by ultrasonography, IV urography, or retrograde pyelography.
- Blood chemistries and a 24-hour urine test should be performed for measurements of calcium, uric acid, creatinine, sodium, pH, and total volume.
- Chemical analysis is performed to determine stone composition.
- Dietary and medication histories and family history of renal stones are obtained to identify predisposing factors.

Medical Management
Basic goals are to eradicate the stone, determine the stone type, prevent nephron destruction, control infection, and relieve any obstruction that may be present. The immediate goal in treating renal or ureteral colic is relief of pain until the cause is eliminated.

Pharmacologic and Nutritional Therapy
- Opioid analgesic agents (to prevent shock and syncope) and nonsteroidal anti-inflammatory drugs (NSAIDs).
- Increased fluid intake to assist in stone passage, unless patient is vomiting or has heart failure; patients with renal stones should drink eight to ten 8-oz glasses of water daily or have IV fluids prescribed to keep the urine dilute.
- For calcium stones: reduced dietary protein and sodium intake; liberal fluid intake; medications to acidify urine, such as ammonium chloride and thiazide diuretics if parathormone production is increased.
- For uric stones: low-purine and limited protein diet; allopurinol (Zyloprim).
- For cystine stones: low-protein diet; alkalinization of urine; increased fluids.
- For oxalate stones: dilute urine; limited oxalate intake (e.g., spinach, strawberries, rhubarb, chocolate, tea, peanuts, and wheat bran).

U

Stone Removal Procedures

If the stone does not pass spontaneously or if complications occur, the following interventions may be used.

- Ureteroscopy: stones fragmented with use of laser, electro-hydraulic lithotripsy, or ultrasound and then removed
- Extracorporeal shock wave lithotripsy (ESWL)
- Percutaneous nephrostomy; endourologic methods
- Electrohydraulic lithotripsy
- Chemolysis (stone dissolution): alternative for those who are poor risks for other therapies, refuse other methods, or have easily dissolved stones (struvite)
- Surgical removal is performed in only 1% to 2% of patients; the surgery performed may be a nephrolithotomy (incision into the kidney with removal of the stone) or a nephrectomy (kidney is removed).

NURSING PROCESS

The Patient With Kidney Stones

Assessment

- Assess for pain and discomfort, including severity, location, and radiation of pain.
- Assess for associated symptoms, including nausea, vomiting, diarrhea, and abdominal distention.
- Observe for signs of UTI (chills, fever, frequency, and hesitancy) and obstruction (frequent urination of small amounts, oliguria, or anuria).
- Observe urine for blood; strain for stones or gravel.
- Focus history on factors that predispose patient to urinary tract stones or that may have precipitated current episode of renal or ureteral colic.
- Assess patient's knowledge about renal stones and measures to prevent recurrence.

Diagnosis

NURSING DIAGNOSES

- Acute pain related to inflammation, obstruction, and abrasion of the urinary tract
- Deficient knowledge regarding prevention of recurrence of renal stones

U

COLLABORATIVE PROBLEMS/POTENTIAL COMPLICATIONS
- Infection and urosepsis (from urinary tract infection and pyelonephritis)
- Obstruction of the urinary tract by a stone or edema, with subsequent acute renal failure

Planning and Goals

Major goals may include relief of pain and discomfort, prevention of recurrence of renal stones, and absence of complications.

Nursing Interventions

RELIEVING PAIN
- Administer opioid analgesics (IV or intramuscular) with IV NSAID as prescribed.
- Encourage and assist patient to assume a position of comfort.
- Assist patient to ambulate to obtain some pain relief.
- Monitor pain closely and promptly report increases in severity.

MONITORING AND MANAGING COMPLICATIONS
- Encourage increased fluid intake and ambulation.
- Begin IV fluids if patient cannot take adequate oral fluids.
- Monitor total urine output and patterns of voiding.
- Encourage ambulation as a means of moving the stone through the urinary tract.
- Strain urine through gauze.
- Crush any blood clots passed in urine, and inspect sides of urinal and bedpan for clinging stones.
- Instruct patient to report decreased urine volume, bloody or cloudy urine, fever, and pain.
- Instruct patient to report any increase in pain.
- Monitor vital signs for early indications of infection; infections should be treated with the appropriate antibiotic agent before efforts are made to dissolve the stone.

PROMOTING HOME- AND COMMUNITY-BASED CARE
Educating Patients about Self-care
- Explain causes of kidney stones and ways to prevent recurrence.
- Encourage patient to follow a regimen to avoid further stone formation, including maintaining a high fluid intake.
- Encourage patient to drink enough to excrete 3,000 to 4,000 mL of urine every 24 hours.

- Recommend that patient have urine cultures every 1 to 2 months the first year and periodically thereafter.
- Recommend that recurrent urinary infection be treated vigorously.
- Encourage increased mobility whenever possible; discourage excessive ingestion of vitamins (especially vitamin D) and minerals.
- If patient had surgery, provide instructions about the signs and symptoms of complications that need to be reported to the physician; emphasize the importance of follow-up to assess kidney function and to ensure the eradication or removal of all kidney stones to the patient and family.
- If patient had ESWL, encourage patient to increase fluid intake to assist in the passage of stone fragments; inform the patient to expect hematuria and possibly a bruise on the treated side of the back; instruct patient to check his or her temperature daily and notify the physician if the temperature is greater than 38°C (about 101°F), or the pain is unrelieved by the prescribed medication.
- Provide instructions for any necessary home care and follow-up.

Providing Home and Follow-up Care After ESWL
- Instruct patient to increase fluid intake to assist passage of stone fragments (may take 6 weeks to several months after procedure).
- Instruct patient about signs and symptoms of complications: fever, decreasing urinary output, and pain.
- Inform patient that hematuria is anticipated but should subside in 24 hours.
- Give appropriate dietary instructions based on composition of stones.
- Encourage regimen to avoid further stone formation; advise patient to adhere to prescribed diet.
- Instruct patient to take sufficient fluids in the evening to prevent urine from becoming too concentrated at night.

Continuing Care
- Closely monitor the patient to ensure that treatment has been effective and that no complications have developed.
- Assess the patient's understanding of ESWL and possible complications; assess the patient's understanding of factors that increase the risk of recurrence of renal calculi and strategies to reduce those risks.

- Assess the patient's ability to monitor urinary pH and interpret the results during follow-up visits.
- Ensure that the patient understands the signs and symptoms of stone formation, obstruction, and infection and the importance of reporting these signs promptly.
- If medications are prescribed for the prevention of stone formation, explain their actions, importance, and side effects to the patient.

Evaluation

EXPECTED PATIENT OUTCOMES

- Reports relief of pain
- States increased knowledge of health-seeking behaviors to prevent recurrence
- Experiences no complications

For more information, see Chapter 55 in Hinkle, J. L., & Cheever, K. H. (2014). *Brunner and Suddarth's Textbook of Medical-Surgical Nursing* (13th ed.). Philadelphia: Lippincott Williams & Wilkins.

U

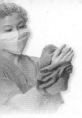

Vein Disorders: Venous Thrombosis, Thrombophlebitis, Phlebothrombosis, and Deep Vein Thrombosis

Vein disorders cause reduction in venous blood flow, causing blood stasis. This may then cause a host of pathologic changes, including coagulation defects, edema formation and tissue breakdown, and an increased susceptibility to infections. Although the vein disorders described here do not necessarily present an identical pathology, for clinical purposes these terms are often used interchangeably.

Pathophysiology

The exact cause of **venous thrombosis** remains unclear, although three factors (Virchow's triad) are believed to play a significant role in its development: venous stasis, endothelial damage, and altered coagulation. Venous thrombosis can occur in any vein but is most frequent in the veins of the lower extremities. Both superficial and deep veins of the legs may be affected.

Thrombophlebitis is an inflammation of the walls of the veins, often accompanied by the formation of a clot. When a clot develops initially in the veins as a result of stasis or hypercoagulability, but *without* inflammation, the process is referred to as *phlebothrombosis*.

Risk Factors

- History of varicose veins, hypercoagulation, neoplastic disease, cardiovascular disease, or recent major surgery or injury
- Direct trauma to the veins from fractures or dislocation, diseases of the veins, and chemical irritation of the vein from IV medications or solutions
- Obesity; pregnancy; advanced age
- Oral contraceptive use, elevated C-reactive protein, abruptly stopping anticoagulant medications, and several blood dyscrasias

723

Clinical Manifestations

Signs and symptoms are nonspecific.

- With affected deep veins, edema and swelling of the extremity result from obstruction of the affected extremity; bilateral swelling may be difficult to detect (owing to a lack of size difference).
- Affected extremity may feel warmer; superficial veins may become more prominent (cordlike venous segment).
- Tenderness occurs later and is detected by gently palpating the affected extremity.
- In some cases, signs of a pulmonary embolus are the first indication of deep vein thrombosis (DVT).
- Thrombus of superficial veins produces pain or tenderness, redness, and warmth in the involved area.
- In massive iliofemoral venous thrombosis (phlegmasia cerulea dolens), the entire extremity becomes massively swollen, tense, painful, and cool to touch.

Assessment and Diagnostic Findings

- Careful assessment in detecting early signs of venous disorders of lower extremities
- History and review of risk factors
- Measuring the circumference of the affected extremity at various levels (e.g., thigh to ankle) with a tape measure and comparing one extremity with the other at same level to determine size differences
- Doppler ultrasonography, duplex ultrasonography, air plethysmography, contrast phlebography (venography)

Prevention

Prevention depends on identifying risk factors for thrombus and on educating the patient about appropriate interventions. Preventive measures include the application of graduated compression stockings; the use of intermittent pneumatic compression devices; and encouragement of early mobilization and leg exercises. Surgical patients should be administered subcutaneous unfractionated or low-molecular-weight heparin (LMWH). Patients should be advised to make lifestyle changes as appropriate, which may include weight loss, smoking cessation, and regular exercise.

Medical Management

Objectives of management are to prevent the thrombus from growing and fragmenting (thus risking pulmonary embolism [PE], recurrent thromboemboli, and postthrombotic syndrome).

Pharmacologic Therapy

- Unfractionated heparin is administered for 5 days by intermittent or continuous IV infusion. Dosage is regulated by monitoring the activated partial thromboplastin time (aPTT), the international normalized ratio (INR), and the platelet count. LMWH is given in one or two injections daily; it is more expensive than unfractionated heparin, but safer.
- Oral anticoagulant agents (e.g., warfarin [Coumadin], a vitamin K antagonist) are given with heparin therapy.
- Factor Xa inhibitors: Fondaparinux (Arixtra) is given subcutaneously for prophylaxis during major orthopedic surgery (e.g., hip replacement). Dabigatran (Pradaxa) given orally twice daily was FDA-approved to reduce the risk of stroke and systemic embolism in patients with nonvalvular atrial fibrillation and for prevention of VTE after planned knee or hip surgery. Rivaroxaban (Xarelto) is another oral factor Xa inhibitor available for DVT prophylaxis once daily, with reduced dosages to patients with renal disorders.
- Thrombolytic (fibrinolytic) therapy (e.g., alteplase [Activase]) is given within the first 3 days after acute thrombosis.
- Throughout therapy, the following are monitored frequently: PTT, prothrombin time (PT), hemoglobin and hematocrit levels, platelet count, and fibrinogen level. Drug therapy is discontinued if bleeding occurs and cannot be stopped.

Endovascular Management

Endovascular management is necessary for DVT when anticoagulant or thrombolytic therapy is contraindicated, when the danger of PE is extreme, or when venous drainage is so severely compromised that permanent damage to the extremity is likely. A thrombectomy may be necessary. A vena cava filter may be placed at the time of the thrombectomy or thrombolysis; this filter traps large emboli and prevents pulmonary emboli. In patients with chronic iliac vein compression (e.g., as is seen in May-Thurner syndrome), balloon angioplasty with stent placement may successfully treat the patient's chronic leg symptoms.

Nursing Management

Assessing and Monitoring Anticoagulant Therapy

- Prevent inadvertent infusion of large volumes of unfractionated heparin, which could cause hemorrhage; administer unfractionated heparin by continuous IV infusion using an electronic infusion device.

- Dosage calculations are based on the patient's weight, and any possible bleeding tendencies are detected by a pretreatment clotting profile; if renal insufficiency exists, lower doses of heparin are required.
- Obtain periodic coagulation tests and hematocrit levels: Heparin is in the effective, or therapeutic, range when the aPTT is one and a half times the control.
- Monitor oral anticoagulants, such as warfarin, by the PT or the INR. Because the full anticoagulant effect of warfarin is delayed for 3 to 5 days, it is usually administered concurrently with heparin until desired anticoagulation has been achieved (i.e., when the PT is one and a half to two times normal or the INR is 2.0 to 3.0).

Monitoring and Managing Potential Complications

- Assess for early signs of spontaneous bleeding (principal complication of anticoagulant therapy): microscopic blood in urine, bruises, nosebleeds, and bleeding gums. Administer IV injections of protamine sulfate to reverse effects of heparin and LMWH (less effective). Administer vitamin K or infuse fresh-frozen plasma or prothrombin concentrate to reverse effects of warfarin.
- Monitor for heparin-induced thrombocytopenia (HIT) by regularly checking platelet counts. Early signs include decreasing platelet count; the need for increasing doses of heparin to maintain the therapeutic level; and thromboembolic or hemorrhagic complications (appearance of skin necrosis, skin discoloration, purpura, and blistering). If thrombocytopenia does occur, the nurse should perform platelet aggregation studies, discontinue heparin, and rapidly initiate alternate anticoagulant therapy.
- Closely monitor the medication schedule, because oral anticoagulants interact with many other medications and herbal and nutritional supplements.

Providing Comfort

- Elevate affected extremity and apply warm, moist packs to reduce discomfort.
- Encourage walking once anticoagulation therapy has been initiated (better than standing or sitting for long periods).
- Recommend bed exercises, such as dorsiflexion of the foot against a footboard.

- Provide additional pain relief with mild analgesic agents as prescribed.
- Initiate compression therapy as prescribed to help improve circulation and increase comfort: graduated compression stockings, external compression devices and wraps (e.g., short stretch elastic wraps, Unna boot, CircAid), intermittent pneumatic compression devices.
- With compression therapy, assess patient for comfort, inspect skin under device for signs of irritation or tenderness, and ensure that prescribed pressures are not exceeded.

> ### Quality and Safety Nursing Alert
>
> Any type of stocking can inadvertently become a tourniquet if applied incorrectly (i.e., rolled tightly at the top). In such instances, the stockings produce, rather than prevent, stasis. For ambulatory patients, graduated compression stockings are removed at night and reapplied before the legs are lowered from the bed to the floor in the morning.

Gerontologic Considerations

Older adult patients may be unable to apply elastic stockings properly. Educate the family member who is to assist the patient in applying the stockings so that there is no undue pressure placed on any part of the feet or legs.

Positioning the Body and Encouraging Exercise

- Periodically elevate the feet and the lower legs above heart level when on bed rest.
- Perform active and passive leg exercises, particularly those involving calf muscles, to increase venous flow preoperatively and postoperatively.
- Provide early ambulation to help prevent venous stasis.
- Encourage deep-breathing exercises because they produce increased negative pressure in the thorax, which assists in emptying the large veins.
- Instruct the patient, once ambulatory, to avoid sitting for more than an hour at a time; encourage patient to walk at least 10 minutes every 1 to 2 hours.
- Educate the patient to perform active and passive leg exercises as frequently as necessary when he or she cannot ambulate (such as during long car, bus, train, and plane rides).

V

Educating Patients About Self-Care

- Educate the patient about how to apply graduated compression stockings and explain the importance of elevating the legs and exercising adequately.
- Educate the patient on the purpose and importance of medication (correct dosage at specific times) and the need for scheduled blood tests to regulate medications.

For more information, see Chapter 30 in Hinkle, J. L., & Cheever, K. H. (2014). *Brunner and Suddarth's textbook of medical-surgical nursing* (13th ed.). Philadelphia: Lippincott Williams & Wilkins.

V

Selected Lab Values

Blood Chemistry		
Test	**Conventional Units**	**SI Units**
Alanine aminotransferase (ALT, formerly SGPT)	Males: 10–40 U/mL Females: 8–35 U/mL	Males: 0.17–0.68 µkat/L Females: 0.14–0.60 µkat/L
Alkaline phosphatase	50–120 U/L	50–120 U/L
Ammonia (plasma)	15–45 µg/dL (varies with method)	11–32 µmol/L
Amylase	60–160 Somogyi U/dL	111–296 U/L
Aspartate amino transferase (AST, formerly SGOT)	Males: 10–40 U/L Females: 15–30 U/L	Males: 0.34–0.68 µkat/L Females: 0.25–0.51 µkat/L
Bicarbonate	24–31 mEq/L	24–31 mmol/L
Bilirubin (total)	0.3–1.0 mg/dL	5–17 µmol/L
Direct	0.1–0.4 mg/dL	1.7–3.7 µmol/L
Indirect	0.1–0.4 mg/dL	3.4–11.2 µmol/L
Blood urea nitrogen (BUN)	10–20 mg/dL	3.6–7.2 mmol/L
Calcium	8.6–10.2 mg/dL	2.15–2.55 mmol/L
Carbon dioxide, arterial (whole blood) partial pressure ($PaCO_2$)	35–45 mm Hg	4.66–5.99 kPa
Chloride	97–107 mEq/L	97–107 mmol/L
Creatine kinase (CK) isoenzymes	MM band present (skeletal muscle); MB band absent (heart muscle)	
Creatinine (serum)	0.7–1.4 mg/dL[†]	62–124 µmol/L[‡]
Gamma-glutamyl-transpeptidase (GGT)	Males: 20–30 U/L Females: 1–24 U/L	0.03–0.5 µkat/L 0.02–0.4 µkat/L
Glucose (blood)	Fasting: 60–110 mg/dL Postprandial (2 h): 65–140 mg/dL	3.3–6.05 mmol/L 3.58–7.7 mmol/L

(continues on page 730)

Blood Chemistry (continued)		
Test	**Conventional Units**	**SI Units**
Glycosylated hemo-globin (HbA$_{1c}$)	4.4%–6.4%	
Lactate dehydroge-nase (LDH)	90–176 mU/mL	90–176 U/L
Cholesterol	150–200 mg/dL	3.9–5.2 mmol/L
Triglycerides	100–200 mg/dL	1.13–3.8 mmol/L
Lipase	<200 U/L	<200 µkat/L
Magnesium	1.3–2.3 mg/dL	0.62–0.95 mmol/L
Osmolality	275–300 mOsm/kg	275–300 mmol/L
Phosphorus (inorganic)	2.5–4.5 mg/dL	0.8–1.45 mmol/L
Potassium	3.5–5.0 mEq/L	3.5–5.0 mmol/L
Prostate-specific antigen (PSA)	0–4 ng/mL	
Protein total	6.0–8.0 gm/dL	60–80 g/L
Albumin	3.5–5.5 g/dL	40–55 g/L
Globulin	1.7–3.3 g/dL	17–33 g/L
Thyroxine (T$_4$) total	5.0–11.0 µg/dL	65–138 mmol/L
Thyroxine, free (FT$_4$)	0.8–2.7 ng/dL	10.3–35 pmol/L
Triiodothyronine (T$_3$) total	70–204 ng/dL	1.08–3.14 nmol/L
Thyroid-binding globulin	10–26 µg/L	100–260 µg/L
Sodium	135–145 mEq/L	135–145 mmol/L
Thyroid-stimulating hormone (TSH)		0.4–4.2 mIU/L
Uric acid	2.5–8 mg/dL	0.15–0.5 mmol/L

†Laboratory and/or method specific

‡Varies with age and muscle mass

Hematology		
Test	Conventional Units	SI Units
Erythrocyte count (RBC count)	Males: 4,600,000–6,200,000/cu mm	Males: 4.6–6.2 × 10^{12}/L
	Females: 4,200,000–5,400,000/cu mm	Females: 4.2–5.4 × 10^{12}/L
Hematocrit (Hct)	Males: 42%–52%	Males: 0.42–0.52
	Females: 35%–47%	Females: 0.35–0.47
Hemoglobin (Hb)	Males: 13–18 gm/dL	Males: 2.02–2.79 mmol/L
	Females: 12–16 gm/dL	Females: 1.86/2.48 mmol/L
Mean corpuscular hemoglobin (MHC)	28–33 pg/cell	28–33 pg
Mean corpuscular hemoglobin concentration (MCHC)	33%–35%	Concentration fraction: 0.33–0.35
Mean corpuscular volume (MCV)	84–96 fL	
Reticulocyte count	0.5%–1.5% of red cells	Number fraction: 0.005–0.015
Leukocyte count (WBC count)	4,500–11,000/cu mm	4.5–11 × 10^9/L
Basophils	0%–1%	Number fraction: 0.00–0.01
Eosinophils	0%–4%	Number fraction: 0.00–0.04
Lymphocytes	20%–40%	Number fraction: 0.2–0.4
Monocytes	2%–8%	Number fraction: 0.02–0.08
Neutrophils	45%–63%	Number fraction: 0.45–0.73

NANDA International Nursing Diagnoses 2012–2014

A

Activity Intolerance
Activity Intolerance, Risk for
Activity Planning, Ineffective
Activity Planning, Risk for Ineffective
Adverse Reaction to Iodinated
    Contrast Media, Risk for
Airway Clearance, Ineffective
Allergy Response, Risk for
Anxiety
Aspiration, Risk for
Attachment, Risk for Impaired
Autonomic Dysreflexia
Autonomic Dysreflexia, Risk for

B

Behavior, Disorganized Infant
Behavior, Readiness for Enhanced
    Organized Infant
Behavior, Risk for Disorganized
    Infant
Bleeding, Risk for
Blood Glucose Level, Risk for
    Unstable
Body Image, Disturbed
Body Temperature, Risk for
    Imbalanced
Breast Milk, Insufficient
Breast-feeding, Ineffective
Breast-feeding, Interrupted
Breast-feeding, Readiness for
    Enhanced
Breathing Pattern, Ineffective

C

Cardiac Output, Decreased
Caregiver Role Strain
Caregiver Role Strain, Risk for

Childbearing Process, Ineffective
Childbearing Process, Readiness for
    Enhanced
Childbearing Process, Risk for
    Ineffective
Comfort, Impaired
Comfort, Readiness for Enhanced
Communication, Readiness for
    Enhanced
Confusion, Acute
Confusion, Chronic
Confusion, Risk for Acute
Constipation
Constipation, Perceived
Constipation, Risk for
Contamination
Contamination, Risk for
Coping, Defensive
Coping, Ineffective
Coping, Readiness for Enhanced
Coping, Ineffective Community
Coping, Readiness for Enhanced
    Community
Coping, Compromised Family
Coping, Disabled Family
Coping, Readiness for Enhanced
    Family

D

Death Anxiety
Decision Making, Readiness for
    Enhanced
Decisional Conflict
Denial, Ineffective
Dentition, Impaired
Development, Risk for Delayed
Diarrhea
Disuse Syndrome, Risk for

Diversional Activity, Deficient
Dry Eye, Risk for

E
Electrolyte Imbalance, Risk for
Energy Field, Disturbed
Environmental Interpretation
    Syndrome, Impaired

F
Failure to Thrive, Adult
Falls, Risk for
Family Processes, Dysfunctional
Family Processes, Interrupted
Family Processes, Readiness for
    Enhanced
Fatigue
Fear
Feeding Pattern, Ineffective Infant
Fluid Balance, Readiness for
    Enhanced
Fluid Volume, Deficient
Fluid Volume, Excess
Fluid Volume, Risk for Deficient
Fluid Volume, Risk for Imbalanced

G
Gas Exchange, Impaired
Gastrointestinal Motility,
    Dysfunctional
Gastrointestinal Motility, Risk For
    Dysfunctional
Gastrointestinal Perfusion, Risk for
    Ineffective
Grieving
Grieving, Complicated
Grieving, Risk for Complicated
Growth, Risk for Disproportionate
Growth and Development, Delayed

H
Health, Deficient Community
Health Behavior, Risk-Prone
Health Maintenance, Ineffective
Home Maintenance, Impaired
Hope, Readiness for Enhanced
Hopelessness
Human Dignity, Risk for Compromised

Hyperthermia
Hypothermia

I
Immunization Status, Readiness for
    Enhanced
Impulse Control, Ineffective
Incontinence, Bowel
Incontinence, Functional Urinary
Incontinence, Overflow Urinary
Incontinence, Reflex Urinary
Incontinence, Stress Urinary
Incontinence, Risk for Urge Urinary
Incontinence, Urge Urinary
Infection, Risk for
Injury, Risk for
Insomnia
Intracranial Adaptive Capacity,
    Decreased

J
Jaundice, Neonatal
Jaundice, Risk for Neonatal

K
Knowledge, Deficient
Knowledge, Readiness for Enhanced

L
Latex Allergy Response
Latex Allergy Response, Risk for
Lifestyle, Sedentary
Liver Function, Risk for Impaired
Loneliness, Risk for

M
Maternal–Fetal Dyad, Risk for
    Disturbed
Memory, Impaired
Mobility, Impaired Bed
Mobility, Impaired Physical
Mobility, Impaired Wheelchair
Moral Distress

N
Nausea
Noncompliance
Nutrition: Less Than Body
    Requirements, Imbalanced

Nutrition: More Than Body Requirements, Imbalanced
Nutrition: More Than Body Requirements, Risk for Imbalanced
Nutrition, Readiness for Enhanced

O
Oral Mucous Membrane, Impaired
Other-Directed Violence, Risk for

P
Pain, Acute
Pain, Chronic
Parenting, Impaired
Parenting, Readiness for Enhanced
Parenting, Risk for Impaired
Perioperative Positioning Injury, Risk for
Peripheral Neurovascular Dysfunction, Risk for
Personal Identity, Disturbed
Personal Identity, Risk for Disturbed
Poisoning, Risk for
Posttrauma Syndrome
Posttrauma Syndrome, Risk for
Power, Readiness for Enhanced
Powerlessness
Powerlessness, Risk for
Protection, Ineffective

R
Rape Trauma Syndrome
Relationship, Ineffective
Relationship, Readiness for Enhanced
Relationship, Risk for Ineffective
Religiosity, Impaired
Religiosity, Readiness for Enhanced
Religiosity, Risk for Impaired
Relocation Stress Syndrome
Relocation Stress Syndrome, Risk for
Renal Perfusion, Risk for Ineffective
Resilience, Impaired Individual
Resilience, Readiness for Enhanced
Resilience, Risk for Compromised

Role Conflict, Parental
Role Performance, Ineffective

S
Self-Care, Readiness for Enhanced
Self-Care Deficit, Bathing
Self-Care Deficit, Dressing
Self-Care Deficit, Feeding
Self-Care Deficit, Toileting
Self-Concept, Readiness for Enhanced
Self-Directed Violence, Risk for
Self-Esteem, Chronic Low
Self-Esteem, Risk for Chronic Low
Self-Esteem, Risk for Situational Low
Self-Esteem, Situational Low
Self-Health Management, Ineffective
Self-Health Management, Readiness for Enhanced
Self-Mutilation
Self-Mutilation, Risk for
Self-Neglect
Sexual Dysfunction
Sexuality Pattern, Ineffective
Shock, Risk for
Skin Integrity, Impaired
Skin Integrity, Risk for Impaired
Sleep Deprivation
Sleep Pattern, Disturbed
Sleep, Readiness for Enhanced
Social Interaction, Impaired
Social Isolation
Sorrow, Chronic
Spiritual Distress
Spiritual Distress, Risk for
Spiritual Well-Being, Readiness for Enhanced
Spontaneous Ventilation, Impaired
Stress Overload
Sudden Infant Death Syndrome, Risk for
Suffocation, Risk for
Suicide, Risk for
Surgical Recovery, Delayed
Swallowing, Impaired

T

Therapeutic Regimen Management, Ineffective Family
Thermal Injury, Risk for
Thermoregulation, Ineffective
Tissue Integrity, Impaired
Tissue Perfusion, Ineffective Peripheral
Tissue Perfusion, Risk for Decreased Cardiac
Tissue Perfusion, Risk for Ineffective Cerebral
Tissue Perfusion, Risk for Ineffective Peripheral
Transfer Ability, Impaired
Trauma, Risk for

U

Unilateral Neglect
Urinary Elimination, Impaired
Urinary Elimination, Readiness for Enhanced
Urinary Retention

V

Vascular Trauma, Risk for
Ventilatory Weaning Response, Dysfunctional
Verbal Communication, Impaired

W

Walking, Impaired
Wandering

Index

A

Abdominal aortic aneurysms, 55
  assessment and diagnostic
    findings, 56
  cause, 55
  clinical manifestations, 56
  gerontologic considerations,
    55–56
  medical management, 57
  prevalence, 55
  surgical management, 57
Abdominal pain
  in abdominal aortic aneurysm,
    57
  in appendicitis, 73
  in cholelithiasis, 234, 237
  in colorectal cancer, 162
  in Crohn's disease, 253
  in diabetic ketoacidosis, 280
  in diverticular disease, 294
  in gastric cancer, 209
  in hepatic cirrhosis, 247
  in large bowel obstruction, 104
ABG analysis. See Arterial blood
    gas (ABG) analysis
Acalculous cholecystitis, 233
Acetabulum fracture, 327
Acetylcholine, 29, 31, 485
Acoustic neuroma, 109
Acquired immunodeficiency
    syndrome (AIDS), 1–16
  assessment and diagnostic
    findings, 4
  clinical manifestations, 2
    cachexia, 2
    depression, 3–4
    gastrointestinal, 2
    gynecologic, 4
    integumentary, 4
    neurologic, 3
    oncologic, 2–3
    respiratory, 2
  complementary and alternative
    modalities, 7
  definition, 1
  HIV transmission in, 1

  and Kaposi's sarcoma, 431
  medical management, 4
    antidepressant therapy, 6–7
    antidiarrheal therapy, 6
    chemotherapy, 6
    nutrition therapy, 7
    opportunistic infections, 4–6
  nursing interventions, 10–16
    activity tolerance, 12
    airway clearance, 12–13
    bowel patterns, 11
    complications management,
      14–15
    continuing care, 16
    feelings of isolation,
      decreasing, 14
    grief management, 14
    home- and community-based
      care, 15–16
    infection prevention, 11
    knowledge on HIV infec-
      tion, 14
    nutritional status, 13–14
    pain management, 13
    self-care, 15–16
    skin integrity maintenance,
      10–11
    thought processes, 12
  nursing process, 8–16
    assessment, 8–9
    diagnosis, 9–10
    evaluation, 16
    interventions, 10–16
    planning and goals, 10
  stages of, 1
  supportive care in, 7–8
Acral-lentiginous melanoma,
    205
Activity tolerance
  in Addison's disease, 27–28
  in AIDS, 12
  in burn injury, 127–128
  in COPD, 242
  in heart failure, 370
  in TB, 701
Acute bacterial prostatitis, 596

Acute coronary syndrome (ACS), 16–22
  assessment methods, 18
  characterization of, 16–17
  clinical manifestations, 17–18
  collaborative problems, 20
  diagnosis, 20
  diagnostic methods, 18
  examination, 19–20
  medical management
    goals, 18
    MIDCAB, 18
  nursing interventions, 20–22
  pharmacologic therapy for, 18–19
Acute fulminant infection, 463
Acute gastritis, 331. *See also* Gastritis
  clinical manifestations, 332
  medical management, 332–333
Acute glomerulonephritis, 338–339
  assessment and diagnostic findings, 338
  clinical manifestations, 338
  medical management, 338–339
  nursing management, 339
  postinfectious causes, 338
Acute kidney failure (AKF), 621–626
  clinical manifestations, 622
  clinical stages, 622
  in elderly people, 623
  fluid and electrolyte balance, 625
  infection prevention, 626
  medical management, 624–625
  metabolic rate, 626
  nursing management, 625
  psychosocial support, 626
  pulmonary function, 626
  skin care, 626
Acute lymphocytic leukemia (ALL), 440–441
  chemotherapy, 441
  clinical manifestations, 440
  medical management, 441
  pathophysiology, 440
Acute myeloid leukemia (AML), 443–445

assessment and diagnostic findings, 444
  blasts in, presence of, 444
  classification, 443
  clinical manifestations, 444
  hematopoietic stem cell transplantation, 445
  medical management, 444
  pathophysiology, 444
  pharmacologic therapy, 444–445
  supportive care, 445
Acute nephritic syndrome, 489–491
  assessment and diagnostic findings, 489
  clinical manifestations, 489
  continuing care, 490–491
  home- and community-based care, 490–491
  hospital care, 490
  medical management, 490
  nursing management, 490
  pathophysiology, 489
  self-care, 490
Acute otitis media, 511–512
  clinical manifestations, 511
  complications, 511
  medical management, 511–512
  myringotomy, 512
Acute pancreatitis, 514–519
  abdominal pain in, 514–515
  causes of, 514
  diagnosis, 515
  gerontologic considerations, 515
  nursing management
    breathing pattern, 517
    continuing care, 519
    fluid and electrolyte disturbance, 518
    multiple organ failure, 518
    nutritional status, 517
    pain and discomfort, 516–517
    pancreatic necrosis, 518
    self-care, 518–519
    shock, 518
    skin integrity, 517–518
  treatment
    acute phase, 515–516
    postacute phase, 516
Acute pharyngitis, 575–576

Acute pulmonary edema, 608–610
  clinical manifestations, 609
  diagnosis, 609
  nursing management, 610
  pharmacologic therapy for, 610
Acute pyelonephritis, 616–618
Acute renal failure (ARF),
      621–626
  clinical manifestations, 622
  clinical stages, 622
  in elderly people, 623
  fluid and electrolyte balance,
      625
  infection prevention, 626
  medical management, 624–625
  metabolic rate, 626
  nursing management, 625
  psychosocial support, 626
  pulmonary function, 626
  skin care, 626
Acute respiratory distress syndrome
      (ARDS), 22–25
  assessment and diagnostic
      findings, 23
  characterization of, 22–23
  clinical manifestations, 23
  factors associated with
      development of, 23
  medical management, 23
  mortality rate, 23
  nursing management, 24–25
Acute respiratory failure, 121
  monitoring and managing, 126
Acute rheumatic fever, 301
Acute thyroiditis, 687–688
Adefovir, in hepatitis B, 384
Adenocarcinoma, 157, 161, 186,
      196, 208, 209
Addison's disease, 25–27
  assessment and diagnostic
      findings, 26
  clinical manifestations, 25
  medical management, 26
  nursing management, 27
Addisonian crisis, 26
ADH. See Antidiuretic hormone
      (ADH) Adjunctive therapy
      for hyperthyroidism, 406
Adrenalectomy, 256
Adrenal enzyme inhibitors, 256

Adrenal glands and Addison's
      disease, 25
Adrenal hypofunction, 258
Adrenocortical insufficiency. See
      Addison's disease
Adrenocorticotropic hormone
      (ACTH), 25
ADT. See Androgen deprivation
      therapy (ADT)
Advanced hypothyroidism,
      416
Aflatoxins, 183
Agitation management, 33
AIDS. See Acquired immunodefi-
      ciency syndrome (AIDS)
Airway management
  in AIDS, 12–13
  in burn injury, 119–120
  in cancer of larynx, 179
  in chronic obstructive pulmonary
      disease, 242
  in increased ICP, 426
  in perioperative nursing, 561
  in pneumonia, 588–589
  in pulmonary tuberculosis,
      700
  in SCI, 658–659
  in traumatic brain injury, 357
  in unconscious patient,
      712–713
Akinetic mutism, 710
Alcohol consumption
  and acute pancreatitis, 514
  and chronic pancreatitis, 519
  and gastritis, 331–333
  and gout, 344
  and peptic ulcer, 536
Alcoholics Anonymous, 379
ALL. See Acute lymphocytic
      leukemia (ALL)
Allopurinol, 596
  in gout, 344
Alpha-adrenergic blocking agents,
      in Guillain-Barré syndrome,
      346
Alpha-interferon, in hepatitis
      B, 384
Alternative therapies
  for PCP, 5
  for pericarditis, 542

Alzheimer's disease (AD), 29–34
    assessment and diagnostic
        findings, 30
    classification, 29
    clinical manifestations, 29–30
    evaluation, 34
    nursing diagnoses, 31
    nursing interventions, 32–34
    risk factors for, 29
    treatment, 30–31
Ambulation, 124, 160, 179, 237,
    243
Amenorrhea, and pituitary tumors,
    581
AML. *See* Acute myeloid leukemia
    (AML)
Ampicillin, in meningitis, 464
Amyotrophic lateral sclerosis
    (ALS), 34–36
    causes of, 34–35
    clinical features of, 35
    diagnosis, 35
    medical management, 35–36
    nursing care, 36
Anagrelide, 595
Anakinra, in gout, 344
Analgesic medications
    for osteoarthritis, 502
    for pericarditis, 542
    for peritonitis, 573
    for pleurisy, 584
    for viral pharyngitis, 575–576
Anaphylactic shock, 643–644
    causes, 643
    characteristics of, 643
    clinical manifestations, 643–644
    medical management, 644
    nursing management, 644
    pathophysiology, 643
    pharmacologic therapy, 644
    risk factors, 643
Anaphylaxis, 36–38
    clinical manifestations, 37
    diagnostic evaluation, 37
    medical management
        CPR, 38
        pharmacologic therapy, 38
    nursing management, 38
    prevention, 37–38
Anastrazole, 152

Androgen deprivation therapy
    (ADT), 198
Anemia, 39–43
    assessment
        GI function, 41
        neurologic deficits, 41
    classification, 39
    collaborative problems, 41
    diagnostic evaluation, 39–40
    evaluation, patient outcomes, 43
    gerontologic considerations, 40
    management, 49
    nursing interventions, 41–42
    symptoms, 39
Anemia, aplastic, 43–44
    clinical manifestations, 43
    diagnosis, 43–44
    etiology, 43
    medical management, 44
    nursing management, 44
Anemia, iron-deficiency, 44–46
    causes of, 44–45
    clinical manifestations, 45
    diagnosis, 45
    medical management, 45
    nursing management, 45–46
Anemia, megaloblastic, 46–49
    assessment and diagnostic
        findings, 47
    clinical manifestations, 47
    medical management, 48
    nursing management, 48–49
    pathophysiology
        folic acid deficiency, 46–47
        vitamin B12 deficiency, 47
Anemia, sickle cell, 49–55
    assessment, 51–52
    assessment and diagnostic
        findings, 50
    clinical manifestations, 50
    collaborative problems, 52
    complications management, 54
    evaluation, patient outcomes, 55
    medical management, 50–51
    nursing diagnoses, 52
    nursing interventions, 53–54
    pathophysiology, 49
Aneurysm, aortic, 55–58
    clinical manifestations, 56
    diagnostic findings, 56–57

gerontologic considerations,
    55–56
medical management, 57
nursing management
    postperative assessment, 58
    preoperative assessment, 57
surgical management, 57
thoracic, 55
Aneurysm, intracranial, 58–63
clinical manifestations, 59
collaborative problems, 61
complications, 62
diagnostic methods for, 59
evaluation, patient outcomes,
    63
medical management, 59–60
neurologic assessment, 60
nursing diagnoses, 60–61
nursing interventions, 61–63
prognosis, 58
Aneurysms
classification, 55
clinical manifestations, 56
Anginal pain, factors affecting,
    63
Angina pectoris, 63–67
assessment, 65
clinical manifestations, 63–64
diagnostic methods for, 65
elderly person with, 64
evaluation, patient outcomes,
    67
medical management, 64–65
nursing diagnoses, 65
nursing interventions, 66–67
potential complications, 65
Angiography, for pulmonary
    embolism, 612
Angiomas, 110
Angiotensin-converting enzyme
    (ACE) inhibitors
in mitral regurgitation, 466
in nephrotic syndrome, 492
Angiotensin receptor blockers
    (ARBs), in mitral
    regurgitation, 466
Angle-closure glaucoma, 335
Anorexia
in hepatitis A, 381
in kidney failure, 627

in peritonitis, 573
in pulmonary arterial hyper-
    tension, 606
in renal failure, 627
in ulcerative colitis, 702
Antacids, 537
Antiarrhythmics, in mitral valve
    prolapse, 468
Antibacterial therapy, in impetigo,
    422
Antibiotics
in acute otitis media, 511
in epididymitis, 305
in hepatic encephalopathy,
    378
in impetigo, 422–423
in lung abscess, 449
in lymphedema, 451
in meningitis, 463
in osteomyelitis, 505
in peptic ulcer, 537
in peritonitis, 574
in prevention of infective
    endocarditis, 299
Anticoagulation therapy
for Guillain-Barré syndrome,
    346
for multiple myeloma, 472
for PE, 613
for pulmonary arterial hyperten-
    sion, 607
for vein disorders, 725–726
Antidepressant therapy, in AIDS,
    6–7
Antidiarrheal therapy, in AIDS, 6
Antiembolism stockings
for Guillain-Barré syndrome,
    346
for PE, 616
for perioperative nursing
    management, 566
for SCI, 657, 661
Antiemetics, in Ménière's disease,
    460
Antihistamines, 596
in Ménière's disease, 460
Antiinflammatory agents, 597
Antiplatelet agents, 571
Antithyroid medications, in
    hyperthyroidism, 405

Anxiety management
  in acute coronary syndrome, 21
  in AD, 33
  after bariatric surgery, 495
  in AIDS, 12
  in angina pectoris, 66
  in breast cancer, 154
  in burn injury, 121
  in cardiomyopathies, 228
  in cervical cancer, 159
  in diabetic ketoacidosis, 283–284
  in gastric cancer, 211
  in gastritis, 333
  in GBS, 348
  in heart failure, 371
  in intracranial aneurysm, 61
  in leukemia, 438
  in malignant melanoma, 207
  in mastoid surgery, 456
  in Ménière's disease, 460
  in PE, 615
  in perioperative nursing, 550
  before prostatectomy, 200
  in toxic epidermal necrolysis, 693
  in ulcerative colitis, 707–708
Aortic insufficiency, 68–69
  causes of, 68
  clinical manifestations, 68
  management, 69
Aortic regurgitation. See Aortic insufficiency
Aortic stenosis, 70–71
Aortic valvuloplasty for aortic regurgitation, 69
Apheresis device, 80
Appendicitis, 71–74
  causes of, 72
  clinical manifestations, 72
  diagnosis, 72–73
  gerontologic considerations, 73
  medical management, 73
  nursing management, 74
Arterial blood gas (ABG) analysis
  in acute pancreatitis, 517
  in AIDS, 8
  in ARDS, 23
  in asthma, 85
  in bronchogenic carcinoma, 188
  in burn injury, 119

  in cirrhosis, 245
  fractures and, 322
  in head injury, 357
  in hyperglycemic hyperosmolar syndrome, 395
  in hypothyroidism, 417
  in PE, 612–613
  in traumatic brain injury, 357
Arterial embolism, 74–76
  diagnostic findings, 75
  medical management, 75–76
  nursing management, 76
  symptoms, 75
Arterial insufficiency of extremities, 570
Arterial thrombosis, 74–76
Arteriography
  for aortic aneurysm, 57
  for arterial embolism, 75
  for atherosclerosis, 78
  for bone tumors, 101
  for cholelithiasis, 234
  for liver cancer, 183
Arthritis, rheumatoid. See Rheumatoid arthritis
Arthroscopy, for fractures, 318
Asterixis
  in hepatic encephalopathy, 377
  in kidney failure, 627
  in renal failure, 627
Asthma, 83–89
  assessment and diagnostic methods for, 85
  clinical manifestations, 84–85
  community-based care, 88–89
  home care, 88–89
  medical management, 85–86
  nursing management, 88–89
  risk factors, 83
  status asthmaticus. See Status asthmaticus
Asymptomatic inflammatory prostatitis, 596
Atherectomy, 65
Atherosclerosis, 77–78
  clinical manifestations, 77
  management, 78
  pathologic processes, 77
  risk factors, 77
Aura, 307

Autoimmune (cell-mediated and
    humoral) attack, 344
Autonomic hyperreflexia, 661
Autotransfusion, 593
Avascular necrosis (AVN) of bone,
    321
Axillary lymph nodes, 151

B

Back pain, low, 92–95
    assessment and diagnostic
        methods, 93
    causes of, 92
    medical management, 93
    nursing management
        assessment, 94
        interventions, 94–95
Bacterial infection
    acute pharyngitis, 575–576
    peritonitis, 572–575
    thyroiditis, 687–688
Bacterial meningitis, 461–462.
    See also Meningitis
Bariatric surgery, 493–498
    assessment and diagnostic
        findings, 493
    medical management, 493–994
    nursing interventions, 495–498
        anxiety reduction, 495
        body image changes, 497
        bowel habits, 497
        complications assessment, 497
        continuing care, 498
        dietary limitations, 495
        fluid and volume balance, 496
        home- and community-based
            care, 497–498
        infection prevention, 496
        nutritional status, 496–497
        pain management, 495–496
        self-care, 497–498
    nursing process, 494–498
        assessment, 494
        diagnosis, 494
        evaluation, 498
        interventions, 495–498
        planning and goals, 495
        potential complications, 495
Barium swallow, in hiatal hernia,
    387

Basophilic tumors, 581
B-cell lymphomas, 3
Bed rest
    in pheochromocytoma, 579
    in viral pharyngitis, 576
Bell's palsy, 95–97
    causes of, 96
    medical management, 96
    nursing management
        eye care, 97
        muscle tone, 97
Benign bone tumors, 100
Benign prostatic hyperplasia
    (BPH), 97–99
    assessment and diagnostic
        methods, 98–99
    clinical manifestations, 98
    medical management, 99
    nursing management, 99
Benzodiazepine antagonists, in
    hepatic encephalopathy,
    378
Beta-adrenergic blocking agents, in
    hyperthyroidism, 405
Beta-blockers, in mitral
    regurgitation, 466
Biliary drainage, in acute
    pancreatitis, 544
Biliopancreatic diversion with
    duodenal switch, 494.
    See also Bariatric surgery
Biopsy
    for ALS, 35
    for bone tumors, 101
    for breast cancer, 151
    for cancer, 132, 133
    for cardiomyopathies, 226
    for cervical cancer, 158
    for colorectal cancer, 162
    for endometrium cancer, 170
    for esophageal cancer, 171
    for exfoliative dermatitis, 266
    for gastric cancer, 209
    for gastritis, 332
    for hepatic cirrhosis, 245
    for Hodgkin lymphoma, 391
    for infective endocarditis, 299
    for Kaposi's sarcoma, 431
    for liver tumors, 183
    for lung cancer, 188

Biopsy (*continued*)
  for malignant melanoma, 205
  for multiple myeloma, 471
  for nephritic syndrome, 489
  for nephrotic syndrome, 491
  for osteomalacia, 503
  for pemphigus, 531
  for peptic ulcer, 536
  for pericarditis, 542
  for pleural effusion, 582
  for pneumothorax, 592
  for thrombocytopenia, 684
  for thyroid cancer, 216
  for vulvar cancer, 219
Bisphosphonates, in multiple
      myeloma, 472
Bladder cancer, 147–148
  assessment and diagnostic
      methods, 147
  clinical manifestations, 147
  medical management, 147
  risk factor for, 147
  surgical management, 148
Bleeding
  in acute pancreatitis, 515
  in epistaxis, 312–313
  from esophageal varices, 314
  in hemophilia, 374
  in kidney failure, 627
  in peptic ulcer, 535
  in renal failure, 627
  and thrombocytopenia, 684–685
  in thrombocytopenia, 685
  in ulcerative colitis, 702, 706
  in vein disorders, 725
Blindness, glaucoma and, 335.
      See also Glaucoma
Blood studies
  for chronic glomerulonephritis,
      341
  for glomerulonephritis, 338
  for peptic ulcer, 537
  for pulmonary embolism, 612
  for systemic lupus erythematosus,
      681
  for ulcerative colitis, 703
Blood transfusions
  for bleeding esophageal varices,
      315
  for unconscious patient, 713

Body mass indices (BMI), 498
Body temperature management
  in chronic pyelonephritis, 619
  in perioperative nursing,
      563–564
  in toxic epidermal necrolysis,
      692–693
  in traumatic brain injury, 359
  in unconscious patient, 714
Bone marrow biopsy
  in Hodgkin lymphoma, 391
  in multiple myeloma, 471
  in non-Hodgkin lymphomas, 453
Bone marrow transplantation. *See*
      Hematopoietic stem cell
      transplantation (HSCT)
Bone pain, in multiple myeloma,
      470
Bone tumors, 100–103
  assessment and diagnostic
      findings, 101
  benign, 100
  clinical manifestations, 101
  malignant, 100–101
  medical management, 101–102
  nursing management, 102–103
  secondary, 101
Bowel decompression, 106
Bowel management
  in Parkinson's disease, 525
  in perioperative nursing, 552
  in SCI, 660
  in unconscious patient, 715
Bowel obstruction, large, 104–105
  clinical manifestations, 104
  medical management, 104–105
  nursing management, 105
Bowel obstruction, small, 105–107
  clinical manifestations, 105–106
  medical management, 106
  nursing management, 106–107
Boxer's fracture, 326
Bradycardia
  and pneumonia, 585, 587
  and spinal cord injury, 655, 657,
      659
Bradykinesia in Parkinson's
      disease, 522
Brain abscess, 107–109
  clinical manifestations, 107

management, medical and
nursing, 108–109
prevention, 107
Brain injury. *See* Head injury;
Traumatic brain injury (TBI)
Brain stem herniation elevated
ICP and, 425
Brain tumors, 109–111
assessment and diagnostic
findings, 111
classification, 109–110
clinical manifestations
focal/localized, 110–111
increased ICP, 110
incidence of, 109
medical treatments, 111
metastasization of, 109
BRCA gene mutation, 150
Breast cancer, 149–157
assessment and diagnostic
findings, 151
clinical manifestations, 150–151
medical management, 151
nursing interventions
home- and community-based
care, 156
postoperative, 154–156
preoperative, 153–154
nursing process, 152–157
assessment, 152
diagnosis, 152–153
evaluation, 156–157
interventions, 153–156
planning and goals, 153
pathophysiology, 149
pharmacologic therapy, 152
prevention strategies, 150
protective factors, 150
radiation therapy, 152
risk factors, 149–150
staging of, 151
surgical management, 151
Breast-conserving surgery, 151
Breathing patterns
in acute pancreatitis, 517
in SCI, 658–659
Breath, shortness of
in acquired immunodeficiency
syndrome, 2
and end-stage kidney disease, 627

and end-stage renal disease, 627
in mitral valve prolapse, 468
and pleural effusion, 582
and pleurisy, 584
and spinal cord injury, 657
Broad-spectrum antibiotics
for pelvic inflammatory disease
(PID), 528
for septic shock, 652
Bronchiectasis, 113–114
causes of, 113
clinical manifestations, 113
medical management, 113–114
Bronchitis, chronic, 239
Bronchogenic carcinoma, 186–190
assessment and diagnostic
methods, 188
causes of, 186
classification, 186
clinical manifestations, 187
managing side effects of
treatment, 189
breathing problems, 189
fatigue, 189
psychological support, 189
medical management, 188–189
radiation therapy, 188
risk factors, 187
surgical management, 188
Bronchopleural fistula, 448
Bronchopneumonia, 585
Brudzinski's sign in meningitis,
462
B symptoms
in CLL patients, 442
in non-Hodgkin lymphomas, 453
Bulbar muscle impairment, 35
Bulbar muscle weakness, 345
Bullectomy for COPD, 241
Bullous impetigo, 422
Burn injury, 114–129
depth of, 114
evaluation, patient outcomes, 129
gerontologic considerations, 115
medical management, 117
nursing interventions
activity tolerance, 127–128
body image and self-concept,
128
potential complications, 128

Burn injury (*continued*)
  nursing management, acute/
      intermediate phase
    assessment, 122
    complications, 124–125
    coping strategies, 125
    fluid balance, 123
    infection, 123
    nutrition, 123
    pain and discomfort, 124
    patient and family processes,
        125
    physical mobility, 124–125
    skin integrity, 123–124
  nursing management, emergent/
      resuscitative phase
    assessment, 118
    body temperature, 120
    fluid and electrolyte balance,
        120
    gas exchange and airway clear-
        ance, 119–120
    pain and anxiety, 121
  planning/goals, 127
  rehabilitation
    assessment, 126–127
    collaborative problems, 127
    nursing diagnoses, 127
  self-care, 128–129
  total body surface area, 118
Burr holes, 353
Butterfly rash, 681

C

Calcium channel blockers, 467,
    469, 607, 621
Calcium intake and osteoporosis,
    518
Calculous cholecystitis, 233
Cancer, 130–147
  clinical manifestations, 131
  definition of, 131
  diagnostic tests, 132
  grading, 132–133
  medical management, 133–134
  nursing management
    biologic response modifiers,
        135–136
    bleeding and hemorrhage,
        139–140

    image and self-esteem,
        137–138
    bone marrow transplantation,
        144–145
    chemotherapy, 143–144
    fatigue, 137
    hyperthermia, 146
    infection prevention, 138–139
    negative feelings, 138
    nutritional problems, 136
    pain, 136–137
    radiation therapy, 142
    septic shock, 139
    surgery, 141–142
    tissue integrity, 134
  pathophysiology, 131
  screening, 132
  self-care, 140
  staging, 132
  types
    bladder, 147–148
    breast, 149–157
    cervical, 157–161
    colon, 161–169
    endometrium, 169–170
    esophageal, 170–172
    kidneys, 173–175
    larynx, 175–182
    liver, 183–186
    lung, 186–190
    oral cavity, 190–191
    ovarian, 192–193
    pancreas, 193–196
    pharynx, 190–191
    prostate, 196–203
    rectum, 161–169
    skin, 204–208
    stomach, 208–213
    testicular, 214–216
    thyroid, 216–217
    urinary bladder, 147–148
    vaginal, 218
    vulva, 219–221
Carcinomas, renal cell, 594
Cardiac arrest, 221–223
Cardiac stress testing
  in heart failure, 368
Cardiac tamponade
  clinical manifestations, 541
  surgical management, 542

Cardiogenic shock, 645–647
  causes of, 645
  clinical manifestations, 645
  fluid administration for, 646–647
  hemodynamic monitoring in,
    646
  medical management, 645–646
  medications for, 646
  prevention, 646
Cardiomyopathies, 223–230
  assessment, 227
  assessment and diagnostic
    methods, 226
  classification, 223
  clinical manifestations, 225
  collaborative problems, 228
  medical management
    surgical intervention, 226
    ventricular assist devices, 226
  nursing diagnoses, 227–228
  nursing interventions
    activity tolerance, 228
    anxiety reduction, 228–229
    cardiac output, 228
    continuing care, 229
    emotional responses, 228–229
    self-care, 229
  pathophysiology, 223
  planning/goals, 228
Cardiomyopathy, in muscular
    dystrophies, 479
Cataract, 230–232
  assessment and diagnostic
    findings, 231
  clinical manifestations, 230
  medical management, 231
  nursing management, 231–232
  pathophysiology, 230
Catheterization, cardiac, 606
Cell-mediated immunity, 688
Cellular degeneration and
    Parkinson's disease, 521
Cephalgia. See Headache
Cephalosporins, 464
Cephulac, 378
Cerebellopontine angle tumors,
    111
Cerebellar tumors, 110
Cerebral angiography
  for brain tumors, 111

  in elevated ICP, 424
  in headaches, 364
  in head injury, 351
  in intracranial aneurysm, 59
  in increased intracranial
    pressure, 424
Cerebral concussion, 351–352
Cerebral contusion, 352
Cerebral edema, 284
Cerebrospinal fluid (CSF) evalua-
    tion, in Guillain-Barré syn-
    drome, 346
Cervical cancer, 157–161
  assessment, 158
  assessment and diagnostic
    findings, 157
  clinical manifestations, 157–158
  complications, 160
  evaluation, patient outcomes,
    161
  medical management, 158
  nursing diagnoses, 159
  nursing interventions, 159–161
  planning/goals, 159
  risk factors, 157
Chemical pleurodesis for pleural
    effusion, 583
Chemotherapy
  for acute myeloid leukemia,
    444–445
  for AIDS, 6
  for bone tumors, 102
  for brain tumors, 111, 112
  for breast cancer, 152
  for bronchogenic carcinoma, 189
  for cancer, 133, 143
  for chronic myeloid leukemia, 447
  for CLL patients, 443
  for gastric cancer, 210
  for Hodgkin lymphoma, 391
  for laryngeal cancer, 176
  for malignant melanoma,
    205–206
  for multiple myeloma, 471, 472
  for non-Hodgkin lymphomas,
    453–454
  for ovarian cancers, 193
  for pancreatic cancer, 195
  for prostate cancer, 199
  for vaginal cancer, 218

Chest pain
  in PE, 611
  in pleural effusion, 582
  in pneumonia, 585–586
  in pulmonary embolism, 611, 615
Chest physiotherapy, 659
  in lung abscess, 449
Chest x-ray
  in heart failure, 368
  in Hodgkin lymphoma, 391
  in lung abscess, 448
Chlamydia trachomatis
  assessment and diagnostic
    findings, 639
  clinical manifestations, 638–639
  complications, 639
  medical management, 639–640
  nursing management, 640
  risk of, 638
Cholelithiasis and cholecystitis,
    233–238
  clinical manifestations, 233–234
  gallstones. See Gallstones
  gerontologic considerations,
    235–236
  nutritional and supportive
    therapy for, 234
  pharmacologic therapy for, 235
  surgical management, 235–236
Cholesteatoma, 455, 512
Christmas disease.
    See Hemophilia B
Chromophobic tumors, 581
Chronic bacterial prostatitis, 596
Chronic gastritis, 331. See also
    Gastritis
  clinical manifestations, 332
  medical management, 333
Chronic glomerulonephritis,
    340–342
  assessment and diagnostic
    findings, 341
  causes, 340
  clinical manifestations, 340
  glomerular damage in, 340
  kidneys in, 340
  medical management, 341
  nursing management, 341–342
  renal insufficiency and chronic
    kidney failure, 340

renal insufficiency and chronic
    renal failure, 340
Chronic kidney failure (CKF),
    626–630
  clinical manifestations, 627
  dialysis, 629
  in elderly people, 628
  nursing management fluid status,
    629
  self-care, 630
  nutritional therapy for, 629
  pharmacologic management,
    628–629
Chronic lymphocytic leukemia
    (CLL), 441–443
  clinical manifestations, 442
  medical management, 442
  pathophysiology, 442
  pharmacologic therapy, 443
Chronic mastoiditis, 455. See also
    Mastoiditis
Chronic myeloid leukemia (CML),
    446–447
  clinical manifestations, 446
  medical management, 446
  pathophysiology, 446
  pharmacologic therapy,
    446–447
  stages, 446
Chronic obstructive pulmonary
    disease (COPD), 113,
    239–244
  and aging, 241
  clinical manifestations, 240
  complications of, 239
  medical management, 241
Chronic otitis media, 512–513
  clinical manifestations, 512
  medical management,
    512–513
  nursing management, 513
Chronic pancreatitis, 519–521
  clinical manifestations, 520
  diabetes mellitus in, 520
  diagnostic methods, 520
  incidence of, 519
  long-term alcohol consumption
    and, 519
  surgery for, 520
  treatment, 520–521

Chronic pharyngitis, 577
Chronic prostatitis/chronic pelvic pain syndrome (CP/CPPS), 596
Chronic pyelonephritis, 618–619
Chronic renal failure (CRF), 626–630
  clinical manifestations, 627
  dialysis, 629
  in elderly people, 628
  nursing management
    fluid status, 629
    self-care, 630
  nutritional therapy for, 629
  pharmacologic management, 628–629
Chronic thyroiditis, 688–689
Chronic ulcers, 534
Chvostek's sign, 413
Cilostazol, 571
Cirrhosis, hepatic, 244–248
  clinical manifestations, 245
  liver function tests, 245
  medical management, 246
  nursing management
    complications, 247
    home- and community-based care, 247–248
    injury risk, 247
    nutritional status, 246
    rest, 246
    skin care, 247
Cirrhosis, hepatitis C and, 385
Clavicle, fracture of, 323–324
CLL. See Chronic lymphocytic leukemia (CLL)
Clonidine suppression test, 579
Closed fracture, 317. See also Fractures
Cluster headaches, 362, 363. See also Headache
CML. See Chronic myeloid leukemia (CML)
Cochlear disease, 459. See also Ménière's disease
Cognitive management
  for multiple sclerosis, 477–478
  for TB, 701
  for traumatic brain injury, 359

Colchicine, in gout, 343
Colles' fracture. See Wrist fractures
Colonoscopy
  for colorectal cancer, 162
  for diverticular disease, 292
  for iron deficiency anemia, 45
  for large bowel obstruction, 104
  for pancreatic cancer, 193
Colorectal cancer, 161–169
  abdominal and rectal examination, 162
  assessment, 164
  CEA studies, 162–163
  clinical manifestations, 162
  collaborative problems/complications, 165
  in elderly people, 163
  evaluation, patient outcomes, 169
  incidence of, 161–162
  medical management, 163
  nursing diagnoses, 164–165
  nursing interventions
    emotional support, 166
    fluid and electrolyte balance, 167
    healthy diet, 166–167
    home- and community-based care, 168
    patient preparation for surgery, 165–166
    planning/goals, 165
  surgical management, 163–164
  survival rates, 162
Coma, 710
Comminuted fractures, 317. See also Fractures
Community-based care
  for ACS, 21–22
  for acute nephritic syndrome, 490–491
  for acute pancreatitis, 518–519
  for Addison's disease, 28
  after mastoid surgery, 458
  for AIDS, 15–16
  for ALS, 34
  for appendicitis, 74
  for asthma, 88–89
  for breast cancer, 156

Community-based care (*continued*)
 for burn injury, 128–129
 for cancer, 140–141
 for cardiomyopathies, 229
 for cataract, 232
 for cervical cancer, 160–161
 for cholelithiasis and cholecystitis, 238
 for chronic kidney failure (CKF), 630
 for chronic renal failure (CRF), 630
 for colorectal cancer, 168
 for COPD, 243–244
 for cystitis (lower UTI), 263
 for diabetes, 277
 for epilepsies, 311–312
 for gastric cancer, 208
 for gastritis, 334
 for glaucoma, 337
 for Guillain-Barré syndrome, 349
 for headache, 366
 for heart failure, 372–373
 for hepatic cirrhosis, 247–248
 for hiatal hernia, 388–389
 for hypertension, 401–402
 for hyperthyroidism, 409
 for hypothyroidism, 418
 for larynx cancer, 181–182
 for leukemia, 438–439
 in multiple myeloma, 472–473
 for multiple sclerosis, 478–479
 for osteomyelitis, 506–507
 for Parkinson's disease, 526–527
 for peptic ulcer, 539–540
 for perioperative nursing, 569
 for peripheral arterial occlusive disease, 572
 for prostate cancer, 203
 for psoriasis, 604–605
 for pulmonary embolism (PE), 616
 for rheumatoid arthritis, 82–83
 for sickle cell anemia, 54
 for traumatic brain injury, 360
 for ulcerative colitis, 709
 for vulvar cancer, 221
Compartment syndrome, fractures and, 320–322

Complete fracture, 317. *See also* Fractures
Complex regional pain syndrome (CRPS), 321, 322
Compression therapy, 727
Computed tomography (CT)
 in acute kidney failure, 623
 in acute pancreatitis, 515
 in acute renal failure, 623
 in chronic glomerulonephritis, 341
 in chronic pancreatitis, 520
 in diffuse axonal injury, 353
 in elevated ICP, 424
 in headaches, 364
 in head injury, 351
 in hiatal hernia, 387
 in Hodgkin lymphoma, 391
 in lung abscess, 448
 in meningitis, 463
 in non-Hodgkin lymphomas, 453
 in Parkinson's disease, 522
 in pericarditis, 541
 in pheochromocytoma, 579
 in pituitary tumors, 581
 in pulmonary embolism, 612
 in spinal cord injury, 655
 in ulcerative colitis, 703
Concussion, 351–352
 grades of, 352
 mechanism of injury, 351–352
 nursing management, 352
Congenital lymphedema, 450.
 See also Lymphedema
Congestive HF. *See* Heart failure (HF)
Conjunctival retraction, 693
Constipation, 248–250
 in appendicitis, 72
 causes, 248
 clinical manifestations, 249
 diagnosis, 249
 in diverticular disease, 292, 294
 and headache, 362
 in large bowel obstruction, 104
 medical management, 250
 in multiple sclerosis, 477
 nursing management, 250

Constipation, in Parkinson's disease, 522
Constructional apraxia, 377
Contact dermatitis, 264–265
  clinical manifestations, 264
  medical management, 264
  nursing management, 265
Continuing care
  for ACS, 22
  for acute nephritic syndrome, 490–491
  for acute pancreatitis, 519
  for Addison's disease, 28
  after bariatric surgery, 498
  for asthma, 89
  for breast cancer, 156
  for cancer, 140–141
  for cardiomyopathies, 229
  for cataract, 232
  for cervical cancer, 161
  for chronic kidney failure (CKF), 630
  for chronic renal failure (CRF), 630
  for colorectal cancer, 168
  for COPD, 244
  for diabetes, 277
  for epilepsies, 312
  for heart failure, 372–373
  for hiatal hernia, 389
  for hypertension, 402
  for hyperthyroidism, 409–410
  for hypothyroidism, 418
  for larynx cancer, 182
  for leukemia, 439
  for lung abscess, 450
  for multiple myeloma, 472–473
  for multiple sclerosis, 478–479
  for osteomyelitis, 507
  for Parkinson's disease, 527
  for peptic ulcer, 540
  for prostate cancer, 203
  for rheumatoid arthritis, 82–83
  for ulcerative colitis, 709
  for vulvar cancer, 221
Contusion, 481. See also Musculoskeletal trauma
Contusions, 352
Coping management
  in psoriasis, 604
  in ulcerative colitis, 708

Corneal integrity in unconscious patient, 714
Coronary artery disease (CAD)
  and acute coronary syndrome, 17
  and diabetes mellitus, 267
  and hypertension, 398
  and ischemic cardiomyopathy, 223
Coronary atherosclerosis and CAD, 251–252
  clinical manifestations, 251–252
  prevention, CHD, 252
  risk factors, 251
Coronary heart disease (CHD)
  prevention, 252
  risk factors, 252
Coronary bypass surgery, 368
Cortical spreading depression (CSD), 362
Corticosteroids
  in elevated ICP, 425
  in gout, 344
  in immune thrombocytopenic purpura, 420
  in multiple myeloma, 472
  in myasthenia gravis, 485
  in osteoarthritis, 502
  in pemphigus, 531
  in pericarditis, 542
  in SLE, 682
Cotton tampon, use of, in epistaxis, 313
Cough
  in acquired immunodeficiency syndrome, 2
  in chronic pharyngitis, 577
  lung abscess and, 448
  in pericarditis, 541
  in pleurisy, 584
  in pneumonia, 585–586
  rib fractures and, 330
  in spinal cord injury, 656
  in TB, 699, 701
Cranial arteritis, 362–364
Crepitus, 318
Crohn's disease, 252–254
  assessment and diagnostic findings, 253–254
  clinical manifestations, 253
  pathophysiology, 253

Cryptococcal meningitis, 5
Cryptococcus neoformans, 3, 642
CT. *See* Computed tomography
(CT)
Cushing's response, 424
Cushing syndrome, 254–259
assessment, 256
causes of, 254
clinical manifestations, 254–255
collaborative problems, 257
diagnostic findings, 255
evaluation, patient outcomes,
259
medical management, 255–256
nursing diagnoses, 256–257
nursing interventions in
body image, 258
patient education, 258–259
rest and activity, 257
risk of injury and infection,
257
skin integrity, 257
planning/goals, 256
Cushing's triad, 424
Cyanosis
in pneumothorax, 593
in Raynaud's phenomenon,
620
Cyclo-oxygenase 2 (COX-2)
enzyme blockers, in osteoarthritis, 502
Cystitis (lower UTI), 259–263
assessment, 256
clinical manifestations, 260
collaborative problems, 252
in elderly patients, 260
evaluation, patient outcomes,
263
nursing diagnoses, 262
nursing interventions
home- and community-based
care, 263
pain management, 262–263
pharmacologic therapy for
acute/long-term, 261
patient education and, 261
planning/goals, 262
Cystine stones, 718
Cytomegalovirus retinitis, 5–6
Cytoprotective agents, 536

D
DAI. *See* Diffuse axonal injury
(DAI)
Danazol, in endometriosis, 303
DASH diet, 399
Decongestant agent, use of, in
epistaxis, 313
Deep vein thrombosis, 561, 723
endovascular management, 725
symptoms, 657
Degenerative joint disease. *See*
Osteoarthritis (OA)
Dehydration
and acute kidney failure, 623
and acute renal failure, 623
and hyperglycemic hyperosmolar
syndrome, 395
and hypovolemic shock, 647
Dementia, and Parkinson's disease,
522
Depression
in AIDS, 3–4
in multiple sclerosis, 474
in Parkinson's disease, 522
Dermatitis
contact (*see* Contact dermatitis)
exfoliative (*see* Exfoliative
dermatitis)
Desmopressin, in hemophilia,
374–375
Dexamethasone, in meningitis,
464
Diabetes insipidus, elevated ICP
and, 425
Dialysis, 624
in chronic glomerulonephritis,
341
Diarrhea
in peptic ulcer, 535
in ulcerative colitis, 705
in urolithiasis, 717
Diabetes insipidus, 278–279
assessment and diagnostic
methods, 278–279
causes of, 278
clinical manifestations, 278
fluid deprivation test, 278–279
nursing management, 279
Diabetes mellitus, 267–277
acute complications of, 267, 270

assessment and diagnostic
   methods, 269–270
chronic complications of, 270
in elderly patients, 270
gestational, 269
medical management, 271
nursing management
   continuing care, 277
   patient education, 273–277
   self-care, 277
nutritional management,
   271–272
prevention, 270
type 1, 268
type 2, 268–269
Diabetic ketoacidosis (DKA),
   279–285
assessment and diagnostic
   findings, 280
causes of, 280
medical management
   acidosis, 281
   dehydration, 281
   electrolyte loss, 281
signs and symptoms of, 256,
   264
Diarrhea, 285–288
assessment and diagnostic
   findings, 286
in Addison's disease, 26
in AIDS, 2, 6, 7, 9, 10
causes of, 285
clinical manifestations, 285–286
complications of, 286
medical management, 286–287
nursing management, 287
types of, 285
DIC. *See* Disseminated intravascular coagulation (DIC)
Dietary management, in peptic
   ulcer, 536–537
Diffuse axonal injury (DAI),
   352–353
Disseminated intravascular coagulation (DIC), 288–291, 321
assessment and diagnostic
   findings, 289
clinical manifestations,
   288–289
diagnosis, 289

medical management
   heparin infusion, 289
   tissue ischemia, 289
nursing management
   fear and anxiety, 291
   fluid volume, 290
   hemodynamic status, 290
   skin integrity, 290
   tissue perfusion, 290–291
pathophysiology of, 288
Diuretics
in lymphedema, 451
in Ménière's disease, 460
in nephrotic syndrome, 492
Diverticular disease, 291–295
assessment and diagnostic
   findings, 292
clinical manifestations, 292
congenital predisposition, 291
dietary and pharmacologic
   management, 292–293
gerontologic considerations, 292
surgical resection of, 293
Diverticulitis
assessment, 293
clinical manifestations, 292
collaborative problems in, 294
dietary and pharmacologic
   management of, 292–293
evaluation, patient outcomes,
   295
nursing diagnoses, 294
nursing interventions, elimination patterns, 294
pain management, 294
for potential complications,
   294–295
planning/goals, 294
Diverticulosis, 291
clinical manifestations, 292
Dizziness
in pericarditis, 543
in pheochromocytoma, 578
in polycythemia vera, 595
Dopamine levels and Parkinson's
   disease, 521
Dual-energy x-ray absorptiometry
   (DEXA), in osteoporosis,
   508
Dural meningioma, 109

Dyspnea
  in PE, 611
  in pleural effusion, 582
  in pulmonary arterial
      hypertension, 606
  in pulmonary embolism, 610
Dysrhythmias
  in cardiogenic shock, 645
  in pulmonary embolism, 613

E
Echocardiography
  in heart failure, 368
  in mitral regurgitation, 465
  in mitral stenosis, 467
  in mitral valve prolapse, 468
Eczema. *See* Contact dermatitis
Edema
  in end-stage kidney disease, 627
  in end-stage renal disease, 627
  nephrotic syndrome and, 491
  in peritonitis, 572
  pulmonary, 608–610
Edrophonium injection
  in myasthenia gravis, 484
Elbow fractures, 324–325
Electrocardiography (ECG)
  in cardiogenic shock, 646
  in chronic glomerulonephritis,
      341
  in heart failure, 368
  in hyperglycemic hyperosmolar
      syndrome, 395
  in mitral stenosis, 467
  in pericarditis, 541
Electroencephalograms (EEGs)
  in epilepsies, 308
  in hepatic encephalopathy, 378
Electroencephalography
  in seizure, 634
Electrolyte management
  in ARF, 625
  in pemphigus, 533
Electromyography (EMG)
  in headaches, 364
  in myasthenia gravis, 484
Electronystagmogram, in Ménière's
      disease, 459
Elephantiasis, 451. *See also*
      Lymphedema

Elimination patterns, normal
  in ulcerative colitis, 706
Embolism
  pulmonary, 610–616
  in spinal cord injury, 657
Emergency thoracotomy, 594
Emotional support
  in chronic glomerulonephritis, 341
  in end-stage kidney disease, 630
  in end-stage renal disease, 630
  in perioperative nursing
      management, 567
Empyema, 296–297
  assessment and diagnostic
      findings, 296
  clinical manifestations, 296
  medical management, 296–297
  nursing management, 297
Endocarditis
  infective, 297–301 (*see also*
      Infective endocarditis)
  rheumatic, 301–302 (*see also*
      Rheumatic endocarditis)
Endolymphatic hydrops, 458
Endometrial cancer, 169–170
  assessment and diagnostic
      findings, 170
  clinical manifestations, 170
  medical management, 170
  pathophysiology, 169
Endometriosis, 302–304
  assessment and diagnostic
      findings, 303
  clinical manifestations, 303
  incidence, 302
  medical management, 303
  nursing management, 304
  pathophysiology, 302–303
  pharmacologic therapy, 303
  surgical management, 304
Endoscopy
  for chronic pancreatitis, 520
  for gastritis, 332
  for peptic ulcer, 536
End-stage kidney disease, 626–630
Enzyme immunoassay, 4
Eosinophilic tumors, 581
Epididymectomy, 305
  in epididymitis, 305
Epididymitis, 304–306

assessment and diagnostic
findings, 305
clinical manifestations, 305
incidence and prevalence, 304
medical management, 305
nursing management, 306
pathophysiology, 305
risk factors, 304
sexually transmitted infections
and, 305
Epidural hematoma, 353
Epilepsies, 306–312
assessment and diagnostic
findings, 308
clinical manifestations, 307
complex partial seizures, 307
generalized seizures, 307
gerontologic considerations, 308
medical management, 308
nursing process, 309–312
assessment, 309
diagnosis, 309
evaluation, 312
nursing interventions,
309–312
planning and goals, 309
pathophysiology, 306–307
pharmacologic therapy, 308
postictal state, 307
primary, 306
secondary, 306
simple partial seizures, 307
status epilepticus, 310
surgical management, 308–309
Epistaxis, 312–314
medical management, 312–313
nursing management, 313
risk factors, 312
self-care in, education for,
313–314
Epsilon aminocaproic acid
(EACA)
in immune thrombocytopenic
purpura, 420
Ergotamine preparations, in
headaches, 365
Erythema, in toxic epidermal
necrolysis, 689
Erythroderma. *See* Exfoliative
dermatitis

Escherichia coli
and epididymitis, 305
and peritonitis, 573
Esophageal cancer, 170–172
assessment and diagnostic
findings, 171
clinical manifestations, 171
medical management, 171
nursing management, 171–172
risk factors, 170–171
Esophageal varices, bleeding,
314–316
assessment and diagnostic
findings, 314
clinical manifestations, 314
medical management, 314–315
nonsurgical treatment, 315
nursing management, 315–316
pharmacologic therapy, 315
risk factors, 314
surgical management, 315
Evoked potential studies, in
Guillain-Barré syndrome,
346
Excisional lymph node biopsy, in
Hodgkin lymphoma, 391
Exercise management
in fractures, 319
for muscular dystrophies, 480
in peripheral arterial occlusive
disease, 571
in vein disorders, 727
Exercise testing, in mitral stenosis,
467
Exfoliative dermatitis, 265–267
assessment and diagnostic
findings, 266
causes, 265
clinical manifestations, 265–266
medical management, 266
nursing management, 267

F

Family and patient education
in chronic glomerulonephritis,
341–342
in hemophilia, 375–376
in hepatitis B, 384
in hypoglycemia, 412
Fasciotomy, 322

Fat embolism syndrome (FES), fractures and, 322
Femoral shaft fractures, 328–329
Fetor hepaticus, 377
Fever
  in acquired immunodeficiency syndrome, 2
  in infective endocarditis, 298
  lung abscess and, 448
  in meningitis, 462
Fiberoptic endoscopy, in gastritis, 333
Fingolimod (FTY720), in multiple sclerosis, 475
Flash pulmonary edema, 608
Fluid balance management
  in acute pancreatitis, 518
  in ARF, 624, 625
  in gastritis, 334
  in heart failure, 370–371
  in hypovolemic shock, 648
  in Ménière's disease, 460
  in pemphigus, 533
  in toxic epidermal necrolysis, 692
  in traumatic brain injury, 358
  in unconscious patient, 713
Fluid intake
  in perioperative nursing, 551
  in ulcerative colitis, 707
Fluid redistribution, 648
Focal seizures, 632
Follicular Lymphoma International Prognostic Index (FLIPI), 453
Fowler's position
  in pancreatitis, 517
  in perioperative nursing management, 568
  in pneumonia, 589
  in pulmonary embolism, 615
Fractures, 317–330
  of acetabulum, 327
  assessment and diagnostic findings, 318
  avascular necrosis (AVN) of bone and, 321
  of clavicle, 323–324
  clinical manifestations, 318
  compartment syndrome and, 320–321

complex regional pain syndrome and, 321
complications, 319–321
  management of, 321–323
definition, 317
and delayed union, 321
disseminated intravascular coagulation and, 321
of elbow, 324–325
emergency management, 318
fat embolism syndrome and, 320
femoral shaft, 328–329
gerontologic considerations, 328
of hand and fingers, 326
of hip, 328
of humeral neck, 324
hypovolemic shock and, 320
immobilization, 319
infections and, 321
maintaining and restoring function, 319
and malunion, 321
nursing management
  closed fractures, 323
  open fractures, 323
  at specific sites, 323–328
pathophysiology, 317
of pelvis, 326–327
of radial and ulnar shaft, 325
of radial head, 325
reduction of, 318
  closed reduction, 319
  open reduction, 319
rib, 330
of thoracolumbar spine, 330
tibia and fibula, 329–330
types, 317
of wrist, 325–326
Fulminant hepatic failure, 379–380
  categories, 379
  causes, 380
  clinical manifestations, 380
  medical management, 380
  nursing management, 380

G

Gait problems, 522
Gastric banding, 493–494. *See also* Bariatric surgery

Gastric cancers, 208–213
  assessment and diagnostic
      findings, 209
  clinical manifestations, 209
  gerontologic considerations,
      210
  medical management, 209–210
  nursing process, 210–213
    assessment, 210–211
    diagnosis, 211
    evaluation, 213
    interventions, 211–213
    planning and goals, 211
  pathophysiology, 209
Gastritis, 331–334
  acute, 331
  assessment and diagnostic
      findings, 332
  chronic, 331
  clinical manifestations, 332
  erosive, 331
  medical management, 332–333
  nonerosive, 331
  nursing management, 333–334
    anxiety, 333
    fluid balance, 334
    home- and community-based
        care, 334
    nutrition, 333–334
    pain, 334
  pathophysiology, 331–332
Gastrointestinal disorder
  hemorrhage, 685
  inflammation
    in ulcerative colitis, 705
GBS. See Guillain-Barré syndrome
      (GBS)
GB virus-C (GBV-C), 386
Generalized seizures, 632
Genetic counseling, in muscular
      dystrophies, 480
Gentamicin injection, in Ménière's
      disease, 460
Gerontologic considerations. See
      also Olders adults
  in acute pancreatitis, 515
  in perioperative nursing
      management, 545, 548, 554,
      557–558, 568–569
  in pneumonia, 587

  in pulmonary tuberculosis, 699
  in septic shock, 652
Glasgow Coma Scale (GCS),
      355
  for unconscious patient, 711
Glatiramer acetate, in multiple
      sclerosis, 475
Glaucoma, 335–337
  assessment and diagnostic
      findings, 336
  clinical manifestations,
      335–336
  medical management, 336
  nursing management, 337
  pathophysiology, 335
  pharmacologic therapy,
      336–337
  surgical management, 337
  types of, 335
Gliomas, 109
Glomerulonephritis, 338
  acute, 338–339 (see also Acute
      glomerulonephritis)
  and acute nephritic syndrome,
      338
  chronic, 340–342 (see also
      Chronic glomerulonephritis)
GnRH agonists, in endometriosis,
      303
Gout, 342–344
  assessment and diagnostic
      findings, 343
  clinical manifestations, 343
  medical management, 343–344
  nursing management, 344
  pathophysiology, 342–343
  primary hyperuricemia and,
      344
  secondary hyperuricemia and,
      344–345
  uric acid deposits in, 342, 343
Gram-negative organisms
  and pneumonia, 585
  and septic shock, 650
Gram-positive organisms, and sep-
      tic shock, 650
Graves' disease. See
      Hyperthyroidism
Greenstick fracture, 317. See also
      Fractures

Guillain-Barré syndrome (GBS),
344–349
assessment and diagnostic
findings, 345–346
clinical manifestations, 345
medical management, 346
nursing interventions, 347–349
communication, 348
fear and anxiety, 348
home- and community-based
care, 348–349
nutrition, 348
physical mobility, 347–348
potential complications,
348–349
respiratory function, 347
nursing process, 346–349
assessment, 346
diagnosis, 347
evaluation, 349
interventions, 347–349
planning and goals, 347
pathophysiology, 345
pharmacologic therapy, 346

H

Hashimoto's thyroiditis. *See*
Chronic thyroiditis
HD. *See* Huntington disease (HD)
Head injury, 350–361
assessment and diagnostic
findings, 351
clinical manifestations, 350–351
concussion after, 351–352
contusions, 352
diffuse axonal injury, 352–353
and elevated ICP, 423
epidural hematoma, 353
intracerebral hemorrhage and
hematoma, 354
intracranial hemorrhage, 353
medical management, 351
nursing management, 352
nursing process, 355–361
scalp and skull injuries, 351
subdural hematoma, 353–354
traumatic brain injury, 350
(*see also* Traumatic brain
injury (TBI))
Headache, 361–366

acute attack, management of,
365
assessment and diagnostic
findings, 364
brain tumors and, 110
clinical manifestations, 362–364
cluster, 362, 363
cranial arteritis, 362–364
home- and community-based
care, 366
medical management, 364–365
in meningitis, 462
migraine, 361–362 (*see also*
Migraine)
nursing management, 365–366
pathophysiology, 361–362
pharmacologic therapy,
364–365
primary, 361
secondary, 361
tension, 362, 363
Hearing and communication
after mastoid surgery, 457
Heart failure (HF), 367–373
assessment and diagnostic
findings, 368
clinical manifestations, 367
left-sided, 367
medical management, 368
nursing interventions,
370–373
activity tolerance, 370
anxiety control, 371
fatigue reduction, 370
fluid volume, 370–371
home- and community-based
care, 372–373
potential problems, 372
sense of powerlessness, 372
nursing process, 369–373
assessment, 369
diagnosis, 369
evaluation, 373
interventions, 370–373
planning and goals, 370
pharmacologic therapy, 368
right-sided, 368
surgical management, 368
Helicobacter pylori
and peptic ulcer, 534

Helicobacter pylori infection
  and gastritis, 331
  immune thrombocytopenic
    purpura and, 420
Hematomas, 353
  in aortic aneurysm, 592
  in brain injury, 353–354
  epidural, 353
  intracerebral, 354
  in perioperative nursing
    management, 592
  subdura, 353–354
Hematopoietic stem cell
    transplantation (HSCT)
  in acute myeloid leukemia, 445
  in chronic myeloid leukemia, 447
  in non-Hodgkin lymphomas, 453
Hematuria
  and pyuria, 717
  and urolithiasis, 721
Hemodynamic status, in spinal
    cord injury, 653
Hemophilia, 373–376
  assessment and diagnostic
    findings, 374
  clinical manifestations, 374
  gerontologic considerations, 376
  hemophilia A, 373
  hemophilia B, 373
  medical management, 374–375
  nursing management, 375–376
Hemophilia A, 373
Hemophilia B, 373
Hemopneumothorax, 591
Hemorrhagic stroke, 662–668
  assessment, 665–666
  assessment and diagnostic
    findings, 664
  clinical manifestations,
    663–664
  collaborative problems/potential
    complications, 666
  community-based care, 668
  complications of, 664
  continuing care, 668
  evaluation, patient outcomes,
    668
  home care, 668
  medical management, 664–665
  nursing diagnoses, 666

  nursing interventions
    anxiety reduction, 667
    cerebral tissue perfusion,
      666–667
    hyponatremia, 668
    potential complications,
      667–668
  pathophysiology of, 663
  patient education, 668
  pharmacologic therapy, 665
  planning and goals, 666
  prevention, 664
  risk factors
    modifiable/treatable, 663
    nonmodifiable, 663
  self-care, 668
  surgical management, 665
Hemothorax, 591–593
Heparin-induced thrombocytope-
    nia, 726
Heparin therapy, for vein disorders,
    725
Hepatic encephalopathy
  ammonia in, role of, 377
  assessment and diagnostic
    findings, 378
  causes, 377
  clinical manifestations, 377
  and hepatic coma, 377–379
  medical management, 378
  nursing management, 378–379
Hepatic failure, fulminant. *See*
    Fulminant hepatic failure
Hepatitis A, 380–382
  assessment and diagnostic
    findings, 381
  causative virus, 380–381
  clinical manifestations, 381
  nursing management, 382
  prevention, 380–381
  recovery from, 381
Hepatitis B, 382–385
  assessment and diagnostic
    findings, 383
  causative virus, 382
  clinical manifestations, 383
  gerontologic considerations, 382
  medical management, 384
  nursing management, 384–385
  prevention, 383–384

Hepatitis C, 385
  risk factors, 385
  triple therapy for, 385
Hepatitis D, 385
Hepatitis E, 385–386
Hepatitis G virus (HGV), 386
Hepatocellular carcinoma (HCC),
  183
Hepsera. See Adefovir
Herniation syndrome, 353
HF. See Heart failure (HF)
HHS. See Hyperglycemic hyperosmolar syndrome (HHS)
Hiatal hernia, 386–389
  assessment and diagnostic
    findings, 387
  clinical manifestations, 386–387
  esophageal condition and reflux
    in, 387–389
    aspiration risk, decreasing, 388
    assessment of, 387
    evaluation, 389
    home- and community-based
      care, 388–389
    nursing diagnoses, 387
    nutritional intake in, 388
    pain management, 388
    planning/goals, 388
  medical management, 387
  paraesophageal, 386–387
  sliding, 386
  surgical management, 387
Hip fractures, 328
  in older adults, 328
HIV encephalopathy, 3
HIV-related peripheral neuropathy, 3
Hodgkin lymphoma, 389–392
  assessment and diagnostic
    findings, 391
  clinical manifestations, 390–391
  medical management, 391
  mixed cellularity subgroup, 390
  nodular sclerosis type, 390
  nursing management, 392
  pathophysiology, 389–390
Hodgkin's disease. See Hodgkin
  lymphoma
Home care
  for acute nephritic syndrome,
    490–491

for acute pancreatitis, 518–519
after mastoid surgery, 458
for chronic kidney failure (CKF),
  630
for chronic renal failure (CRF),
  630
for gastritis, 334
for glaucoma, 337
Guillain-Barré syndrome, 349
for headache, 366
for heart failure, 372–373
in hiatal hernia, 388–389
in hyperthyroidism, 409
in hypothyroidism, 418
for leukemia, 438–439
for multiple myeloma, 472–473
in Parkinson's disease, 525–527
for peptic ulcer, 539–540
for perioperative nursing, 569
for peripheral arterial occlusive
  disease, 572
for peripheral arterial occlusive
  disease, 572
for psoriasis, 604–605
for pulmonary embolism (PE),
  616
in traumatic brain injury, 360
for ulcerative colitis, 709
Hormone therapy, thyroid, 689
H2-receptor antagonists, 536
HSCT. See Hematopoietic stem
  cell transplantation (HSCT)
Human immunodeficiency virus
  (HIV) infection, 1. See also
  Acquired immunodeficiency
  syndrome (AIDS)
Humeral neck, fracture of, 324
Humidified oxygen, 686
Huntingtin, 393
Huntington disease (HD),
  392–394
  assessment and diagnostic
    findings, 393
  clinical manifestations, 392–393
  medical management, 393
  nursing management, 394
Hydrocortisone, 686
  in hypothyroidism, 417
Hypercalcemia, in peptic ulcer,
  534

Hyperglycemic hyperosmolar
    syndrome (HHS), 394–396
  assessment and diagnostic
      findings, 395
  causes, 394
  clinical manifestations, 395
  medical management, 395
  nursing management, 395–396
  pathophysiology, 394–395
Hyperlipidemia
  in acute pancreatitis, 514
  in end-stage kidney disease, 626
  in end-stage renal disease, 626
Hypertension
  assessment and diagnostic
      findings, 398–399
  classification, 396
  clinical manifestations, 398
  definition, 396
  gerontologic considerations,
      398–400
  home- and community-based
      care, 401–402
  and hypertensive crisis,
      396–403
  medical management, 399
  nursing process, 400–403
    assessment, 400
    diagnosis, 400–401
    evaluation, 403
    interventions, 401–403
    older adults, and medication
        regimen, 402
    planning and goals, 401
  pathophysiology, 397–398
  pharmacologic therapy, 399
  prehypertension, 396
  primary, 396
  secondary, 396
Hypertensive emergency, 396, 397.
      See also Hypertension
Hypertensive urgency, 396, 397.
      See also Hypertension
Hyperthyroidism, 403–410
  assessment and diagnostic
      findings, 404–405
  causes, 404
  clinical manifestations, 404
  gerontologic considerations,
      406

  medical management, 405–406
    adjunctive therapy, 406
    antithyroid medications, 405
    radioactive iodine, 405
  nursing interventions
    body temperature, 408
    coping measures, 408
    home- and community-based
        care, 409–410
    nutrition, 407–408
    potential complications, 409
    self-esteem, improving, 408
  nursing process, 407–410
    assessment, 407
    diagnosis, 407
    evaluation, 410
    interventions, 407–410
    planning and goals, 407
  surgical management, 406
  in thyroid storm, 686
Hypocalcemia
  in acute pancreatitis, 515
  in cardiogenic shock, 645
Hypoglycemia, 410–412
  assessment and diagnostic
      findings, 411
  clinical manifestations, 411
  definition, 410
  gerontologic considerations,
      410–411
  late afternoon, 410
  medical management, 411–412
    in conscious patient, 411–412
    in unconscious patient, 412
  middle-of-the-night, 410
  midmorning, 410
  mild, 411
  moderate, 411
  nursing management, 412
  pathophysiology, 410
  severe, 411
Hypokinesia in Parkinson's
      disease, 522
Hypoparathyroidism, 413–414
  assessment and diagnostic
      findings, 413
  clinical manifestations, 413
  medical management, 413–414
  nursing management, 414
Hypopituitarism, 414–415

Hyporeflexia
in Guillain-Barré syndrome, 345
Hypotension, in PE, 612
Hypothermia, in hypothyroidism, 416
Hypothermia prevention, in toxic epidermal necrolysis, 692–693
Hypothyroidism, 415–418
causes, 415
central, 415
clinical manifestations, 416
cretinism, 416
gerontologic considerations, 416
hypothalamic, 415
medical management, 417
medication interactions, prevention of, 417
myxedema, 415
nursing management, 418
pharmacologic therapy, 417
primary, 415
secondary, 415
Hypovolemic shock, 320–322, 647–649
causes of, 647
clinical manifestations, 647
medical management, 647–648
nursing management, 648–649
pharmacologic therapy for, 648

I

Idiopathic thrombocytopenic purpura. See Immune thrombocytopenic purpura (ITP)
Immune globulin vaccination, hepatitis A and, 381
Immune thrombocytopenia. See Immune thrombocytopenic purpura (ITP)
Immune thrombocytopenic purpura (ITP), 419–421
assessment and diagnostic findings, 419–420
causes, 419
clinical manifestations, 419
medical management, 420
nursing management, 420–421
pathophysiology, 419
pharmacologic therapy, 420

primary, 419
secondary, 419
Immunosuppressive therapy
in immune thrombocytopenic purpura, 420
in myasthenia gravis, 485
for pemphigus, 531
for SLE, 682
Impetigo, 421–423
clinical manifestations, 421–422
medical management, 422–423
nursing management, 423
pathophysiology, 422
pharmacologic therapy, 422–423
Increased intracranial pressure (ICP). See Intracranial pressure (ICP), increased
Infection prevention
after bariatric surgery, 496
in AIDS, 11
in ARF, 626
in mastoid surgery, 457
in osteomyelitis, 506
Infective endocarditis, 297–301
assessment and diagnostic findings, 299
clinical manifestations, 298–299
medical management, 300
nursing management, 301
pathophysiology, 298
patient populations at risk of, 297–298
prevention, 299–300
surgical management, 300–301
Influenza, 429–430
management, 430
prevention, 429–430
Informed consent, 549–550
Injury prevention
after mastoid surgery, 457
in Ménière's disease, 460
in multiple sclerosis, 477
in osteoporosis, 510
Insulin reaction. See Hypoglycemia
Integumentary system, 681
Intercostal nerve block, 584
Interferon alpha

in hepatitis D viral infection, 385
in Kaposi's sarcoma, 432
Interferon beta-1a, in multiple sclerosis, 475
Interferon beta-1b, in multiple sclerosis, 475
Internal fixation devices, 319
The International League Against Epilepsy (ILAE), 632
International Prognostic Index (IPI), 453
Intestinal decompression, 656
Intra-aortic balloon counterpulsation, 647
Intra-articular fracture, 317. *See also* Fractures
Intracerebral hematoma, 354
Intracranial pressure (ICP), increased, 423–429
  assessment and diagnostic findings, 424
  clinical manifestations, 424
  complications, 425
  medical management, 425
  nursing interventions
    breathing pattern, 427
    cerebral tissue perfusion, 427
    infection prevention, 428
    negative fluid balance, 427–428
    patent airway maintenance, 426
    potential complications, 428–429
  nursing process, 425–429
    assessment, 425–426
    diagnosis, 426
    evaluation, 429
    interventions, 426–429
    planning and goals, 426
  pathophysiology, 423
  pharmacologic therapy, 425
Intraocular pressure (IOP), in glaucoma, 335
Intravenous gamma globulin
  in immune thrombocytopenic purpura, 420
Intravenous immunoglobulin (IVIG)
  in Guillain-Barré syndrome, 346

in myasthenia gravis, 485
for toxic epidermal necrolysis, 691
Ischemic stroke, 669–679
  acute phase, 672–673
  assessment, 672–673
  assessment and diagnostic findings, 671
  clinical manifestations
    cognitive impairment and psychological effects, 670–671
    communication loss, 670
    disturbances and sensory loss, 670
    motor loss, 670
  collaborative problems/potential complications, 674
  complications, 672
  evaluation, patient outcomes, 679
  home- and community-based care
    continuing care, 679
    self-care, 678
  medical management, 671
  nursing diagnoses, 673
  nursing interventions
    ambulation, 675
    bladder and bowel control, 677
    communication, 677
    discomfort, 676
    exercise program, 674–675
    family support, 678
    mobility and joint deformities prevention, 674
    nutrition, 676–677
    self-care, 675–676
    sensory-perceptual difficulties, 676
    sexual dysfunction, 678
    shoulder pain prevention, 675
    skin integrity, 678
    structured training program, 677
  pathophysiology, 669
  pharmacologic therapy, 671
  planning and goals, 674
  postacute phase, 673
  prevention, 671
  risk factors
    modifiable or treatable, 669–670
    nonmodifiable, 669
  surgical management, 672

ITP. *See* Immune thrombocytopenic purpura (ITP)
IV glucose,
  in hepatic encephalopathy, 378

J

Janeway lesions in infective endocarditis, 298
Jaundice
  in cholelithiasis, 234
  in fulminant hepatic failure, 379, 380
  in hepatic cirrhosis, 245, 246
  in hepatitis A, 381, 382
  in hepatitis E, 386
  in Hodgkin lymphoma, 390
  in liver cancer, 183
  in megaloblastic anemia, 47
  in pancreatic cancer, 194, 195
  in sickle cell anemia, 50
Joint arthroplasty, 502
Joint dislocations, 481–482. *See also* Musculoskeletal trauma
Joint integrity in unconscious patient, 714

K

Kaposi's sarcoma (KS), 2, 431–432
  in AIDS patients, 431
  assessment and diagnostic findings, 431
  clinical manifestations, 431
  medical management, 431–432
  nursing management, 432
  pharmacologic therapy, 432
Kernig's sign, in meningitis, 462
Kidney biopsy
  in glomerulonephritis, 338
  in nephritic syndrome, 489
  in nephrotic syndrome, 491
Kidney cancer, 173–175
  assessment and diagnostic findings, 173
  clinical manifestations, 173
  medical management, 173–174
  nursing management, 174–175.
    See also Renal cancer
Kidney stones
  assessment, 719

collaborative problems/ complications, 720
diagnosis, 719
evaluation, patient outcomes, 722
nursing interventions
  continuing care, 721–722
  fluid intake and ambulation, 720
  home care, 721
  pain management, 720
  self-care, 720–721
Klebsiella species, 531
KS. *See* Kaposi's sarcoma (KS)

L

Laboratory studies
  in acute myeloid leukemia, 444
  in headaches, 364
  in heart failure, 368
  in hemophilia, 374
  in Hodgkin lymphoma, 391
  in hyperglycemic hyperosmolar syndrome, 395
  in hypertension, 399
  in hypoparathyroidism, 413
  in osteomalacia, 503
  in osteoporosis, 508
Lactulose (Cephulac)
  in hepatic encephalopathy, 378
Lamivudine (Epivir), in hepatitis B, 384
Laparoscopy, for endometriosis, 303
Laryngeal cancer, 175–182
  assessment and diagnostic findings, 176
  clinical manifestations, 175
  laryngectomy, 177–182
  medical management, 176
  surgical management, 176–177
Laryngectomy, 177–182
  assessment, 177
  diagnosis, 177–178
  evaluation, 182
  gerontologic considerations, 181
  home- and community-based care, 181–182
  nursing interventions, 178–181
  planning and goals, 178

Laser surgery, for endometriosis, 303
Laser trabeculoplasty, for glaucoma, 337
Latent tetany, 413
Lentigo-maligna melanoma, 205
Lesions
  in ulcerative colitis, 702
  uremic GI, 622
Leukemia, 433–439
  acute lymphocytic (*see* Acute lymphocytic leukemia (ALL))
  acute myeloid (*see* Acute myeloid leukemia (AML))
  assessment and diagnostic findings, 434
  chronic lymphocytic (*see* Chronic lymphocytic leukemia (CLL))
  chronic myeloid (*see* Chronic myeloid leukemia (CML))
  classification, 433
  clinical manifestations, 433
  nursing interventions, 435–439
    anxiety and grief management, 438
    bleeding prevention, 435
    continuing care, 439
    fatigue reduction, 437–438
    fluid and electrolyte balance, 438
    infection prevention, 435–436
    mucositis management, 436
    nutritional intake, 437
    pain management, 437
    self-care, 438–439
    spiritual and religious practices, 438
    terminal care, 439
  nursing process, 434–439
    assessment, 434
    diagnosis, 434–435
    evaluation, 436
    interventions, 435–439
    planning and goals, 435
  pathophysiology, 433
Level of consciousness (LOC), altered, in brain injury, 351
Lifestyle modifications
  in hypertension, 399
  for obesity treatment, 499

Lifestyle recommendations, in heart failure, 368
Liver cancer, 183–186
  assessment and diagnostic findings, 183–184
  clinical manifestations, 183
  medical management, 184
  nursing management, 185–186
  surgical management, 185
Liver cancer, hepatitis C and, 385
Liver function tests
  for bleeding esophageal varices, 315
Liver transplantation, in fulminant hepatic failure, 380
Locked-in syndrome, 710
Lorcaserin (Belviq)
  in obesity treatment, 500
Lung abscess, 447–450
  assessment and diagnostic findings, 449
  clinical manifestations, 448
  continuing care, 449–450
  home- and community-based care, 449–450
  medical management, 449
  nursing management, 449
  organisms associated with, 448
  pathophysiology, 448
  self-care, 449–450
Lymphadenopathy, in CLL patients, 442
Lymphedema
  congenital, 450
  and elephantiasis, 450–452
  medical management, 451
  nursing management, 451–452
  pathophysiology, 450–451
  pharmacologic therapy, 451
  primary, 450
  secondary, 450
  surgical management, 451
Lymphedema praecox. *See* Congenital lymphedema
Lymphomas, non-Hodgkin. *See* Non-Hodgkin lymphomas (NHLs)
Lynch II syndrome, 169

M

Magnetic resonance imaging (MRI)
  in acute kidney failure, 623
  in acute renal failure, 623
  in chronic glomerulonephritis, 341
  in diffuse axonal injury, 353
  in elevated ICP, 424
  in epilepsies, 308
  in fractures, 318
  in headaches, 364
  in head injury, 351
  in meningitis, 463
  in multiple sclerosis, 474
  in myasthenia gravis, 484
  in osteomyelitis, 505
  in seizure, 634
  in spinal cord injury, 655
  in ulcerative colitis, 703
Malignant bone tumors, 100–101
Malignant melanoma, 204–208
  assessment and diagnostic findings, 205
  clinical manifestations, 204–205
  medical management, 205–206
  nursing process, 206–208
    assessment, 206
    diagnosis, 206–207
    evaluation, 208
    home- and community-based care, 208
    nursing interventions, 207–208
    planning and goals, 207
  risk factors, 204
  surgical management, 206
Mannitol (Osmitrol)
  in fulminant hepatic failure, 380
Mastoiditis, 455–458
  chronic, 455
  clinical manifestations, 455
  mastoid surgery, nursing process and, 455–458 (see also Mastoid surgery)
  medical management, 455
  surgical management, 455
Mastoid surgery
  assessment, 455
  evaluation, 458
  nursing diagnoses, 456

nursing interventions
  anxiety reduction, 456
  hearing and communication, 457
  home- and community-based care, 457
  infection prevention, 457
  injury prevention, 457
  pain management, 456–457
  sensory perception, altered, 457
  planning and goals for, 456
MedicAlert bracelets, 376
Medical management
  of abdominal aortic aneurysms, 57
  of acute gastritis, 332–333
  of acute glomerulonephritis, 338–339
  of acute lymphocytic leukemia, 441
  of acute myeloid leukemia, 444
  of acute nephritic syndrome, 490
  of acute otitis media, 511–512
  of AIDS, 4–7
  bariatric surgery and, 493–994
  of breast cancer, 151
  of burn injury, 117
  of chronic gastritis, 333
  of chronic glomerulonephritis, 341
  of chronic lymphocytic leukemia, 442
  of chronic myeloid leukemia, 446
  of chronic otitis media, 512–513
  of contact dermatitis, 264
  of empyema, 296–297
  of endometrial cancer, 170
  of endometriosis, 303
  of epididymitis, 305
  of epilepsies, 308
  of epistaxis, 312–313
  of esophageal cancer, 171
  of esophageal varices, bleeding, 314–315
  of exfoliative dermatitis, 266
  of fractures, 318
  of fulminant hepatic failure, 380
  of gastritis, 332–333
  of glaucoma, 336
  of gout, 343–344

of Guillain-Barré syndrome, 346
of headache, 364–365
of head injury, 351
of heart failure, 368
of hemophilia, 374–375
of hepatic encephalopathy, 378
of hepatitis B, 384
of hiatal hernia, 387
of Hodgkin lymphoma, 391
of Huntington disease (HD), 393
of hyperglycemic hyperosmolar syndrome, 395
of hypertension, 399
of hyperthyroidism, 405–406
of hypoglycemia, 411–412
of hypoparathyroidism, 413–414
of hypothyroidism, 417
of immune thrombocytopenic purpura, 420
of impetigo, 422–423
of increased intracranial pressure, 425
of infective endocarditis, 300
of Kaposi's sarcoma (KS), 431–432
of liver cancer, 184
of lung abscess, 449
of lymphedema, 451
of mastoiditis, 455
of Ménière's disease, 459
of meningitis, 463
of mitral regurgitation (insufficiency), 465–466
of mitral stenosis, 467
of mitral valve prolapse, 468–469
of morbid obesity, 499
of multiple myeloma, 471
of multiple sclerosis, 474
of muscular dystrophies, 479–480
of musculoskeletal trauma, 482–483
of myasthenia gravis, 484–485
of myocarditis, 487–488
of nephritic syndrome, 490
of nephrotic syndrome, 491–492
of non-Hodgkin lymphomas (NHLs), 453

of osteoarthritis, 501
of osteomalacia, 503–504
of osteomyelitis, 504
of osteoporosis, 508–509
of status asthmaticus, 90
of thoracic aortic aneurysms, 57
Ménière's disease, 458–461
    assessment and diagnostic findings, 459
    clinical manifestations, 459
    cochlear disease, 459
    dietary management, 459
    medical management, 459
    pharmacologic therapy, 460
    surgical management, 460
    and vertigo, 460–461
        anxiety reduction, 460
        disability adjustment, 460
        fluid volume maintenance, 460
        injury prevention, 460
    vestibular disease, 459
Meningiomas, 109
Meningitis, 461–464
    aseptic form, 461
    assessment and diagnostic findings, 463
    clinical manifestations, 462–463
    medical management, 463
    nursing management, 464
    pathophysiology, 462
    pharmacologic therapy, 463–464
    prevention, 463
    septic form, 461
Mental status assessment, 564
Metacarpal fracture, 326
Metastatic bone disease, 101
Methotrexate, 603
Methylprednisolone
    in multiple sclerosis, 475
MG. See Myasthenia gravis (MG)
Migraine, 361–362
    cause, 362
    clinical manifestations, 362
        aura phase, 362–363
        headache phase, 363
        prodrome phase, 362
        recovery phase, 363
    incidence, 362
    pharmacologic therapy, 365

Mitoxantrone, in multiple
  sclerosis, 475
Mitral regurgitation (insuffi-
    ciency), 465–466
  assessment and diagnostic
    findings, 465
  clinical manifestations, 465
  medical management, 465–466
  pathophysiology, 465
  surgical management, 466
Mitral stenosis, 466–467
  assessment and diagnostic
    findings, 467
  clinical manifestations, 466–467
  medical management, 467
  pathophysiology, 466
  prevention, 467
  surgical management, 467
Mitral (systolic) click, 468
Mitral valve prolapse, 468–469
  assessment and diagnostic
    findings, 468
  clinical manifestations, 468
  medical management, 468–469
  nursing management, 469
  pathophysiology, 468
Mobility management
  Parkinson's disease, 525
  in perioperative nursing, 551
  in SCI, 659
Morbid obesity, 498–500
  assessment and diagnostic
    findings, 499
  lifestyle modifications, 499
  medical management, 499
  nursing management, 500
  pathophysiology, 499
  pharmacologic therapy, 499–500
  surgical management, 500 (see
    also Bariatric surgery)
MRI. See Magnetic resonance
  imaging (MRI)
MS. See Multiple sclerosis (MS)
Multiple myeloma, 469–473
  assessment and diagnostic
    findings, 471
  clinical manifestations, 470–471
  gerontologic considerations, 471
  home- and community-based
    care, 472–473

nursing management, 472
pathophysiology, 470
pharmacologic therapy, 472
Multiple sclerosis (MS), 473–479
  assessment and diagnostic
    findings, 474
  bowel and bladder problems
    related to, 475
  clinical manifestations, 474
  courses, 473–474
  demyelination in, 473
  exacerbations and remissions,
    474
  medical management, 474
  nursing interventions
    bladder and bowel control, 477
    continuing care, 478–479
    coping mechanisms, 478
    home management, 478
    injury prevention, 477
    physical mobility, 476–477
    self-care, 478
    sensory and cognitive function,
      477–478
    sexual dysfunction, 478
    speech and swallowing
      difficulties, 477
  nursing process, 475–479
    assessment, 475–476
    diagnosis, 476
    evaluation, 479
    interventions, 476–479
    planning and goals, 476
  pathophysiology, 473
  pharmacologic therapy
    disease modification, 475
    symptom management, 475
  prevalence, 473
  secondary manifestations related
    to complications, 474
Muscular dystrophies, 479–481
  clinical manifestations, 479
  medical management, 479–480
  nursing management, 480–481
Musculoskeletal system, in SLE,
  681
Musculoskeletal trauma, 481–483
  assessment and diagnostic
    findings, 482
  clinical manifestations, 482

medical management, 482–483
nursing management, 483
pathophysiology, 481–482
Myasthenia gravis (MG), 483–487
assessment and diagnostic
findings, 484
clinical manifestations, 484
complications, 484
medical management, 484–485
nursing management, 485–487
pharmacologic therapy, 485
Myasthenic crisis, 484
Mycobacterium avium, 642
Mycobacterium avium complex
disease, 5
Mycotic aneurysms, 55
Myocarditis, 487–488
assessment and diagnostic
findings, 487
clinical manifestations, 487
medical management, 487–488
nursing management, 488
Myringotomy, 512
Myxedema, 415. *See also*
Hypothyroidism
Myxedema coma, 416

N

Nasal sponge, 313
Nasal sprays, 577
Neisseria gonorrhoeae
assessment and diagnostic
findings, 639
clinical manifestations, 638–639
complications, 639
medical management, 639–640
nursing management, 640
pelvic inflammatory disease, 638
Neisseria meningitidis, and
meningitis, 461
Nephritic syndrome, acute, 489–491
assessment and diagnostic
findings, 489
clinical manifestations, 489
continuing care, 490–491
home- and community-based
care, 490–491
hospital care, 490
medical management, 490
nursing management, 490

pathophysiology, 489
self-care, 490
Nephrolithiasis. *See* Urolithiasis
Nephrotic syndrome, 491–492
assessment and diagnostic
findings, 491
clinical manifestations, 491
medical management, 491–492
nursing management, 492
Neurogenic shock, 649–650
clinical manifestations, 649–650
medical management, 650
nursing management, 650
pathophysiology, 649
risk factors, 649
Neurologic assessment, in traumatic brain injury, 355–356
Neurologic signs
in elevated ICP, 424
in hyperglycemic hyperosmolar
syndrome, 395
Neurosensory changes, in chronic
glomerulonephritis, 340
NHLs. *See* Non-Hodgkin lymphomas (NHLs)
Nodular melanoma, 205
Non-Hodgkin lymphomas (NHLs),
452–454
assessment and diagnostic findings, 453
clinical manifestations, 452–453
incidence, 452
medical management, 453
nursing management, 454
pathophysiology, 452
pharmacologic therapy, 453–454
prognosis, 454
Nonsteroidal anti-inflammatory
drugs (NSAIDs)
in endometriosis, 303
in gout, 343
in Kaposi's sarcoma, 432
in multiple myeloma, 472
in osteoarthritis, 502
for peptic ulcer, 534
for pericarditis, 542
for SLE, 682
for subacute thyroiditis, 688
for systemic lupus erythematosus,
682

Nosebleed. *See* Epistaxis
NSAIDs. *See* Nonsteroidal
    anti-inflammatory drugs
    (NSAIDs)
Nuchal rigidity, in meningitis,
    462
Numbness
  in peripheral arterial occlusive
    disease, 570
Nursing management
  in acute glomerulonephritis, 339
  in acute kidney failure, 625
  in acute nephritic syndrome, 490
  in acute pancreatitis, 517–519
  in acute pulmonary edema, 610
  in acute renal failure, 625
  in acute respiratory distress
    syndrome, 24–25
  in Addison's disease, 27
  in ALS, 36
  in anaphylactic shock, 644
  in anaphylaxis, 38
  in anemia, 44, 45, 48
  in aortic aneurysm, 57
  in aortic Insufficiency, 69
  in appendicitis, 74
  in arterial embolism and arterial
    thrombosis, 76
  in asthma, 88
  in bone tumors, 102–103
  in brain abscess, 108
  in brain tumors, 112
  in chronic glomerulonephritis,
    341–342
  in chronic kidney failure,
    629–630
  in chronic otitis media, 513
  in chronic renal failure, 629–630
  in concussion, 352
  in contact dermatitis, 265
  in empyema, 297
  in endometriosis, 304
  in epididymitis, 306
  in epistaxis, 313
  in esophageal cancer, 171–172
  in esophageal varices, 315–316
  in fractures, 323–328
  in fulminant hepatic failure,
    380
  in gastritis, 333–334

  in glaucoma, 337
  in gout, 344
  in headache, 365–366
  in head injury, 352
  in hemophilia, 375–376
  in hepatic encephalopathy,
    378–379
  in hepatitis A, 382
  in hepatitis B, 384–385
  in Hodgkin lymphoma, 392
  in Huntington disease, 394
  in hyperglycemic hyperosmolar
    syndrome, 395–396
  in hypoglycemia, 412
  in hypoparathyroidism, 414
  in hypothyroidism, 418
  in hypovolemic shock, 648–649
  in immune thrombocytopenic
    purpura, 420–421
  in impetigo, 423
  in infective endocarditis, 301
  in Kaposi's sarcoma, 432
  in kidney cancer, 174–175
  in large bowel obstruction, 105
  in liver cancer, 185–186
  in low back pain, 94
  in lung abscess, 449
  in lymphedema, 451–452
  in meningitis, 464
  in mitral valve prolapse, 469
  in morbid obesity, 500
  in multiple myeloma, 472
  in muscular dystrophies, 480–481
  in musculoskeletal trauma, 483
  in myasthenia gravis, 485–487
  in myocarditis, 488
  in nephritic syndrome, 490
  in nephrotic syndrome, 492
  in neurogenic shock, 650
  in non-Hodgkin lymphomas,
    454
  in osteoarthritis, 502
  in ovarian cancer, 193
  in pancreatic cancer, 195–196
  in pelvic inflammatory disease,
    528–529
  perioperative, 544–569
  in peritonitis, 574–575
  in pheochromocytoma, 580
  in pleural effusion, 583

in polycythemia, 596
in postanesthesia care unit,
    555–556
in prostatitis, 598
in pruritus, 600
in pulmonary arterial hyper-
    tension, 608
in pulmonary embolism,
    614–616
in pulmonary tuberculosis,
    700–701
in Raynaud's phenomenon, 621
in renal cancer, 174–175
in seborrheic dermatoses, 632
in sexually transmitted infec-
    tion, 638
in small bowel obstruction,
    106–107
in status asthmaticus, 91
in syphilis, 638
in systemic lupus erythematosus,
    682–683
in testicular cancer, 215–216
in thyroid cancer, 217
in thyroid storm, 687
in transient ischemic attack,
    696
in tuberculosis, 700–701
in vulvar cancer, 220
Nursing process
    vertebral fracture related to
        osteoporosis, 509–511
Nutrition management
    in acute pancreatitis, 517
    in AIDS, 7
    in chronic glomerulonephritis,
        341
    in chronic kidney failure (CKF),
        629
    in chronic renal failure (CRF),
        629
    in gastritis, 333–334
    in hiatal hernia, 388
    in Parkinson's disease, 525–526
    in perioperative nursing,
        550–551, 564–565
    in traumatic brain injury, 358
    in ulcerative colitis, 703
    in unconscious patient, 713
    in urolithiasis, 718

O

OA. *See* Osteoarthritis (OA)
Obesity, 493–498
    morbid (*see* Morbid obesity)
    and osteoarthritis, 501
    and pituitary tumors, 581
    surgery for (*see* Bariatric surgery)
    and vein disorders, 723
Older adults
    delirium in, 328
    hemophilia in, 376
    hepatitis B and, 382
    hip fractures in, 328
    in hyperglycemic hyperosmolar
        syndrome, 394–396
    hypertension, 399–400
    hyperthyroidism in, 406
    hypoglycemia in, 410–411
    hypothyroidism in, 416
    isolated systolic hypertension
        in, 398
    multiple myeloma in, 471
    osteoporosis and, 508
    seizures in, 308
Open fracture, 317. *See also*
    Fractures
Opioid analgesic agents, 718
Opioids, in Kaposi's sarcoma, 432
Opportunistic infections
    prevention of, 6
    treatment of, 4
        cryptococcal meningitis, 5
        cytomegalovirus retinitis, 5–6
        Mycobacterium avium complex
            disease, 5
        pneumocystis pneumonia, 4–5
Optic nerve, damage of, in
    glaucoma, 335, 336
Optic nerve demyelination, 345
Oral anticoagulants, 726
Oral care, for infective
    endocarditis prevention, 300
Oral cavity and pharynx, cancer
    of, 190–191
Oral contraceptives, for
    endometriosis, 303
Oral hygiene management, in
    pemphigus, 532
OraQuick Rapid HIV-1 antibody
    test, 4

OraSure saliva test, 4
Orlistat (Xenical), in obesity
    treatment, 500
Orthostatic hypotension, 661
Osler nodes, in infective
    endocarditis, 298
Osmotic diuresis, 395
Osmotic diuretic agents, in
    elevated ICP, 425
Osteoarthritis (OA), 500–502
    assessment and diagnostic
        findings, 501
    clinical manifestations, 501
    conservative measures, 501
    medical management, 501
    nursing management, 502
    pharmacologic therapy, 502
    prevention, 501
    primary, 501
    risk factors for, 500–501
    secondary, 501
    surgical management, 502
Osteoarthrosis. See Osteoarthritis
    (OA)
Osteomalacia, 502–504
    assessment and diagnostic
        findings, 503
    clinical manifestations, 503
    gerontologic considerations, 503
    medical management, 503–504
    risk factors, 503
Osteomyelitis, 504–507
    assessment and diagnostic
        findings, 505
    clinical manifestations, 504
    home- and community-based
        care, 506–507
    infection prevention, 506
    medical management, 504
    nursing process, 505–507
        assessment, 505
        continuing care, 507
        diagnosis, 505–506
        evaluation, 507
        interventions, 506–507
        planning and goals, 506
        self care, 506–507
    pain management, 506
    physical mobility, improvement
        in, 506

Osteoporosis, 507–511
    assessment and diagnostic
        findings, 508
    gerontologic considerations, 508
    medical management, 508–509
    risk factors, 508
    secondary, 508
    vertebral fracture related to,
        509–511
        assessment, 509
        diagnosis, 509
        evaluation, 510–511
        interventions, 510
        planning and goals, 509
Osteotomy, 502
Otitis media
    acute (see Acute otitis media)
    chronic (see Chronic otitis
        media)
    infection of, 455 (see also
        Mastoiditis)
Ovarian cancer, 192–193
    assessment and diagnostic
        findings, 192
    clinical manifestations, 192
    medical management, 192–193
    nursing management, 193
    pathophysiology, 192
Overt tetany, 413
Oxalate stones, 718
Oxygenation
    cerebral, 609–610
    of heart muscle, 646
Oxygen therapy, 615
    for PE, 615
    for peritonitis, 574
    for SCI, 656

P
Pain management
    in acute pancreatitis, 516–517
    after bariatric surgery, 495–496
    in AIDS, 13
    in gastritis, 334
    in headaches, 365–366
    in hiatal hernia, 388
    in mastoid surgery, 456–457
    in osteomyelitis, 506
    in osteoporosis, 510
    in peptic ulcer, 538

in pericarditis, 543
in perioperative nursing, 562–563
in toxic epidermal necrolysis, 693
in ulcerative colitis, 706–707
Pancreatic cancer, 193–196
assessment and diagnostic findings, 194–195
clinical manifestations, 194
medical management, 195
nursing management, 195–196
Pancreatic enzyme replacement therapy, 520
Pancreatic necrosis, 518
Pancreatitis, 514–521
Paraesophageal hernia, 386–387. *See also* Hiatal hernia
Parenteral nutrition (PN), in traumatic brain injury, 358
Paresthesias, in Guillain-Barré syndrome, 345
Parkinson's disease, 521–527
assessment, 522–523
cardinal signs of, 522
diagnostic methods, 522–523
evaluation, patient outcomes, 527
idiopathic form, 521
nursing diagnoses, 524
nursing interventions
bowel elimination, 525
communication improvement, 526
continuing care, 527
coping abilities, 526
mobility, 525
nutritional needs, 526
self-care, 525–527
swallowing of food, 525–526
use of assistive devices, 526
pathophysiology, 521
pharmacologic therapy for, 523
planning/goals, 525
surgical management, 523
Passive limb movement, resistance to, 522
Patient education, psoriasis, 604
Pelvic fractures, 326–327

Pelvic infection. *See* Pelvic inflammatory disease (PID)
Pelvic inflammatory disease (PID), 527–529
broad-spectrum antibiotic therapy for, 528
clinical manifestations, 528
complications, 528
nursing management, 528–529
pathophysiology, 527–528
risk factors, 528
Pemphigus, 530–534
assessment, 531
clinical manifestations, 530
corticosteroids for, 531
diagnosis, 531
evaluation, patient outcomes, 533–534
immunosuppressive agents for, 531
nursing diagnoses, 531–532
nursing interventions
fluid and electrolyte balance, 532–533
oral hygiene, 532
positive body image, promoting, 532
potential complications, 532–533
skin integrity, 532
pathophysiology, 530
planning/goals, 532
Pentoxifylline, 571
Peptic ulcer, 534–540
anxiety reduction in, 538
assessment, 535–536
causes of, 534
clinical manifestations, 535
collaborative problems/complications, 538
complications
dizziness and nausea, 538
perforation and penetration, 539
continuing care in, 540
diagnostic tests for, 536
evaluation, patient outcomes, 540
and gastrinoma
nursing diagnoses, 537

Peptic ulcer (*continued*)
    pain reduction in, 538
    pharmacologic therapy for, 536
    planning/goals, 538
    predisposing factors, 534
    self-care in, 539–540
    surgical management, 537
Percutaneous transluminal
        coronary angioplasty
        (PTCA), 368
Perianal care, 708
Pericardial effusion in pericarditis,
        544
Pericarditis, 540–544
    assessment, 542–543
    causes of, 540
    classification, 540
    clinical manifestations, 541
    diagnosis, 541
    evaluation, patient outcomes,
        544
    nursing diagnoses, 543
    pain management in, 543
    pericardial effusion in, 544
    pharmacologic therapy for, 542
    planning/goals, 543
Perioperative nursing management,
        544–569
    active body movement, 551
    airway management, 556
    anxiety reduction, 550
    assessment
        ambulatory surgery, 547–548
    body temperature, 563–564
    bowel preparation for surgery,
        552
    cardiovascular stability, 556–557
    emotional support to patient and
        family, 567
    evaluation, patient outcomes,
        554, 569
    family's needs, 554
    fluid intake, 550
    gerontologic considerations, 548
    GI function, 564–565
    hepatic and renal function, 551
    home- and community-based
        care, 559–560
    informed consent, 549–550
    mental status assessment, 564

    mobility, 551
    nursing diagnoses, 548
    nutrition, 550–551, 564–565
    operating room, 553
    pain management, 552, 562–563
    physical mobility, 565–566
    planning/goals, 548
    in postanesthesia care unit
        documentation of information,
            555
        gerontologic considerations,
            568–569
        PACU nurse, 556
    preoperative patient education
        ambulatory surgical patient,
            549
        preparation procedures,
            548–549
    psychosocial support, 550
    respiratory and cardiovascular
        status, 551
    in same-day surgery, 558–559
    skin preparation for surgery,
        552
    spiritual help, 552
    wound complications
        infection, 568
    wound dehiscence and
        evisceration, 568
Peripheral arterial occlusive
        disease, 570–572
    clinical manifestations, 570
    diagnosis, 570
    home- and community-based
        care, 572
    pharmacotherapy for, 571
    postoperative management
        circulation through arterial
            repair, 571
        edema, 572
        fluid imbalances, 571
    surgery for, 571
Peritoneal fluid, 515
Peritonitis, 572–575
    clinical features, 573
    medical management, 573–574
    nursing management, 574–575
    pathophysiology, 572–573
PET. *See* Positron emission
        tomography (PET)

Pharmacologic management
of chronic kidney failure (CKF),
528–529
of chronic renal failure (CRF),
528–529
Pharmacologic therapy
for acute myeloid leukemia
(AML), 444–445
for acute pulmonary edema, 610
for breast cancer, 152
for chronic lymphocytic leukemia (CLL), 443
for chronic myeloid leukemia
(CML), 446–447
for endometriosis, 303
for epilepsies, 308
for esophageal varices, bleeding, 315
for glaucoma, 336–337
for Guillain-Barré syndrome
(GBS), 346
for heart failure (HF), 368
for hypertension, 399
for hypothyroidism, 417
for hypovolemic shock, 648
for immune thrombocytopenic
purpura, 420
for impetigo, 422–423
for increased intracranial
pressure, 425
for Kaposi's sarcoma, 432
for lymphedema, 451
for Ménière's disease, 460
for meningitis, 463–464
for migraine, 365
for morbid obesity, 499–500
for multiple myeloma, 472
for multiple sclerosis, 475
for myasthenia gravis (MG), 485
for non-Hodgkin lymphomas,
453–454
for osteoarthritis, 502
for Parkinson's disease, 523
for peptic ulcer, 536
for peripheral arterial occlusive
disease, 571
for pulmonary tuberculosis, 700
for SLE, 682
for trigeminal neuralgia, 697
for ulcerative colitis, 703–704

for urolithiasis, 718
for vein disorders, 725
Pharyngitis
acute, 575–576
chronic, 577
Pheochromocytoma, 578–580
clinical manifestations, 578
diagnostic methods for, 579
incidence of, 578
medical management, 579
nursing management, 580
Phlebothrombosis. See Vein disorders
Phlebotomy, 595
Photochemotherapy for psoriasis,
603
Photophobia, in meningitis, 462
Physical mobility
in perioperative nursing, 551
Pituitary adenomas, 109
Pituitary tumors, 580–582
Plasmacytomas, 470
Plasmapheresis
in hemophilia, 374
in multiple myeloma, 471
in myasthenia gravis, 485
Pleural effusion, 582–583
clinical manifestations, 582
nursing management, 583
treatment modalities, 583
Pleural fluid, drainage of, 296–297
Pleurisy, 584
Pneumocystis jiroveci, 642
Pneumocystis pneumonia, 4–5
Pneumonia, 585–591
antibiotics for, 586
assessment, 586
classification, 585
clinical manifestations, 585–586
collaborative problems/
complications, 588
in elderly patients, 587
nursing diagnoses, 588
nursing interventions
airway patency, 588–589
fluid intake, 589
patient education, 589
rest, 589
self-care, 590–591
pathophysiology, 585
planning/goals, 588

Pneumothorax, 591–594
  clinical manifestations, 593
  medical management, 593–594
  simple, 592
  tension, 592
  traumatic, 592
Polycythemia, 594–596
  classification, 594–595
  clinical manifestations, 595
  medical management, 595–596
  nursing management, 596
Polycythemia vera, 595
Polyradiculoneuritis. *See* Guillain-
    Barré syndrome (GBS)
Polyuria, in hyperglycemic hyper-
    osmolar syndrome, 395
Portosystemic encephalopathy
    (PSE). *See* Hepatic encepha-
    lopathy
Positron emission tomography
    (PET)
  in elevated ICP, 424
  in Hodgkin lymphoma, 391
  in non-Hodgkin lymphomas, 453
  in unconscious patient, 710
Postanesthesia care, 555
Postanesthesia care unit (PACU)
  cardiovascular stability,
    556–557
  documentation of information,
    555
  home care nurse and, 559–560
  nursing management in,
    555–556
  patient's readiness for discharge
    from, 558
  same-day surgery, discharge from,
    558–559
Postoperative complications
  hematoma, 567–568
  venous thromboembolism, 567
  wound dehiscence and eviscera-
    tion, 568
  wound sepsis, 568
Postoperative nursing management
  bladder distention, 565
  cardiovascular stability, 556–557
  care unit, 555–556
  in clinical unit, 555
  deep vein thrombosis, 561

  emotional support to patient and
    family, 567
  family's needs, 554
  GI function, 564–565
  hemorrhage, 564
  hyperthermia, 564
  hypothermia, 564
  mental status assessment, 564
  mobility, 551
  nutrition, 564–565
  pain management, 562–563
  patient's physiologic equilibrium,
    555
  postanesthesia care, 555–556
  in same-day surgery, 558–559
Potassium
  in hyperglycemic hyperosmolar
    syndrome, 395
Preoperative patient education
  ambulatory surgical patient, 549
  patient education, 548–549
Primary open-angle glaucoma
    (POAG), 335
Primary pulmonary hypertension,
    605
Primary syphilis, 637
Probenecid, in gout, 344
Progressive multifocal leukoen-
    cephalopathy, 3
Prophylactic antimicrobial therapy,
    618
Propylthiouracil (PTU), 686
Prostate cancer, 196–203
  advanced stage, 197
  assessment and diagnostic
    findings, 197
  clinical manifestations, 197
  hormone therapy, 198–199
  medical management, 197
  pathophysiology, 196
  prostatectomy, and nusing pro-
    cess, 199–203
  radiation therapy, 198
  surgical management, 197–198
Prostatitis, 596–598
  causes of, 596
  clinical manifestations, 597
  nursing management, 598
  treatment goals, 597
  types of, 596

Pruritus, 598–600
  causes of, 598
  clinical manifestations, 599
  medical management, 599–600
  nursing management, 600
Psoralens and ultraviolet A
    (PUVA) therapy, 603
Psoriasis, 601–605
  assessment, 603
  clinical manifestations, 601
  complications, 601–602
  diagnostic methods for, 602
  medical management
    photochemotherapy, 603
    removal of scales, 602
    systemic therapy, 603
    topical therapy, 602
  nursing interventions
    coping strategies, 604
    patient education, 604
    self-care, 604–605
    skin integrity, 604
  pathophysiology, 601
Psychiatric changes in Parkinson's
    disease, 522
Psychosocial support, in ARF, 626
Psychotherapy, in Huntington
    disease, 393
Pulmonary arterial hypertension,
    605–608
  anticoagulation therapy for, 607
  clinical manifestations, 606
  diagnostic evaluation, 606
  lung transplantation, 607
  nursing management, 608
  pathophysiology, 605–606
  primary, 605
  secondary, 605
Pulmonary edema, acute. See Acute
    pulmonary edema
Pulmonary embolism (PE), 610–616
  clinical manifestations, 611
  diagnostic methods for, 612
  medical management
    anticoagulation therapy, 613
    cardiopulmonary system stabi-
      lization, 612–613
    surgical management, 614
    thrombolytic therapy, 613–614
  nursing management

  anxiety reduction, 615
  chest pain, 615
  invasive procedures, 614
  oxygen therapy, 615
  postoperative nursing care, 615
  self-care, 616
  thrombus formation
    prevention, 614
  prevention, 612
Pulmonary resection, in lung
    abscess, 449
Pulmonary tuberculosis, 698–701
  adherence to treatment regimen
    for, 700–701
  assessment and diagnostic
    methods, 699
  clinical manifestations, 699
  in elderly people, 699
  mode of transmission, 698
  nursing management, 700–701
  nutritional regimen for, 701
  pharmacologic therapy for, 700
  preventing spreading of, 701
  risk factors, 699
Pupillary block. See Angle-closure
    glaucoma
Pyelonephritis
  acute, 616–618
  chronic, 618–619
Pyridostigmine bromide, in myas-
    thenia gravis, 485

R
Radial and ulnar shaft fractures, 325
Radial head fractures, 325
Radiation therapy
  in Kaposi's sarcoma, 431–432
  in multiple myeloma, 471
  in non-Hodgkin lymphomas, 453
  in pituitary tumors, 582
Radioactive iodine therapy, in
    hyperthyroidism, 405
Radiographic examination, for
    fractures, 318
Radioisotope bone scans, in
    osteomyelitis, 505
Rash, in meningitis, 462
Raynaud's phenomenon, 620–621
  clinical manifestations, 620–621
  medical management, 621

Raynaud's phenomenon (*continued*)
  nursing management, 621
  prognosis for, 620
Red man syndrome, 265
Reed–Sternberg cell, 389–390
Regional enteritis, 252–254
  assessment and diagnostic
      findings, 253–254
  clinical manifestations, 253
  pathophysiology, 253
Renal cancer, 173–175
  assessment and diagnostic
      findings, 173
  clinical manifestations, 173
  medical management, 173–174
  nursing management, 174–175
Renal failure. *See* Acute kidney failure
      and chronic kidney failure
Respiratory therapy, in Guillain-
      Barré syndrome, 346
Resting tremors, 522
Restlessness
  in hepatic encephalopathy, 377
  in traumatic brain injury, 358
Retinal findings, in chronic
      glomerulonephritis, 340
Rheumatic endocarditis, 301–302
  causative agents, 301–302
  rheumatic fever and, 301–302
  treatment, 302
Rheumatoid arthritis, 78–83
  assessment and diagnostic
      findings, 79
  body image, 82
  clinical manifestations, 78
  fatigue, 81
  medical management, 79
  mobility, 81
  nursing management, 80
  pain, 80
  self-care, 81
Rib fractures, 330
Richter's lymphoma, 442
Roth spots, in infective endocar-
      ditis, 298
Roux-en-Y gastric bypass, 493.
      See also Bariatric surgery

S

Scalp trauma, 351
Seborrhea, 631

Seborrheic dermatoses, 631–632
  dry form of, 631
  genetic predisposition for, 631
  medical management, 631–632
  nursing management, 632
  oily form of, 631
Secondary polycythemia, 594
Secondary pulmonary hyperten-
      sion, 605
Secondary syphilis, 637
Secondary thrombocytopenia, 685
Seizures, 632–635
  causes of, 633
  chlamydia and gonorrhea, 638–640
  clinical manifestations, 633
  epileptic, 306 (*see also* Epilepsies)
  in meningitis, 462
  pathophysiology, 633
Self-care, 709
  in ACS, 22
  in acute nephritic syndrome, 490
  in acute pancreatitis, 518–519
  in Addison's disease, 28
  after bariatric surgery, 497–498
  in AIDS, 15–16
  in asthma, 88–89
  in breast cancer, 156
  in cancer, 140–141
  in cardiomyopathies, 229
  in cataract, 232
  in cervical cancer, 160–161
  in cholelithiasis and
      cholecystitis, 238
  in chronic kidney failure (CKF),
      630
  in chronic renal failure (CRF), 630
  in colorectal cancer, 168
  in COPD, 243–244
  in cystitis (lower UTI), 263
  in diabetes, 277
  in epilepsies, 311
  in gastritis, 334
  in glaucoma, 337
  in Guillain-Barré syndrome, 349
  in headache, 366
  in heart failure, 372–373
  in hiatal hernia, 388–389
  in hypertension, 401–402
  in hyperthyroidism, 409
  in hypothyroidism, 418
  in larynx cancer, 181–182

in leukemia, 438–439
in lung abscess, 449–450
in multiple myeloma, 472
in multiple sclerosis, 478
in osteomyelitis, 506–507
in Parkinson's disease, 525–527
in peptic ulcer, 539–540
in prostate cancer, 203
in psoriasis, 604–605
in rheumatoid arthritis, 82
in traumatic brain injury, 360
in ulcerative colitis, 709
in vulvar cancer, 221
Sensory stimulation
in unconscious patient, 715
in urolithiasis, 715
Sepsis, 693
Septic shock, 650–653
clinical manifestations, 651
in elderly persons, 652
pathophysiology, 651
risk factors, 650
Sequential compression boots in
Guillain-Barré syndrome, 346
Serum amylase levels, 515
Serum lipase levels, 515
Severe hypothyroidism, 416
Sexually transmitted infection
(STI), 635–642
assessment, 640
assessment and diagnostic
findings, 637
collaborative problems/potential
complications, 641
evaluation, patient outcomes,
642
medical management, 637–638
monitoring and managing
potential complications
congenital infections, 642
gonococcal arthritis, 642
gonococcal meningitis, 642
human immunodeficiency
virus, 642
neurosyphilis, 642
risk of ectopic pregnancy, 642
syphilitic aortitis, 642
nursing diagnoses, 640
nursing interventions
anxiety reduction, 641
increasing compliance, 641–642

knowledge and, 641
preventing spread of disease, 641
nursing management, 638
nursing care, 634–635
other diseases, 636
pathophysiology, 636
pharmacologic therapy, 638
planning and goals, 641
prevention of, 636
risk of, 636
sites of, 636
syphilis, 637
types of, 632
Shock. See Anaphylactic shock;
Cardiogenic shock;
Hypovolemic shock;
Neurogenic shock; Septic
shock
Shock, in acute pancreatitis, 518
Sibutramine HCl, in obesity
treatment, 499
Simple pneumothorax, 592, 593
Single-drug therapy, for epilepsies,
308
Single photon emission tomography (SPECT)
in elevated ICP, 424
Skin care, in ARF, 626
Skin integrity
in acute pancreatitis, 517–518
in pemphigus, 532
in psoriasis, 604
in SCI, 660
in toxic epidermal necrolysis, 692
in unconscious patient, 714
Skin lesions, in ulcerative colitis,
702
Skull fractures, 351
Sleeve gastrectomy, 493. See also
Bariatric surgery
Sliding hernia, 386. See also Hiatal
hernia
Smoking
cessation, 536
and chronic pancreatitis, 519
Spinal cord injuries (SCI), 653–662
assessment, 657–658
assessment and diagnostic
methods, 655
categorization of, 654
causes of, 653

Spinal cord injuries (SCI) (*continued*)
  collaborative problems/
    complications, 658
  complications
    deep vein thrombosis, 657
    spinal and neurogenic shock,
      656
    spinal shock, 655
  emergency management, 655
  evaluation, patient outcomes,
    662
  incomplete, 654
  medical management
    high-dose corticosteroids,
      655–656
    oxygenation, 656
    surgery, 656
  neurologic level, 654
  nursing diagnoses, 658
  nursing interventions
    adaptation to disturbed sensory
      perception, 659–660
    autonomic hyperreflexia, 661
    bowel function, 660
    breathing and airway clear-
      ance, 658–659
    comfort measures, 660–661
    home- and community-based
      care, 661–662
    mobility improvement, 659
    orthostatic hypotension, 661
    skin integrity, 660
  planning/goals, 658
  respiratory problems in, 655
  risk factors, 654
Splenectomy, 420
Spontaneous bleeding, 726
Sprain, 481. *See also*
    Musculoskeletal trauma
Sputum culture
  in lung abscess, 448
Staphylococcus aureus
  and bone infections, 504
  and bullous impetigo, 422
Statin therapy, 571
Status asthmaticus, 89–91
  assessment and diagnostic
    findings, 90
  clinical manifestations, 90
  medical management, 90

nursing management, 91
pathophysiology, 90
Status epilepticus, 310
Stereotactic radiation therapy, for
    pituitary tumors, 582
Stevens-Johnson syndrome,
    689–694
STI. *See* Sexually transmitted
    infection (STI)
Stool analysis, in hepatitis A, 381
Strain, 481. *See also*
    Musculoskeletal trauma
Streptococcus pneumoniae, and
    meningitis, 461
Stress ulcer, 534. *See also* Peptic
    ulcer
Stroke. *See* Hemorrhagic stroke;
    Ischemic stroke
Subacute thyroiditis, 688
Subdural hematoma, 353–354
Subluxation, 482
Superficial spreading melanoma,
    204–205
Supportive care, in AIDS, 7
Surgical management
  of abdominal aortic aneurysms, 57
  of chronic pancreatitis, 520
  of endometriosis, 304
  of epilepsies, 308–309
  of esophageal varices, 315
  of glaucoma, 337
  of heart failure, 368
  of hiatal hernia, 387
  of hyperthyroidism, 406
  of infective endocarditis, 300–301
  of liver cancer, 185
  of lymphedema, 451
  of mastoiditis, 455
  of Ménière's disease, 460
  of mitral regurgitation
    (insufficiency), 466
  of mitral stenosis, 467
  of osteoarthritis, 502
  of Parkinson's disease, 523
  of peptic ulcer, 537
  of peripheral arterial occlusive
    disease, 571
  of pheochromocytoma, 579
  of pituitary tumors, 582
  of pulmonary embolism (PE), 614

of SCI, 656
of trigeminal neuralgia, 697
of ulcerative colitis, 704
Sympathectomy, 621
Sympathetic innervation, 656
Sympatholytic agents, 686
Syndrome of inappropriate antidiuretic hormone (SIADH),
679–680
elevated ICP and, 425
Synthetic levothyroxine, in
hypothyroidism, 417
Syphilis
assessment and diagnostic
findings, 637
causes of, 637
medical management, 637–638
nursing management, 638
pharmacologic therapy, 638
serologic tests, 637
stages, 637
Systemic lupus erythematosus
(SLE), 680–683
clinical manifestations, 681
diagnosis, 681–682
nursing management, 682–683
pathophysiology of, 680–681
pharmacologic therapy for, 682
Systemic therapy for psoriasis, 603

T

TBI. See Traumatic brain injury
(TBI)
Tension pneumothorax, 592, 593
Tension-type headache, 362, 363.
See also Headache
Terminal care, in leukemia, 439
Tertiary syphilis, 637
Testicular cancer, 214–216
assessment and diagnostic
findings, 214–215
clinical manifestations, 214
medical management, 215
nursing management, 215–216
pathophysiology, 214
Tetrabenazine (Xenazine)
in Huntington disease, 393
Thoracic aortic aneurysms, 55
assessment and diagnostic
findings, 56

clinical manifestations, 56
medical management, 57
Thoracolumbar spine, fractures
of, 330
Thrombocytopenia, 684–685
Thrombolytic therapy, 614
Thrombophlebitis, 723
Thrombopoietin receptor agonists
in immune thrombocytope-
nic purpura, 420
Thrombus formation prevention,
614
Thymectomy, in myasthenia
gravis, 485
Thyroid cancer, 216–217
assessment and diagnostic
findings, 216
clinical manifestations, 216
medical management, 216–217
nursing management, 217
Thyroid hormone therapy, 689
Thyroid storm, 685–687
clinical manifestations, 686
medical management, 686
nursing management, 687
Thyroiditis. See Acute thyroiditis;
Chronic thyroiditis
TIA. See Transient ischemic attack
(TIA)
Tibia and fibula fractures, 329–330
Tic douloureux. See Trigeminal
neuralgia
Tonsillectomy, 577
Topical corticosteroid cream, 632
Topical therapy for psoriasis, 602
Toxic epidermal necrolysis, 689–694
assessment and diagnostic
findings, 690
assessment of, 691
clinical manifestations, 689–690
collaborative problems/
complications, 692
complications, 689, 690
evaluation, patient outcomes, 694
medical management, 690–691
nursing diagnoses, 691–692
nursing interventions
anxiety management, 693
conjunctival retraction, 693
fluid balance, 692

Toxic epidermal necrolysis
(*continued*)
  hypothermia prevention,
    692–693
  pain management, 693
  sepsis, 693
  skin and mucous membrane
    integrity, 692
  planning/goals, 692
Trabectome surgery, for glaucoma,
  337
Transcranial Doppler, in elevated
  ICP, 424
Transesophageal echocardiography
  (TEE)
  in mitral regurgitation, 465
Transient ischemic attack (TIA),
  694–696
  assessment and diagnostic
    findings, 695
  clinical manifestations, 695
  medical management, 695
  nursing management, 696
  pathophysiology, 695
  pharmacologic therapy, 695–696
  prevention, 695
  risk factors, 695
Trauma
  abdominal, 592
  blunt, 592
  multiple organ, 534
Traumatic brain injury (TBI), 350.
    See also Head injury
  causes, 350
  mild, 351
  motor functions, assessment of,
    355
  neurologic signs, 355–356
  nursing interventions
    airway maintenance, 357
    body temperature mainte-
      nance, 359
    cognitive functioning, 359
    family coping, 359–360
    fluid and electrolyte balance,
      358
    home- and community-based
      care, 360–361
    injury prevention, 358–359
    neurologic function, 357
  nutrition, 358
  potential complications, 360
  skin integrity, 359
  sleep pattern disturbance,
    prevention of, 359
  nursing process, 355–361
    assessment, 355–356
    diagnosis, 356
    evaluation, 361
    interventions, 357–361
    planning and goals, 357
  primary injury, 350
  secondary injury, 350
  vital signs in, monitoring of, 355
Traumatic pneumothorax, 592
Tremor at rest, 522
Trendelenburg position, 648
Trigeminal neuralgia, 696–698
  clinical manifestations, 696
  nursing interventions, 697–698
  pathophysiology, 696
  pharmacologic therapy for, 697
  surgical management, 697
Trimethoprim-sulfamethoxazole
  (TMP-SMZ), 597
Trousseau's sign, 413
Tuberculosis, pulmonary, 698–701
  adherence to treatment regimen
    for, 700–701
  assessment and diagnostic
    methods, 699
  clinical manifestations, 699
  in elderly people, 699
  mode of transmission, 698
  nursing management, 700–701
  nutritional regimen for, 701
  pharmacologic therapy for, 700
  preventing spreading of, 701
  risk factors, 699
Tumors
  malignant, 680
  neoplastic, 582
Tympanotomy. *See* Myringotomy

U

Ulcerative colitis, 702–710
  assessment and diagnostic
    methods, 703
  assessment findings, 705
  bleeding in, 702

clinical manifestations, 702
collaborative problems/
  complications, 706
evaluation, patient outcomes,
  709–710
nursing diagnoses, 705–706
nursing interventions
  anxiety management, 707–708
  continuing care, 709
  coping measures, 708
  fluid intake, 707
  normal elimination patterns,
    706
  pain management, 706–707
  perianal care, 708
  potential complications, 708
  rest, 707
  self-care, 709
nutritional therapy for, 703
pharmacologic therapy for,
  703–704
planning/goals, 706
surgical management, 704
Ulcers
  acute, 535
  asymptomatic, 535
  esophageal, 534
  oral, 681
Ultraviolet B (UVB) light therapy,
  603
Uncal herniation, 353
Unconscious patient, 710–716
  assessment, 711
  assessment and diagnostic
    methods, 710–711
  collaborative problems/
    complications, 712
  evaluation, patient outcomes,
    716
  medical management, 711
  nursing diagnoses, 711–712
  nursing interventions
    airway maintenance, 712–713
    body temperature manage-
      ment, 714
    bowel function, 715
    corneal integrity, 714
    fluid balance, 713
    mouth care, 713–714
    nutritional needs, 713

patient protection, 713
potential complications, 716
sensory stimulation, 715
skin and joint integrity, 714
urinary retention prevention, 715
planning/goals, 712
Unknown seizures, 632
Upper respiratory infection (URI),
  429. See also Influenza
Ureteral colic, 717
Uric acid, 342. See also Gout
Uricosuric agents, in gout, 344
Uric stones, 718
Urinalysis, in chronic glomerulonephritis, 341
Urinary retention prevention, 715
Urolithiasis, 717–722. See also
  Kidney stones
  assessment and diagnostic
    methods, 718
  in bladder, 718
  factors favoring formation of, 717
  pharmacologic and nutritional
    therapy for, 718
  in renal pelvis, 717
  stone removal procedures, 719

V
Vaccinations
  hepatitis A and, 381
  hepatitis B and, 384
  influenza, 429–430
  meningitis, 463
Vaginal cancer, 218
Vaginal candidiasis, HIV infection
  and, 4
Vagus nerve demyelination, 345
Valvuloplasty, 467
Vein disorders, 723–728
  anticoagulant therapy for,
    725–726
  assessment and diagnostic
    methods, 724
  clinical manifestations, 724
  endovascular management, 725
  heparin-induced thrombo-
    cytopenia, 726
  pharmacologic therapy for, 725
  prevention, 724
  risk factors for, 723

Vein disorders (*continued*)
  self-care for, 728
  spontaneous bleeding, 726
Venous thrombosis, 723
Vertebroplasty, in multiple
    myeloma, 471
Vertical-banded gastroplasty, 494.
    See also Bariatric surgery
Vestibular disease, 459. *See also*
    Ménière's disease
Viral hepatitis, and fulminant
    hepatic failure, 380
Viral infections
  Guillain-Barré syndrome, 345
  pharyngitis, 575–576
Viral load tests, 4
Viral pharyngitis, 575–576
Virchow's triad, 723
Visual disturbances, in multiple
    sclerosis, 474
Vulvar cancer, 219–221
  assessment and diagnostic
      findings, 219
  clinical manifestations, 219
  medical management, 219
  nursing interventions
    home- and community-based
        care, 221
    postoperative, 220–221
    preoperative, 220
  nursing management, 220
  pathophysiology, 219

W
Warfarin, 725
Wasting syndrome, AIDS and, 2
Weakness
  in Guillain-Barré syndrome, 345
  in multiple sclerosis, 474
  in muscular dystrophies, 479
  in myasthenia gravis, 484
  in osteomalacia, 503
Weber's test, in Ménière's disease,
    459
Western blot assay, 4
Wound bacteria, 692
Wound drainage specimens, 652
Wound drainage systems, 562
Wound swelling, 568
Wrist fractures, 325–326

X
Xenical, 500
Xenon-enhanced CT scan, 671
X-ray
  in head injury, 351
  in hiatal hernia, 387
  in musculoskeletal trauma, 482
  in osteoarthritis, 501
  in osteomalacia, 503
  in osteomyelitis, 505
  in osteoporosis, 508

Z
Zollinger-Ellison syndrome, 534